Head Injury

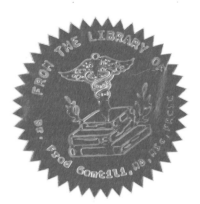

Head Injury

Paul R. Cooper, M. D., Editor

Associate Professor of Neurosurgery
New York University
School of Medicine
New York, N.Y.

WILLIAMS & WILKINS
Baltimore/London

Made in the United States of America

Library of Congress Cataloging in Publication Data

Main entry under title:

Management of head injuries.

   Includes index.
   1. Head—Wounds and injuries. I. Cooper, Paul R. [DNLM: 1. Head injuries—Therapy. WE 706 M266]
RD521.M33   617′.51044   81-15990
ISBN 0-683-02106-0   AACR2

Composed and printed at the
Waverly Press, Inc.
Mt. Royal and Guilford Aves.
Baltimore, MD 21202, U.S.A.

To
LFC

Preface

There have been dramatic advances in the diagnosis and treatment of patients with head injury in the last 15 years. Increased understanding of the mechanisms of trauma has allowed therapy to be applied in a more rational fashion. Awareness of the importance of elevations of intracranial pressure in the postoperative period and in those patients who have nonoperative lesions has resulted in significant improvement in care. From a diagnostic point of view, the advent of the CT scanner has led to a more rapid and accurate evaluation of patients with severe head injury and has had a greater impact in improving the management of the severely head-injured patient than it has in perhaps any other area of neurosurgical practice. Cognizance of the role of medical complications in influencing outcome and increased skill in treating these problems represents a less dramatic but probably no less significant event.

These advances have led to a very real improvement in outcome when applied by aggressive and interested neurosurgeons in large centers as well as community hospitals. Accurate data collection of clinical and physiological parameters, cooperative studies, and more sophisticated statistical techniques now allow early and accurate prediction of outcome in a substantial number of severely head-injured patients. In spite of these changes there is now no up-to-date multi-authored book on the management of head injury available in the English language. I hope that this volume, with chapters by 24 American contributors, will fill this void.

This book has been written primarily for the practicing neurosurgeon and contains the latest theoretical and practical information that is relevant to the management of head injury. Neurologists, emergency room physicians, general surgeons, and others who are called upon to render initial care to the head injured will also find this book an aid in managing head injuries. The content has been organized so that a physician confronted with a specific problem can quickly find a concise and authoritative answer to questions of diagnosis and treatment as well as the theoretical basis for actions taken. Insofar as possible, a balanced, eclectic point of view has been presented and individual authors have interpreted controversial issues for the reader in a dispassionate fashion. Copious references have been provided to substantiate points of view and to provide the reader with a guide for further study.

Acknowledgment

The editor gratefully acknowledges the assistance of Ms. Carol Meinhofer, Ms. Jill Backenroth and Ms. Christine Capuano in manuscript preparation.

Contributors

Harold P. Adams, Jr., M.D., Associate Professor of Neurology, University of Iowa, Iowa City, Iowa

Daniel C. Baker, M.D., Assistant Professor of Surgery, (Plastic Surgery) New York University School of Medicine, Attending Surgeon, Institute of Reconstructive Plastic Surgery New York University Medical Center and Manhattan Eye, Ear and Throat Hospital, New York, New York

David J. Boarini, M.D., Resident, Neurosurgery, University of Iowa, Iowa City, Iowa

Thomas J. Boll, Ph.D., Professor of Psychology, Pediatrics and Neurological Surgery; Director, Medical Psychology Program, University of Alabama, Birmingham, Alabama

Sharon A. Bowers, B.S.N., Manager, Comprehensive Central Nervous System Injury Center, University of California, School of Medicine San Diego, San Diego, California

Derek A. Bruce, M.B., Ch.B., Associate Professor of Neurosurgery and Pediatrics, University of Pennsylvania, School of Medicine, Philadelphia, Pennsylvania

Barry B. Ceverha, M.D., Clinical Instructor of Neurological Surgery, University of Southern California, School of Medicine, Los Angeles, California

Raymond A. Clasen, M.D., Associate Professor of Pathology, Rush Medical School, Chicago, Illinois

Paul R. Cooper, M.D., Associate Professor of Neurosurgery, New York University School of Medicine, New York, New York

Thomas A. Gennarelli, M.D., Assistant Professor of Neurosurgery, University of Pennsylvania, School of Medicine, Philadelphia, Pennsylvania

Harold Gewirtz, M.D., Clinical Instructor of Surgery, (Plastic Surgery) New York University Medical School, Chief Resident in Plastic Surgery, Institute of Reconstructive Plastic Surgery, New York University Medical Center, New York, New York

Steven L. Giannotta, M.D., Assistant Professor of Neurological Surgery, University of Southern California, School of Medicine, Los Angeles, California

Neal F. Kassell, M.D., Associate Professor of Neurosurgery, University of Iowa School of Medicine, Iowa City, Iowa

P. R. S. Kishore, M.D., Professor of Radiology, Chief of Neuroradiology, Medical College of Virginia, Richmond, Virginia

Sheldon H. Landesman, M.D., Assistant Professor of Medicine, Infectious Disease Division, State University of New York, Downstate Medical Center, Brooklyn, New York

Anthony Marmarou, Ph.D., Associate Professor, Department of Neurosurgery, Albert Einstein College of Medicine, Bronx, New York

Lawrence F. Marshall, M.D., Associate Professor of Surgery (Neurosurgery), University of California School of Medicine, San Diego, California

Raj Murali, M.D., Assistant Professor of Clinical Neurosurgery, New York University School of Medicine, New York, New York

Richard D. Penn, M.D., Associate Professor of Neurosurgery, Rush Medical School, Chicago, Illinois

Lawrence H. Pitts, M.D., Associate Professor of Neurosurgery, University of California at San Francisco, San Francisco, California

Richard Rovit, M.D., Professor of Clinical Neurosurgery, New York University School of Medicine, New York, New York

Kamran Tabaddor, M.D., Associate Professor of Neurosurgery, Albert Einstein College of Medicine, Bronx, New York

Erwin R. Thal, M.D., Professor, Department of Surgery, Southwestern Medical School, University of Texas Health Science Center at Dallas, Dallas, Texas

John M. Weiner, Dr. P.H., Associate Professor of Medicine, University of Southern California, School of Medicine, Los Angeles, California

Harold A. Wilkinson, M.D., Ph.D., Professor and Chairman, Department of Neurosurgery, University of Massachusetts, Worcester, Massachusetts

Contents

Epidemiology of Head Injury

PAUL R. COOPER

PROBLEMS IN DATA COLLECTION

Epidemiologic information is of great importance in the allocation of resources for treatment and in formulating policy designed to reduce the incidence, morbidity, and mortality of head injury. In the United States at this time much epidemiologic data regarding head injury does not exist, is hard to find, or is inaccurate. The reasons for this are several. There is no centrally run health care system in this country and head injuries are managed in a wide variety of municipal, voluntary, and federal hospitals. Although data is accumulated at the state level, the quality of record keeping and the types of data obtained vary widely. Because of the heterogeneity of geography and population, extrapolations based on head injury patterns in one state or region are not necessarily valid on a national basis. The national health statistics compiled in the Vital Statistics of the United States[38] give incomplete information regarding head injuries. While it is possible to determine mortality from cancer or heart disease or a number of other illnesses from the Vital Statistics of the United States, the same is not true for head injury. Accidental deaths are catalogued as to *etiology* (for example death from falls, motor vehicles, etc.) and there is no information available as to the part of the body injured. Although some states do keep records on the frequency of head injury this is not uniformly the case.

In an attempt to obtain accurate statistics on a current basis, the National Center for Health Statistics collects information from a nationwide sample of households on a continuous basis.[39] Forty thousand households with 116,000 persons were interviewed in 1976. Data obtained from these interviews are assumed to represent a statistically accurate cross-section of the population.

The incidence of head injury and certain other disease entities, estimated by extrapolating from the data obtained in the health interview survey, is incomplete and head injuries are included within a mixed group entitled "other current injuries." However, more specific data on head injuries may be obtained from the National Center for Health Statistics (Table 1.1). It is emphasized that the data in Table 1.1 are an estimate only. Moreover, there is no information regarding mortality and, for several of the categories, the sample is too small to ensure statistical reliability.

In 1977, 8,779,000 people were estimated to have sustained "head injuries" (including laceration and contusions of the face and head) in the United States (Table 1.1). The incidence of skull fracture and intracranial injury is approximately one-fourth of this total or about 2,211,000. The incidence of all non-fatal cranial and intracranial injuries in the United States based on the health interview survey is about 1%. Klauber *et al*[20], in an epidemiologic survey in San Diego, reported an incidence of 0.3% for serious head injury. Annegers and Kur-

1

Table 1.1

Number of Persons Injured by Class of Accident and Type of Head Injury: United States, 1977[40] (Incidence in Thousands)

Diagnosis	ICDA 8th Revision N Codes	Total	Moving Motor Vehicle		While at Work	Home	Other
			Total	Traffic			
Skull fracture and intracranial injury	N800, 801, 803, 850, 854	2,211	536[a]	536[a]	301[a]	1,058	472[a]
Other and unspecified laceration of head	N873	5,234	475[a]	475[a]	139[a]	3,220	1,602
Contusion of face, scalp, and neck, except eye	N920	1,333	239[a]	194[a]	94[a]	815	231[a]
All head injuries	N800, 801, 803, 850– 854, 873, 920	8,779	1,251	1,205	534[a]	5,093	2,305

[a] Figures do not meet standards of reliability or precision.

land[2] reported a similar incidence. From their data, it is apparent that only 30% of all head injuries are serious ones.

Data on hospital utilization is obtained by similar sampling techniques. Twenty-four thousand medical record abstracts were analyzed from 423 representative "non-institutional civilian hospitals" and an estimate of hospital discharges was obtained.[41] Intracranial injuries are included as a distinct category. Thus, it is possible to gain a reasonably accurate estimate of the number of patients *discharged from the hospital* with head injuries exclusive of skull fractures (skull fractures are included with fractures from other parts of the body). It is not possible to determine how sick these patients were or how many needed neurosurgical operations. Similarly, it is not possible to directly determine what percentage of the total number of patients with head injury are hospitalized. Nevertheless, given these limitations, a pattern of the epidemiology of head injury in the United States may be drawn.

ACCIDENTAL DEATH AND INJURY IN THE UNITED STATES

Based on data from the National Center for Health Statistics, the National Safety Council[26] estimates that the average number of persons injured annually in the United States for the years 1974–1976 totals over 65,000,000, or almost one-third of the entire population. Most of these injuries are minor. Nevertheless, in 1977 10,400,000 people were disabled and 104,000 died from their injuries.

That accidents form a major public health problem can be seen from the mortality figures compiled in the Vital Statistics of the United States[38] (Table 1.2). Accidents are the fourth most common cause of death for all ages with a mortality rate of 48/100,000 persons per year. However, accidents are by far the single largest cause of death in persons between the ages of 1 and 34. It is not until age 35 that deaths from malignancy exceed those from accidents. Statistics compiled by the World Health Organization[46] show similar data for other industrialized nations. In developing nations, infectious disease remains the major cause of mortality.

Table 1.2

Mortality Rate (per 100,000 Population) United States 1975[38]

Heart disease	336
Malignant neoplasms	172
Cerebrovascular disease	91
All accidents	48
Motor vehicle accidents	21.5
All other causes	26.8

HEAD INJURY DEMOGRAPHY

Head Injury in Relationship to All Trauma

The statistics regarding mortality and morbidity from accidental death quoted above give no information regarding mortality from head injuries in relationship to all accidental deaths.

Canadian statistics are quite helpful in this regard.[10] In 1965, there were 10,978 deaths from trauma of all kinds in Canada. Over 4,100, or about 40%, resulted from head injuries. In 1950, 34% of the 7,607 trauma deaths were a result of head injury. The reasons for this changing percentage are not clear, but it may be due to better and more rapid treatment of systemic injuries without a concomitant improvement in head injury care. In addition, during the period from 1950–1965, total trauma deaths increased by 50% but deaths from motor vehicle accidents increased by almost 125%. Thus, more recently a greater percentage of deaths were from vehicular trauma which is more likely to result in severe head injury. If deaths from head injury in the United States are estimated to represent 40% of all accidental deaths, the head injury mortality rate is 19.2/100,000. This is similar to the 22.3/100,000 rate calculated by Klauber et al[20] on the basis of their epidemiologic study in San Diego.

Fifty percent of all accidental deaths result from motor vehicle accidents. Head injury was the cause of death in 62% of motor vehicle occupant fatalities.[26] In a study of over 1,000 traffic fatalities, Tonge et al[37] confirmed that in over 50% of all victims there was evidence of "brain injury" and in 60% there was evidence of "intracranial hemorrhage." There is obviously some overlap between these two categories, but it is likely that over three-quarters of all fatally injured persons involved in motor vehicle accidents have an intracranial injury. It is not clear from this latter study how often the head injury was a *cause of death*. However, data from Japan[32] show that 74% of all motor vehicle fatalities in Tokyo resulted from head in-

jury. Abdominal injuries were next in frequency, being responsible for only 10% of all deaths. In a study of multiply injured patients admitted to the hospital in Switzerland,[45] one-half of all deaths resulted from head injury. In interpreting these data, it must be remembered that the series are not strictly comprable: the Swiss series includes only hospitalized patients, the data of Tonge et al[37] and Sano[32] include only patients injured in motor vehicle accidents. It does seem clear, however, that the head is the part of the body most likely to be injured in motor vehicle accidents and is more likely to result in fatalities than injuries to other parts of the body.

The National Safety Council[27] has complied statistics from a number of sources confirming that the head is the commonest part of the body injured in automobile accidents. The relative frequency of injuries to all body parts in adults is seen in Table 1.3. However, only 5% of all head injuries were fatal (Table 1.4) and most were probably relatively mild, consisting of concussions or soft tissue injuries.

Table 1.3
Frequency of Body Area Injured[27]

Body Area Injured	%[a]	Rank
Head	70	1
Neck and cervical spine	9	6
Thorax and thoracic spine	39	3
Abdomen, pelvis, lumbar spine	16	5
Upper extremities	35	4
Lower extremities	48	2

[a] Total percentage adds up to greater than 100% because many patients sustained injury to two or more parts of their body.

Table 1.4
Percentage of Injuries Which Were Fatal, By Body Area[27]

Body Area	%	Rank
Head	5	3
Neck and cervical spine	16	1
Thorax and thoracic spine	6	2
Abdomen, pelvis, lumbar spine	4	4
Upper extremities	<0.5	6
Lower extremities	<0.5	5

The Influence of Sex and Age

That head injury is more frequent in males has been universally noted. Male predominance varies from 81% reported by Kerr et al[19] in England to a low of 59% in the United States reported by Kraus.[22]

The relationship of head injury morbidity and mortality to age can be examined in several ways: total numbers of injuries in each age group, the age-specific incidence, and the relationship of head injury incidence to other causes of mortality. All studies show that in absolute numbers, head injuries are most frequent in younger age groups. Age specific morbidity and mortality rates, however, are higher in the elderly.

The estimated incidence of skull fracture or intracranial injury in the United States in 1977 is seen in Table 1.5. In England and Wales, 10% of hospitals were queried as to the ages and numbers of patients discharged with a diagnosis of head injury.[7] These data were extrapolated to obtain an estimate of the total number of hospital discharges (Table 1.6) and probably accurately represent the incidence of moderate and severe head injuries. Over one-half of all patients admitted were under the age of

Table 1.5
Incidence of Skull Fracture and Intracranial Injury by Age: United States 1977[40]

Age	Incidence
Under 6	226,000
6–16	516,000
17–44	1,123,000
45–64	213,000

Table 1.6
Hospital Discharge for Head Injury: England and Wales, 1972[7]

Age	Total Patients
0–4	19,392
5–14	34,519
15–19	18,355
20–24	15,149
25–34	15,234
35–44	9,454
45–64	17,168
65–74	6,571
75 and over	6,174
Total all ages	142,016

20. Field[7] believed that the proportion of children seen in the emergency room is even higher than that admitted to hospital.

Age-specific mortality figures for head injury are not available for the United States. However, the National Safety Council[26] has published data which give the age-specific death rate for *all* accidents occurring in the United States in 1977. Deaths from head injury are estimated to make up 40% of the total number of trauma deaths. Extrapolating from this 40% figure, there were almost 42,000 deaths from head injury in 1977 in the United States. An estimated 9,600 head injury deaths occurred in the 15–24 age group and only one-third as many or 6,000 in the 65–74 age group. However, the age-specific death rate is 24 per 100,000 in the 15–24 age group and 68 per 100,000 in the 65–74 age group. Although there are smaller numbers of head injury deaths in the elderly, the number of deaths in proportion to the population at risk is much higher than that for the younger groups.

Because the overall death rate in younger patients is low, deaths from head injury of other accidents ranks first as a cause of mortality. In the elderly, the death rates from vascular disease, stroke, cancer, etc, are so high that the incidence of death from accidents ranks sixth after these other causes.

The older patient is less likely to survive a severe head injury than a younger one. In a study of 1,500 cases of head injury,[15] 6% of all head injured patients admitted to hospital were over the age of 50. However, 38% of all deaths were in the over 50 age group. Klauber et al[20] reported a case mortality rate of 17.5% in older patients which was over twice the rate for their series at large. Selecki et al[33] reported similar findings. They speculate that associated medical diseases may be the reason for higher death rates. It is also likely that a larger number of children are admitted with minor injuries for observation thus lowering the case mortality rate for this group.

Influence of Day and Time

Because motor vehicle accidents are by far the single largest cause of head injuries, an examination of motor vehicle deaths in relation to the time of day, week, and year is of interest. In absolute terms, motor vehicle deaths are slightly more common at night than in the day but the death rate (per 100,000,000 miles) is sharply higher at night—6.62 at night versus 2.11 during the day.

The time of occurrence of weekend and weekday fatalities differs considerably and is graphically represented in Figure 1.1. These data are similar to the Canadian experience reported by Klonoff and Thompson[21] who found that patients admitted to hospital emergency rooms had the greatest chance of sustaining an injury between 5 PM and midnight. As might be expected, Friday through Sunday are the peak days for motor vehicle deaths with 21% occurring on Saturday and 54% occurring between Friday and Sunday. June through August are the peak months with about 29% of all injuries occurring during this period.

Alcohol

Alcohol consumption is a significant contributing factor in patients sustaining trauma and, in particular, in those sustaining head injury. The National Safety Council[26] estimates that in the United States "drinking is indicated as a factor in at least half of the fatal motor vehicle accidents." In Finland, Honkanen and Visuri[14] noted an overall incidence of alcohol ingestion in 37% of over 1,000 injury victims. When the incidence of alcohol ingestion is narrowed to patients with head injury Honkanen and Visuri[14] found 47% of emergency room patients had ingested alcohol. Rutherford[31] reported that 42% of a consecutive series of patients with mild head injuries had positive blood alcohol tests. Galbraith et al[9] found detectable blood alcohol levels (greater than 5 mg %) in 62% of head injured males and 27% of head injured women.

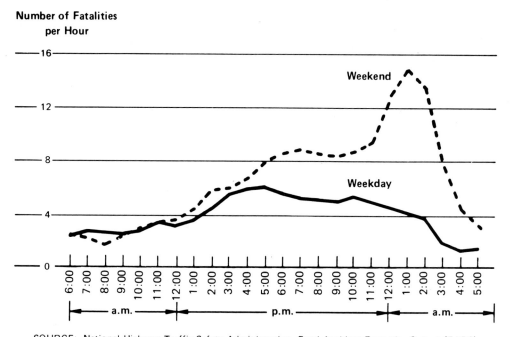

SOURCE: National Highway Traffic Safety Administration, Fatal Accident Reporting System (FARS)

NOTE: Weekend crashes (6 p.m. Friday - 12 p.m. Sunday) produce many more fatalities in the evening and early morning hours than do weekday crashes. This is primarily a result of increased recreational driving on weekend nights and associated increased use of alcohol.

Figure 1.1. Graph shows number of motor vehicle fatalities by hour.

ETIOLOGIC FACTORS

Motor Vehicle Accidents

In industrialized countries, and increasingly in developing nations, motor vehicle accidents are the most frequent cause of head injury. The mortality rate for motor vehicle accidents in 1977 in the United States was 22.9/100,000.[26]

The relative frequency of causes of head injury for the United States cannot be determined from the Vital Statistics of the United States,[38] but it is likely that about almost one-half of all head injury deaths were related to vehicular accidents. In San Diego, it has been reported that 53% of all head injuries occurred as a result of motor vehicle accidents.[20] The relative frequency of causes of head injury from a number of representative series is seen in Table 1.7. Several conclusions may be drawn from these series: among adults motor vehicle accidents represent the single most common cause of head injury; in small children, falls are the most frequent cause of head injury and motor vehicle accidents are second in importance. Data from several large pediatric series show that children tend to sustain head injuries as pedestrians or while on bicycles. Over 80% of all motor vehicle accident head injuries occurred this way in the series of Hendrick et al[12] and 98% in this fashion in the series of Rowbotham et al.[30]

When motor vehicle fatalities in the United States are compared with those from Canada and Western Europe, several interesting patterns emerge (Table 1.8). Because the population of the United States is larger than any of these countries, the total number of United States fatalities is by far the largest. However, the fatality rate per 100,000 population in the United States is exceeded by three other countries, and the number of fatalities per 100,000 passenger cars and per 100,000 kilometers travelled are the lowest of all the nations studied.

Within the United States, there is a wide geographic variation in deaths from motor vehicle accidents. The death rates for selected states are listed in Table 1.9. In general, the most densely populated urban states have the lowest death rates, the fewest deaths per 10,000 motor vehicle registrations, and the lowest death rates per mile travelled.

Seat Belts. Because head injuries account for one-half of all automobile fatalities, anything that will prevent a passenger from striking the interior of an automobile, or being ejected from the vehicle, will reduce head injury deaths. It has been noted that "belted occupants are rarely killed except in high speed accidents; a given severity of injury needs an average speed 12 miles per hour (19 kilometers per hour) greater if the occupant is belted than if he is unbelted."[35] Similarly Tonge et al[37] noted that "car occupants wearing seat belts properly fitted and worn, seldom become fatalities unless involved in impact with severe deformation of the vehicle or entrusion into the occupants area." Bohlin[4] studied 28,000 automobile accidents and could find no fatalities where the vehicle was traveling at less than 100 kilometers per hour and upper torso restraints were used.

Table 1.7
Relative Frequency of Causes of Head Injury (in Percent)

Author	MVA	Domestic	Sport	Work	Assault	Fall	Other
Barr and Ralston[3]	67	11	11	9	2		
Selecki[33]	31	6	12	5	7		29
Jennett[17]	58			2	17	17	6
Klonoff and Thompson[21] [a]	53		3	11	4	23	7
Maloney[25]	64	12	6	9	11		8
Hendrick et al[12] [b]	32					53	15
Craft[6]	33	27.5			7		33

[a] Hospitalized patients only.
[b] Children only.

Table 1.8
Automobile Fatality Rate for the United States and Selected Foreign Countries 1975[42]

Country	Fatalities per 100,000 Population	Fatalities per 100,000 Passenger Cars	Fatalities per 100 Million Vehicle Kilometers (Passenger Cars)
Belgium	23.9	89	8.5
Canada	26.6	72	3.5
Finland (1974)	18.4	90	7.0
Germany	24.1	83	6.0
Netherlands	17.0	69	4.5
Norway	13.4	58	4.5
Spain	16.4	128	14.0
Sweden	14.3	43	3.0
United States	20.9	43	3.0

Table 1.9
Motor Vehicle Death Rate of Selected States, 1977[26]

	Death Rate[a]	Registration Death Rate[b]	Mileage Death Rates[c]
New York	13.6	3.1	3.6
California	22.6	3.2	3.4
Michigan	21.4	3.1	3.1
Georgia	28.9	4.1	3.4
Wyoming	61.3	6.2	5.4
District of Columbia	12[d]		1.9[d]
U.S. Average	22.9	3.32	3.38

[a] Deaths per 100,000 population.
[b] Motor vehicle death/10,000 motor vehicles.
[c] Motor vehicle death/100,000,000 vehicle miles.
[d] 1976.

When restraints were not used, fatalities occurred at speeds as low as 20 kilometers per hour. Although all new automobiles in the United States are now equipped with seat belts, only a small percentage of automobile occupants use safety belt restraint systems. In 1976–1977 model year automobiles, only 24.9% of subcompact occupants and 13% of luxury car occupants used seat belts.[43] The frequency of seat belt use was somewhat higher in the 1974–1975 models because interlock systems made it impossible to start an automobile if seat belts were not fastened.

A law making it compulsory to wear seat belts was introduced in New South Wales, Australia at the end of 1971. A survey showed that approximately 75% of front seat passengers complied with the law.[11] A calculation of automobile deaths in 1972 showed a 25% drop from the expected rate. Aldman[1] estimated that at least "50% of

serious injuries to car occupants can be prevented by the use of proper restraining devices." Christian[5] studied injury patterns in almost 2,000 driver and front seat passengers with non-fatal injuries. All categories of injuries (legs, pelvis, ribs, arms, spine, head) were decreased in seat belt wearers as compared to non-wearers. Only injuries to the clavicle were higher in seat belt wearers. The percentage decrease in injury as a result of seat belt wearing was greatest for skull and facial fractures—8.2% of non-wearers and 3.5% of wearers who were involved in accidents sustaining such injuries.

It is clear that head injuries are decreased by seat belt usage. Are the risks for seat belt wearers increased in other ways? An increase in clavicular fractures has already been mentioned. Being trapped by seat belts in a burning car is of concern but fire occurs in less than 0.5% of accidents.[35] The fear of being trapped by seat belts and injured in a crushed automobile when the occupant might have been ejected safely is a myth. Automobile occupants have a 25% risk of being killed when ejected and over half of all automobile fatalities occurred when occupants were ejected. Of 2,879 occupants studied by Hobbs,[13] none would have fared better without seat belts.

Motorcycle Accidents

Motorcycle accidents represent a specialized form of motor vehicle accident and deserve special comment. Motorcycle accidents are most likely to occur at 4 PM–6 PM, on dry roads, at relatively low speeds (20–30 miles per hour) and as a result of collision with other vehicles. The injured tend to be almost exclusively males (90%) under the age of 25 who have had licenses for less than one year. In 40% of fatalities, there was a detectable blood alcohol level.

In 1977, motorcycles comprised 3.4% of all vehicle registrations in the United States.[29] Motorcycles represented 1.6% of the total number of vehicles involved in accidents. Motorcycle involvement in accidents would appear to be less than might

be expected. However, motorcycles were involved in 6.5% of all fatal vehicle accidents. The vulnerability of motorcycle drivers and passengers is even more apparent when the mileage death rate is examined. In 1979, the mileage death rate for all motor vehicles was 3.4/100,000,000 miles but for motorcycles was 17/100,000,000 miles. Thus, motorcyclists run five times the risk of a fatal accident per mile travelled. The total lack of crash protection afforded by motorcycles places the motorcyclist at an 80–90% risk of death or injury in any accident. The risk of death or injury for all types of motor vehicle accidents is only 8.1%. It is estimated that 430,000 injuries to motorcyclists occurred in 1977. This figure may be a significant underestimate. A California study[24] would indicate that police reports identify less than 40% of all injured motorcyclists.

Implicit in any discussion of motorcycle accidents is the fact that the head is the part of the body most likely to be injured. Jamieson and Kelly[16] recorded minor or major head injury in over two-thirds of all injured motorcyclists. Two-thirds of motorcycle riders killed in Illinois suffered a skull fracture.[29] Knowledge of these and similar

Head Injury Rates Per 1000 Crash-Involved Helmeted and Non-Helmeted Riders

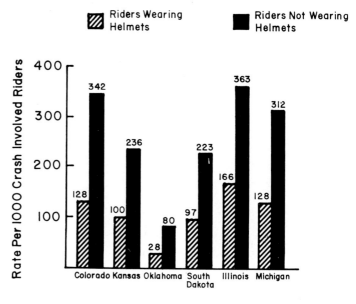

Figure 1.2 Graph compares head injury rates in helmeted and non-helmeted motorcyclists. Head injury rate for non-helmeted riders is at least double that for helmeted ones.

statistics has resulted in the passage of laws mandating helmet usage. In Kansas, 93% of non-helmeted motorcyclist fatalities resulted from head injury. When helmets were worn, only one-third of fatalities were caused by head injuries. The dramatic effect of crash helmets in reducing motorcycle related head injuries may be seen in Figure 1.2. In each of the six states shown, head injury in helmeted riders was reduced by at least 60%. When fatal head injuries are examined, the decrease in mortality is even more dramatic (Fig. 1.3). By 1975, as a result of Department of Transportation directives, 47 states had adopted laws requiring motorcyclists to wear helmets. In 1976, legislation was passed by Congress forbidding the federal government to withhold funds from states failing to require compulsory helmet wearing. As a result, 26 states repealed or weakened their helmet laws between 1976 and 1978. Figure 1.4 shows the effect of this legislation on motorcycle fatalities. Until 1975, motorcycle registration increased at a much faster rate than fatalities. There was a particularly significant drop in fatalities from 1974–1975 as a result of helmet legislation. The rapid increase in motorcycle deaths since 1975 is almost certainly due to the repeal of helmet laws. Watson et al[44] estimate that repeal of helmet laws resulted in a 40% increase in motorcycle-related fatalities.

The Department of Transportation[43] has summarized the relationship of head injury and helmet wearing: 1) Motorcyclists unprotected by helmets have twice as many head injuries and 3 to 4 times the number of fatal injuries as helmet wearers. 2) In states where laws require helmet usage, 90–100% of motorcyclists comply. The usage rate falls to less than 60% with repeal of these laws. 3) Helmets do not reduce hearing or visibility in a way that would lead to accidents.

Pedestrian Injuries

Specific data regarding the frequency of death from injury to pedestrians has been compiled by the National Safety Council.[26]

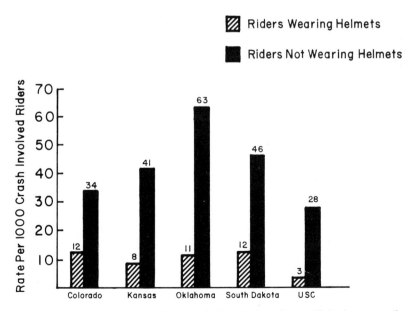

Fatal Head Injury Rate Per 1000 Helmeted and Non-Helmeted Riders

Figure 1.3. Fatal head injury rate in non-helmeted motorcyclists is many times that for helmeted riders.

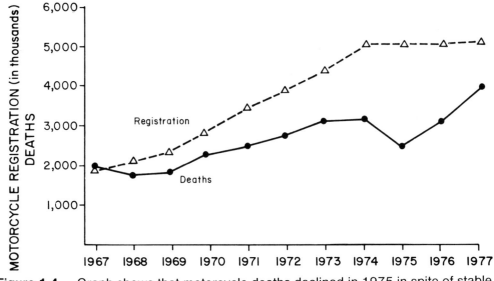

Figure 1.4. Graph shows that motorcycle deaths declined in 1975 in spite of stable or slightly increasing motorcycle registration. Rise in deaths thereafter is a reflection of the repeal of motorcycle helmet laws in many states.

In 1977, 8,600 pedestrians were killed. They accounted for 20% of all motor vehicle-related fatalities and 110,000 non-fatal injuries. Two-thirds of deaths occur in urban areas and two-thirds of the urban injuries occur at crossing intersections.

Other Causes

Head injuries also result from occupational accidents, falls, assaults, gunshot wounds, and sporting accidents. Data compiled by Field[7] in Canada and Europe would indicate that these factors account for 20 to 25% of all head injuries. In the United States, gunshot wounds cause 2,000 deaths[26] per year, but it is impossible to state the percentage dying as a result of head injury.

EMERGENCY CARE

Pre-hospital Mortality

One-half or more of all patients who die of head injuries never reach hospitals and they make few demands on medical resources. Tonge et al[37] in Australia established that 49% of patients who eventually succumbed to their head injuries died within an hour of the accident. In Texas (North Central Texas Council of Governments: 1980, unpublished data), 70% of the total number of patients who died from head injury did so before reaching the hospital. Klauber et al[20] in San Diego found that 48% of all fatalities in males occurred at the accident scene and 18% died en route to the hospital or in the emergency room. Thus, two-thirds of patients who went on to die did so before being admitted to the hospital.

Emergency Room

The numbers of patients presenting with head injury in hospital emergency rooms is determined by the frequency of head injury in the community, the proximity of the emergency room to population centers, the availability of transport, the patient's perception of his need for care, and the availability of primary care physicians to treat the patient with relatively minor injuries. In particular, the availability of primary care physicians will tend to decrease total emergency room visits.

In an analysis of head injuries in Scottish hospitals, Strang et al[36] found that 11% of all patients visiting emergency rooms had head injuries. Extrapolating from this data, it is estimated that one million patients with head injury will attend British emergency rooms each year. Twenty percent of patients seen in metropolitan area emergency rooms were admitted. Thirty-five percent of patients seen in hospitals more than 30 miles away from large cities were admitted. Because most patients are self-referred, the proportion of patients with minor injuries is high. Eighty percent had no evidence of altered consciousness at any time. Fifteen percent gave a history of altered consciousness but had a normal emergency room examination. Only 5% had evidence of altered consciousness at the time of examination in the emergency room.

One-half of all head-injured patients arrived between 5 PM and midnight and over one-third came on Fridays and Saturdays. Forty-four percent of patients presenting were under 14 years of age and 54% were less than 20.

HOSPITALIZATION

Incidence

Almost 36 million patients were hospitalized in the United States in 1977. Head injury patients represent 1% of this total, although it is likely this underestimates the number of head injured for the reasons previously given. In 1977, 383,000 people in the United States were discharged from short-stay general and specialty hospitals, with a diagnosis of intracranial injury.[41] This is an incidence of 18 discharges per 10,000 population. The average length of stay was greatly influenced by the number of patients admitted with minor injuries and was 5.3 days for the United States as a whole. This compares to an average of almost 12 days of hospitalization reported from India[18] and over 13 days in Australia.[34] Both these series were from large referral centers and it is likely that only the more serious injuries were referred to these institutions. In Glasgow where all patients with post-traumatic amnesia are admitted to the hospital (although not generally cared for by neurosurgeons), 85% of patients were discharged within 48 hours and only 5% stayed longer than one week.[8] In Great Britain, 142,000 patients in a population of 49,000,000 were admitted with head injury in 1972.[7] The actual number of admissions in both Great Britain and the United States is influenced (in addition to the incidence of head injury) by the availability of hospital beds and the personal feelings of the individual physicians regarding the medical necessity for admission. In the United States, legal and economic considerations also play a role.

In England and Wales, there has been a decline in deaths from head injury since 1966.[7] In spite of this, since 1966 head injury admissions have increased from 116,000 to 142,000 per year. It is possible that there has been a real increase in non-lethal head injuries. It is more likely that admission policies have changed with regard to head injury or that there have been changes in the methods of classifying head injury. In support of this latter contention is the fact that the number of skull fractures has remained remarkably constant while there has been a large increase in the number of patients with "other and unspecified cranial injury."

Frequency of Neurosurgical Care

Whether patients with head injury are seen by neurosurgical specialists is determined by the severity of the patient's injury and by the distribution of neurosurgeons within the medical community. In the United States, where there is approximately one neurosurgeon for every 80,000 persons, patients admitted to hospital with head injury generally receive neurosurgical consultation. In Great Britain, where there are many fewer neurosurgeons in relation to the population, neurosurgical care is reserved for the most seriously injured patients. Lesser injuries are cared for by general practicioners, general surgeons, or emergency room physicians. Of 918 patients admitted to a Scottish teaching hospital, only 41 (4%) had neurosurgical consultation.[8] In Canada, where there are greater numbers of neurosurgeons in relation to the population than in Britain (but fewer than in the United States), 58% of in-hospital head-injured patients had neurosurgical care or consultation.

Frequency of Operation

Only a small proportion of patients hospitalized with head injury require surgical therapy. The exact percentage will depend on the frequency of admission of patients with minor head injury. Craft et al,[6] in a hospital series of pediatric head injury, noted that only 8 of 200 patients required operation. Operation was necessary in 12.4% of 4,465 pedestrian head injuries reported by Hendrick et al[12] and in 21% of patients in Rowbotham's series.[30] However, in this latter series most operations were for the treatment of depressed fractures or scalp lacerations. Less than half of all operations were for treatment of intracranial hematoma.

Case-fatality Ratio

The case-fatality ratio is derived from the ratio of deaths to the total number of persons sustaining head injuries. The case fatality ratio for the United States cannot be obtained from the health interview survey because fatal cases are excluded. However, in San Diego County, data compiled by Klauber et al[20] indicate that 7.5% of head injured patients died. The case-fatality rate for *hospitalized* patients in this same study was 3%. It has been emphasized, however, that case-fatality rates are very difficult to compare because of "failure to classify patients with head injury in a consistent and standard way."[23]

The case fatality rate also varies markedly according to the etiology of the head injury. Thus, persons who sustained head injury in motorcycle accidents had a 22.6% case fatality rate, whereas those involved in non-vehicular accidents had 4.6% rate.[23] It is apparent from these data, then, that the head injuries sustained in motorcycle accidents are much more severe than those sustained in non-vehicular accidents.

TRENDS IN HEAD INJURY INCIDENCE AND MORTALITY

Because the automobile is responsible for one-half of all head-injury deaths in the United States, trends in automobile fatality rates will have a significant influence on head injury mortality. The total number of motor vehicle deaths has increased little since 1965. This has occurred while the number of vehicle miles travelled and the number of registered vehicles was increasing. Thus, deaths per registered vehicle and deaths per vehicle mile have decreased.

A National Safety Council analysis[26] indicates that speed reduction has accounted for a significant decrease in motor vehicle-related deaths since 1973. Seat belt use is not responsible for this decline, as the number of occupants using seat belts has decreased. The increasing use of interstate roads with their lower fatality rates contributes significantly to this decrease. Data from Texas would indicate that the development of systems employing skilled emergency medical technicians and paramedics and well-defined trauma centers has resulted in a 31% decrease in motor vehicle related fatalities (North Central Texas Council of Governments: 1980, unpublished data).

ECONOMIC ASPECTS OF HEAD INJURY

Costs of Hospitalization

In the United States in 1977, 2,000,000 hospital days (383,000 patients hospitalized for an average of 5.3 days) were spent by patients with head injury.[41] At an average per day cost for hospital rooms of $150.00, the cost for hospitalization was $3,000,000,000 a year. This does not include the price of diagnostic tests, physician's fees, emergency room charges for patients not admitted, or the cost of follow-up care. When all factors are considered, it is likely that the combined medical costs for head injury are at least $6,000,000,000 a year.

Long-term Costs

The exact cost of the sequelae of head injury (death, days lost from work) is difficult to determine (see also Chapter 19). In Barr and Ralston's series,[3] only 62% of patients had returned to work by the end of the first month, even though the vast majority had trivial injuries. By seven months, however, only 4% of patients had not returned to work. Rowbotham et al[30] analyzed 1,000 patients hospitalized with head injury. They queried 250 patients as to their employment status several years after the injury. Two-hundred thirty-six patients re-

Table 1.10
Employment Status of Head-Injured Patients[30]

Number of Patients	%	Average Time from Discharge to Return to Work (Weeks)	Work Status
169	72	10.5	Normal work
38	16	27	Light work then normal work
19	8	32	Permanent light work
10	4	16	Irregular work

plied to the questionnaire. Results are seen in Table 1.10.

Approximately 200,000 *adults* are hospitalized each year in the United States with head injury. If their median income is $15,000, these patients sustained an income loss of over $750,000,000 a year extrapolating from Rowbotham's figures. Loss of income over an expected lifetime for the 42,-000 patients dying of head injury is more difficult to calculate because of the unknown factor of inflation. If it is assumed that half of all deaths occur in patients below the age of 20, with an average of 40 years earning potential, and that for patients over 20 there is an average of 30 working years left, the income lost from head-injury deaths in 1977 in the United States is about 22 billion dollars.

References

1. Aldman, B.: Road accidents in Sweden. J. Trauma, 10:921–925, 1970.
2. Annegers, J.F., Kurland, L.T.: The epidemiology of central nervous system trauma. In: Central Nervous System Trauma Research Status Report. Ed. Odom, G.L., Washington, D.C., National Institute of Health, 1979.
3. Barr, J.R., Ralston, G.J.: Head injuries in a peripheral hospital. A five year survey. Lancet, 2:519–522, 1964.
4. Bohlin, N.I.: A statistical analysis of 28,000 accident cases with emphasis on occupant restraint value. In: Proceedings of Eleventh Stapp Car Crash Conference. New York, Society of Automotive Engineers, Inc., 1967, pp. 455–478.
5. Christian, M.S.: Non-fatal injuries sustained by seatbelt wearers: a comparative study. Br. Med. J., 2:1310–1311, 1976.
6. Craft, A.W., Shaw, D.A., Cartlidge, N.E.F.: Head injuries in children. Br. Med. J., 4:200–203, 1972.
7. Field, J.H.: Epidemiology of Head Injuries in England and Wales. Her Majesty's Stationery Office, London, 1976.
8. Galbraith, S., Murray, W.R., Patel, A.R.: Head injury admissions to a teaching hospital. Scot. Med. J., 22:129–132, 1977.
9. Galbraith, S., Murray, W.R., Patel, A.R., Knill-Jones, R.: The relationship between alcohol and head injury and its effect on the conscious level. Br. J. Surg., 63:128–130, 1976.
10. Hay, R.K.: Neurosurgical aspects of traffic accidents. Can. Med. Assoc. J., 97:1364–1368, 1967.
11. Henderson, M., Wood, R.: Compulsory wearing of seat belts in New South Wales, Australia. An evaluation of its effect on vehicle occupant deaths in the first year. Med. J. Aust., 2:797–801, 1973.
12. Hendrick, E.B., Harwood-Hash, D.C.F., Hudson, A.R.: Head injuries in children: a survey of 4465 consecutive cases at the hospital for sick children, Toronto, Canada. Clin. Neurosurg., 11:46–65, 1964.
13. Hobbs, C.A.: The effectiveness of seat belts in reducing injuries to car occupants. Laboratory report 811. Crowthorne, Transport and Road Research Laboratory, 1978.
14. Honkanen, R., Visuri, T.: Blood alcohol levels in a series of injured patients with special reference to accident and type of injury. Ann. Chirurg. Gynaecol., 65:287–294, 1976.
15. Jain, S.P., Kankanady, V.D.: A study of 1500 cases of head injury in Delhi. J. Indian Med. Assoc., 52:204–211, 1969.
16. Jamieson, K.G., Kelly, D.: Crash helmets reduce head injuries. Med. J. Aus , 2:806–809, 1973.
17. Jennett, B., Murray, A., McMillan, R., MacFarlane, J., Bentify, C., String, I., Hawthorne, V.: Head injuries in Scottish hospitals. Lancet, 2:696–698, 1977.
18. Kalyanaraman, S., Ramamurthi, B.: The pattern of head injury at Madras. Int. Surg., 51:479–487, 1969.
19. Kerr, T.A., Kay, D.W.K., Lacman, L.P.: Characteristics of patients, type of accident, and mortality in a consecutive series of head injuries admitted to a neurosurgical unit. Br. J. Prev. Soc. Med., 25:179–185, 1971.
20. Klauber, M.R., Barrett-Connor, E., Marshall, L.F., Bowers, S.A.: Epidemiology of head injury: a prospective study of an entire community, San Diego, California. Am. J. Epidemiol., 113:500–509, 1981.
21. Klonoff, H., Thompson, G.B.: Epidemiology of head injuries in adults: a pilot study. Can. Med. Assoc. J., 100:235–241, 1969.

22. Kraus, J.F.: Epidemiologic features of head and spinal cord injury. Adv. Neurol., 19:261–279, 1978.

23. Kraus, J.F.: Injury to the head and spinal cord. The epidemiological relevance of the medical literature published from 1960 to 1978. J. Neurosurg., 53:S3–S10, 1980.

24. Kraus, J.F., Riggins, R.S., Franti, C.E.: Some epidemiologic features of motorcycle collision injuries. Am. J. Epidemiol., 102:74–98, 1975.

25. Maloney, A.F.J., Whatmore, W.J.: Clinical and pathological observations in fatal head injuries. A 5-year survey of 173 cases. Br. J. Surg., 1:23–31, 1969.

26. National Safety Council: Accident facts. National Safety Council, Chicago, 1978.

27. National Safety Council: Body area of motor vehicle occupant injured in motor vehicle accident. National Safety Council, Chicago, 1966.

28. National Safety Council: Factors contributing to the decrease in motor-vehicle fatalities. National Safety Council, Chicago, 1979.

29. National Safety Council: Motorcycle facts. National Safety Council, Chicago, 1978.

30. Rowbotham, G.F., Maciver, I.N., Dickson, J., Bousfield, M.E.: Analysis of 1,400 cases of acute injury to the head. Br. Med. J., 1:726–730, 1954.

31. Rutherford, W.H.: Diagnosis of alcohol ingestion in mild head injuries. Lancet, 1:1021–1023, 1977.

32. Sano, K.: Survey of the organization of services for the treatment of acute head injury in Japan. Exp. Med. Int. Congr. Ser. 93:33–37, 1965.

33. Selecki, B.R., Gonski, L., Gonski, A., Blum, P.W., Matheson, J.M., Poulgrain, P.: Retrospective survey of neurotraumatic admissions to a teaching hospital. Med. J. Aust., 2:232–274, 1978.

34. Selecki, B.R., Hoy, R.J., Ness, P.: A retrospective survey of neuro-traumatic admissions to a teaching hospital. 1. General aspects. Med. J. Aust., 2:113–117, 1967.

35. Special Correspondent: A modern epidemic. Road accidents-seat belts and the safe car. Br. Med. J., 2:1695–1698, 1978.

36. Strang, I., MacMillan, R., Jennett, B.: Head injuries in accident and emergency departments at Scottish hospitals. Injury, 10:154–159, 1978.

37. Tonge, J.I., O'Reilly, M.J.J., Davison, A., Johnston, N.G., Wilkey, I.S.: Traffic-crash fatalities (1968–73): injury patterns and other factors. Med. Sci. Law, 17:9–24, 1977.

38. U.S. Dept. of Health, Education, Welfare: National Center for Health Statistics. Vital Statistics of the United States 1975, Hyattsville, Md., 1979.

39. U.S. Dept. of Health, Education, Welfare: Current Estimates from the Health Interview Survey. National Center for Health Statistics, Series 10, Number 119, Hyattsville, Md., 1977.

40. U.S. Dept. Health, Education, Welfare: Unpublished data from the Health Interview Survey, 1980.

41. U.S. Dept. Health, Education, Welfare: Public Health Service Office of Health Research, Statistics and Technology. Utilization of short-story hospitals. Annual Summary of the United States, 1977, Series 13, Number 41, National Center for Health Statistics, Hyattsville, Md., 1979.

42. U.S. Dept. of Transportation. National Highway Traffic Safety Administration. Motor Vehicle Safety. U.S. Government Printing Office Wash., D.C., 1977.

43. U.S. Dept. of Transportation. National Highway Traffic Safety Administration: The effect of motorcycle helmet usage on head injuries, and the effect of usage laws on helmet wearing rates. A preliminary report, 1979.

44. Watson, G.S., Zador, P.L., Wilks, A.: The repeal of helmet use laws and increased motorcyclist mortality in the United States, 1975–1978. Am. J. Pub. Health, 70:579–585, 1980.

45. Weibel, M.A., Suter, P.M.: Comparaison des patients polyblessés en 1970 et 1976: pathologie dominante et causes de mortalité. Rév. Chir. Orthoped., 64:205–211, 1978.

46. World Health Organization: World Health Statistics Annual (1973–1976) World Health Organization, Geneva, 1976.

2

Emergency Care; Initial Evaluation

KAMRAN TABADDOR

Despite an extensive effort to provide care to victims of head injury over the past decade, the in-hospital mortality rate has not been significantly reduced.[48] A large number of patients still die before reaching the hospital. Field,[25] reported that 60% of all deaths from head injury in England occurred before admission to the hospital, 40% were dead at the scene of the accident, and 20% died in the emergency ward. A higher proportion of pre-hospital head trauma mortality (74%) was observed in an epidemiologic study of head and spinal cord injury conducted in the Bronx, N.Y., area served by the head injury service at my institution. These figures indicate that greater attention must be paid to the role of emergency medical services in the pre-hospital phase of care for head trauma. Recent studies in various countries suggest that approximately 20% of motor vehicle accident victims could be saved with better treatment before arrival in the emergency room. Waters and Wells[93] claimed that a 24% reduction in auto accident mortality could be obtained by instituting an advance life-support system during this pre-hospital phase. This conclusion was reached by comparing mortality figures before and after implementation of emergency medical services. The 24% reduction in mortality included a 9% reduction from pre-hospital care, and 15% reduction from improved emergency room resuscitative measures. Although these reports are encouraging, it is difficult to evaluate the impact of pre-

hospital care unless the mortality and morbidity of the pre-hospital and in-hospital phases are studied as a whole. As the emergency medical services response time shortens, and the care provided by emergency technicians improves, some trauma victims who would have died on the street may now reach the hospital alive. These patients, however, may die several hours later in the emergency room or the intensive care unit thereby artificially inflating the in-hospital mortality and reducing the pre-hospital mortality.

PRE-HOSPITAL MANAGEMENT OF THE PATIENT WITH HEAD TRAUMA

The goal of the early management of the head injured patient is to prevent secondary damage and to facilitate the recovery process by providing the brain with an optimal physiologic environment. This includes restoration and maintenance of effective cerebral oxygenation and perfusion. Correcting any derangement in oxygen delivery takes precedence over the neurological assessment since the result of the assessment cannot be interpreted in the presence of shock or hypoxia.

Early Airway Management

Several laboratory studies suggest that impact of sufficient force to produce unconsciousness is always associated with apnea.[10, 94] Miller et al.[62] reported an increase in mortality when head injury is associated

15

with hypoxia, supporting the role of early resuscitation of head trauma victims. With the exception of some case reports, however, there has been no clinical study which could determine to what extent the outcome of patients with severe head injury could be improved by early respiratory resuscitation.[49, 71]

Upper respiratory tract obstruction is the most common cause of impaired ventilation in comatose, head-injured patients. Obstruction may occur as the tongue falls backward or when the mouth and oropharynx are occluded by hemorrhage from facial injuries. Upper airway obstruction may also occur as a result of aspiration of gastric contents. Initially, the mouth and oropharynx should be digitally cleared of foreign objects and food fragments. The trachea should then be suctioned in order to remove the aspirated material. In the patient with a depressed level of consciousness, the patency of the upper airway can best be maintained by insertion of an esophageal airway which will prevent the regurgitation of stomach contents and preclude inflation of the stomach when respirations are assisted or maintained by a face mask and ambu bag. The esophageal airway also obviates the need for turning the patient to a lateral position to maintain an adequate airway. When there is a need for ventilatory assistance by face mask and bag, satisfactory oxygenation and mild hypocarbia can be achieved by bagging at a rate of 24 breaths per minute. When convenient, a cuffed endotracheal tube is inserted and the esophageal airway removed. (See also Chapter 3.)

Hypotension

After an adequate airway is established, attention should be directed toward maintenance of cerebral perfusion. Although *transient* hypotension after head injury is not an infrequent occurrence,[62] sustained post-traumatic hypotension in *adults* is almost always secondary to extracranial causes. Neurogenic hypotension is a preterminal event and does not occur until brain stem reflexes disappear and spontaneous respirations cease. Hypotension in patients with head injury may occur from blood loss from a compound wound of the dural venous sinuses or scalp lacerations. In both cases, bleeding can be controlled by digital compression of the source of hemorrhage. It is only in infants and children (under the age of two) that sustained hypotension may occur as a result of severe head injury. Because the circulating blood volume in these patients is relatively small, intracranial hematomas (particularly if associated with subgaleal hemorrhage) may result in loss of a significant proportion of the patient's circulating blood volume.

Respiratory Insufficiency

The adequacy of ventilation can be determined by obtaining arterial blood gases. If the earlier measures to maintain adequate blood oxygenation are ineffective, endotracheal intubation must be considered. Intubation should be performed in all comatose patients with an arterial PaO_2 of less than 70 torr or a $PaCO_2$ of greater than 45 torr. When intubation becomes necessary prior to assessing the stability of the cervical spine, neck extension should be avoided by using a nasotracheal tube. In the obtunded patient with intact pharyngeal reflexes, intubation may provoke bucking which can cause a dangerous rise in intracranial pressure. This reaction can be prevented by the use of a topical anesthetic or the intravenous administration of a short-acting barbiturate.

A distended stomach is common after severe head injury and can compromise respiration by limiting diaphragmatic excursion. It also places the patient at risk of vomiting and aspiration. These potential complications can be minimized by emptying the stomach with a nasogastric tube. Because the passage of the nasogastric tube may cause regurgitation and aspiration, insertion should be performed after intubation with an endotracheal tube with an inflated cuff.

Respirations may also be compromised by primary central nervous system dysfunction with decreased respiratory frequency and excursion.[28, 68] Inadequate ventilation may also result from hypothalamic injury causing a massive sympathetic discharge and neurogenic pulmonary edema. Irrespective of their origin, these respiratory difficulties are associated with hypoxemia which necessitates assisted or controlled ventilation.

Hypoxia secondary to neurogenic pulmonary shunting is a common finding in severe head injury and usually responds to positive end-expiratory pressure (PEEP). PEEP, however, increases intrathoracic pressure, decreases cerebral venous return and may thereby elevate the intracranial pressure (ICP).[1, 36] This untoward effect of PEEP can be reduced by elevating the head to 30°, which facilitates intracranial venous drainage. A PEEP of 5–10 cm H_2O can then be tolerated without significant effect on ICP.[28] If increased pulmonary shunting is secondary to fluid overload, it can be corrected with a loop diuretic such as furosemide. Osmotic diuretics such as mannitol should be avoided in this situation.

Hypovolemia

In the emergency department, hypovolemic hypotension must be vigorously treated by hemostasis and volume replacement (see Chapter 3). Administration of crystalloid will expand the circulating vascular volume and the simultaneous transfusion of packed red blood cells will increase the oxygen-carrying capacity of the circulation.

Effect of Decreased Cerebral Oxygen Delivery on Outcome

Oxygen delivery to cerebral parenchyma in the early post-traumatic period plays an important part in determining the eventual outcome of patients with brain and multiple systems injuries. Miller et al (62) have shown that there is an increase in morbidity and mortality when the head injured patient presents with hypoxia (arterial PaO_2 less than 65 torr), hypercarbia ($PaCO_2$ greater than 45 torr), anemia (hematocrit less than 30%) or hypotension (systolic blood pressure of less than 95 mm Hg) as a result of systemic injuries. Forty-four percent of patients with severe head injury had one or more of these insults present prior to admission. For the patients with diffuse brain injury, the presence of one of these insults resulted in a statistically significant increase in unsatisfactory outcome (36 vs 13% for those in whom no insult was present).

NEUROLOGICAL ASSESSMENT

The baseline neurological assessment is obtained only after cardiopulmonary resuscitation is completed. The initial evaluation should include such information as time, location, and mechanism of injury and can be obtained from paramedics, policemen, relatives, or other witnesses.

Indeed, the occurrence of head injury is often not suspected and depression of the level of consciousness may be falsely attributed to alcoholism or stroke. Galbraith[29] has pointed out that altered consciousness is unlikely to be secondary to alcohol consumption when the blood alcohol level is less than 200 mg %. Cerebral infarction from occulusion of the vessels of the anterior portion of the Circle of Willis does not usually produce a depressed level of consciousness. When there is depression of consciousness, it generally occurs several days after the ictus as a result of cerebral swelling.

Patients with epilepsy may present a particular problem in diagnosis. Epileptics may sustain head injury resulting in intracranial hemorrhage with minimal external evidence of injury. Depression of the level of consciousness may be wrongly attributed to the post-ictal state. However, intracranial hematoma should be suspected whenever post-ical focal deficit, focal seizures, or status epilepticus are observed in an epileptic without a previous history of such seizure patterns.[82]

The temporal course of the patient's level of consciousness is particularly relevant; a history of a lucid interval in a patient who presents unconscious, strongly suggests an expanding intracranial hematoma and excludes the diagnosis of diffuse brain injury. The mechanism of injury is also significant since direct blows to the head are more likely to cause epidural hematomas, whereas acceleration-deceleration injuries are more commonly associated with diffuse cerebral damage.[12, 58] Neurological examination of head injured patients must be succinct and reproducible when performed sequentially and over a period of time by different observers. The patient's level of consciousness is the single most important clinical sign in the assessment of the severity of injury. The use of the terms "stupor," "semi-comatose," or "obtunded" to describe the level of consciousness have different connotations to different examiners, are imprecise, and should be avoided.

The challenge has been to quantitate the level of neurological function and level of consciousness in a manner that would correlate with the severity of injury and the patient's ultimate outcome. To a large extent, the Glasgow Coma Score (GCS) (Fig. 2.1) objectively quantifies the level of consciousness and correlates well with recovery from injury.[45, 85, 87]

This scale consists of three components: eye opening, motor response, and verbal response. The most sensitive of the three components is the motor response. Extensive clinical data indicates that this component correlates with both the extent of injury and outcome.[66, 87] This is particularly true for severe injuries where the motor score is four or less.

Although the GCS provides a very useful quantitative assessment of the severity of neurological dysfunction, there are certain circumstances where it may be inaccurate, or cannot be used. Patients who are in shock, hypoxic, intoxicated, or post-ictal may have a GCS that does not accurately reflect the degree of brain damage. Associated injury such as bilateral orbital trauma or cervical spinal cord damage may interfere with the use of this scale. In the agitated, uncooperative, dysphasic or intubated patient, accurate scoring may be impossible.[6] The GCS cannot be applied to pre-verbal children. Furthermore, since the motor score is recorded from the side with the *best* response, it fails to reflect unilateral deterioration. This can be avoided by recording the motor response of both sides. Although the GCS is a useful quantitative measure of consciousness, it is not a substitute for a detailed neurological assessment. Nevertheless, the coma scale is a practical and useful tool for neurological evaluation by paramedical personnel, physicians, or nurses. The use of the scale does not require intensive training or a medical background and there is a high degree of correlation between the scores obtained by physicians, nursing staff, and paramedics.[8, 86] By objectifying and standardizing assessments of the level of consciousness, the GCS also permits the design of various treatment protocols for use by emergency medical and paramedical personnel.[94] The routine use of this scale by trauma centers allows for inter-center comparison and/or multi-center investigation of different aspects of head injury.[48, 87]

A complete neurological examination can only be performed in an alert and coopera-

Verbal Response:	
None	1
Incomprehensible sounds	2
Inappropriate words	3
Confused	4
Oriented	5
Eye Opening:	
None	1
To pain	2
To speech	3
Spontaneously	4
Motor Response:	
None	1
Abnormal extensor	2
Abnormal flexion	3
Withdraws	4
Localizes	5
Obeys	6

Figure 2.1. The Glasgow Coma Score (GCS) evaluates the patient's level of consciousness in three ways: verbal response, eye opening, and motor response. The GCS is obtained by adding the individual scores for each of the three components. A fully oriented, alert patient would receive a maximum score of 15. A mute, flaccid patient who has no eye opening to any stimuli would receive a score of three.

tive patient. In patients with head injury, the examination is abbreviated and adapted to the patient's level of consciousness. After the patient is initially evaluated using the GCS, the position, movement, shape, size of the eyes and the reaction of the pupils should be noted and recorded. Spontaneous eye movements in lighter stages of coma are usually roving and may be conjugate or dysconjugate. Horizontal roving eye movements indicate only that the midbrain and pontine tegmentum are intact. In deep coma, there are no spontaneous eye movements and the integrity of brain stem function can be tested with the oculovestibular or the oculocephalic reflex (Fig. 2.2), but the latter should not be done until the stability of the cervical spine has been determined. Oculovestibular reflexes gener-

ally persist after oculocephalic reflexes have disappeared. Therefore, if the oculocephalic reflexes are absent, oculovestibular testing must be performed. When either reflex is present and normal, it is likely that the pons and midbrain (through which the afferent and efferent arcs of this reflex traverse) are structurally intact.

The pupillary light reflex is an important diagnostic test in comatose patients. Brain injury severe enough to render patients deeply comatose and decerebrate is usually associated with unresponsive or poorly responsive pupils, whereas patients in deep coma from metabolic disease have sparing of the pupillary light reflex.[69] Abnormal pupillary light reactions may have a localizing value. Small, but reactive pupils, are seen in diencephalic injury and/or meta-

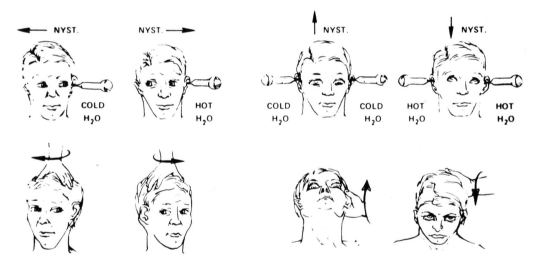

Figure 2.2. *Top row*: In the awake patient, cold water introduced into the external auditory canal produces nystagmus with the quick component away from the stimulated ear. In the comatose, head-injured patient with an intact brain stem, cold water will cause tonic deviation of the eyes toward the side of the stimulus. Bilateral instillation of cold water produces upward nystagmus in the conscious patient and downward tonic deviation in the unconscious patient with an intact brain stem. Warm water produces movements in the opposite direction from cold water. When the brain stem has been injured, eye movements will be dysconjugate or absent in response to caloric stimuli. *Bottom row*: Drawings demonstrate the oculocephalic response. In the comatose patient with an intact brain stem, the eyes will deviate as indicated in response to rotation or flexion of the head. If brain stem injury is present, the eye responses will be absent or dysconjugate. Oculocephalic responses are never present in conscious patients. (Reproduced with permission: Posner, J.B.: Clinical evaluation of the unconscious patient. Clinical Neurosurgery, 22:281–301, 1975.)

bolic disorders. Small, reactive pupils may sometimes be observed during early phases of cerebral herniation. At this stage, patients are usually responding appropriately to painful stimuli, but as the coma deepens, the pupils become fixed and dilated. This phenomenon has been explained by hypothalamic compression in early stages of herniation with resultant Horner's syndrome.[16, 69] If the process of herniation is not reversed by decompression of the expanding mass, the brain stem will be irreversibly damaged. Pinpoint pupils generally occur with pontine hemorrhages and are believed to result from simultaneous sympathetic interruption and parasympathetic irritation. Pinpoint pupils may also be seen in patients who have not had significant head trauma as a result of narcotic ingestion. Midbrain damage may produce midposition, non-reactive pupils with spontaneous fluctuation of size (hippus).[68]

A unilaterally dilated and fixed pupil is usually indicative of a supratentorial expanding mass with midline shift, uncal herniation, and compression of the third cranial nerve. Rarely, uncal herniation with a third nerve palsy may occur in an awake patient. The third nerve is occasionally damaged directly by orbital trauma but in this circumstance there is commonly an associated fourth and sixth nerve injury as well. In the presence of a fixed, dilated pupil, optic nerve injury must also be considered. If the optic nerve has been injured, the pupil will not react directly to light although the consensual light reflex will be preserved. The consensual and direct light reflex are absent in third nerve injury.

Other neurological findings such as hemiparesis and dysphasia are evidence of hemispheric lesions and their progression may reflect an expanding intracranial mass. Hemiplegia is usually contralateral to the side of the brain injury and third nerve paresis is ipsilateral to the lesion. On occasion, however, motor deficit is seen ipsilateral to the side of the lesion. This occurs as a result of rapid shift of the brain stem by the medial temporal lobe with compression of the contralateral cerebral peduncle against the opposite tentorial edge. For the most part, the side of the third nerve palsy is a more reliable indicator than is the hemiparesis in localizing the site of the mass lesion. Clinical localization of the side of an expanding intracranial hematoma may be important in cases where there is rapid deterioration of the patient's neurological status, mandating operative exploration without diagnostic studies (see also Chapter 11).

Other abnormalities of the motor examination include decortication and decerebration. Decortication (or decorticate rigidity) is an abnormal flexion of the arm and hand and extension, internal rotation, and plantar flexion of the lower extremity. Decerebration (or decerebrate rigidity) is abnormal extension and pronation of the arm with extension of the lower extremities accompanied by plantar flexion.[68] Both are frequently seen in patients with severe head injury and may be observed to occur spontaneously or only with noxious stimuli. Decortication has been thought to result from injury to the corticospinal tract in the internal capsule or rostral cerebral peduncle.[68] Decerebration has been thought to occur from injury to the region of the rostral midbrain. Recent pathological studies, however, indicate that such correlation between decerebrate posturing and structural brain damage does not always exist.[9]

Ataxia, nystagmus, or abnormalities of lower cranial nerves are generally uncommon after head injury. If seen, they should raise suspicion of an infratentorial injury or a growing mass lesion. Evidence of a direct occipital blow (scalp laceration, fracture involving the foramen magnum) will help to confirm the posterior fossa as the site of injury.

Examination of the Head

Scalp contusions and lacerations not only provide proof of head trauma, but can also, in certain circumstances, overlie the site of the lesion (*e.g.*, depressed fractures). Since hair and dirt are usually driven into the wound, liberal irrigation and thorough debridement of devitalized tissue and debris are essential. Initially, hemostasis can be accomplished by digital pressure on the wound margins. Ligation of bleeding vessels is rarely necessary. Before repairing the scalp laceration, hair should be shaved at least one inch on both sides of the wound. Small scalp avulsions may be repaired primarily by undermining the galea but larger avulsions commonly require rotation of a scalp flap (see Chapter 15). An assiduous search for a depressed skull fracture beneath the laceration should be made. Accurate identification of compound depressed fractures is facilitated by self-retaining retractors, high-intensity lighting, and hemostasis. In suspected cases of depressed fracture, skull roentgenograms will confirm the presence of the injury. When a compound-depressed fracture is found, the fracture should be elevated and the wound closed in the operating room. Early debridement is essential as the dura is frequently torn in compound injuries and elevation of the fracture after 24 hours results in a significant increase in infectious complications.[42, 60] Care must be taken not to manipulate depressed skull fractures in the emergency room, as fragments may be tamponading a lacerated vessel or a dural sinus and their removal may result in uncontrolled hemorrhage. The same principle applies to penetrating objects (ice picks, spikes, knives) which protrude from the skull. The offending object must be protected from any movement during transportation of the patient from the emergency room to the X-ray department and operating room. Radiographic views of the object within the skull are helpful in planning the surgical exposure. If the object is lying close to where a large vessel is expected to be, angiography is indicated before the object is removed.

Hemotympanum, ecchymosis over the mastoid area (Battle's sign), or periorbital ecchymosis are valuable clues to the presence of a basal skull fracture. In these conditions, one should be cognizant of the increased incidence of meningitis and CSF fistulae. Any patient with these signs and/ or suspected cerebrospinal fluid fistula should be admitted for observation. In a majority of cases, CSF rhinorrhea appears in the first 48 hours after injury. Delayed forms may also occur from several days to several months later. It is therefore important for the emergency room examiner to alert the patient to such potential complications should he decide to discharge the patient. In order to confirm the diagnosis of CSF rhinorrhea, the fluid discharge from the nose or ear must contain more than 30 mg % of glucose. Dextrostix may give a positive reaction with as little as 5 mg % of glucose. The reaction may be positive in as many as 75% of patients with normal nasal secretion but a negative reaction can reliably rule out the presence of cerebrospinal fluid (see also Chapter 5).

MANAGEMENT OF INTRACRANIAL HYPERTENSION IN THE EMERGENCY ROOM

Although more than half of all head injury mortality is associated with intracranial hypertension,[63, 89] the role of various levels of ICP elevation on the outcome of head injured patients is unclear.[59, 88, 91] Significant intracranial hypertension may reduce the cerebral perfusion pressure below the critical level required to maintain normal cerebral metabolism. In order to prevent secondary brain damage, intracranial hypertension must be detected and controlled early. This may have to be done in appropriate cases soon after the patient is resuscitated and before diagnostic studies are completed.

Patients who enter with a dilated pupil and contralateral hemiparesis or who develop these findings in the emergency room almost certainly have elevations of ICP from an expanding intracranial hematoma. However, it is usually impossible on the basis of the clinical examination to identify with certainty those patients who have elevations of ICP. Patients who enter bilaterally decerebrate may have sustained a diffuse brain injury without elevation of ICP or they may have decerebration on the basis of a large mass which is compressing brain stem structures. Under these circumstances, the clinician has two choices. He may insert any one of a number of ICP monitoring devices (described in Chapter

10) *or* make the assumption that the patient has elevated ICP and treat him appropriately. It is obviously preferable to monitor the ICP and treat the patient according to values obtained (levels greater than 15 mm Hg are generally considered elevated). However, neurosurgical assistance in placing the monitor may not be immediately available. Whatever the case, whether the patient has suspected or confirmed elevation of ICP, hyperventilation is the most effective method for the rapid reduction of elevated pressure. This should be begun immediately and the arterial $PaCO_2$ should be lowered to 25–30 torr. Mannitol (0.5–1.0 g per kg) should be given in a rapid intravenous infusion over 15–20 minutes and a Foley catheter should be inserted. These and other methods to lower ICP are detailed in Chapter 9.

MANAGEMENT OF POST-TRAUMATIC EPILEPSY IN THE EMERGENCY ROOM

Post-traumatic epilepsy has been implicated as one of the avoidable causes of death in patients who die from complications of head injury.[41] The incidence of early post-traumatic epilepsy in closed head injury is about 4%.[39] This incidence rises to about 10% when the head injury is associated with a depressed skull fracture.[43] Laceration of the dura and the brain further increase the chance of post-traumatic seizures. In penetrating injuries and gunshot wounds, the incidence of seizures is even higher. Other contributing factors are intracranial hematomas, retained intracerebral foreign bodies, infectious processes, and the location of injury.[17, 18] The role of the prophylactic use of anti-convulsants in preventing seizures is unclear.[17, 72, 95] The importance of prompt control of post-traumatic seizures, however, cannot be overemphasized. Seizure activity may not only cause respiratory embarassment, but also increase cerebral blood flow and cerebral blood volume resulting in elevation of ICP. The risk of complications is markedly higher when seizures become repetitive and progress to status epilepticus. The initial treatment consists of rapid infusion of intravenous diazepam (0.2 mg per kg). The duration of the anti-epileptic activity of this agent is short and has to be supplemented by a longer acting medication. Intravenous phenytoin is the drug of choice to achieve a sustained anti-convulsant effect.[20, 21] Phenytoin should be infused at a rate of 50 mg per minute for a total dose of 15 mg per kg. This slow rate of infusion is required to avoid cardiovascular complications. With this regimen, an adequate blood level is obtained within several minutes. Intravenous phenobarbital may also be used for this purpose, but in order to achieve a satisfactory anti-convulsant effect in a short time, sedative doses are required. This effect is not always desirable and may compromise the value of subsequent neurological examinations.

DIAGNOSTIC STUDIES

After cardiopulmonary resuscitation is completed, and before any other neuroradiologic procedures are performed, stability of the cervical spine must be determined by a lateral radiographic view of the neck. In reviewing the X-rays, one should make certain to visualize the entire cervical spine as an incomplete study may not reveal fractures of the lower cervical vertebrae.[77] This is particularly important in patients with multiple injuries and in victims of motor vehicle accidents in whom the risk of injury is high (Fig. 2.3).

The technical aspects of the neuroradiologic evaluation of the patient with head injury are extensively discussed in Chapter 4. Nevertheless, the physician in the emergency room is frequently confronted with the need to make decisions regarding the *necessity* for special diagnostic studies and the *types* of studies which will provide useful information. An algorithm that may be helpful in guiding the clinician in his selection of diagnostic studies is seen in Figure 2.4.

The overall importance of skull roentgenography has been the subject of considerable controversy. Skull roentgenograms are obtained in the following circumstances: 1) suspicion of a depressed skull fracture, 2) gunshot wounds or other penetrating inju-

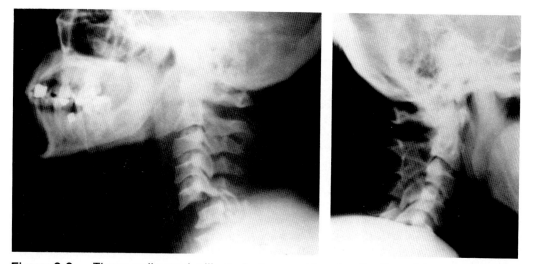

Figure 2.3. These radiographs illustrate the need for visualization of the entire cervical spine. Initial X-rays in this patient (*right*) failed to show the C5-6 fracture dislocation which was visualized only after shoulders were pulled down (*left*).

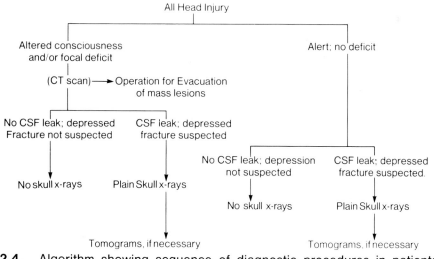

Figure 2.4. Algorithm showing sequence of diagnostic procedures in patients with head injury.

ries, and 3) suspicion of a basal skull fracture or cerebrospinal fluid leak. All patients with gunshot wounds, focal neurological deficit, or altered states of consciousness should have CT scans. Angiography is used only when the CT scan is unavailable or vascular injury is suspected. In the absence of CT scanning, twist drill ventriculograms may also be used for delineation of the side of the mass lesion (this technique is discussed more fully in Chapter 4).

Hypocloidal tomography of the skull base is performed in all patients with cerebrospinal fluid fistulae or pneumocephalus.

CRITERIA FOR ADMISSION TO THE HOSPITAL

While all seriously injured patients are admitted to the hospital without question, decision-making regarding admission of the patient with a minor head injury is more difficult and controversial. The patient who is neurologically intact at the time of presentation in the emergency room and who has had no loss of consciousness, does not require admission. Patients who have been unconscious for 10 minutes or more are admitted even though they may be intact at the time of presentation. This time limit is clearly an arbitrary one and there are no statistics to prove or disprove the efficacy of this policy. In addition, we also admit: 1) patients who have any degree of focal neurological deficit, 2) patients with post-traumatic seizures without a previous history of seizure activity or those who develop new patterns of seizures, 3) all patients with depressed skull fractures or penetrating wounds, 4) patients who are not fully alert or those in whom drug or alcohol ingestion makes neurological evaluation difficult 5) all patients with basal skull fractures and/or cerebrospinal fluid fistulae, and 6) patients in whom there is any doubt about the first five criteria.

References

1. Aidinis, S.J., Lafferty, J., Shapiro, H.M.: Intracranial response to PEEP. Anesthesiology, 45:275–286, 1976.
2. Baratham, G., Dennyson, W.G.: Delayed traumatic intracerebral hemorrhage. J. Neurol. Neurosurg. Psychiatry, 35:698–706, 1972.
3. Becker, D.P., Miller, J.D., Sweet, R.C., et al.: Head Injury Management. In: Neural Trauma (Seminars in Neurological Surgery), Eds. A. John Popp, Robert S. Bourke, Louis R. Nelson, Harold K. Kimelberg. Raven Press, New York, 1978, pp. 313–328.
4. Becker, D.P., Miller, J.D., Ward, J.D., et al.: The outcome from severe head injury with early diagnosis and intensive management. J. Neurosurg., 47:491–502, 1977.
5. Bergeron, R.T., Rumbaugh, C.: Non space-occupying sequelae of head trauma. Radiol. Clin. North Am., 12:315–331, 1974.
6. Bouzarth, W.F.: Coma scale (letter). J. Neurosurg., 49:477–478, 1978.
7. Braakman, R.: Survey and follow-up of 225 consecutive patients with a depressed skull fracture. J. Neurol. Neurosurg. Psychiatry, 34:106, 1971.
8. Braakman, R., Avezaat, C.J., Maas, A.I., et al.: Inter observer agreement in the assessment of the motor response of the Glasgow Coma Scale. Clin. Neurol. Neurosurg., 80:100–106, 1977.
9. Bricolo, A., Turazzi, S., Alexandre, A., et al.: Decerebrate rigidity in acute head injury. J. Neurosurg., 47:680–698, 1977.
10. Brown, G.W., Brown, M.L., Hines, H.M.: Effects of experimental concussion on blood flow, arterial pressure and cardiac rate. Am. J. Physiol., 170:294–300, 1952.
11. Brown, F.D., Mullan, S., Duda, E.E.: Delayed traumatic intracerebral hematoma. J. Neurosurg., 48:1019–1022, 1978.
12. Bruce, D.A., Gennarelli, T.A., Langfitt, T.W.: Resuscitation from coma due to head injury. Crit. Care Med., 6:254–269, 1978.
13. Bruce, D.A., Schut, L., Bruno, L.A., et al.: Outcome following severe head injuries in children. J. Neurosurg., 48:679–688, 1978.
14. Buckell, M.: Blood changes on intravenous administration of mannitol or urea for reduction of intracranial pressure in neurosurgical patients. Clin. Sci., 27:223–227, 1964.
15. Busch, E.A.V.:Brain stem contusions: Differential diagnosis, therapy, and prognosis. Clin. Neurosurg., 9:18–33, 1963.
16. Caronna, J.J., Simon, R.P.: The comatose patient: A diagnostic approach and treatment. Int. Anesthesiol. Clin., 17:3–18, 1979.
17. Caveness, W.F., Meirowsky, A.M., Rish, B.L., et al.: The nature of post-traumatic epilepsy. J. Neurosurg., 50:545–553, 1979.
18. Caviness, V.S., Jr.: Epilepsy and craniocerebral injury of warfare. In: Head Injury Conference Proceedings. Eds.: W.F. Caveness, A.E. Walker. J.B. Lippincott, Philadelphia, 1966, pp. 220–234.
19. Cooper, P.R., Moody, S., Clark, W.K.: Dexamethasone and severe head injury. A prospective double-blind study. J. Neurosurg., 51:307–316, 1979.
20. Cranford, R.E., Leppik, I.E., Patrick, B., et al.: Intravenous phenytoin: clinical and pharmacokinetic aspects. Neurology 28:874–880, 1978.
21. Cranford, R.E., Leppik, I.E., Patrick, B., et al.: Intravenous phenytoin in acute treatment of seizures. Neurology, 29:1474–1479, 1979.
22. Diaz, F.G., Yock, D.H., Larson, D., et al.: Early diagnosis of delayed post-traumatic intracerebral hematomas. J. Neurosurg., 50:217–223, 1979.
23. Dodge, P.R., Meirowsky, A.M.: Tangential wounds of scalp and skull. J. Neurosurg., 9:472–483, 1952.
24. Faupel, G., Reulen, H.J., Muller, D., et al.: Double-blind study on the effects of steroids on severe closed head injury. Eds. H.M. Papius, W. Feindel. In: Dynamics of Brain Edema. Springer-Verlag, Berlin, 1976, pp. 337–343.
25. Field, J.H.: Epidemiology of Head Injuries in England and Wales (The Field Report), London, HMSO, 1976.
26. Fishman, R.A.: Brain edema. N. Engl. J. Med., 293:706–711, 1975.
27. French, B.N., Dublin, A.B.: The value of computerizing tomography in the management of 1000 consecutive head injuries. Surg. Neurol., 7:171–183, 1977.
28. Frost, E.A.M.: The physiopathology of respiration in neurosurgical patients. J. Neurosurg., 50:699–714, 1979.
29. Galbraith, S.: Misdiagnosis and delayed diagnosis in traumatic intracranial haematoma. Br. Med. J., 1:1438–1439, 1976.
30. Galicich, J.H., French, L.A.: Use of dexametha-

sone in the treatment of cerebral edema resulting from brain tumors and brain surgery. Am. Pract., 12:169–174, 1961.

31. Garde, A.: Experience with dexamethasone treatment of intracranial pressure caused by brain tumors. Acta Neurol. Scand. Suppl., 13:439–443, 1965.

32. Gobiet, W., Bock, W.J., Liesegang, J., et al.: Treatment of acute cerebral edema with high dose of dexamethasone. Eds. J.W.F. Beks, D.A. Bosch, M. Brock. In: Intracranial Pressure III. Springer-Verlag, Berlin, 1976, pp. 231–235.

33. Goodnight, S.H., Kenoyer, G., Rapaport, S.I., et al.: Defibrination after brain-tissue destruction. A serious complication of head injury. N. Engl. J. Med., 290:1043–1047, 1974.

34. Gudeman, S.K., Miller, J.D., Becker, D.P.: Failure of high-dose steroid therapy to influence intracranial pressure in patients with severe head injury. J. Neurosurg., 51:301–306, 1979.

35. Hubschmann, O., Shapiro, K., Baden, M., et al.: Craniocerebral gunshot injuries in civilian practice—prognostic criteria and surgical management: experience with 82 cases. J. Trauma, 19:6–12, 1979.

36. Huseby, J.S., Pavlin, E.G., Butler, J.: Effect of positive end-expiratory pressure on intracranial pressure in dogs. J. Appl. Physiol., 44:25–27, 1978.

37. Jamieson, K.: The toll of the road: Clinical aspects. Med. J. Aust., 23:157–160, 1969.

38. Jennett, B.: Assessment of the severity of head injury. J. Neurol. Neurosurg. Psychiatry, 39:647–655, 1976.

39. Jennett, B.: Epilepsy after non-missile head injuries. Scot. Med. J., 18:8–13, 1973.

40. Jennett, B.: Prognosis after head injury. Handbook of Clin. Neurol., 24:669–681, 1976.

41. Jennett, B., Carlin, J.: Preventable mortality and morbidity after head injury. Injury, 10:31–39, 1978.

42. Jennett, B., Miller, J.D.: Infection after depressed fracture of skull. Implications for management of non-missile injuries. J. Neurosurg., 36:333–339, 1972.

43. Jennett, B., Miller, J.D., Braakman, R.: Epilepsy after non-missile depressed skull fracture. J. Neurosurg., 41:208–216, 1974.

44. Jennett, B., Teasdale, G., Braakman, R., et al.: Predicting outcome in individual patients after severe head injury. Lancet 1:1031–1034, 1976.

45. Jennett, B., Teasdale, G., Galbraith, S., et al.: Severe head injuries in three countries. J. Neurol. Neurosurg. Psychiatry, 40:291–298, 1973.

46. Keimowitz, R.M., Annis, B.L.: Disseminated intervascular coagulation associated with massive brain injury. J. Neurosurg., 39:178–180, 1973.

47. Laver, M.B., Lowenstein, E.: Lung function following trauma in man. Clin. Neurosurg., 19:133–174, 1972.

48. Langfitt, T.W.: Measuring the outcome from head injuries. J. Neurosurg., 48:673–678, 1978.

49. Langfitt, T.W., Weinstein, J.D., Kassell, N.F., Jackson, J.L.F.: Contributions of trauma, anoxia and arterial hypertension to experimental acute brain swelling. Trans. Am. Neurolog. Assoc.,

92:267–259, 1967.

50. Long, D.M., Hartmann, J.F., French, L.A.: The response of experimental cerebral edema to glucosteroid administration. J. Neurosurg., 24:843–854, 1966.

51. Lundberg, N.: Continuous recording and control of ventricular fluid pressure in neurosurgical practice. Acta Psychiat. Scand., 36 (Suppl. 149):1–193, 1960.

52. Lundberg, N., Kjallquist, A., Kullberg, G., et al.: Non-operative management of intracranial hypertension. In: Advances and technical standards in neurosurgery. Eds. H. Krayenbuhl, et al. Springer Wien, New York, 1974.

53. Marino deVillasante, J., Taveras, J.M.: Computerized tomography (CT) in acute head trauma. Am. J. Roentgenol., 126:765–778, 1976.

54. Maxwell, R.E., Long, D.M., French, L.A.: The effects of glucosteroids on experimental cold-induced brain edema. J. Neurosurg., 34:477–487, 1971.

55. McDonald, E.J., Winestock, D.P., Hoff, J.T.: The value of repeat cerebral arteriography in the evaluation of trauma. Am. J. Roentgenol., 126:792–797, 1967.

56. McGauley, J.L., Miller, C.A., Penner, J.A.: Diagnosis and treatment of diffuse intravascular coagulation following cerebral trauma. J. Neurosurg., 43:374–376, 1975.

57. Meinig, G., Aulich, A., Wende, S., et al.: The effect of dexamethasone and diuretics on peritumor brain edema: Comparative study of tissue water content and CT. In: Dynamics of Brain Edema. Eds. H.M. Pappius, W. Feindel. Springer-Verlag, Berlin, 1976, pp. 301–305.

58. Miller, J.D., Becker, D.P., Rosner, M.J., et al.: Implications of intracranial mass lesions for outcome of severe head injury. In: Neural Trauma. Eds. A.J. Popp, et al. Raven Press, New York, 1978, pp. 173–180 .

59. Miller, J.D., Becker, D.P., Ward, J.D., et al.: Significance of intracranial hypertension in severe head injury. J. Neurosurg., 47:503–516, 1977.

60. Miller, J.D., Jennett, W.B.: Complications of depressed skull fracture. Lancet, 2:991–995, 1968.

61. Miller, J.D., Leech, P.: Effects of Mannitol and steroid therapy on intracranial volume-pressure relationships in patients. J. Neurosurg., 42:274–281, 1975.

62. Miller, J.D., Sweet, R.C., Narayan, R., et al.: Early insults to the injured brain. J.A.M.A., 240:439–442, 1978.

63. Mitchell, D.E., Adams, J.H.: Primary focal impact damage to the brainstem in blunt head injuries. Does it exist? Lancet 2:215–218, 1973.

64. North, J.B., Jennett, S.: Abnormal breathing patterns associated with acute brain damage. Arch. Neurol., 31:338–344, 1974.

65. Obrist, W.D., Gennarelli, T.A., Segawa, H., et al.: Relation of cerebral blood flow to neurological status and outcome in head-injured patients. J. Neurosurg., 51:292–300, 1979.

66. Overgaard, J., Hvid-Hansen, O., Land, A.M., et al.: Prognosis after head injury based on early clinical

examination. Lancet, 2:631–635, 1963.

67. Oxbury, J.M., Whitty, C.W.M.: Causes and consequences of status epilepticus in adults. Brain, 94:733–744, 1971.

68. Plum, F., Posner, J.B.: The diagnosis of stupor and coma, 2nd Ed., F.A. Davis, Philadelphia, 1972.

69. Posner, J.B.: Clinical evaluation of the unconscious patient. Clin. Neurosurg., 22:281–301, 1975.

70. Preston, F.E., Malia, R.G., Sworn, M.J., et al.: Disseminated intravascular coagulation as a consequence of cerebral damage. J. Neurol. Neurosurg. Psychiatry, 37:241–248, 1974.

71. Price, D.J., Murray, A.: The influence of hypoxia and hypotension on recovery from head injury. Injury, 3:218–224, 1972.

72. Rapport, R.L., Penry, J.K.: A survey of attitudes toward the pharmacological prophylaxis of posttraumatic epilepsy. J. Neurosurg., 38:159–166, 1974.

73. Reilly, P.L., Adams, J.H., Graham, D.I., et al.: Patients with head injury who talk and die. Lancet, 2:375–377, 1975.

74. Roberson, F.C., Kishore, P.R.S., Miller, J.D., et al.: The value of serial computerized tomography in the management of severe head injury. Surg. Neurol., 12:161–167, 1979.

75. Rose, J., Valtonen, S., Jennett, B.: Avoidable factors contributing to death after head injury. Br. Med. J., 2:615–618, 1977.

76. Rosner, M.J., Becker, D.P.: ICP monitoring: Complications and associated factors. Clin. Neurosurg., 23:494–519, 1976.

77. Scher, A.T.: A plea for routine radiographic examination of the cervical spine after head injury. S. Afr. Med. J., 51:885–887, 1977.

78. Sherrington, C.S.: Decerebrate rigidity and reflex coordination of movement. J. Physiol., 22:319–332, 1898.

79. Sundbärg, G., Kjällquist, Å., Lundberg, N., et al.: Complications due to prolonged ventricular fluid pressure recording in clinical practice. In: Intracranial Pressure. Eds. M. Brock, H. Dietz. Springer-Verlag, Berlin, 1972, pp. 348–352.

80. Sweet, R.C. Miller, J.D., Lipper, M., et al.: Significance of bilateral abnormalities on the CT scan in patients with severe head injury. Neurosurgery, 3:16–21, 1978.

81. Tabaddor, K.: Is ICP monitoring useful in head injury? Paper presented at Congress of Neurological Surgeons Meeting, Houston, Texas, 1980.

82. Tabaddor, K., Balagura, S.: Acute epidural hematoma following epileptic seizures. Arch. Neurol., 38:198–199, 1981.

83. Tabaddor, K., Bhushan, C., Pevsner, P.H., et al.: Prognostic value of cerebral blood flow (CBF) and cerebral metabolic rate of oxygen (CMRO$_2$) in acute head trauma. J. Trauma, 12:1053–1055, 1972.

84. Teasdale, G., Galbraith, S., Jennett, B.: Operate or observe? ICP and the management of the "silent" traumatic intracranial haematoma. In: Intracranial Pressure IV. Eds. K. Shulman, A. Marmarou, J.D. Miller, et al. Springer-Verlag, Berlin, 1980, pp. 36–38.

85. Teasdale, G., Jennett, B.: Assessment of coma and impaired consciousness. A practical scale. Lancet, 2:81–83, 1974.

86. Teasdale, G., Knill-Jones, R., Van der Sande, J.: Observer variability in assessing impaired consciousness and coma. J. Neurol. Neurosurg. Psychiatry, 41:603–610, 1978.

87. Teasdale, G., Murray, G., Parker, L., et al.: Adding up the Glasgow Coma Score. Acta Neurochirurg. Suppl., 28:13–16, 1979.

88. Tindall, G.T., Fleischer, A.S.: Intracranial pressure (ICP) monitoring and prognosis in closed head injury. In: Head Injuries. Second Chicago Symposium on Neural Trauma. Ed. R.L. McLaurin. Grune & Stratton, New York, 1976, pp. 31–34.

89. Troupp, H.: Intraventricular pressure in patients with severe brain injuries. J. Trauma, 5:373–378, 1965.

90. Van der Sande, J.J., Veltkamp, J.J., Boekhout-Mussert, R.J., et al.: Head injury and coagulation disorders. J. Neurosurg., 49:357–365, 1978.

91. Vapalahti, M., Troupp, H.: Prognosis for patients with severe brain injuries. Br. Med. J., 3:404–407, 1971.

92. Waters, J., Wells, C.: The effects of a modern Emergency Medical Care System in reducing automobile crash death. J. Trauma, 13:645–647, 1973.

93. White, J.C., Brook, J.R., Goldthwait, J.D., et al.: Changes in brain volume and blood content after experimental concussion. Ann. Surg., 118:619–634, 1943.

94. Winston, S.R.: Preliminary communication: EMT and the Glasgow Coma Scale. J. Iowa Med. Soc., 69:393–398, 1979.

95. Wohns, R.N.W., Wyler, A.R.: Prophylactic phenytoin in severe head injuries. J. Neurosurg., 51:507–509, 1979.

96. Zimmerman, R.A., Bilaniuk, L.T., Bruce, D., et al.: Computed tomography of pediatric head trauma: Acute general cerebral swelling. Radiology, 126:403–408, 1978.

Initial Management of the Multiply Injured Patient

ERWIN R. THAL

Accidental injury, the leading cause of death in the first four decades of life, permanently disables nearly four hundred thousand people annually at a cost that is estimated to be in excess of seventy-five billion dollars. Initial evaluation, resuscitation, stabilization, and treatment now available to the over ten million people who are temporarily incapacitated have been considerably improved by the development of sophisticated emergency medical service (EMS) systems. Pre-hospital care provided by emergency medical technicians and paramedics trained in the skills of basic and advanced life support, coupled with advanced field communications and better organized transportation systems, have extended the services of the hospital emergency room.

These advanced EMS systems provide a greater challenge to physicians who are now seeing more critically injured patients. Therefore, an effective, organized approach coupled with an appreciation of the natural history of the trauma patient and the potential for serious sequelae, serves as the background for this discussion.

ASSESSMENT AND STABILIZATION

When the injured patient is first seen, a rapid evaluation is made to determine the severity of injury. The initial assessment, stabilization, and definitive treatment frequently necessitate the simultaneous activity of several people, all under the direction of one physician, usually a general surgeon, who assumes the responsibility for total patient care. Consultative services are provided as indicated. Although neurologic injury may be significant, priorities are determined according to acute physiologic changes.

In the more seriously injured patient, immediate attention is directed toward airway management, treatment of shock, and control of hemorrhage. Those injuries that pose an immediate threat to life, such as cardiac tamponade, tension pneumothorax, impaired airway, or exsanguinating hemorrhage are immediately assessed and stabilized.

If it is not possible to stabilize these parameters, diagnostic studies are deferred and immediate operative intervention is undertaken. If these life-threatening conditions are controlled, a judicious diagnostic evaluation may be pursued. These patients must be closely observed and the work-up terminated at the first sign of deterioration. This principle is frequently overlooked and, in an ambitious attempt to gain as much information as possible, precious time may be lost and irreversible conditions allowed to develop. Mature clinical judgment may have to supercede sophisticated time-consuming diagnostic procedures. Although CT scans are invaluable, a study may have

Grateful acknowledgement is made to Mr. Thomas Sims and Mr. Anthony Pazos for their art work.

to be abandoned in a patient who is exsanguinating from a chest or abdominal injury associated with serious head injury. Once the patient's acute problem has been stabilized, a more leisurely work-up may be resumed.

Many patients will present with occult injuries, requiring all the expertise of the experienced physician to avoid overlooking a potential problem. These patients often appear uninjured and their condition will remain stable for several hours or, in some instances, several days. Information concerning the mechanism of injury and circumstances surrounding the accident coupled with repeat evaluation, preferably by the same examiner, will lessen the chance of overlooking many serious but obscure problems.

Airway

Hypoxia is suspected in all patients who are apprehensive, anxious, combative, or uncooperative. The most common causes of upper airway obstruction are the tongue, presence of foreign objects or material, edema of the glottic area or injury to the vocal cords. Frequently clearing the upper airway by simple maneuvers such as removing debris, dentures, or secretions will restore adequate ventilation. Any manual maneuver, such as the chin lift, jaw lift, or jaw thrust which moves the mandible anteriorly will also move the tongue and help open the airway. Mechanical methods of maintaining an open airway include the use of an oropharyngeal airway, nasopharyngeal airway, esophageal obturator airway, or standard endotracheal tube.

Cervical spine injuries should be suspected when patients complain of neck pain, give a history of falling from a height greater than 10 feet, or arrive at the hospital unconscious. In cases of suspected or proven cervical spine instability, nasotracheal intubation or tracheostomy is preferred and endotracheal intubation and the cervical manipulation it entails should be avoided.

Occasionally, patients will be intubated at the scene of their injury with an esophageal obturator airway. Since these patients will invariably vomit when the esophageal airway is removed, it is necessary to provide protection from aspiration (especially in the unconscious patient). If intubation is still indicated, this may be accomplished by inserting a standard endotracheal tube around the esophageal obturator tube before it is removed (Fig. 3.1).

If manual and mechanical maneuvers are unsuccessful, or edema of the glottis is present, it may be impossible to successfully intubate the patient. If a laryngeal fracture is suspected because of crepitation, soft tissue air on X-ray, or inability to speak, endotracheal intubation is specifically contraindicated. In these cases, cricothyroidotomy should be considered. Emergency tracheostomy is rarely indicated as it is a

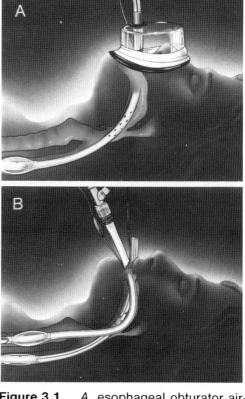

Figure 3.1.   *A,* esophageal obturator airway with face mask, pharyngeal holes and inflated balloon. Inflated balloon occludes esophagus and holes in airway permit reliable ventilation without tracheal intubation. *B,* endotracheal tube in place before removal of esophageal obturator.

time-consuming, difficult procedure associated with excessive bleeding.

Cricothyroidotomy may be readily performed by making an incision through the cricothyroid membrane and inserting a small tracheostomy tube. A formal tracheostomy may then be performed, if needed, on a leisurely basis 24 to 48 hours later.

Shock

Simeone[32] defined shock as a "clinical condition characterized by signs and symptoms which arise when the cardiac output is insufficient to fill the arterial tree with blood under sufficient pressure to provide organs and tissues with adequate blood flow." This definition emphasizes the two major manifestations of shock, namely low cardiac output and inadequate tissue perfusion which leads to the low-flow state.

Blalock[5] described four etiologic categories of shock: 1) hematogenic, 2) neurogenic, 3) vasogenic, and 4) cardiogenic. Shock generally occurs as a result of failure of one or more of the following factors: 1) the pump (heart), 2) fluid which is pumped (blood), 3) arterial resistance, and 4) venous capacitance. When evaluating the hypotensive patient, it is important to consider all etiologic factors. Whereas hemorrhagic or hypovolemic shock predominates in the trauma patient, occasionally multiple causes may be present. Motor vehicle accidents may occur as a result of unconsciousness secondary to myocardial infarction. These patients may sustain multiple injuries resulting in hypotension due either to hypovolemia or spinal cord injury and possibly complicated by cardiogenic shock as well. It is important to be aware of the multiple causes of hypotension so that each can be treated appropriately.

A systolic blood pressure below 100 mm Hg is commonly accepted as evidence of shock. However, in hypertensive patients, alert apprehensive patients, and older patients, a systolic blood pressure less than 110 mm Hg following trauma should be worrisome. It is important to assess the pulse rate, amount of blood loss, and response to positional change (tilt test) when evaluating patients for hemodynamic instability.

The presence of hypotension secondary to spinal cord injury is frequently overlooked in the multiply injured patient. It occurs as a result of massive vasodilation and is relatively easy to differentiate from hemorrhagic shock (Table 3.1).

Hypotension does not occur secondary to closed head injuries in adults. In infants with open cranial sutures, a significant proportion of the circulating blood volume may be lost intracranially and result in hypotension. Low blood pressure in older children and adult patients with head injuries is nearly always due to systemic blood loss. This usually occurs in either the chest or abdominal cavities or in conjunction with pelvic or long bone fractures. A rapid attempt is made to identify the source of blood loss in these patients. Needle thoracentesis, abdominal paracentesis, or peritoneal lavage is indicated in an unconscious patient who remains hypotensive.

The treatment of shock begins with fluid administration. Replacement of the depleted extracellular fluid by an electrolyte solution such as Ringer's lactate, which is similar to extracellular fluid, has been shown to be of significant benefit in the cellular response to hypovolemic shock.[8, 31] It has also been shown to be of clinical benefit in a large number of patients.[29]

Resuscitation is begun with the insertion of a large bore 14 to 16 gauge catheter and the rapid infusion of two liters of crystalloid solution such as Ringer's lactate. Because of complications such as pneumothorax, hydrothorax, air embolism, and bacterial contamination, the subclavian route is not gen-

Table 3.1

	Hemorrhagic Shock	Hypotension from Spinal Cord Injury
Pulse	Increased	Normal—decreased
Neurologic deficit	Absent	Present
Skin	Cool and clammy	Dry and warm
Mentation	May be altered	Unchanged
Urine output	Decreased	Frequently normal

erally used in the emergency room unless no other site is available. All intravenous lines inserted in the field or emergency room should be removed within the first 24 hours because of the increased incidence of contamination. Saphenous vein cutdowns are acceptable as long as at least one intravenous site is also present in the upper extremity.

Central venous pressure (CVP) catheters are inserted in severely injured patients via veins in the upper extremity. J wires may be passed through the external jugular vein as a guide for an alternate CVP route.

It is emphasized that fluid resuscitation should not be withheld in patients with multiple injures and evidence of blood loss, even though associated head injuries may be present. Frequently, restoration of adequate circulating blood volume will reverse some neurologic manifestations and prevent irreversible ischemic injury from lack of perfusion. In patients with isolated head injuries, fluids are administered judiciously to minimize the occurrence of cerebral edema.

If the patient remains hypotensive after receiving two liters of fluid, a rapid assessment of other causes of hypotension should be made. If there is no evidence of cardiogenic or vasogenic shock, blood replacement is indicated. Ideally typed and crossmatched blood will be available, but if time does not permit, type-specific or O-negative blood may be used. Micropore filters and blood warmers are routinely used with blood administration.

The MAST (medical anti-shock trouser) garment is now available for use in sustaining the blood pressure in selected patients. The garment is best used when transporting patients, but may be used if there is uncontrollable delay in instituting definitive treatment.[3, 7, 15, 19, 20, 25] Inflation of the garment results in an increase in total peripheral resistance and is contraindicated in those patients whose condition would be harmed by increasing afterload.[12] Specific contraindications include congestive heart failure or pulmonary edema. The use of this garment is safe with head injury patients, as there is no significant increase in intracranial pressure when it is inflated. In patients with significant chest injuries, it is recommended that only the lower extremities be inflated unless the patients are intubated and adequately ventilated.

As the garment is deflated, the vital signs should be closely monitored. Deflation should begin with the abdominal compartment and each subsequent compartment should be deflated slowly and individually. If the blood pressure falls, the garment should be re-inflated and maintained until either the circulation is stabilized or hemorrhage is controlled in the operating room.

Pharmacologic support of the blood pressure is rarely indicated and there is no place for vasopressors in patients who are hypovolemic. Similarly, other agents such as mannitol and diuretics should be withheld until the volume deficits are restored and stabilized.

General Management

Following initial assessment, and as fluids are begun, Levin tubes and Foley catheters are inserted. The Levin tube serves to assess injury to the upper gastrointestinal tract, as well as evacuate stomach contents and prevent aspiration. Antacids (30–60 cc) are given via the nasogastric tube to neutralize the stomach contents in the event that aspiration occurs.

Exception to the routine use of Levin tubes is a potential vascular injury at the base of the neck. If a clot becomes dislodged with the retching associated with its insertion, it may become difficult to gain control of an injured subclavian vessel. If pressure is applied to an injured carotid vessel for a prolonged period, cerebral ischemia may result. The tube should not be inserted in patients with suspected fractures at the base of the frontal fossa. Intracranial passage of a nasogastric tube has been reported and is associated with a fatal outcome (see also Chapter 5).

A Foley catheter should be inserted in all severely injured patients. In addition to detecting injury to the genitourinary system, it provides a guide to the adequacy of fluid resuscitation. An exception to the routine use of the Foley catheter is a suspected urethral injury. Blood at the tip of the meatus or evidence of a perineal or scrotal hematoma, is frequently seen with this injury and is an indication for urethrography.

Laboratory determinations and X-ray studies are obtained as indicated. All attempts should be made to individualize the studies ordered for each patient. Increased emphasis should be placed on clinical evaluation and less on expensive, non-productive laboratory tests and X-rays. At a minimum, however, a CBC, urinalysis, and amylase determination are required on all multiply injured patients. A clot is sent to the blood bank and patients typed and cross-matched for at least four to six units of whole blood.

A baseline determination of arterial blood gases is obtained. Tetanus toxoid is given if the patient's immunization is not current. Hypertet is given simultaneously with the toxoid if the patient has not received the basic series (1).

Following initial assessment and stabilization, attention is directed to the management of specific injuries. In patients with head injuries or an altered state of consciousness, the detection of these injuries may be difficult.

SPECIFIC INJURY MANAGEMENT

Maxillofacial Trauma

There are two areas of concern in evaluating patients with maxillofacial injuries: airway patency and management of hemorrhage.

Some facial fractures such as a displaced mandible may cause impingement on the oral or nasal airway. Similarly, the soft tissues of the tongue and floor of the mouth may cause airway compromise by posterior displacement. Mid-face fractures of the LeFort type may cause displacement of both the mid-facial bony structures and soft tissue of the pharyngeal areas and palate, leading to obstruction of the nasal airway.

Restoration of the airway is accomplished by rapid suctioning of the oral and nasal passages. An examining finger is moved quickly across the dorsum of the tongue into the posterior pharyngeal airway. Any foreign material causing airway obstruction is readily removed. Having secured the airway, manipulation of the fractures may provide temporary stabilization and restoration of the airway.

Nasal hemorrhage can be life-threatening. Placement of an anterior and/or posterior nasal pack may be required to control acute nasal bleeding secondary to severe mid-facial fractures (Fig. 3.2).

Hemorrhage of the tongue is evaluated, and if branches of the lingual artery are identified, they may be ligated. Bleeding associated with fractures of the maxillary or mandibular bones can be stabilized and bleeding controlled with pressure dressings (Fig. 3.3). Severe swelling of the pharyngeal wall and tongue is frequently seen with maxillofacial trauma. Of special concern are patients who sustain gunshot wounds which traverse the soft tissues near the oral and nasal airway. These patients frequently require early tracheostomy if swelling appears rapidly.

Penetrating Neck Injuries

The management of penetrating neck injuries is currently undergoing re-evaluation.

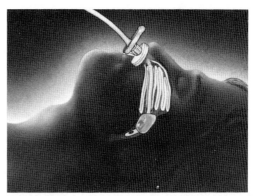

Figure 3.2. Anterior and posterior nasal pack to control hemorrhage.

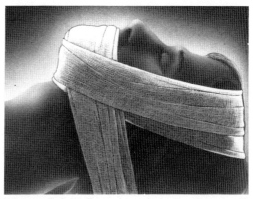

Figure 3.3. Pressure dressing for maxillary or mandibular fractures.

Many centers recommend mandatory exploration for all wounds that violate the platysma muscle. With the advent of better diagnostic procedures, selective management following careful evaluation is now becoming more popular. Physical examination is invaluable and occasionally an arteriovenous fistula will be detected by auscultation. A delayed expanding hematoma may occur with compromise of the airway several hours after injury.

Unless there is exsanguinating hemorrhage or airway obstruction requiring immediate attention, arteriography is recommended for most penetrating neck injuries. This is especially important if the missile trajectory or injury is in proximity to the carotid or vertebral vessels. Complete evaluation warrants a four vessel multiplane study, including adequate visualization of the artery proximal to the injury and complete visualization of the cerebral circulation. Arteriography delineates the site of injury and helps in the planning of the appropriate operative approach.[11]

Potential esophageal injuries are carefully evaluated by endoscopy and radio-opaque studies.

Aspiration

Aspiration is a common complication in the patient with multiple injuries. This usually occurs prior to arrival at the hospital and is frequently seen in the unconscious patient. Early diagnosis and vigorous treatment with bronchoscopy and suction will reduce the effects of this potentially fatal complication. The use of steroids is somewhat controversial and convincing data is still lacking regarding its efficacy.

Penetrating Chest Trauma

Injuries to the chest are frequently associated with hypoxia. This may confuse the neurologic assessment but rapid stabilization will often lead to better oxygenation and improvement in the neurologic status. Careful physical examination, supplemented by good quality, erect PA, and lateral chest films at frequent intervals will provide optimum diagnostic yield. Both inspiratory and expiratory films are obtained to better detect subtle abnormalities.

Gunshot wounds are difficult to manage because of their tendency to take an erratic course. Wounds below the nipple line may cause intra-abdominal injuries, whereas those above the nipple line may injure the subclavian and axillary vessels.

Thoracotomy is performed when the missile trajectory passes in proximity to the heart. This will occasionally necessitate an urgent procedure and is sometimes performed in the emergency room. Indications for emergency room thoracotomy include exsanguinating hemorrhage from the chest and inability to adequately perform cardiopulmonary resuscitation in a salvageable patient with serious chest trauma. Thoracotomies are occasionally performed in patients who are hemodynamically unstable and suspected of having a significant intra-abdominal hemorrhage.[16] This hemorrhage may be controlled by opening the chest and cross clamping the aorta prior to opening the abdomen. The survival rate after emergency room thoracotomy[22] is not great. Baker et al[2] recently reported a 6.6% survival rate in 91 patients who had no vital signs upon arrival with cardio-respiratory arrest of recent onset but with signs of life at the scene of the injury. Four of 20 patients in that series who survived were agonal upon admission (i.e., they had attempted respiration with a very thready pulse but no palpable blood pressure). Mattox et al[22] reported an 8% overall survival following thoracotomy in patients who were agonal or who had no vital signs upon admission. Several precautions are necessary when performing emergency thoracotomy. Care should be taken to avoid transection of the coronary arteries when doing the pericardiotomy. Posterior cardiac wounds may bleed precipitiously, causing sudden cardiac arrest when the heart is manipulated. Blind clamping of the aorta may cause additional injury to the vessel or esophagus in addition to the primary injury. Mature judgment will determine which patients qualify for these heroic procedures.

Stab wounds of the chest between the second and fifth intercostal space, without evidence of intra-thoracic injury, are best observed a minimum of six hours, then reevaluated with inspiratory and expiratory films. These patients are instructed to return for re-evaluation in 24 hours.

Pneumothorax. Pneumothorax is frequently seen with both penetrating and blunt trauma. It may occur at the time of injury or several hours later and may or may not be associated with rib injuries. Pneumothorax may also occasionally develop as a complication of subclavian catheter insertion. Minimal deflation of the lung (less than 10%), may be aspirated by thoracentesis. As a rule, however, closed tube thoracostomy is the treatment of choice. If a chest tube is not inserted, frequent evaluation is necessary. If the pneumothorax recurs following thoracentesis, it is best treated with an anterior chest tube. Single tubes are placed in the second intercostal space in the mid-clavicular line. Tubes placed in the fourth intercostal space laterally may, however, give a better cosmetic result. Regardless of where the tube is placed, the tip is directed superiorly and anteriorly as this is where air will accumulate in the bed-ridden patient.

Tension pneumothorax may occur if a flap or ball-valve injury occurs. This is an acute surgical emergency and will cause a shift of the mediastinum which is associated with a decreased venous return and decreased cardiac output. Unrecognized and untreated tension pneumothorax can quickly lead to death. This condition must be immediately reversed and needle thoracentesis may be a life-saving procedure. It is important to be aware of this potential complication in all patients with pneumothorax and particularly in those patients whose condition suddenly deteriorate. If it becomes necessary to move a patient from one facility to another, chest tubes should be inserted prior to transport.

Subcutaneous emphysema may be present when pneumothorax occurs. Chest tubes are not indicated if subcutaneous emphysema is detected in the absence of pneumothorax. These patients are best managed by repeated and frequent clinical evaluation.

Hemothorax. Hemothorax may occur as a result of penetrating or blunt trauma.[4] The accumulation of blood may be rapid, but in some instances, is very gradual. Careful auscultation and percussion will generally be sufficient to make this diagnosis and is confirmed by upright or lateral decubitus chest films. If time does not permit a chest film to be obtained, needle thoracentesis will generally confirm the presence of blood in the pleural cavity.

Hemothorax is best drained by a large caliber tube inserted in the seventh or eighth intercostal space in the mid-axillary line, directed posteriorly and inferiorly. Evacuation of blood from the pleural cavity and re-expansion of the lung will stop most parenchymal bleeding. Patients with hemopneumothorax are best treated with both anterior and posterior chest tubes (Fig. 3.4). However, if the blood loss is in excess of 1500 ml, or if the rate of bleeding continues at greater than 200 ml per hour, a formal thoracotomy is indicated. In these cases, the internal mammary artery or an intercostal artery is usually the cause of persistent bleeding. Injury to larger vessels generally produces exsanguinating hemorrhage prior to arrival at the hospital.

Jones *et al*[14] have recently described the technique of emergency thoracoscopy as an adjunctive procedure in the evaluation of patients with penetrating chest trauma. The procedure is performed under local anesthesia and provides an anatomic definition of the injury. The efficacy of this technique is yet to be determined in a large series of patients.

Sucking Chest Wounds. Sucking chest wounds are initially treated by the use of an occlusive, non-circumferential dressing. Primary suture of the wound will facilitate subsequent care. These wounds are invariably associated with pneumo- or hemopneumothorax and should be treated with appropriate chest tubes.

Cardiac Tamponade. Cardiac tamponade is an immediate threat to survival and should be suspected in any patient with a penetrating injury in the vicinity of the heart, especially when associated with resistant hypotension, distended neck veins, elevated central venous pressure, distant and muffled heart sounds, or a narrow pulse pressure.

Immediate pericardiocentesis via the subxyphoid route can be a life saving pro-

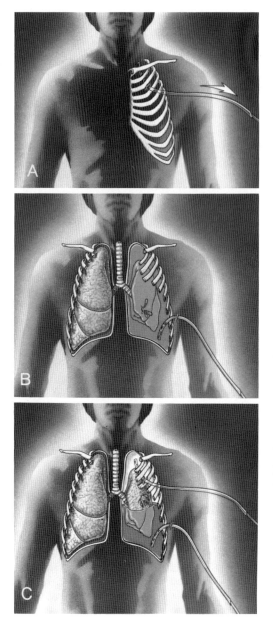

cedure in patients with cardiac tamponade (Fig. 3.5). An alligator clip is attached to an 18-gauge needle, allowing electrocardiographic monitoring during the aspiration. Removal of just a few milliliters of blood will generally reverse this syndrome. Although life-saving, this procedure is usually a temporizing measure and is best followed by immediate thoracotomy. If blood re-accumulates rapidly, a plastic intravenous type catheter is inserted through the pericardium to facilitate continuous or intermittent aspiration.

Diaphragmatic Injuries. A diaphragmatic defect may be difficult to recognize, especially if the injury is small and the wound has sealed. Nevertheless, these injuries may be troublesome and will occasionally lead to an incarcerated hernia at a later time. Peritoneal lavage and routine X-rays may fail to identify this injury in the absence of significant bleeding.

When a combined thoraco-abdominal injury is suspected, a prophylactic anterior chest tube may prevent unsuspected pneumothorax from developing during abdominal exploration.

Blunt Chest Trauma

The general assessment of patients with blunt chest trauma includes a thorough physical examination followed by appropriate X-rays, electrocardiogram, and special

Figure 3.4. *A*, single tube for pneumothorax inserted in second intercostal space in the mid-clavicular line. Tube is directed superiorly. *B*, single tube for hemothorax inserted in the seventh intercostal space in the mid-axillary line. Tube is directed inferiorly. *C*, anterior and posterior tubes for hemo-pneumothorax.

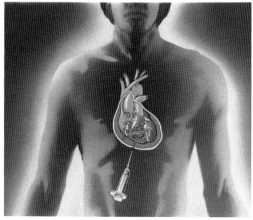

Figure 3.5. Illustration showing pericardiocentesis via the subxyphoid approach.

studies as indicated. The more common injuries sustained with blunt trauma include flail chest, traumatic aortic aneurysm, contusion and aspiration.[17]

Flail Chest. This condition occurs when more than two ribs are broken and each rib is fractured in two places (Fig. 3.6). In essence, a segment of the chest wall becomes totally disconnected from the rest of the bony thorax. This causes paradoxical respiration which is easily visible when the patient is observed from the head or foot of the examining table. A major flail segment should be aggressively treated lest pulmonary insufficiency occur. Patients with flail chest have considerable pain due to the broken ribs and will not ventilate adequately without assistance. Analgesics tend to further suppress the respiratory effect.

Initial stabilization may be accomplished by placing a sandbag or heavy object on the flail segment. Although many methods of treatment have been described, intubation with positive pressure breathing will provide optimum support. Prolonged ventilatory assistance frequently requires tracheostomy. Even though tracheostomy is anticipated, it is better to intubate initially, delaying the tracheostomy to a time when

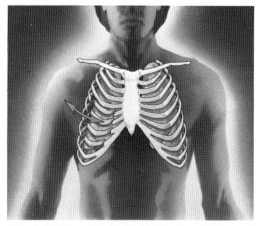

Figure 3.6. Diagram illustrates how multiple fractures can result in a portion of the chest wall that is disconnected from the remainder of the bony thorax. With inspiration this segment moves paradoxically inward.

it can be performed in the operating room under optimum conditions.

Traumatic Aortic Aneurysm. Patients sustaining a traumatic aortic aneurysm have a mortality rate of 60 to 80%. This injury occurs almost exclusively in the thoracic aorta and is usually located just distal to the subclavian artery where the vessel is relatively fixed by the ligamentum arteriosum.

The definitive diagnosis is made by aortography (Fig. 3.7). The more readily acceptable radiographic indications for arch aortography include a widening of the superior mediastinum (greater than 8 cm), fractured sternum, multiple rib fractures with crushed chest, first rib fracture, a posteriorly displaced clavicular fracture, recurrent large or continuing left hemothorax, tracheal displacement to the right and depression of the left main stem bronchus.[21] A history of a rapid decceleration accident with evidence of chest wall abrasions is an indication for arteriography even in the absence of classic X-ray findings. Ten to 15% of patients with this injury will not have the typical X-ray findings. Some clinicians prefer to follow these patients with serial chest X-rays, but the morbidity and mortality of this injury far surpass the morbidity and mortality of a negative arteriogram.

Contusion. Pulmonary contusion is frequently associated with blunt trauma to the chest. Early recognition and pulmonary support may lessen the ravages of the acute respiratory insufficiency syndrome. Serial blood gases combined with physical examination and X-ray findings will generally confirm the diagnosis. Occasionally, radiographic evidence of pulmonary contusion will lag behind the clinical manifestations.

Thoracoabdominal Injury

The diaphragm rises as high as the fourth to fifth intercostal space anteriorly, the fifth to sixth intercostal space laterally, and the sixth to seventh intercostal space posteriorly. All penetrating wounds at or below this level are evaluated for abdominal injury as well as chest injuries.

Gunshot Wounds. All patients with gunshot injuries and a wound of entrance

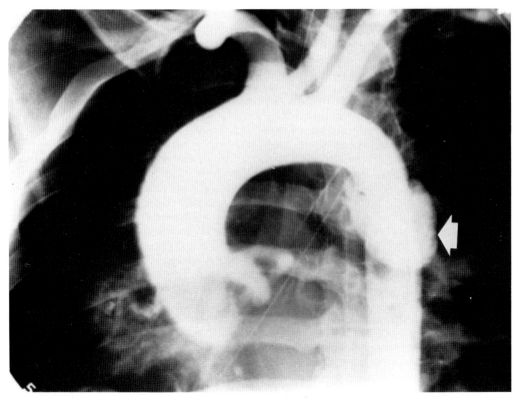

Figure 3.7.   Photograph illustrates traumatic thoracic aortic aneurysm (*arrow*).

or exit at or below these landmarks are taken to the operating room for an exploratory celiotomy. Because of the unpredictable course of the missile, it is not possible to draw a straight line between the entrance and exit wound or entrance wounds and missile location. It is not uncommon for a bullet to penetrate the diaphragm and return to the thoracic cavity. Occasionally, depending upon the caliber of the bullet and the distance at which the missile was fired, blast effect will injure intra-abdominal organs without actual penetration of the peritoneal cavity.

Physical examination is unreliable in detecting early intra-abdominal injury in 10 to 20% of these cases. A recent review of this subject at Parkland Memorial Hospital in Dallas revealed that 25% of patients with gunshot wounds to the lower chest also had intra-abdominal injuries.[34]

Stab Wounds. Patients with stab wounds to the lower chest may be managed more selectively. The path of the stab wound is more predictable than that of a gunshot wound. If any sign of peritoneal irritation or evidence of injury is present, the patient is prepared for celiotomy. If, however, an anterior stab wound is located between the two posterior axillary lines and below the nipple line, and the abdominal examination is considered negative, peritoneal lavage is performed (see section on blunt trauma).[33] If the lavage is positive (RBC>100,000; WBC>500; presence of amylase, bile or bacteria), celiotomy is performed. There is currently considerable debate concerning the number of red cells that should be considered significant. Although this has not been resolved, a red cell count of 100,000 as originally described by Root *et al.*,[26] is equal to about 20 cc of blood. Using this value, the incidence of false negative lavages remains 1–2% and appears to detect virtually all significant injuries. The presence of a negative peritoneal lavage does not preclude the need for continued close observation. If lavage is negative, the patient is admitted to the hospital and observed for 24 hours.

Abdominal Injury

Penetrating Abdominal Trauma. Patients sustaining gunshot wounds to the lower chest and abdomen are managed aggressively. Blast effect may cause injury to intraperitoneal viscera without actual penetration of the peritoneal cavity. If peritoneal penetration occurs, 90 to 95% of these patients will sustain an intra-abdominal injury. Adjunctive studies used in the evaluation of patients with stab wounds and blunt trauma are not applicable in the evaluation of these patients.

Peritoneal lavage was recently evaluated as a predictor of intra-abdominal injury in patients with gunshot wounds to the lower chest and abdomen. Fifteen of 59 patients with a negative lavage had significant visceral injuries at operation including nine colon injuries, six small bowel injuries, two stomach injuries, one pancreatic injury, and one aortic injury. Although there was little blood in the abdominal cavity, the procedure failed to predict these injuries. Likewise, physical examination was inaccurate in 15 to 20% of patients.[34]

Because of the unpredictable missile trajectory and high incidence of visceral injury, virtually all patients sustaining gunshot wounds to the lower chest and abdomen are taken to the operating room for exploratory celiotomy following stabilization. The mortality rate following a negative celiotomy for trauma is extremely low.[18] In a collected series of over 800 negative operations for trauma, the mortality rate was 0.25%. The added morbidity and mortality of missed injuries in this group of patients far outweighs the risk of an occasional negative celiotomy.

Patients sustaining stab wounds may be safely managed on a more selective basis[24, 27] although a few authors still recommend mandatory exploration.[6] Small innocuous wounds may occasionally cause devastating injuries. Physical examination is generally reliable but again, can be misleading in 10 to 15% of patients. Adjunctive

diagnostic studies are more reliable in these patients than in patients with gunshot wounds. Such techniques as local wound exploration, injection of radio-opaque contrast material into the wound and peritoneal lavage have been advocated.

Local wound exploration is a useful technique for patients sustaining stab wounds to the abdomen, flank, or back that are located below the lower rib margins. In the absence of peritoneal signs and obvious indications for celiotomy, local exploration of the stab wound helps determine the depth of injury. This technique will differentiate superficial abdominal wounds from deeper penetrating injuries. Approximately 15 to 20% of patients sustaining stab wounds to the abdomen will have superficial wounds that do not require operative exploration. The skin is prepared, infiltrated with local anesthesia, and the wound extended. Using retractors the entire wound is inspected under direct vision and, if the end of the tract is seen and does not extend beyond the posterior rectus fascia, the wound is partially closed, drained, and the patient discharged. However, if the depth of the wound is not seen, or the tract enters the peritoneal cavity, and the physical examination is considered clinically negative, peritoneal lavage is performed. If the lavage is negative, the patient is admitted to the hospital and observed for 24 hours. Some authors do not recommend admission of these patients, following a negative lavage. However, complications do occur and observation is strongly recommended. With a positive lavage, the patient is taken directly to the operating room for celiotomy.

The role of lavage in stab wounds of the flank and back is less clearly defined.[13] The accuracy of lavage is not as great with injuries in the retroperitoneal space. Whereas lavage may pick up an occasional intraperitoneal injury in patients sustaining stab wounds to the back, it is less frequently used. These patients may be closely observed and evaluated with adjunctive studies such as intravenous pyelograms and gastrointestinal contrast studies. It is important to remember, however, that retroperitoneal injuries may be difficult to detect and will produce signs of peritoneal irritation less frequently than injuries within the peritoneal cavity.

Blunt Abdominal Trauma. Patients sustaining blunt abdominal trauma are among the most difficult to evaluate in clinical medicine. Frequently signs and symptoms of injury are not manifest for several hours and in some cases of pancreatic and other retroperitoneal injuries, not for several days. Associated injuries such as chest or extremity trauma, and head injury further complicate this problem. Often, the patient is unconscious because of alcoholism, shock, or head injury. Seemingly minor trauma or relatively trivial injuries on occasion may cause significant damage including rupture of abdominal viscera; hence, the index of suspicion must be high if diagnostic errors are to be avoided.

Evaluation begins with a careful history and physical examination. Knowledge of the mechanism of the injury may be helpful. Factors such as rapid deceleration, impaling forces, and seat belt restraints make the abdominal viscera prone to injury.

Physical examination of the alert patient remains the most reliable method of diagnosing intra-abdominal injury, and yet this may be misleading in 10 to 20% of cases. Abdominal pain, guarding and rigidity, loss of bowel sounds, and unexplained shock are all parameters that are associated with the acute surgical abdomen. The diagnosis of intra-abdominal bleeding may be difficult as some patients experience exquisite pain with blood in the peritoneal cavity, while others report very little discomfort. When the diagnosis is doubtful, one must depend upon repeated frequent examinations, preferrably by the same examiner, and adjunctive studies such as paracentesis, peritoneal lavage, and arteriography.

Paracentesis using either a bilateral flank approach, or a four quadrant abdominal approach, is still a good procedure. If the aspirate is positive, it is extremely reliable. However, the false negative rate is 40 to 60%. It is less time-consuming and associated with fewer complications than the more frequently used peritoneal lavage. When paracentesis is negative, lavage is performed because of its greater accuracy.

Culdocentesis may be considered in female patients.

Peritoneal lavage is very reliable and the incidence of false negative and positive results is low (1–2% for each) in numerous series.[10, 35] Lavage is an invasive procedure and is not indicated in all patients with blunt abdominal trauma. If there is an altered state of consciousness, equivocal abdominal findings, or the patient is going to be anesthetized for another operative procedure, lavage should be considered. Numerous techniques have been described but most authors agree that the safest approach is to make an incision down to the peritoneum and introduce the catheter under direct vision (Fig. 3.8). Early lavage may not detect injury to retroperitoneal structures, particularly if the posterior peritoneum remains intact.

Arteriography is frequently used when assessing potential injury to the renal artery. Selective catheterization has been useful in patients with lower abdominal bleeding secondary to pelvic fractures. The site of bleeding is easily determined and may frequently be controlled by using vasospastic agents or embolizing autologous clot.

While liver and spleen scans are avail-

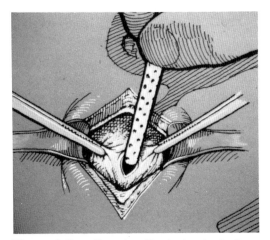

Figure 3.8. Drawing illustrates technique for peritoneal lavage. An incision is made in the abdomen down to the peritoneum which is grasped by hemostats. The peritoneum is incised and lavage catheter is inserted under direct vision.

able, these modalities are seldom employed. Laporoscopy has been described, but it is rarely used and not recommended for the multiply injured patient. It does not provide the necessary exposure to rule out all significant intra-abdominal injuries. The role of the newer, non-invasive studies such as sonography and computerized tomography is unclear and, at present, they are seldom used.

Genitourinary Trauma

The presence of a bruise over the ribs or flank, or a mass in the loin should suggest the possibility of trauma to the kidney. Examination of the urine should be performed in all patients sustaining either blunt or penetrating trauma. When gross or microscopic hematuria (more than 4–6 RBC's per high power field) is present, an intravenous pyelogram, cystogram, and voiding cystourethrogram is indicated. If the patient's condition is precarious, a single five-minute film taken after the intravenous contrast material injection will usually provide sufficient information.

If the intravenous pyelogram does not visualize a kidney on one side or function is significantly delayed, arteriography is indicated. Penetrating renal injuries are generally surgically explored. A stable patient following blunt trauma may be managed conservatively.

Testicular torsion frequently occurs in young males following seemingly minor trauma. On physical examination, the patient suspected of torsion may be differentiated from the patient with epididymal orchitis as the patient with torsion usually obtains no relief by elevation of the testis. Physical examination may disclose pain and tenderness confined to the scrotal area. The testis often is located high in the scrotum, but a mass, the twisted cord, can sometimes be palpated superiorly.

Pediatric Trauma

Accidental injury continues to be the leading cause of death and disability in children. The absence of external signs of trauma may impose undesirable delays in management, while a severely contused ab-

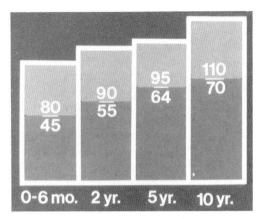

Figure 3.9. Figure illustrates lower limits of normal pediatric blood pressures.

dominal wall may precipitate unnecessary surgical intervention.

Trivial accidents, such as falls against furniture and bicycle handlebars, will often produce serious, but difficult to diagnose injuries. Child abuse is an increasingly common problem and may be the etiology of many cases of pediatric trauma.

It is emphasized that children cannot be treated as small adults nor evaluated as such. Because normal blood pressure varies with age it is important to be familiar with normal values (Fig. 3.9). In small children, more accurate pressures can be obtained with a doppler than with a stethoscope or by palpation. Children have a much lower margin of reserve with respect to blood loss than do adults. Blood loss greater than 10% is considered significant and, therefore, a rapid loss of 200 cc in a young child can produce clinical shock, and acute blood loss exceeding 400 cc may cause death.

Liberal use of paracentesis and peritoneal lavage will help detect occult abdominal injuries. Because evisceration may occur when performing lavage in infants, a purse string suture should be placed in the peritoneum and tied as soon as the catheter is removed lessening the chance of this complication.

When performing lavage in small children, 10–15 ml per kg of fluid is infused. The criteria for positive lavage in adults is based on a 1 liter infusion. The actual dilution factor in children will vary according to the volume of infusate and the red blood cell count must be extrapolated for a one liter infusion.

Orthopedic Injuries

Orthopedic injuries have a lower priority in the multiply injured patient with life-threatening problems. Splinting is usually done in the field, but should be maintained or instituted in all cases of fracture or dislocation. Extensions that can be added to emergency room carts facilitate extremity stabilization.

When it is necessary to delay operative treatment of an open fracture, the wound is covered with sterile dressings, antibiotics are begun and the bones are adequately splinted. Digital examination is not recommended because of the high risk of infection and bleeding. Frequent assessment of the circulation to the distal segment of the injured limb is made and recorded.

Rapid reduction of dislocated joints is advocated in most instances. Frequently, this is accomplished in the emergency room with local analgesia. Both pre- and post-reduction films are essential and continued monitoring of the neurovascular status is important.

The initial assessment of hand injuries is made under sterile conditions. The extent of skin loss and injury is determined by inspection. Damage to tendons, nerves, and arteries is best assessed by functional examination of the digits, without wound probing. Bleeding from the wound is controlled by pressure and elevation with no attempt to clamp arteries. Amputated parts are cleansed under sterile conditions, wrapped in a sterile saline-soaked gauze and placed in a sterile plastic bag which is covered with ice, or refrigerated until surgical replantation. X-rays of both the amputated and remaining parts are obtained to assess the extent of bone and joint damage.

Vascular Injuries

Vascular injuries are seen frequently in penetrating trauma but may also occur as a result of blunt trauma. When associated with blunt trauma, they occur secondary to fractures or from the fracturing of atheromatous plaques. The baseline examination should include assessment of bruits and peripheral pulses. The presence of a cold, pulseless extremity constitutes an acute emergency and valuable time should not be wasted with sophisticated diagnostic studies. Distal pulses may be palpable in the presence of proximal injuries including complete occlusion in some instances. This has been reported in 10–30% of patients with vascular injuries.

Suspected vascular injuries should not be probed or digitally examined since uncontrollable hemorrhage may ensue if a thrombus is inadvertently dislodged. Doppler examination is quite helpful in determining distal flow. The appearance of a bruit may indicate an A-V fistula or external compression of the vessel because of soft tissue swelling. Its disappearance may be misleading if a clot forms between the injured vessels. If the viability of an extremity is not in jeopardy, preoperative arteriography and venography are quite helpful and are a reliable guide to the site of injury and necessity for operative intervention.

Other indications for early exploration and repair include an expanding hematoma, history of arterial bleeding, absent pulses, related neurologic deficit and the presence of a bruit or thrill.

SUMMARY

An effective, organized approach to the multiply injured patient integrating the expertise of paramedical personnel, ancillary services and the experience of consultative services, will provide optimum care for the seriously injured patient. An awareness of the mechanism of injury, the natural history of traumatic injuries and a well-equipped modern emergency room will help the physician meet the challenge the trauma patient presents.

References

1. American College of Surgeons Committee on Trauma: Early Care of the Injured Patient. 2nd Ed. W.B. Saunders Company, Philadelphia, 1976.
2. Baker, C.C., Thomas, A.N., Trunkey, D.D.: The role of emergency room thoracotomy in trauma. J. Trauma, 20:848–855, 1980.

3. Batalden, D.J., Wickstrom, P.H., Ruiz, E., Gustilo, R.B.: Value of the g suit in patients with severe pelvic fracture. Controlling hemorrhagic shock. Arch. Surg., 109:326–328, 1974.
4. Beal, A.C., Crawford, H.W., DeBakey, M.E.: Considerations in the management of acute traumatic hemothorax. J. Thoracic Cardiovasc. Surg., 52:351–360, 1966.
5. Blalock, A.: Shock: further studies with particular reference to effects of hemorrhage. Arch. Surg., 29:837, 1937.
6. Bull, J.C. Jr., Mathewson, C. Jr.: Exploratory laparotomy in patients with penetrating wounds of the abdomen. Am. J. Surg., 116:223–228, 1968.
7. Burdick, J.F., Warshaw, A.L., Abbott, W.M.: External counterpressure to control postoperative intra-abdominal hemorrhage. Am. J. Surg., 129:369–373, 1975.
8. Canizaro, P.C., Prager, M.D., Shires, G.T.: The infusion of Ringer's lactate solution during shock. Changes in lactate, excess lactate, and pH. Am. J. Surg., 122:494–501, 1971.
9. Cunningham, J.N. Jr., Shires, G.T., Wagner, Y.: Changes in intracellular sodium and potassium content of red blood cells in trauma and shock. Am. J. Surg., 122:650–654, 1971.
10. Fisher, R.P., Beverlin, B.C., Engrav, L.H., et al: Diagnostic peritoneal lavage fourteen years and 2,568 patients later. Am. J. Surg., 136:701–704, 1978.
11. Fry, R.E., Fry, W.J.: Extracranial carotid artery injuries. Surgery, 88:581–587, 1980.
12. Gaffney, A.F., Thal, E.R., Taylor, W.F., Bastian, B.C., Weigelt, J.A., Atkins, J.M., Blomquist, C.G.: Hemodynamic effects of anti-shock trousers. J. Trauma, 21:931–937, 1981.
13. Jackson, G.L., Thal, E.R.: Management of stab wounds to the back and flank. J. Trauma, 19:660–664, 1979.
14. Jones, J.W., Kitahamba, A., Webb, W.R., McSwain, N.: Emergency thoracoscopy: a logical approach to chest trauma management. J. Trauma, 21:280–284, 1981.
15. Kaplan, B.C., Civetta, J.M., Nagel, E.L., Nussenfeld, S.R., Hirschman, J.C.: The military antishock trouser in civilian pre-hospital emergency care. J. Trauma, 13:843–848, 1973.
16. Kirsh, G., Kozloff, L., Joseph, W.L., Adkins, P.C.: Indications for early thoracotomy in the management of chest trauma. Ann. Thoracic Surg., 22:23–28, 1976.
17. Kirsh, M.M., Sloan, H.: Blunt Chest Trauma. Little, Brown and Company, New York, 1977.
18. Lowe, R.J., Boyd, D.R., Folk, F.A., Baker, R.J.: The negative laparotomy for abdominal trauma. J. Trauma, 12:853–861, 1972.
19. McSwain, N.E.: Pneumatic trousers and the management of shock. J. Trauma, 17:719–724, 1977.
20. McSwain, N.E. Jr.: G-suits and shock: a non-invasive transfusion technique. J. Kans. Med. Soc., 77:438–441, 1976.
21. Marsh, D.G., Sturm, J.T.: Traumatic aortic rupture: roentgenographic indications for angiography. Ann. Thoracic Surg., 21:337–340, 1976.
22. Mattox, K.D., Beall, A.C., Jordan, G.C., DeBakey, M.E.: Cardiorrhaphy in the emergency center. J. Thoracic Cardiovasc. Surg., 68:886–895, 1974.
23. Middleton, E.S., Mathews, R., Shires, G.T.: Radiosulphate as a measure of the extracellular fluid in acute hemorrhagic shock. Ann. Surg., 170:174–186, 1969.
24. Nance, F.C., Wennar, M.H., Johnson, L.W., Ingram, J.C. Jr., Cohn, I. Jr.: Surgical judgement in the management of penetrating wounds of the abdomen: experience with 2,212 patients. Ann. Surg., 179:639–646, 1974.
25. Pelligra, R., Sandberg, E.C.: Control of intractable abdominal bleeding by external counterpressure. J.A.M.A., 241:708–713, 1979.
26. Root, H.D., Hauser, C.W., McKinley, C.R., et al: Diagnostic peritoneal lavage. Surgery, 57:633–637, 1965.
27. Shaftan, G.W.: Indications for operation in abdominal trauma. Am. J. Surg., 99:657–664, 1960.
28. Shires, G.T., Cunningham, J.N., Baker, C.R.F., Reeder, S.F., Illner, H., Wagner, I.Y., Maher, J.: Alterations in cellular membrane function during hemorrhagic shock in primates. Ann. Surg., 176:288–295, 1972.
29. Shires, G.T.: Care of the Trauma Patient. McGraw Hill, New York, 1979.
30. Shires, G.T., Carrico, C.J.: Current status of the shock problem. Curr. Probl. Surg., March, 1966.
31. Shires, T., Coln, D., Carrico, J., Lightfoot, S.: Fluid therapy in hemorrhagic shock. Arch. Surg., 88:688–693, 1964.
32. Simeone, F.A.: Shock. In: Christopher's Textbook of Surgery. W.B. Saunders Company, Philadelphia, 1964, pp. 58–62.
33. Thal, E.R.: Evaluation of peritoneal lavage and local exploration in lower chest and abdominal stab wounds. J. Trauma, 17:642–648, 1977.
34. Thal, E.R., May, R.A., Beesinger, D.: Peritoneal lavage. Its unreliability in gunshot wounds of the lower chest and abdomen. Arch. Surg. 115:430–433, 1980.
35. Thal, E.R., Shires, G.T.: Peritoneal lavage in blunt abdominal trauma. Am. J. Surg., 125:64–69, 1973.

4

Radiographic Evaluation

P. R. S. KISHORE

CT SCANNING

Indications

Computerized tomography (CT) plays an important role in the early recognition of intracranial traumatic lesions requiring surgical intervention. Because it is safe, rapid, and non-invasive, CT has become the radiological investigation of choice for the evaluation of patients with head injury.[3, 18, 41, 50, 62, 71, 80,] Newer CT scanners with shortened scanning and reconstruction times enable the clinician to diagnose intracranial mass lesions within minutes after the patient is brought into the scanner suite. If the patient is suspected of having other organ injuries in addition to a severe brain injury, the time consumed for cranial CT can be minimized by limiting the CT examination to one section at the level of the lateral ventricles to detect the presence of a life-threatening intracranial mass lesion. The patient can then be treated for other organ injuries if no abnormality is seen on the CT scan. In patients with life-threatening systemic trauma with uncontrolled hemorrhage, treatment of these injuries takes precedence over CT diagnosis of intracranial masses.

Obviously, if the patient has sustained only minor head trauma and does not have neurological dysfunction or history of loss of consciousness, the CT examination can be deferred until systemic injuries are treated (see Chapter 2).

If a CT scanner is not available because of equipment malfunction or other causes, and if the patient is suspected of harboring a significant intracranial mass lesion, ventriculography may be performed in the emergency room by instilling 8–10 ml of air into the lateral ventricle via a twist drill craniotomy.[7] Such a study provides adequate information as to midline shift and helps in the rapid localization of a mass lesion. Other investigators advocate the performance of "one shot angiogram" in similar emergency situations.[64] A percutaneous common carotid arteriogram can be performed using portable X-ray equipment and obtaining antero-posterior and lateral films to detect significant hemispheric mass lesion. A CT can be obtained subsequently to confirm the angiographic findings and identify additional traumatic lesions. One should be aware of the pitfalls of such limited studies, which include false positive diagnosis of extracerebral hematomas (see below).

Technical Considerations

CT is a very sensitive examination for the detection of acute intra- and extra-axial hemorrhagic lesions. Extravasated blood or hematoma in the acute stage has a high attenuation effect on the X-ray beam with Hounsfield (H) numbers between 60 and 90. It is, therefore, seen as increased density compared to the brain, whose H numbers range from 20 to 45—the white matter having less of an attenuation effect than the grey matter.

The high attenuation of extravasated

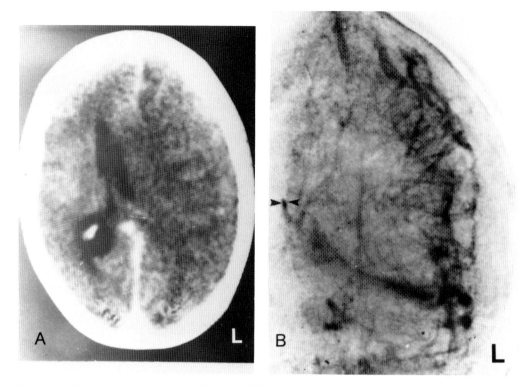

Figure 4.1. *A,* post-contrast CT of a 46-year-old man showing midline displacement and distortion of left lateral ventricle without apparent cause for the mass effect in a patient with a hemoglobin of 10.0 g/100 ml. *B,* carotid angiography revealed an extracerebral hematoma. At operation, 100 ml of freshly clotted subdural hematoma was found. (Reproduced with permission from Smith, W.P., *et al.*: Am. J. Neuroradiol. 2:37–40, 1981.)

blood is believed to result from the globin content of hemoglobin.[54] The density of a hematoma on CT depends upon its size and location and whether or not the hemorrhage is mixed with CSF or traumatized brain. The time elapsed between injury and the performance of CT will also affect the density of the hematoma. A less common factor in determining the density of a hematoma is the patient's hematocrit. Since the density of a hematoma depends primarily upon the globin content of hemoglobin in extravasated blood, in severely anemic patients the hematoma may appear isodense or less dense than adjacent brain[67] (Fig. 4.1).

Size and Location of Hemorrhage and CT Density. Recent hemorrhages may not be seen on CT if they are too small for CT resolution. Even hemorrhages as large as 1.5 cm may go undetected if they are not located in the center of the CT slice because of the partial volume effect (see below).

A typical epidural hematoma developing after trauma can be expected to have a relatively high density compared to an acute subdural hematoma of similar size, because the subdural hematoma is more likely to be mixed with CSF and traumatized brain, resulting in relatively low density of the lesion. Similarly, a contusion has a heterogeneously increased density due to small hemorrhages mixed with areas of traumatized brain and edema. In addition to the poorly defined margins, it has a relatively low density compared to a "pure" intracerebral hematoma.

Time Interval between Injury and CT. The density of a hematoma on CT also depends upon the time elapsed between the injury and the performance of CT. The high attenuation of an acute hematoma gradually decreases with time as resorption of the clot occurs. Depending upon its initial size and location, it may reach the density of adjacent brain in a few days to weeks.[9] Further resolution of hemorrhagic lesions leads to lower density than brain (H numbers 15–25) and the lesion may take on an appearance similar to edema. Thus, a resolving hemorrhagic contusion may be mistaken for "edema" on a CT done only a few days after injury. As pointed out by French and Dublin[27] over 70% of patients undergoing CT within the first 24 hours following trauma were considered to have a contusion, whereas over 80% of the patients whose CT's were performed after 24 hours had apparent edema on CT. After several weeks or months, a hematoma may leave a residual density, similar to that of CSF (H numbers 6–10) (Fig. 4.2).

Partial Volume Effect. The partial volume effect is an inherent technical limitation present in all CT systems. The density on the CT image at a given point is the representation of the average of the attenuation coefficients of all the elements within the voxel (*i.e.*, the tissue block of 1.3 cm (slice thickness) × 1.5 mm × 1.5 mm, using the first generation EMI scanner with a 160 × 160 matrix).[12, 47] Therefore, depending upon the thickness of the slice, which is usually 1.3 cm, a small lesion less than 1.5 cm in diameter, if it is not in the center of the slice thickness, may be completely missed. A high density lesion like hemorrhage may appear isodense to the adjacent brain parenchyma for the same reason. The partial volume effect may also be responsible for the failure to visualize small, acute extracerebral hematomas[45, 69] because of the location of the hematoma adjacent to bone with very high attenuation values (around 1,000 H numbers). The experience of finding a larger than expected hematoma at operation,[27] may be due in part to the partial volume effect. This effect also plays a role in obscuring small hemorrhages that are associated with low attenuation components like lipids, necrosis and cavitation.[42]

CT Appearance of Specific Traumatic Entities

The post-traumatic mass lesions are fully discussed in Chapters 11 and 12. This section is specifically concerned with the CT appearance of these entities.

Edema. Cerebral edema is usually seen as an area of low density (H = 15–25) when compared to brain parenchyma although all areas of low density do not represent post-traumatic edema (see Chapter 12). Ischemic infarction is also seen as an area of low density in the initial stages and cannot be differentiated from post-traumatic edema on conventional CT. If the low density zone does not conform to arterial distribution, it can be taken as evidence for the presence of edema.[18] In our own experience, it appears that "post-traumatic edema," not associated with hemorrhagic lesions, is probably not as common as it was once believed.[53] Therefore, caution should be exercised in making the diagnosis of edema on CT based upon low density appearance alone.

Contusion. Contusions may be single or multiple and usually occur in the anterior frontal and temporal lobes (Fig. 11.18). They appear as areas of non-homogeneous high density zones with attenuation values of 50–60 H due to the presence of multiple small areas of hemorrhage within the brain substance associated with areas of edema and tissue necrosis. Contusions may have varying proportions of dense and lucent areas, depending upon the extent of hemorrhage, degree of edema, and the time elapsed since injury. During the first 24 hours, increased density predominates; but with resolution of the hemorrhage, the amount of low density increases progressively until an appearance similar to that of edema is seen.

A contusion usually has a poorly defined margin that is often surrounded by a low density zone of edema. These areas may be single or multiple and often exert a mass effect with ventricular compression, distortion, and displacement. Occasionally, the contusion may increase in size as increasing

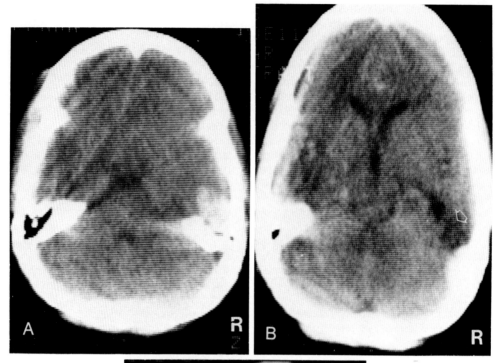

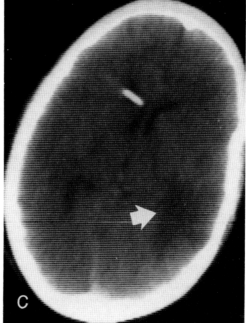

Figure 4.2. *A*, CT performed on day of admission shows a small right posterior temporal contusion. *B*, CT performed 3 days following trauma shows a decrease in the density of the contusion (arrow). *C*, CT at one year on the same patient shows a low density similar to that of CSF in the area of contusion (*arrow*).

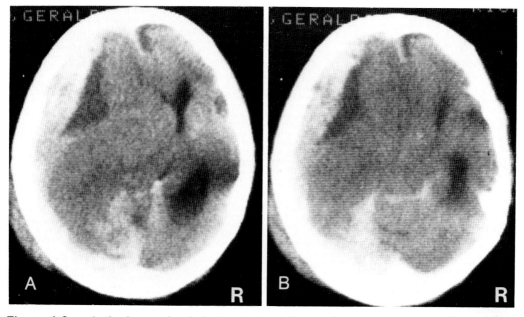

Figure 4.3.   *A,* the hemorrhagic lesion in the left occipital lobe cannot be differentiated from a contusion. *B,* lower level CT reveals that this lesion is an intracerebral hematoma contiguous with the subdural hematoma.

hemorrhage occurs. Usually, however, the initial high density and size of contusion gradually decrease and complete CT resolution of the contusion usually occurs by six weeks, leaving no residual changes or changes similar to porencephaly or focal atrophy.

Difficulty may occasionally arise in differentiating an extracerebral hematoma with intracerebral extension from a cerebral contusion, (Fig. 4.3). Approximately 15% of patients with severe head injury can be expected to have both extra and intracerebral hemorrhages.[40]

Intracerebral Hematoma. The CT appearance of an intracerebral hematoma is that of a high density area with sharply defined margins (Fig. 11.20). The attenuation values in H numbers range from the 40's to the 80's, depending upon the time elapsed since injury. Traumatic intracerebral hematomas tend to be multiple and occur anywhere in the brain, including the corpus callosum and brain stem. Hypertensive hemorrhages, on the other hand, are usually limited to one area and most often involve the basal ganglia.

Isolated brain stem injuries are uncommon and were reported to occur in less than 1% of all types of head injury.[71] When large, hemorrhagic lesions may be detected by the widely used first and second generation CT scanners (Fig. 4.4), but smaller ones may not be seen on CT because of the artifacts in the posterior fossa images. However, in a series reported by Tsai *et al.,*[71] less than 20% of brain stem lesions were hemorrhagic on CT, increasing the difficulty of recognition. The presence of hemorrhage in the subarachnoid spaces around the brain stem on CT may be the only evidence of brain stem injury (Fig. 4.5). The recognition of brain stem injury has important prognostic implications as patients with CT-documentated brain stem injury have a poor outcome.[71, 19]

Other uncommon hematomas are those located in the corpus callosum (Fig. 11.19). These are believed to be the result of diffuse shearing injury of white matter and are associated with a grave prognosis.[41] Nearly 90% of patients reported with this lesion die or remain in a persistent vegetative state.

Depending upon their size, intracerebral

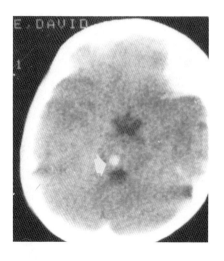

Figure 4.4. CT shows a small well-circumscribed hematoma (*arrow*) in the midbrain of a child who sustained a severe head injury.

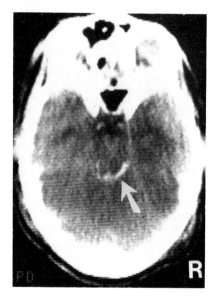

Figure 4.5. Increased density in the quadrigeminal cistern (*arrow*) is the only evidence of mid-brain hemorrhage following trauma. At autopsy a mid-brain hemorrhage was found.

hematomas may reach an isodense stage as early as two weeks and may or may not leave a residual change detectable by CT scan.[9, 82] The absence of high density on CT does not mean that the intraparenchymal hematoma has completely resolved[52] and contrast enhanced CT (CECT) may help in detecting otherwise unnoticeable isodense hemorrhage.[82] The peripheral enhancement of intracerebral hematomas on CECT may occur as early as six days and may persist six months after hemorrhage. This enhancement phenomenon is believed to be a result of extravasation of contrast medium secondary to a breakdown of the blood-brain barrier.[28] Intravascular pooling of iodine in granulation tissue also appears to play a significant role in such enhancement.[37, 82] The enhancement may be the only clue for the detection of a hematoma in a head injury patient who presents several days following injury (Fig. 4.6).

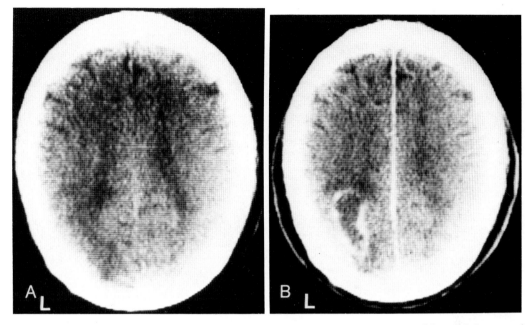

Figure 4.6. *A,* non-contrast CT of a patient with previous history of head injury and residual left hemispheric symptoms shows no apparent abnormality. *B,* CECT reveals the area of previous hemorrhage. Peripheral enhancement defines the margins of resolving hemorrhage.

Subdural Hematoma. The majority of acute subdural hematomas are clearly visualized on CT as high attenuation collections (H numbers ranging from 50–80).[3, 5, 41, 65, 80] The medial margin tends to be concave because the hematoma expands in the subdural space along the brain surface. The acute subdural hematoma is usually associated with a mass effect appropriate for its size with a midline shift and/or ipsilateral ventricular distortion (Fig. 11.12). If such secondary changes are not evident, one should suspect a contralateral abnormality. The adjacent brain may or may not show evidence of parenchymal damage, but the incidence of parenchymal injury associated with subdural hematoma is higher than that seen with epidural hematoma.

Some correlation exists between the density of the hematoma and time elapsed since injury. A majority of the high density hematomas are seen in patients who undergo CT during the first week after injury.[65] High density hematomas are also known to have an increased incidence of associated mass effect compared to low attenuation subdural hematomas. In one report, 95% of the high density subdural hematomas were associated with ventricular deformity compared to only 55% with low density collections.[26] While these reports suggest that one may be able to classify subdural hematomas as acute or chronic, depending upon the CT density, caution should be exercised in making such a determination using CT density alone. For example, a patient with a recent hemorrhage into a pre-existing low density subdural collection may not show a density which can be discerned from the adjacent brain parenchyma, because the mixture of a high density clot and low density collection may result in an isodense lesion. Such a patient with a significant mass effect causing ventricular compression and midline shift is considered to have an acute subdural hematoma for therapeutic purposes. Rarely, an acute isodense hematoma may be encountered in head injury patients with severe anemia (see above).

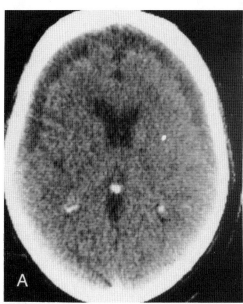

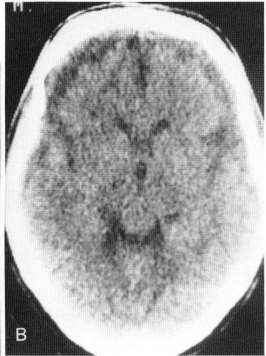

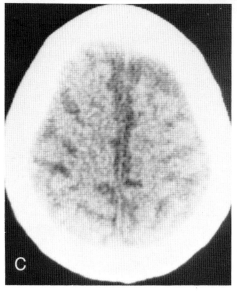

Figure 4.7 *A,* CT images at the ventricular level reveal bilateral low density extracerebral collections simulating low attenuation hematomas. *B* and *C,* CT images of the same patient at a lower level and over the convexity clearly reveal that the low attenuation collections are continuous with the sylvian fissures and the sulci consistent with atrophy.

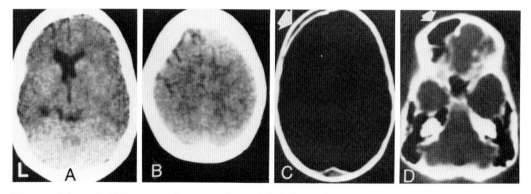

Figure 4.8. *A,* CT scan shows enlarged left lateral ventricle with ipsilateral midline displacement of the third ventricle and septum pellucidum in a patient with cerebral hemiatrophy mimicking the CT appearance of an isodense hematoma on the contralateral side. *B,* higher cut shows prominent sulci seen with this entity. *C,* bone window setting shows thickening of the calvarium (*arrow*). *D,* lower cuts with bone window setting shows small anterior and middle cranial fossae on the left and enlargement of the paranasal sinuses (*arrow*), a manifestation of small hemicronium. (Reproduced by permission from A. Zilkha: Am. J. Neuroradiol. 1:255–258, 1980.)

Occasionally, patients with markedly dilated subarachnoid spaces secondary to cortical atrophy may be mistaken for harboring a low density subdural hematoma (Fig. 4.7). Such a misdiagnosis can be avoided on careful scrutiny of CT. In such cases, the other subarachnoid spaces (*e.g.,* the sylvian fissures) are also enlarged and the mass effect, as evidenced by ventricular distortion, is absent.

The CT image of an isodense subdural hematoma can simulate hemiatrophy (Fig. 4.8). However, the calvarial thickening associated with hemiatrophy can be appreciated on CT.[11, 35, 79] CECT may be helpful in visualizing isodense subdural hematomas (see below).

Epidural Hematoma. Epidural hematoma is seen as a high density, extracerebral collection with attenuation values somewhat higher than those of subdural hematoma. The hematoma usually has a convex medial margin because the firm dural attachment to the inner table limits the peripheral expansion of the hematoma. The midline shift is relatively small compared to a subdural hematoma unless there is associated parenchymal injury (Fig. 11.14).

Although the majority of epidural hematomas occur shortly after injury, some may not be manifest for many hours or days[44] (Fig. 4.9). It may not always be possible to localize the hemorrhage to the subdural or epidural space based upon CT alone. This is especially so if there is a concommitant parenchymal injury. Approximately 20% of patients can be expected to have hemorrhage in both the subdural and epidural spaces following trauma.[36]

Intraventricular Hemorrhage. Posttraumatic intraventricular hemorrhage (IVH) is frequently associated with intracerebral hematomas (Fig. 4.10). CT has greatly facilitated the management of patients with intraventricular hemorrhage.[27, 57, 62] The incidence of IVH is reported to range from 2–3%,[50, 57] but it is probably more common in severe head injury than these figures indicate. For the optimal detection of IVH, CT must be performed as soon as possible after injury. Our own experience with 100 consecutive severe head injury patients, who had CT scanning within hours of head injury, shows that at least 5% can be expected to have intraventricular hemorrhage.[62] Increased experience with CT shows that IVH does not necessarily imply a grave prognosis as was previously believed.[27, 62]

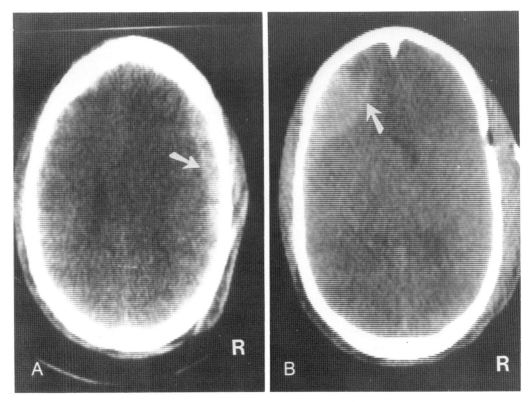

Figure 4.9. *A,* admission CT shows a right subdural hematoma (*arrow*). *B,* twenty-four hours after evacuation of subdural hematoma the patient developed a contralateral epidural hematoma (*arrow*) along the left frontal convexity.

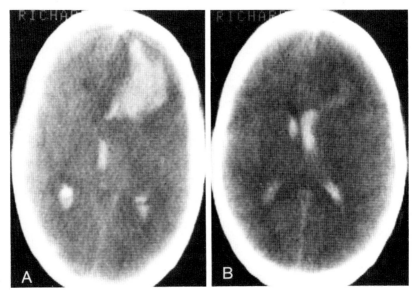

Figure 4.10. *A* and *B,* CT showing intraventricular hemorrhage following head injury. Hemorrhage is present in both lateral ventricles and the third ventricle resulting from extension of the right frontal intracerebral hematoma into the anterior horn.

Subarachnoid Hemorrhage. Subarachnoid hemorrhage is seen on CT as a zone of high density within the various intracranial subarachnoid spaces (the basal cisterns, sylvian fissures, and interhemispheric fissures, etc.) (Fig. 4.5). Nearly 50% of head injury patients with CT evidence of subarachnoid hemorrhage have associated intracranial hemorrhagic lesions.[24]

Serial CT Scanning in Severe Head Injury

A repeat CT during the first week, preferably on the third day or earlier, should be obtained on severe head injured patients who do not show improvement in their neurological status. Several reports emphasize the value of such a CT for the detection of new lesions.[16, 18, 32, 70] The new lesions may be hemorrhagic or nonhemorrhagic and are reported to occur in over 50% of the patients with severe head injury.[18] Two-thirds of the patients deteriorating neurologically after the first 48 hours had new lesions on repeat CT in one series.[16] The delayed hemorrhagic lesions are frequently intra-parenchymal, but may also occur extracerebrally.[16, 46] The delayed parenchymal hematoma may not be heralded by clinical deterioration or elevation of ICP and a majority appear to develop during the first 48 hours.[32] Delayed hemorrhage appears to be associated with poor outcome.[16, 18] Early recognition of these lesions is important for proper management because clinical improvement has been noted in some patients following surgical evacuation.[13, 23]

Although 25% of delayed hemorrhages were found to develop in patients with a normal initial CT, over 50% of the patients developing delayed lesions had initial hemorrhagic lesions and underwent decompressive surgery.[16, 32] Thus, a repeat CT on the third day (or earlier, if necessary) will result in the detection of lesions in many patients who do not improve neurologically during the first 48 hours following surgery for pre-existing lesions.

The Role of CECT in Acute Head Injury

CECT is usually performed following intravenous administration of radiodinated contrast medium like Renografin and Hypaque containing approximately 41 g iodine. Others have advocated the use of higher or double dose (80 g) of iodine for CECT if the patient's renal status permits.[34]

The need for CECT in patients with acute head injury is controversial. Tsai *et al.*[71] reported that CECT was beneficial in visualizing additional abnormalities in 46% of the patients presenting with acute head injury. The additional information consisted of better visualization of extracerebral hematomas and associated damaged cortical areas. It was suggested that CECT be performed routinely on acute head injury patients for diagnostic and prognostic purposes. Forbes and his associates,[26] however, commented that contrast enhancement has not been helpful in diagnosing subdural hematomas in acute head injury. They felt that nothing is gained by using contrast medium if the patient has a normal unenhanced CT.

The routine use of contrast enhancement is unnecessary in patients with head injury who have hemorrhagic lesions consistent with their neurological status. However, if a patient has neurological deficit and non-contrast CT reveals no abnormality or minimal abnormality such as ventricular distortion, CECT may visualize an isodense hematoma.[4, 51] A CECT may reveal the enhancement of the membrane around a chronic subdural hematoma (Fig. 4.11). It may also show extravasation of contrast medium into the subdural hematoma on CT.[52] On delayed CT done four to six hours after intravenous injection of contrast medium, Amendola and Ostrum[4] were able to visualize isodense lesions in nearly 50% of patients with such lesions. Others have suggested that scanning be performed during the latter part of infusion to detect cortical venous displacement caused by isodense extracerebral collections.[39]

The rapid high dose technique advocated by Hayman *et al.*[34] consists of injecting 41 g iodinated contrast material in less than two minutes followed by rapid infusion of another 41 g in six to nine minutes. This technique is far more effective than the others described above. A correct diagnosis of the presence or absence of isodense SDH was made in all of the patients studied by

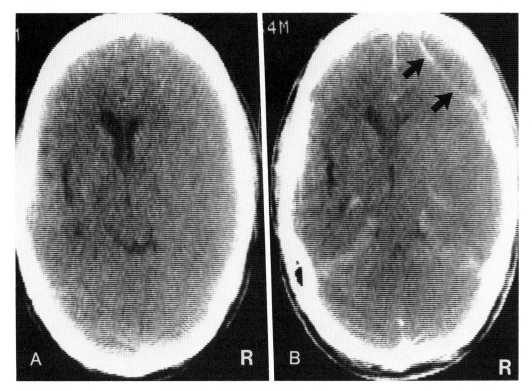

Figure 4.11. *A,* non-contrast CT shows right to left midline displacement without evidence of intra- or extra-axial lesion in a patient with left hemiparesis. *B,* following the intravenous injection of contrast CT reveals enhancement of the membrane (*arrow*) around an isodense subdural hematoma. (Courtesy: A.K. Girevendulis, M.D., Richmond, Virginia.)

the rapid high dose method. By using this technique, angiography may be avoided for the diagnosis of isodense lesions. In the absence of hemiatrophy, if there is ventricular distortion without evidence of focal parenchymal abnormality on CECT in a patient with suspected head trauma, one should be suspicious of the presence of an isodense subdural hematoma. In addition to its value in detecting isodense mass lesions, CECT is also helpful in visualizing infarctions[56, 78] and unsuspected high density tumors, like meningiomas, that may simulate a resolving hematoma.

SKULL RADIOGRAPHY IN HEAD INJURY

The role of skull radiography and the significance of the detection of linear frac-tures in head injured patients has been the subject of much controversy[8, 20, 22, 49, 63, 72] (see also Chapter 5). Although the presence of a linear fracture alone may not alter the management of head-injured patients, it is a measure of the severity of injury sustained by the calvarium. In one series, 80% of the fatal head injury victims were found to have fractures.[1] Sixty-seven percent of the hospitalized patients with skull fractures had associated significant intracranial lesions.[80]

Routine skull radiography includes films done in the lateral, Towne view (inclined antero-posterior projection), straight antero-posterior, and Caldwell projections. In head trauma, however, depending upon the clinical situation and the availability of the CT scanner, the radiographic examination can be limited to a single lateral projection

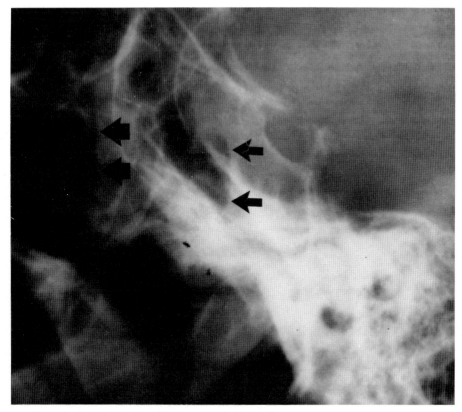

Figure 4.12.   Lateral skull radiograph taken in the supine position in a patient with a history of head trauma shows air-fluid levels in the sphenoid and maxillary sinuses (*arrows*) suggestive of fractures of the skull base and facial skeleton.

with the patient in the supine position. A frontal radiograph in the Towne projection may help identify an occipital fracture. A lateral supine radiograph is also useful in providing indirect evidence of fractures of the base of the skull or facial skeleton by demonstrating air-fluid levels (representing blood or CSF) in the sphenoid and/or maxillary sinuses (Fig. 4.12).

A linear fracture is easily recognized by the presence of a straight lucent line with sharp margins across the calvarium. Occasionally, sutures or vascular grooves may be confused with a fracture. However, fractures tend to be more lucent and have sharper margins than vascular grooves.

Depressed fractures may be detected on CT, especially if the window level and window width are adjusted appropriately (Fig. 4.13). The exact location of an intracranial bony fragment as well as the degree of depression can be evaluated by CT. However, plain skull radiography, with tangential views of the area, may be necessary if the depression is minimal. Depressed fractures, located near the venous sinuses along the high convexity, may not be detected on conventional CT. Skull films may be the only means for detecting these lesions which may lead to compression or obstruction of the venous sinuses.

Only 20% of fractures of the skull base can be diagnosed on plain skull radiography.[33] When a basal skull fracture is suspected because of the presence of CSF rhinorrhea or otorrhea, a Battles sign, or facial nerve palsy, complex motion tomography may be necessary (Fig. 5.8). High resolution CT scanners may delineate fractures of the skull base and eliminate the need for com-

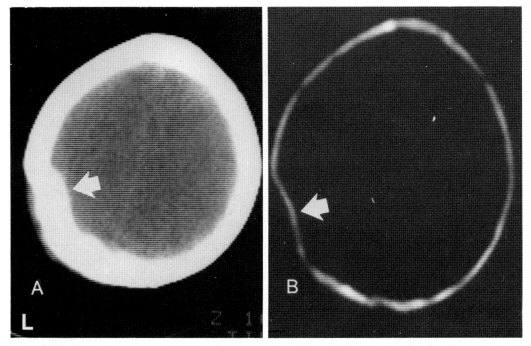

Figure 4.13. *A,* CT of a 5-year-old child following head injury reveals slight irregularity of the calvarium (*arrow*) posteriorly on the left side. *B,* wide windowing technique shows the extent of depression of the fractured fragment (*arrow*).

plex motion tomography in the future[29] (Fig. 4.14). Complex motion tomography, however, may be the only means of detecting undisplaced linear fractures involving the temporal bone and bony canals and ossicular chain disruption.

Metrizamide CT cisternography is also useful in identifying the location of the CSF leak following injury to the base of the skull[29] (Fig. 4.15). Following intrathecal administration of 6 to 8 ml Metrizamide (220 mgI/ml), the patient's head is placed in the CT scanner in a position (in the appropriate lateral decubitus position for otorrhea or in the prone position for rhinorrhea) to facilitate the identification of the site of leakage.

RADIOLOGIC EVALUATION OF THE CERVICAL SPINE

The incidence of cervical spine injury associated with head trauma varies considerably in different series.[2, 66] However, in the autopsy studies reported by Alker *et al.*[2] as many as 17% of fatal vehicular accident victims had isolated upper cervical spine injuries and an additional 8% had associated head injury. While this incidence is higher than that encountered in patients presenting with head injury in the emergency room, it is nevertheless important that all patients with severe head injuries have radiographic examination of the cervical spine or have the neck adequately immobilized before the patient is moved for other diagnostic investigations.

Routine radiographic evaluation of the cervical spine consists of at least five radiographs obtained in different projections: a lateral view, two oblique views, an antero-posterior view of the upper cervical spine with the patient's mouth open for the evaluation of the atlanto-axial area, and a second antero-posterior view for the rest of the cervical spine. However, these views should not be routinely performed on all patients suspected of cervical spine or spinal cord trauma for fear of further injuring the cord. One should, instead, obtain a single lateral

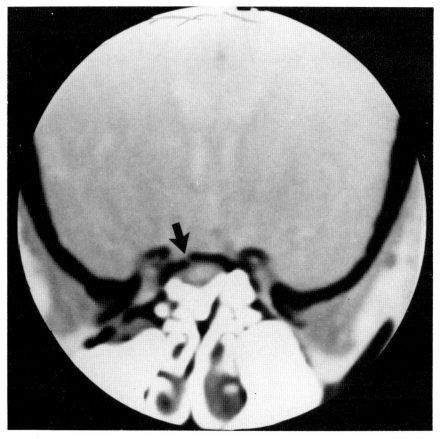

Figure 4.14.   A coronal CT section (in reverse image) through the planum sphenoidale demonstrates a fracture (*arrow*) with herniation of the arachnoid into the sphenoid sinus. (Reproduced by permission of K. Ghoshhajra, Krishna C.V.G. Rao, CT: J. Comput. Tomog., 4:271–276, 1980.)

radiograph of the entire cervical spine with the patient in the supine position before the patient is manipulated for further evaluation. A well-performed radiograph in this position is adequate to demonstrate most of the dislocations and clinically significant fractures of the cervical spine. When evaluating the cervical spine, attention should be paid to the position of the pre-vertebral fat stripe[74] and the size of the pre-vertebral soft tissue. The soft tissue normally measures 5.0 mm or less in the neutral position in the upper cervical spine and does not exceed 7.0 mm in adults on radiographs done at a 40″ film distance.[61] In the lower cervical spine, it is usually 1.5 cm wide but is not more than 2 cm. If the fat stripe displacement exceeds these measurements, this should be considered indirect evidence of cervical spine injury.

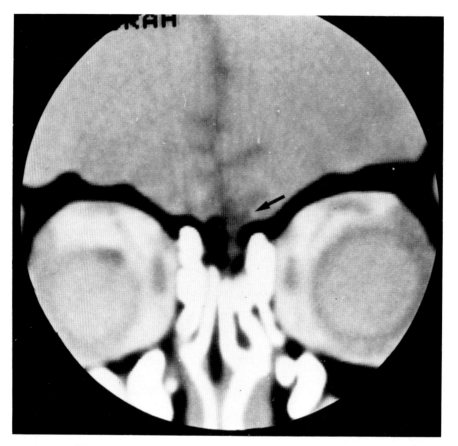

Figure 4.15. A CT cisternogram in the coronal projection (in reverse image) through the cribriform plate shows a diastatic fracture with concentration of Metrizamide at the fracture site (*arrow*) demonstrating the leakage of CSF. (Reprinted by permission of K. Ghoshhajra and Raven Press: J. Assist. Tomog. 4:309, 1980.)

Fractures of the cervical spine most frequently involve the second to sixth vertebrae. If a fracture is suspected, but not detected on conventional radiography, tomography should be performed. This is preferable to manipulating the patient for radiographs in various oblique projections, thereby increasing the risk of spinal cord injury.

If the patient's neurological status permits, spinal trauma can also be evaluated with CT scanners.[17, 38, 43] Using high resolution scanners, this method is reported to identify even undisplaced linear fractures of the vertebral body and neural arch[30] (Fig. 4.16). It is also useful for the demonstration of the spinal canal and detection of bony fragments causing compression of the spinal cord. With the newer scanners, the spinal canal can also be evaluated in the

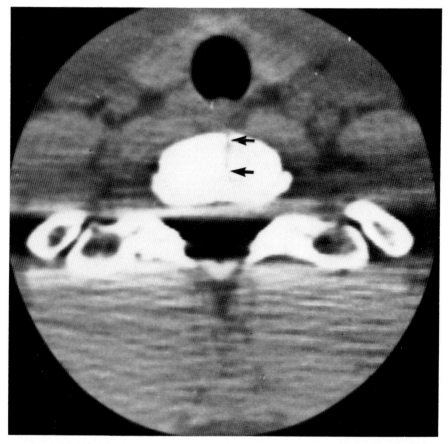

Figure 4.16. CT of upper thoracic spine revealing a linear fracture through the body of T-1 extending anteroposteriorly (*arrow*). (Reproduced by permission of K. Ghoshhajra, *et al.*: CT: J. Comput. Tomog. 4:309, 1980.)

sagittal plane using reconstruction techniques without moving the patient.[17]

Spinal cord injury may occur without demonstrable fractures of the spine. Myelography may be the only method to demonstrate contusion or compression of the cord. Compression of the spinal cord may also be due to herniated disc fragment, an epidural hematoma, or less commonly a subdural hematoma.[59]

ANGIOGRAPHIC EVALUATION IN HEAD INJURY

For the most part, angiography has been replaced by CT for the evaluation of intracranial mass lesions in patients with acute head injury. Its role in the diagnosis of intracranial space occupying masses is lim-

ited to the diagnosis of isodense lesions, which are not demonstrable by any other means. For example, a patient who shows significant midline shift without evidence of parenchymal swelling or hemorrhage or enhancing lesions on CECT, can best be evaluated by angiography for the detection of isodense subdural hematomas. The only pitfall of angiography for the detection of SDH occurs in patients who may appear to have SDH because of failure of the distal branches to reach the inner table due to atrophy or occlusion of the middle cerebral arterial branches[25] (Fig. 4.17).

Angiography still remains essential to demonstrate vascular injuries, whether they involve extracranial cephalic arteries or the intracranial vascular tree. A full dis-

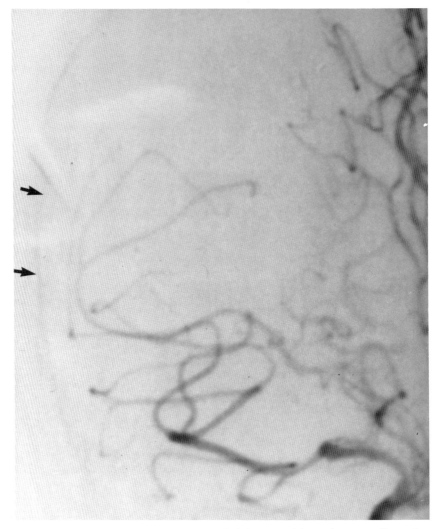

Figure 4.17. Antero-posterior projection of right carotid angiogram. Branches of the right middle cerebral artery fail to reach the inner table (*arrows*) leaving an avascular space suggestive of extracerebral hemorrhage. The avascular zone, however, is a result of occlusion of middle cerebral arterial branches from embolism.

cussion of vascular lesions is the subject of Chapter 14.

When evaluating vascular injury of the extracranial internal carotid artery, one should be careful not to mistake non-opacification of the intracranial circulation as evidence of traumatic occlusion of the internal carotid artery (Fig. 4.18). Such nonvisualization may be secondary to marked intracranial hypertension. In these latter cases, if filming is carried out for a prolonged period of time, with angiography one may be able to demonstrate slow progression of contrast material intracranially.[21] Contrast material is often found to layer along the posterior wall of the carotid artery in such instances on late films. A relatively non-invasive way of diagnosing such a pseudo-occlusion of the internal carotid artery secondary to intracranial hypertension is by dynamic radionuclide scanning.[10] This technique can be performed at the bedside using a scintillation gamma camera following IV administration of radionuclide and when necessary is helpful in documenting the lack of cerebral perfusion

(Fig. 4.19).

Complete evaluation of traumatic lesions like aneurysms, arteriovenous fistulae, or venous thrombosis can be made only by angiography. Although traumatic arterio-venous fistulae, like carotid cavernous fistulae, are detected on contrast enhanced CT, angiography is essential for evaluating the hemodynamics of the fistula and the precise identification of the vascular anat-

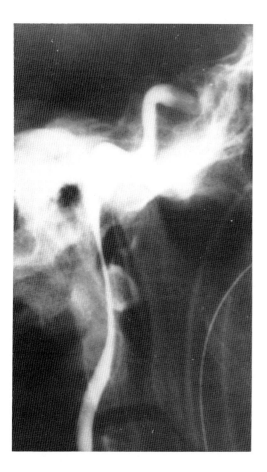

Figure 4.18.   Apparent occlusion of internal carotid artery near the supra-clinoid portion due to markedly raised intracranial pressure.

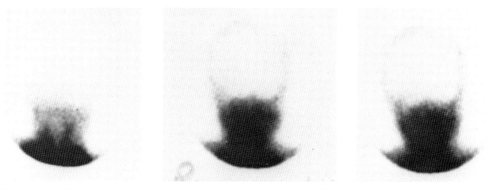

Figure 4.19.   "Radioisotope angiography" using Tc^{m}99, administered intravenously, shows no intracranial radioactivity after several seconds consistent with lack of significant cerebral perfusion in a patient with elevated ICP.

omy. Similarly, infarction occurring following trauma can be adequately demonstrated on CT, but the etiology of infarction
and the exact site of vascular occlusion can
be defined only by angiography.

Arterial spasm may develop following
head injury[55] and in one series was found in
40% of patients following trauma.[48] It may
be present with or without evidence of focal
ischemic damage in the brain and may or
may not be associated with slowing of circulation secondary to spasm. Such spasm
may be present in association with an intracranial hematoma.

CT signs have been described for the
detection of transtentorial herniation and
consist of distortion of the cisterns around
the brain stem.[58] Angiography, however,
remains the preferred method for diagnosing transtentorial herniation as demonstrated by displacement of the anterior cho-
roidal and posterior cerebral arteries and
the basal vein.

The presence of venous sinus thrombosis
or occlusion can be suspected on CECT[14] if
a filling defect is seen in the sinus. Others
have reported that sinus thrombosis can be
diagnosed on non-contrast CT if an area of
high attenuation density measuring 50–60
H numbers[60, 73] is seen in the sinus. However, caution is necessary in making such a
diagnosis in the region of the sagittal sinus
(see above) where a focal increased falx
density may simulate thrombosis of the
sinuses. Radioisotopic studies are also useful in making the diagnosis if lack of activity
in a certain area of the sinus is noted.[6, 31, 76]
Angiography is usually necessary to make
a definite diagnosis of sinus thrombosis or
occlusion.

Dynamic computed tomography using
newer generation scanners with improved
software was reported to have the potential
for evaluating relative cerebral perfusion[55, 77] resulting from spasm. However, the
underlying or causative vascular lesion like
aneurysm can best be evaluated by angiography. Furthermore, when the cause of intracerebral hematoma is unclear because of
questionable history, angiography may be
necessary to detect the etiology.

The newly introduced digital subtraction
angiography or intravenous angiography[15]

or computerized fluoroscopy[68] offers great
promise as another relatively non-invasive
technique in neuroradiology. Using the digital subtraction system, radioiodinated contrast medium injected intravenously with a
power injector is shown to opacify the cerebrovascular tree adequately. This technique requires only a 2–3% concentration of
the contrast medium in the artery as compared with a concentration of 40–50% for
conventional angiography. This non-invasive procedure can soon be expected to be
widely used for the evaluation of stenosis
or occlusion, and other vascular lesions including those resulting from trauma.

References

1. Adams, J.H.: The neuropathology of head injuries.
   In: Handbook of Clinical Neurology, Vol. 23: Injuries of the Brain and Skull Part 1, Eds. P.J.
   Vinken, G.W. Bruyn. North-Holland Publishing
   Co., Amsterdam, Oxford, 1975, pp. 35–65.
2. Alker, G.J., Jr., Young, S., Leslie, E.V.: High cervical spine and cranio-cervical junction injuries in
   fatal traffic accidents: A radiologic study. Orthoped. Clin. North Am., 9:1003–1010, 1978.
3. Ambrose, J., Gooding, M.R., Uttley, D.: EMI scan
   in the management of head injuries. Lancet,
   1:847–848, 1976.
4. Amendola, M.A., Ostrum, B.J.: Diagnosis of isodense subdural hematomas by computed tomography. Am. J. Roentgenol. 129:693–697, 1977.
5. Baker, H.L., Campbell, J.K., Houser, O.W., Reese,
   D.F., Sheedy, P.F., Holman, C.B., Kurland, R.L.:
   Computed assisted tomography of the head: an
   early evaluation. Mayo Clin. Proc., 49:17–27, 1974.
6. Barnes, B.D., Winestock, D.P.: Dynamic radionuclide scanning in the diagnosis of thrombosis of
   the superior sagittal sinus. Neurology, 27:656–661,
   1977.
7. Becker, D.P., Miller, J.D., Ward, J.D., Greenberg,
   R.P., Young, H.F., Sakalas, R.: The outcome from
   severe head injury with early diagnosis and intensive management. J. Neurosurg., 47:491–502, 1977.
8. Bell, R.S., Loop, J.W.: The utility and futility of
   radiographic skull examinations for trauma. N.
   Engl. J. Med., 284:236–239, 1971.
9. Bergstrom, M., Ericson, K., Levander, B., et al.:
   Computed tomography of cranial subdural and
   epidural hematomas: variation of attenuation related to time and clinical events such as rebleeding.
   J. Comp. Assist. Tomog., 1:449–455, 1977.
10. Braunstein, P., Korein, J., Kricheff, I., Corey, K.,
    Chase, N.: A simple bedside evaluation for cerebral
    blood flow in the study of cerebral death: a pro-
    spective study on 34 deeply comatose patients.
    Am. J. Roentgenol. Radium Ther. Nucl. Med.,
    118:757–767, 1973.
11. Brennan, R.E., Stratt, B.J., Lee, K.F.: Computed

tomographic findings in cerebral hemiatrophy. Neuroradiology, 17:17–20, 1978.
12. Brooks, R.A., DiChiro, G.: Principles of computer assisted tomography (CAT) in radiographic radioisotope imaging. Phys. Med. Biol., 21:689–732, 1976.
13. Brown, F.D., Mullan, S., Duda, E.E.: Delayed traumatic intracerebral hematomas. Report of 3 cases. J. Neurosurg., 48:1019–1022, 1978.
14. Buonanno, F.S., Moody, D.M., Ball, M.R., Laster, D.W.: Computed cranial tomographic findings in cerebral sinovenous occlusion. J. Comp. Assist. Tomog., 2:281–290, 1978.
15. Christenson, P.C., Ovitt, T.W., Fisher, H.D. III, Frost, M.M., Nudelman, S., Roehrig, H.: Intravenous angiography using digital video subtraction: intravenous cervicocerebrovascular angiography. A.J.N.R., 1:379–386, 1980.
16. Clifton, G.L., Grossman, R.G., Makela, M.E., Miner, M.E., Handel, S., Sadhu, V.: Neurological course and correlated computerized tomography findings after severe closed head injury. J. Neurosurg., 52:611–624, 1980.
17. Coin, C.G., Pennink, M., Ahmad, W.D., Keranen, V.J.: Diving-type injury of the cervical spine: contribution of computed tomography to management. J. Comp. Assist. Tomog., 3:362–372, 1979.
18. Cooper, P.R., Maravilla, K., Moody, S., Clark, W.K.: Serial computerized tomographic scanning and the prognosis of severe head injury. Neurosurgery, 5:566–569, 1979.
19. Cooper, P.R., Maravilla, K., Kirkpatrick, J., Moody, S.F., Sklar, F.H., Diehl, J., Clark, W.K.: Traumatically induced brain stem hemorrhage and the computerized tomographic scan: clinical, pathological, and experimental observations. Neurosurgery, 4:115–124, 1979.
20. Cummins, R.O.: Clinicians' reasons for overuse of skull radiographs. A.J.N.R., 1:339–342, 1980.
21. Davies, E.R., Sutton, D.: Pseudo-occlusion of the internal carotid artery in raised intracranial pressure. Clin. Radiol., 18:245–252, 1967.
22. DeSmet, A.A., Fryback, D.G., Thornbury, J.R.: A second look at the utility of radiographic skull examination for trauma. Am. J. Roentgenol., 132:95–99, 1979.
23. Diaz, F.G., Yock, D.H. Jr., Larson, D., Rockswold, G.L.: Early diagnosis of delayed posttraumatic intracerebral hematomas. J. Neurosurg., 50:217–223, 1979.
24. Dolinskas, C.A., Zimmerman, R.A., Bilaniuk, L.T.: A sign of subarachnoid bleeding on cranial computed tomograms of pediatric head trauma patients. Radiology, 126:409–411, 1978.
25. Ferris, E.J., Lehrer, H., Shapiro, J.H.: Pseudosubdural hematoma. Radiology, 88:75–84, 1967.
26. Forbes, G.S., Sheedy, P.F., Piepgras, D.G., Houser, O.W.: Computed tomography in the evaluation of subdural hematomas. Radiology, 126:143–148, 1978.
27. French, B.N., Dublin, A.B.: The value of computerized tomography in the management of 1000 consecutive head injuries. Surg. Neurol., 7:171–183, 1977.
28. Gado, M.H., Phelps, M.E., Coleman, R.E.: An extravascular component of contrast enhancement in cranial computed tomography. Radiology, 117:589–593, 1975.
29. Ghoshhajra, K.: CT in trauma of the base of the skull and its complications. J. Computed Tomog., 4:271–276, 1980.
30. Ghoshhajra, K., Rao, C.V.G.: CT in spinal trauma. J. Computed Tomog., 4:309–318, 1980.
31. Go, R.T., Chiu, C.L., Neuman, L.A.: Diagnosis of superior sagittal sinus thrombosis by dynamic and sequential brain scanning. Report of one case. Neurology, 23:1199–1204, 1973.
32. Gudeman, S.K., Kishore, P.R.S., Miller, J.D., Girevendulis, A.K., Lipper, M.H., Becker, D.P.: The genesis and significance of delayed traumatic intracerebral hematoma. Neurosurgery, 5:309–313, 1979.
33. Harwood-Nash, D.C.: Fractures of the petrous and tympanic parts of the temporal bone in children; a tomographic study of 35 cases. Am. J. Roentgenol. Radium Ther. Nucl. Med., 110:598, 1970.
34. Hayman, L.A., Evans, R.A., Hinck, V.C.: Rapid-high-dose contrast computed tomography of isodense subdural hematoma and cerebral swelling. Radiology, 131:381–383, 1979.
35. Jacoby, C.G., Go, R.T., Hahn, F.J.: Computed tomography in cerebral hemiatrophy. Am. J. Roentgenol., 129:5–9, 1977.
36. Jamieson, K.G., Yelland, J.D.N.: Extradural hematoma. Report of 167 cases. J. Neurosurg., 29:13–23, 1968.
37. Jeffries, B.F., Kishore, P.R.S., Singh, K.S., Ghatak, N.R., Krempa, J.: Contrast enhancement in the postoperative brain. Radiology, 139:409–413, 1981.
38. Kershner, M.S., Goodman, G.A., Perlmutter, G.S.: Computed tomography in the diagnosis of an atlas fracture. Am. J. Roentgenol., 128:688–689, 1977.
39. Kim, K.S., Hemmati, M., Weinberg, P.E.: Computed tomography in isodense subdural hematoma. Radiology, 128:71–74, 1978.
40. Kishore, P.R.S., Lipper, M.H., Becker, D.P., Domingues da Silva, A.A., Narayan, R.K.: The significance of CT in head injury: correlation with intracranial pressure. A.J.N.R., 2:307–311, 1981.
41. Koo, A.H., La Roque, R.L.: Evaluation of head trauma by computed tomography. Radiology, 123:345–350, 1977.
42. Lanksch, W., Oettinger, W., Baethmann, A., Kazner, E.: CT findings in brain edema compared with direct chemical analysis of tissue samples. In: Dynamics of Brain Edema, Eds. H.M. Pappius, W. Feindel. Springer-Verlag, New York, 1976, pp. 283–287.
43. Lee, B.C.P., Kazam, E., Newman, A.D.: Computed tomography of the spine and spinal cord. Radiology, 128:95–102, 1978.
44. Lee, S.H., Kishore, P.R.S.: Delayed development of epidural hematomas A.J.N.R. (in press).
45. Levander, B., Stattin, S., Svendsen, P.: Computer tomography of traumatic intra and extracerebral lesions. Acta Radiol. (Suppl. 346) 107–118, 1975.
46. Lipper, M.H., Kishore, P.R.S., Girevendulis, A.K., Miller, J.D., Becker, D.P.: Delayed intracranial hematoma in patients with severe head injury.

Radiology, 133:645–649, 1979.

47. McCullough, E.C., Baker, H.L., Houser, O.W., Reese, D.F.: An evaluation of the quantitative and radiation features of a scanning x-ray transverse axial tomography. The EMI scanner. Radiology, 111:709–716, 1974.

48. MacPherson, P., Graham, D.I.: Arterial spasm and slowing of the cerebral circulation in the ischemia of head injury. J. Neurol. Neurosurg. Psych., 36:1069–1072, 1973.

49. Masters, S.J.: Evaluation of head trauma: efficacy of skull films. A.J.N.R., 1:329–338, 1980.

50. Merino-de Villasante, J., Taveras, J.M.: Computerized tomography (CT) in acute head trauma. Am. J. Roentgenol., 126:765–778, 1976.

51. Messina, A.V.: Computed tomography: contrast media in subdural hematoma. A preliminary report. Radiology, 119:725–726, 1976.

52. Messina, A.V., Chernik, N.L.: Computed tomography: the "resolving" intracerebral hemorrhage. Radiology, 118:609–613, 1976.

53. Miller, J.D., Gudeman, S.K., Kishore, P.R.S., Becker, D.P.: Computed tomography in brain edema due to trauma. In: Advances in Neurology, Vol. 28, Eds., J. Cervos-Navarro, R. Ferszt. Raven Press, New York, 1980, pp. 413–422.

54. New, P.F., Aronow, S.: Attenuation measurements of whole blood and blood fractions in computed tomography. Radiology, 121:635–640, 1970.

55. Norman, D., Axel, L., Berninger, W.H., Edwards, M.S., Christopher, C.E., Redington, R.W., Cox, L.: Dynamic computed tomography of the brain: techniques, data analysis, and applications. A.J.N.R., 2:1–12, 1981.

56. Norton, G.A., Kishore, P.R.S., Lin, J.: CT contrast enhancement in cerebral infarctions. Am. J. Roentgenol., 131:881–885, 1978.

57. Oliff, M., Fried, A.M., Young, A.B.: Intraventricular hemorrhage in blunt head trauma. J. Comp. Assist. Tomog., 2:625–629, 1978.

58. Osborn, A.G., Heaston, D.K., Wing, S.D.: Diagnosis of ascending transtentorial herniation by cranial computed tomography. Am. J. Roentgenol., 130:755–760, 1978.

59. Paredes, E.S.D., Kishore, P.R.S., Ward, J.D.: Cervical spinal subdural hematoma. Surg. Neurol., 15:477–479, 1981.

60. Patronas, N.J., Duda, E.E., Mirfakhraee, M., Wollmann, R.L.: Superior sagittal sinus thrombosis diagnosed by computed tomography. Surg. Neurol., 15:11–14, 1981.

61. Penning, L.: Prevertebral hematoma in cervical spine injury: incidence and etiologic significance. A.J.N.R., 1:557–565, 1980.

62. Roberson, F.C., Kishore, P.R.S., Miller, J.D., Lipper, M.H., Becker, D.P.: The value of serial computerized tomography in the management of severe head injury. Surg. Neurol., 12:161–167, 1979.

63. Roberts, F., Shopfner, C.E.: Plain skull roentgenograms in children with head trauma. Am. J. Roentgenol., 114:230–240, 1972.

64. Saul, T.G., Ducker, T.B.: Management of severe head injuries. Maryland State Med. J., 30:45–48, 1981.

65. Scotti, G., Terbrugge, K., Melancon, D., Belanger, G.: Evaluation of the age of subdural hematomas by computerized tomography. J. Neurosurg., 47:311–315, 1977.

66. Shrago, G.G.: Cervical spine injuries; association with head trauma: a review of 50 patients. Am. J. Roentgenol., 118:670–673, 1973.

67. Smith, W.P. Jr., Batnitzky, S., Rengachary, S.S.: Acute isodense subdural hematomas: a problem in anemic patients. A.J.N.R., 2:37–40, 1981.

68. Strother, C.M., Sackett, J.F., Crummy, A.B., Lilleas, F.G., Zwiebel, W.J., Turnipseed, W.D., Javid, M., Mistretta, C.A., Kruger, R.A., Ergun, D.L., Shaw, C.G.: Clinical applications of computerized fluoroscopy. Radiology, 136:781–783, 1980.

69. Svendsen, P.: Computer tomography of traumatic extracerebral lesions. Br. J. Radiol., 49:1004–1012, 1976.

70. Sweet, R.C., Miller, J.D., Lipper, M., Kishore, P.R.S., Becker, D.P.: Significance of bilateral abnormalities on the CT scan in patients with severe head injury. Neurosurgery, 3:16–21, 1978.

71. Tsai, F.Y., Huprich, J.E., Gardner, F.C., Segall, H.D., Teal, J.S.: Diagnostic and prognostic implications of computed tomography of head trauma. J. Comp. Assist. Tomog., 2:323–331, 1978.

72. Weinstein, M.A., Alfidi, R.J., Duchesneau, P.M.: Computed tomography versus skull radiography. Am. J. Roentgenol., 128:873, 1977.

73. Wendling, L.R.: Intracranial venous sinus thrombosis: diagnosis suggested by computed tomography. Am. J. Roentgenol. Rad. Ther. Nucl. Med., 130:978–980, 1978.

74. Whalen, J.P., Woodruff, C.L.: The cervical prevertebral fat stripe—a new aid in evaluating the prevertebral soft tissue space. Am. J. Roentgenol., 109:445–451, 1970.

75. Wilkins, R.H., Odom, G.L.: Intracranial arterial spasm associated with craniocerebral trauma. J. Neurosurg., 32:626–633, 1970.

76. Williamson, B.E., Teates, C.D., Bray, S.T., Riddlevold, H.O., Lee, R.F., Wakefield, J.A.: Radionuclide brain scan findings in superior sagittal sinus thrombosis. Clin. Nucl. Med., 3:184–187, 1978.

77. Wing, S.D., Anderson, R.E., Osborn, A.G.: Dynamic cranial computed tomography: Preliminary results. A.J.N.R., 1:135–140, 1980.

78. Yock, D.H., Marshall, W.H.: Recent ischemic brain infarcts at computed tomography: appearances pre- and post contrast infusion. Radiology, 117:599–608, 1975.

79. Zilkha, A.: CT of cerebral hemiatrophy. A.J.N.R., 1:255–258, 1980.

80. Zimmerman, R.A., Bilaniuk, L.T., Gennarelli, T., Bruce, D., Dolinskas, C., Uzzell, B.: Cranial computed tomography in diagnosis and management of acute head trauma. Am. J. Roentgenol., 131:27–34, 1978.

81. Zimmerman, R.A., Bilaniuk, L.T., Gennarelli, T.: Computed tomography of shearing injuries of the cerebral white matter. Radiology, 127:393–396, 1978.

82. Zimmerman, R.D., Leeds, N.E., Naidich, T.P.: Ring blush associated with intracerebral hematoma. Radiology, 122:707–711, 1977.

Skull Fracture and Traumatic Cerebrospinal Fluid Fistulas

PAUL R. COOPER

LINEAR SKULL FRACTURE: DIAGNOSIS AND SIGNIFICANCE

The significance of a linear fracture of the cranial vault in adults has been exaggerated. When the skull has been fractured, it can be assumed that the head has been struck by a blow containing considerable energy (Fig. 5.1). Nevertheless, patients with a skull fracture may have no signs or symptoms of central nervous system injury. Conversely, severe neural injury may occur in the absence of skull fracture. The patient's symptoms and signs of neural injury and not the presence of a linear fracture should determine the diagnostic and therapeutic plan.

The presence of a skull fracture has been thought to correlate with occult intracranial hematomas which may result in delayed neurologic deterioration. This is a major reason why a careful search is made for a linear skull fracture and why neurologically intact patients with a linear fracture are admitted for observation in many neurological centers.

This policy raises several questions. First, are excessive numbers of skull roentgenograms performed in an attempt to identify this asymptomatic group of patients and are there clinical criteria that might select out for examination those patients most likely to have a skull fracture? Second, what is the evidence that admitting asympto-

matic patients with a linear skull fracture is a medically and economically effective policy for the early detection of occult intracranial hematomas?

In an attempt to formulate rational and cost effective guidelines for the performance of skull X-ray examinations, Bell and Loop[1] reviewed 1,500 emergency room skull X-ray examinations performed following head injury. Ninety-three factors were identified. There were 21 factors that were associated with a high risk of fracture (Table 5.1). If the presence of at least one of these findings was made a condition for obtaining skull radiographs, 434 patients would not have had studies performed. In only one of these 434 patients would a skull fracture have been missed. The emergency room physician's evaluation of the severity of the patient's injury was the best predictor of the likelihood of finding a skull fracture. If the physician's "overall impression" was that the patient's injury was "trivial," a skull fracture was never found. If the head injury was judged to be mild, only 1 in 40 patients was discovered to have a fracture. It is of more than passing interest that two-thirds of all X-rays were performed on patients with injuries judged to be mild or trivial.

Phillips[31] formulated additional criteria for performing radiographic examination in head injured patients: unconsciousness, decreasing level of consciousness, hemotym-

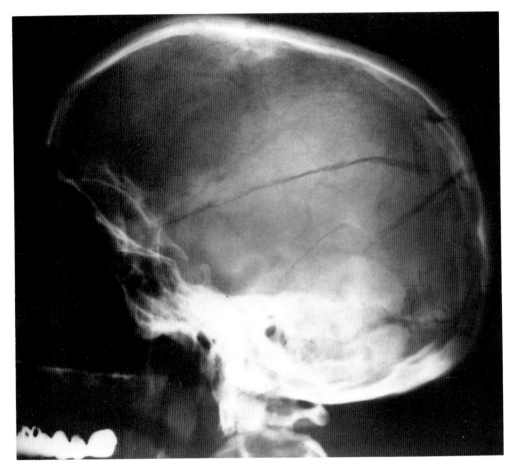

Figure 5.1.   Lateral X-ray of skull showing massively comminuted skull fractures in a patient with severe neural injury. Although there is no consistent correlation between simple linear skull fracture and neural injury, comminuted skull fractures like those seen in this illustration result from severe impact injury and are likely to be associated with neural injury.

Table 5.1
High Yield Findings for Skull Fracture[a]

Source	1 Fracture/No. of Examinations	Percent of Fractures Associated with Finding	p value
History			
>5 min of unconsciousness	1/8	41	<0.001
>5 min of retrograde amnesia	1/7	44	<0.001
Vomiting	1/8	20	<0.001
Nonvisual focal symptoms	1/9	16	<0.02
Accident at work or gunshot wound	1/5	15	<0.001
Physical examination:			
Palpable bony malignment	1/6	15	<0.001
Discharge from ear	1/3	30	<0.001
Discharge from nose	1/9	14	<0.05
Ear-drum discoloration	1/4	23	<0.001
Bilateral black eyes	1/7	8	<0.001
Neurologic examination:			
Stupor, semiconsciousness or coma	1/6	43	<0.001
Breathing irregular or apneic	1/4	16	<0.001
Babinski reflex present	1/5	24	<0.001
Other reflex abnormality	1/7	18	<0.001
Focal weakness	1/9	15	<0.01
Sensory abnormality	1/9	10	<0.08
Anisocoria	1/7	19	<0.001
Other cranial-nerve abnormality	1/5	21	<0.001
Physical evaluation:			
Injury considered "severe"	1/2.5	35	<0.001
Odds for fracture "50:50", or "9:1 certain"	1/3	67	<0.001
Examination because "fracture seriously suspected"	1/7	76	<0.001

[a] Twenty-one findings associated with high yield of skull fractures (From Bell, R.S., and Loop, J.W.: The Utility and Futility of Radiographic Skull Examination for Trauma. N. Engl. J. Med., 284:236–239, 1971. Reprinted with permission.)

panum or fluid discharge from the ear, cerebrospinal fluid rhinorrhea, Battle's sign, bilateral orbital ecchymosis, and palpable skull depression. Strict adherence to these criteria before performing skull X-rays would have eliminated 88% of 1,472 radiographic examinations of the skull in the nine-month period surveyed. These high-yield criteria were not infallible and 29% of fractures would have been missed had the criteria been used. However, retrospective chart review revealed that failure to detect these fractures would have had little effect on the management of these patients.

Harwood-Nash et al.[14] reviewed the records of 4,465 children with head injuries and identified skull fractures in over 27%. The presence or absence of a skull fracture was not a reliable predictor of an intracranial hematoma. An identical proportion of patients[15] with and without skull fracture were found to have epidural hematomas. Twice the percentage of patients *without* skull fractures had subdural hematomas when compared to patients with a fracture. Although the incidence of "brain damage" was four times greater in those with skull fracture than those without fracture (8 *vs.* 2%), it is hardly likely that the physicians caring for these patients needed skull films to tell them which patients had sustained a neurological injury. Eyes and Evans[8] also concluded that post-traumatic skull radiographs were not helpful in the management of the head injured. They could find no correlation between radiographic findings and the need for hospitalization and little correlation between radiographic findings and presenting signs and symptoms.

The predominant current opinion[1, 8, 14, 31] has been challenged by Jennett[22] who feels that the presence of a skull fracture is reason for admission even though the patient may be intact at the time of examination in the emergency room. In support of this argument, he states, "that when dangerous complications develop after initially mild injuries there is usually a skull fracture." In a review of the medico-legal aspects of acute head injury, Jennett[22] notes that most lawsuits arising out of head trauma in Great Britain involved patients who deteriorated after mild injury. The failure to take, correctly interpret, or convey the skull X-ray report was a feature in 63% of the cases involving hospitalized patients and "In every one of the patients sent home from hospitals there was some irregularity about the skull X-ray picture." Galbraith and Smith[11] from Jennett's group, reviewed 307 post-traumatic intracranial hematomas and found that only 57 (19%) did *not* have a skull fracture. Forty-three of these 57 patients without skull fracture had signs or symptoms immediately after injury. The more important question, of course, is how many patients were initially neurologically intact and were admitted to hospitals *solely* because of the finding of a skull fracture and then went on to deteriorate? This question has not been answered. On the other hand, when the traumatic etiology of the depressed level of consciousness is not clear, skull films may be useful. Galbraith[10] examined the records of 33 patients with intracranial hematomas who were initially misdiagnosed as having suffered cerebrovascular accidents. Twenty-nine of these 33 incorrectly diagnosed patients had skull fractures.

The clinician can arrive at a rational *modus operandi* in spite of the conflicting data regarding the usefulness of skull roentgenography following head trauma. An algorithm we have found useful in determining when skull X-rays should be performed and their relationship to other neurodiagnostic studies is seen in Figure 2.4. For the patient with a head injury with a depressed level of consciousness or focal neurological abnormality, the problem is relatively easy and plain films have little place in the initial management. Because the skull fracture (if any) is less important than the extent of the brain injury and the presence of intracranial mass lesions, a CT scan is the initial procedure of choice.

For the less severely injured patient, the search for a skull fracture is indicated only if the clinician finds evidence on physical examination suggestive of a depressed fracture or if a basal skull fracture is suspected. In both these situations the skull film findings may provide information that will directly influence patient management.

It has been our practice not to obtain skull films in *neurologically intact patients* unless a cerebrospinal fluid fistula or depressed fracture is suspected. This is admittedly a controversial subject and in other centers roentgenographic examinations are performed in such patients if they give a history of loss of consciousness. If a fracture is found, the patient is admitted and observed for 24 hours for the development of an intracranial hematoma. This policy will lead to the admission of large numbers of patients with relatively mild head trauma. There is no data regarding the frequency of neurological deterioration under observation or of the relationship of the costs to possible benefits. We would agree with the statement that "linear, nondepressed, closed skull fractures rarely require specific treatment and further, that knowledge of the presence of such a fracture rarely alters or influences management of the patient."[13]

DEPRESSED SKULL FRACTURE

A depressed skull fracture occurs when a small object with a relatively large amount of kinetic energy makes contact with the skull. The dissipation of this energy over a small area results in a depression of the bone at the point of contact. Thus, depressed skull fractures are most likely to occur when the head is struck with objects such as a pool cue, baseball bat, golf ball, or the edge of a brick.

It is generally accepted that clinically

Figure 5.2 CT scan shows left-sided depressed skull fracture (arrow) and subjacent intraparenchymal hematoma.

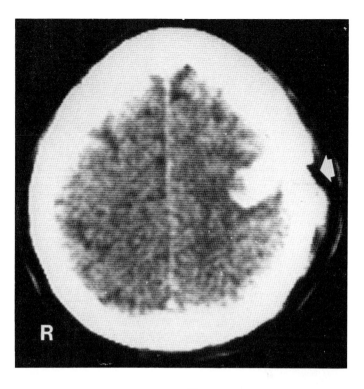

significant skull fractures include those injuries where a bone fragment is depressed below the inner table to a depth greater than the thickness of the skull.

Braakman[3] estimated the incidence of depressed skull fracture to be 20/1,000,000/year. Eighty-five percent of patients are males. Most are below the age of 30. The associated mortality rate is low (11%) and related for the most part to the severity of the central nervous system injury rather than to the depression itself, although infectious complications of the fracture may occasionally result in mortality. Eleven percent of patients are left with persistent neurological deficits. Between 5 and 7% have a co-existing intracranial hematoma (Fig. 5.2) and 12% have involvement of an underlying venous sinus.[13]

Diagnosis

The complications and sequelae of depressed fracture are minimized by early diagnosis and appropriate treatment. Often, however, there is no concomitant neurological injury so skull films are not taken and a depressed fracture is initially missed. Jen-

nett and Miller[23] analyzed the records of 28 patients who presented to hospital emergency rooms soon after injury but in whom the presence of a depressed skull fracture was not initially recognized. In 19 of these 28, skull X-rays were not taken at the time of presentation or the fracture was missed. They emphasize that because the scalp is so mobile, the area of depression may not underlie the laceration and visual exploration of the skull through the scalp laceration may fail to reveal a fracture. Moreover, the inner table may separate from the outer and the depth of depression may not be appreciated on inspection. To accurately identify depressed fractures X-rays must be taken in both the AP and lateral planes (Fig. 5.3). X-ray views tangential to the location of the fracture are useful if a fracture is suspected but not visualized on standard projections. Depressed skull fractures are classified as closed (simple) when there is no laceration of the scalp overlying the area of injury. Fractures present beneath or adjacent to a scalp laceration are considered to be compound or open. Braakman[2] reported that 85% of the depressed frac-

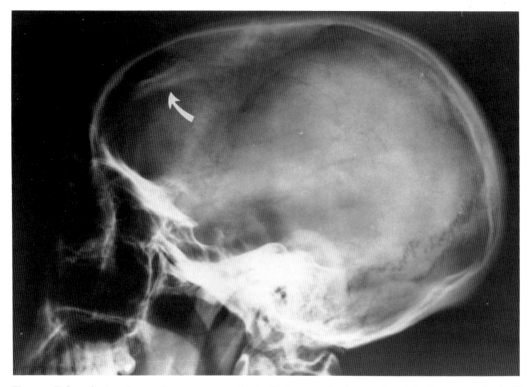

Figure 5.3. Lateral roentgenogram of skull demonstrates a frontal depressed skull fracture (*arrow*). There is an increase in radiodensity of the fragments because of their rotation in relationship to the X-ray beam.

tures in his series were of the compound variety. Similar figures confirming the preponderance of compound injuries have been presented by others.[19, 29]

Treatment

When the scalp overlying a fracture is intact and infection is unlikely, it has been generally accepted practice to elevate depressed fragments on an elective basis to reduce the incidence of post-traumatic seizures. In spite of the advocacy of elevation of *closed* depressed fractures there is no data that shows that elevation reduces the incidence of late epilepsy. Indeed, Jennett *et al.*[24] have presented data showing that there is no difference in the incidence of late epilepsy when patients with closed depressed fractures treated with elevation are compared to those receiving no operative therapy. They state that "how the fracture is treated has no obvious effect on the incidence of epilepsy and it seems likely that the frequency of traumatic epilepsy could

be reduced by improved or different management of the depressed fracture." Braakman[3] has taken a progressively more conservative approach to closed fractures. If the patient is conscious and without neurological deficit, closed depressed fractures are not elevated. Elevation of closed fractures has also been proposed as a means of ameliorating neurological deficit. This seems unlikely unless the depressed fragment is exceedingly large and is acting to compress a large area of the cerebral hemisphere. Glaser and Shafer[12] state that "the force of the blow struck, and not the existence of a simple rounded depressed area of bone, is responsible for the underlying brain damage." On our service we consider it appropriate not to elevate closed depressed fractures unless the fracture creates an unacceptable cosmetic deformity.

Compound depressed skull fractures are a different situation. Because of the danger of infection, these fractures should be explored and elevated at the time of presen-

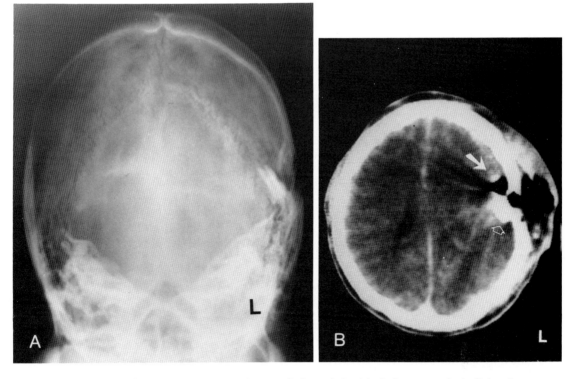

Figure 5.4. *A,* AP roentgenogram shows obvious left-sided depressed skull fracture. There was a large laceration overlying the fracture. The scalp wound was closed and when skull films revealed a depressed fracture the patient refused further treatment. *B,* the patient presented two days later with headache, fever, and a fluctuant scalp mass. CT scan shows a large scalp mass. *Open arrow* delineates depressed fracture. *Closed arrow* shows a small intracerebral hematoma and intracerebral gas collection. At operation Clostridia were cultured from a scalp abscess. A brain abscess was found which also grew Clostridia.

tation to minimize the risk of central nervous system infection (Fig. 5.4). A CT scan is performed preoperatively to identify intracranial hematomas that may need evacuation (Fig. 5.2).

The operation is carried out under local or general anesthesia. After the scalp is widely shaved and prepared, ragged or devitalized skin edges are debrided. Adequate exposure of the depression may be achieved by spreading the debrided laceration with a self-retaining retractor. If this is not possible, the laceration is extended at either end to form an S-shaped incision. If the laceration and fracture are located over the forehead, enlarging the incision in this fashion may result in an unsightly scar. In this situation, it may be necessary to fashion a coronal incision behind the hairline to gain exposure of the fracture. The depressed fracture may be elevated by wedging an instrument below one of the fragments. If this is not possible, a burr hole is placed adjacent to the fracture and bone is rongeured from the burr hole to the depressed fragments. When this is done the fragments may then be grasped with an instrument and removed. The dura is visualized and if a tear is present it is repaired. A dural graft is usually not necessary, but if the dural edges cannot be approximated a piece of pericranium will achieve a watertight closure.

The fragments of bone are soaked in an antibiotic solution and cleansed of hair, devitalized tissue, and foreign bodies. The fragments are replaced unless the operation is carried out greater than 24 hours following injury, the wound is grossly contaminated, or a watertight dural closure cannot be obtained. Replacement of bone fragments precludes the need for a second operation to perform a cranioplasty. Our own experience has convinced us that replacing bone fragments does not result in an increased incidence of infection. Jennett and Miller[23] and Braakman[3] noted no significant difference in the rate of infection when patients in whom the bone was removed were compared with those in whom it was replaced.

Although antibiotics are frequently used prophylactically in the management of compound depressed fractures, there is no evidence to show that their administration reduces the rate of infection. We use antibiotics only for established infections.

Open depressed fractures overlying the transverse or sagittal sinus present the surgeon with a therapeutic dilemma. It is desirable to remove bone fragments and repair the dura for reasons that have previously been given. However, if the sinus has been lacerated by a fragment of indriven bone, removal may be associated with massive hemorrhage that is difficult to control. While the relationship of a depressed fracture to the midline sagittal sinus may be fairly confidently established by examination of the patient and by roentgenographic studies, the position of the transverse sinus is less constant. Cerebral angiography with particular attention to the late venous phase will reveal the relationship of the fracture to the transverse sinus. When it is established that the fracture overlies a venous sinus, the scalp over the fracture is debrided, but the depressed fragments should be left in place. The patients are observed in hospital for five to seven days for the development of a wound infection or meningitis. They are also followed with CT scans at two-week intervals for the first six weeks following injury in order to identify formation of a brain abscess. For the remainder of the first year following injury, an additional one or two CT scans will suffice. Although the risk of abscess formation from retained intracerebral bone

fragments probably persists for the life of the patient, experience with retained fragments following gunshot wounds indicates that this risk is greatest in the first months after the injury.

If infection should occur, cerebral angiography will demonstrate whether or not the sinus is patent. The operative strategy consists of wide bone exposure so that sinus bleeding may be controlled, removal of indriven bone fragments, and evacuation of the abscess. Generally, late exploration in the region of the sinus is associated with less risk of sinus hemorrhage than in the acute situation as thrombus is organized and the tear in the sinus wall may have been sealed as a result of the deposition of fibrous tissue.

Epilepsy

The impact that causes a depressed skull fracture may result in brain injury and epilepsy. The incidence of late epilepsy after depressed fracture has been reported as 7.1 and 9.5% in two large series.[2, 24] The incidence is influenced by the duration of post-traumatic amnesia which is, in turn, a reflection of the severity of the central nervous system injury. When the duration of post-traumatic amnesia is less than 24 hours, the incidence of late epilepsy is 5.4%. With an amnestic interval of greater than 24 hours, the incidence rises to almost 22%.[2] In a study of epilepsy after non-missile head injuries[21] it was found that when depressed skull fracture was present, the factors resulting in a significant increase in the risk of late epilepsy included the presence of a focal deficit, dural tear, early epilepsy, and post-traumatic amnesia greater than 24 hours. These factors interact with each other and the presence of several factors in the same patient increases the risk considerably. For example, the presence of a dural tear is associated with an incidence of epilepsy of 22%. However, when post-traumatic amnesia greater than 24 hours *and* early epilepsy are also present, the risk is over 60%. The influence of combined factors on the development of epilepsy is seen in Table 5.2. Anti-convulsant prophylaxis should be given when the risk of late epilepsy is greater than 20%. This is an arbi-

Table 5.2

The Influence of Combined Factors on the Development of Epilepsy after Depressed Skull Fracture[a]

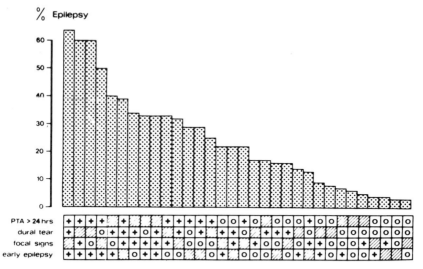

[a] From Jennett, B.: Epilepsy after non-missile head injuries. London: A William Heinemann Medical Books, 1975. Reprinted with permission.

trary figure and may be adjusted in either direction depending on the patient's occupation and social circumstances.

BASAL SKULL FRACTURE AND TRAUMATIC CEREBROSPINAL FLUID FISTULA

The five bones forming the base of the skull (cribriform plate of the ethmoid bone, orbital plate of the frontal bone, the sphenoid bone, the petrous and squamous portion of the temporal bone, and the occipital bone) are frequently fractured following head injury. Lewin and Cairns[26] noted an incidence of basal skull fracture of 7.2% in 1,000 consecutive patients with non-missile head injury. Brawley and Kelly[4] noted an incidence of 24% in 1,250 head injuries. Einhorn and Mizrahi[7] in a study of over 1,300 pediatric head injuries of all degrees and severity reported an incidence of basal fracture of 3.5%. Because the base of the skull cannot be visualized on clinical examination, and is examined radiographically only with a great deal of difficulty, many basal fractures remain undiagnosed and the reported incidence will depend on the care with which a search is made for clinical and roentgenographic signs of fracture. Although the presence of a linear skull fracture involving the cranial vault is very often of no clinical significance, the same is not true of fractures of the base. Basal fractures are of special significance because the dura may be torn adjacent to the fracture site, placing the CNS in contact with the contaminated or potentially contaminated paranasal sinuses. If the dura is torn, the possibility exists that a cerebrospinal fluid fistula may occur. Whether or not there is a cerebrospinal fluid fistula, the dural tear and basal skull fracture will predispose the patient to meningitis.

The clinical signs leading the physician to suspect a fracture of the petrous portion of the temporal bone include: hemotympanum or tympanic membrane perforation with blood within the external auditory canal, hearing loss, evidence of vestibular dysfunction, facial nerve palsy of a peripheral type, ecchymosis of the scalp overlying the mastoid bone (Battle's sign), or cerebrospinal fluid otorrhea. Anosmia, bilateral periorbital ecchymosis, and cerebrospinal

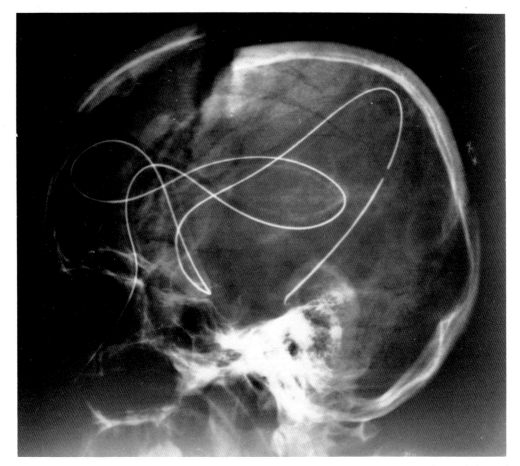

Figure 5.5. Lateral roentgenogram showing massive skull fracture of cranial vault. Basal fractures were not recognized and a nasogastric tube was introduced into the intracranial compartment with fatal consequences.

fluid rhinorrhea are manifestations of a basal fracture involving the sphenoid, frontal or ethmoid bones.

Basal Skull Fracture Without Cerebrospinal Fluid Fistula

If a basal skull fracture is suspected on clinical grounds, plain skull films may be useful. A nasogastric tube must not be used when a fracture of the floor of the frontal fossa is suspected or demonstrated radiographically. Intracranial passage of the nasogastric tube with disastrous outcome has been reported in this situation[9, 34] (Fig. 5.5). If there is extensive comminution, or spicules of bone penetrate upward into the brain, the fracture may be easily recognized on plain film studies. However, linear frac-

tures involving the floor of the frontal fossa or petrous bone are difficult to detect and are often not seen. If there is no cerebrospinal fluid fistula and a fracture is not seen on plain films in spite of clinical signs suggesting a fracture, additional radiographic or other diagnostic studies are not indicated.

The medical and surgical management of patients with basal skull fractures without cerebrospinal fluid fistula remains controversial. Antibiotic prophylaxis for five days has been proposed by Brawley and Kelly[4] to suppress organisms in the paranasal sinuses and nasopharynx until there is healing of the dural tear and the nervous system is sealed from the external environment. However, Einhorn and Mizrahi[7] emphasized that infection never occurred in their series of 46 children with basal skull fractures regardless of whether antibiotics were given or withheld. In a prospective analysis of 129 patients with basal skull fracture, Ignelzi and VanderArk[18] concluded that antibiotics did nothing to prevent infection and may have been harmful. Not a single patient treated without antibiotics became infected, whereas two of 54 patients to whom antibiotic prophylaxis was given developed meningitis. Hoff et al.[16] also prospectively studied 160 patients with basal skull fracture without cerebrospinal fluid leak. Patients were treated with no therapy, low dose penicillin (1.2 million units daily for three days), or high dose penicillin (20 million units daily for three days). No patient in any of the treatment groups developed signs or symptoms of central nervous system infection. The authors concluded that antibiotics were not necessary for the treatment of basal fractures without cerebrospinal fluid leaks.

On our service all patients with clinical or radiographic evidence of basal skull fracture are admitted for three to five days to be observed for the development of a cerebrospinal fluid fistula or evidence of central nervous system infection. If the period of hospital observation passes without complications, they are followed as outpatients.

We have not administered prophylactic antibiotics to patients with basal skull fractures. The literature would indicate that the incidence of infection is low and that antibiotics will not prevent infection. Moreover, antibiotics such as ampicillin or cephalothin, which are effective for the most part against gram-positive organisms will cause a change of the normal nasopharyngeal flora and result in colonization with predominantly gram-negative organisms.[18]

Basal Skull Fracture with Cerebrospinal Fluid Rhinorrhea

Cerebrospinal fluid fistulas occur in 2–3% of all patients with head injury and in over 11% of patients with basal skull fractures.[2, 27] MacGee et al.[28] estimated that there were 150,000 cases of traumatic rhinorrhea yearly in the United States.

The diagnosis of cerebrospinal fluid rhinorrhea following trauma is generally not difficult to make. The nasal discharge is watery and non-mucoid and contains glucose. When cerebrospinal fluid drainage from the nose is mixed with blood, the diagnosis may be overlooked but blood will generally disappear from the nasal discharge within two to three days of trauma. Moreover, if there is a significant amount of blood mixed with the nasal discharge, a false positive test for glucose may be obtained. If there is no blood mixed with the nasal discharge, the presence of glucose may be ascertained using a commercially available paper tape which reacts with glucose.

Generally, patients with cerebrospinal fluid rhinorrhea have sustained a dural tear and fracture of the ethmoid or sphenoid bone or orbital plate of the frontal bone. Very occasionally, with a fracture of the petrous portion of the temporal bone, cerebrospinal fluid may gain entrance to the eustachian tube and, if the tympanic membrane is intact, cerebrospinal fluid will drain from the nose.[15] This phenomenon, otorhinorrhea, is unusual but should be kept in mind when difficulty is encountered in localizing the site of the rhinorrhea.

The clinical examination may be useful in localizing the site of the fracture causing the rhinorrhea. When the rhinorrhea is unilateral, the side of the leak will accurately predict the side of the dural tear and fracture over 95% of the time.[27] However, with bilateral rhinorrhea, only one-half of patients will have bilateral tears. Anosmia is difficult to evaluate in patients with nasal and facial trauma but has been reported to occur in almost 80% of patients with rhinorrhea and, when present, is suggestive of a fracture in the region of the ethmoid bone. In the absence of anosmia, it is highly unlikely that the dural tear overlies the ethmoid bone and the fistula most likely involves the sphenoid bone or orbital plate of the frontal bone.

Plain skull films should be taken on admission and may reveal fractures of the base. In addition the presence of fluid or air-fluid levels within the paranasal sinuses will give important clues to the site of the fracture. Prophylactic antibiotics are not used in patients with cerebrospinal fluid fistulas who do not have meningitis. The reasons are identical to those discussed in the section on basal fracture without cerebrospinal fluid leaks.

There is no agreement regarding the operative management of the leak. Lewin[27] believed that all patients who develop a cerebrospinal fluid fistula (even one of brief duration) should have a craniotomy and dural repair. He felt that the body's repair of the dural tear leading to a cerebrospinal fluid fistula was always imperfect. Of 26 patients with transient cerebrospinal fluid rhinorrhea in whom operation was not performed, six who were followed from three to nine years developed meningitis. In a subsequent report,[20] Jefferson and Reilly postulated that dural healing is permanently prevented by the interposition of damaged brain between the torn dural edges. Although the leak will stop in most cases, the opening to the external environment persists and the patient remains at risk of meningitis for the rest of his life. Jefferson and Reilly[20] believe that operation may even be indicated in basal fractures without cerebrospinal fluid fistula and that "dangerous fractures exist in the absence of cerebrospinal fluid rhinorrhea." They suspect a basal fracture in every patient with a vault fracture below the hairline or with a comminuted anterior temporal fracture. These patients have tomography of the frontal and middle fossa. When the tomograms and/or plain films show that there has been a major injury to the floor of the frontal fossa, craniotomy and dural repair are performed. Using these criteria as a basis for operation, the authors report a high rate of negative exploration (14 of 87 patients). Although there were no cases of late meningitis in the patients who underwent repair, there was no control group available for comparison.

A more conservative approach to cerebrospinal fluid rhinorrhea than the one advocated by Jefferson and Reilly[20] and Lewin[27] has been proposed by others. Leech and Paterson[25] performed operative repair only if a fistula persisted for more than seven days. Mincy[30] advocated a similar approach and noted that in 85% of his patients the fistulous drainage ceased spontaneously within one week and the incidence of infection during this time was low (11%). Brawley and Kelly[4] reported that in all 35 patients with traumatic cerebrospinal fluid fistulas, the leak ceased within two weeks.

In general, our own policy has been to defer operation in patients with cerebrospinal fluid rhinorrhea. However, operation is performed without delay when there is radiographic evidence of elevation of a spicule of bone penetrating the brain or there is a large defect in the floor of the frontal fossa with herniation of brain into one of the paranasal sinuses (Fig. 5.6). In both these situations, the risk of infection is great and the leak should be treated by early operation. Operation is also performed in any patient who develops meningitis, although repair is delayed until after the meningitis is treated with appropriate antibiotic therapy.

All other patients are placed at bed rest in a position that minimizes the leak or causes it to cease. There is no single position that will work for all leaks and the best position will usually have to be determined empirically. If the fistulous drainage has not stopped within 72 hours, the patient is placed on spinal drainage. About 150 ml of cerebrospinal fluid is removed each day for a two to three day period after which the catheter is removed. While there is some theoretical objection that removal of large volumes of cerebrospinal fluid will decrease the flow through the fistula and cause bacteria to pass through the fistulous tract into the central nervous system, there is no evidence that this occurs.

If the fistula persists seven days after injury, non-operative treatment is abandoned. Polytomography is performed to locate the site of the basal fracture and fistula. Although we do not perform polytomographic examination until a decision has been made that operative therapy is indicated, Brawley and Kelly[4] advocate polytomography in all patients admitted with an acute cerebrospinal fluid leak, anosmia, nasal bleeding, or plain film findings, suggesting that a fracture extends into the

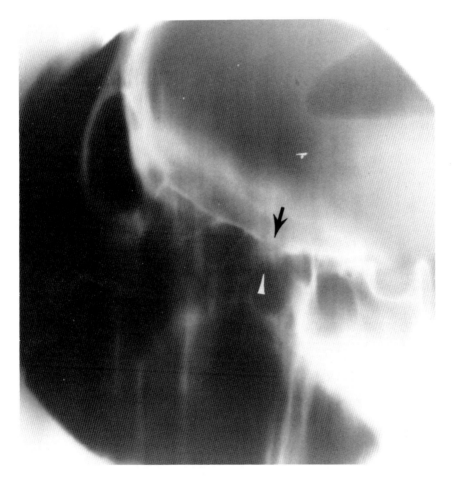

Figure 5.6. Lateral tomogram of skull showing defect in the ethmoid bone (*black arrows*) and soft tissue density (brain) within the ethmoid sinus (*white arrowhead*).

paranasal sinuses. They believe that this policy enables them to identify complex fractures with large frontal floor defects and brain hernias that are likely to seal imperfectly and expose the patient to the risk of meningitis in the future. Tomographic cuts of the floor of the anterior fossa are performed at 3-mm intervals in both AP and lateral projections. AP cuts should extend posteriorly to include the sella turcica.

Occasionally plain films and tomography of the anterior fossa cannot localize the site of the basal fracture. Ray and Bergland[33] reported that they were unable to localize the site of the basal fracture in over 20% of their cases using plain films and tomography of the anterior fossa. This figure is undoubtedly lower now that hypocycloidal polytomography is available. When the site of the leak cannot be determined radiographically, it has been proposed that radio-iodinated serum albumin or dyes such as fluoroscein or indigocarmine be introduced into the spinal subarachnoid space to locate the site of the fistula. Pledgets are then placed in the anterior and posterior roof of the nose, sphenoethmoidal recess, and middle meatus. The radioactivity or dye content of the pledgets may be measured to determine if there is a cerebrospinal fluid fistula. If the anterior nasal roof is stained or radioactive, the cribriform plate or anterior ethmoid bone may be the site of the leak. Similarly, evidence of dye or radioactive cerebrospinal fluid in the posterior nasal roof and spheno-ethmoidal recess implies that the posterior sphenoid or ethmoid bone is involved. Staining of the posterior pharyngeal wall means that cerebrospinal fluid is entering *via* the eustachian tube.[5] Although these isotope dye tests may be helpful in establishing the *presence* of a leak, they have not been useful, in our experience, to determine the location of the leak and we do not use them for that purpose.

Most recently we have begun to use the CT scan to locate the site of cerebrospinal fluid fistulas. After metrizamide is introduced into the lumbar subarachnoid space, the patient is scanned in the coronal plane. Contrast material will be seen in the paranasal sinuses adjacent to the fistulous tract.

We now believe that this is the diagnostic procedure of choice for the localization of cerebrospinal fluid leaks.

When the site of the cerebrospinal fluid fistula has been identified by preoperative studies, is unilateral, and involves the floor of the frontal fossa, a frontal bone flap is fashioned on the side of the leak. Mannitol is administered as the scalp incision is made and provides relaxation of the brain insuring that minimal retraction will be necessary for exposure of the frontal fossa. After the dura is opened, intradural exploration of the floor of the frontal fossa is performed. An extradural search for the site of the fistula is avoided as this technique may create factitious dural tears indistinguishable from those created at the time of the initial trauma. Once the tear is located, intradural repair may be difficult—particularly when the laceration is located medially and posteriorly in the frontal fossa. If this is the case, the dura is dissected off the floor of the frontal fossa and is repaired from an extradural exposure. If primary repair is not possible, a graft of pericranium or fascia lata is used. If necessary, the bony defect is repaired with a piece of wire mesh.

When there are bilateral fractures or the site of the fracture cannot be determined by diagnostic studies, a coronal scalp flap and bifrontal bone flap are fashioned. The most anterior portion of the sagittal sinus is doubly ligated and cut. The falx is cut as well. Bilateral exploration and repair are carried out as described above. If the dural tear cannot be located after intradural exploration, a piece of fascia lata or pericranium is placed intradurally to cover the floor of the entire anterior fossa. Post-operatively, all patients are placed on spinal drainage for 48–72 hours to further reduce the chances of recurrent fistulae. In 25% of patients, the leak may persist although reoperation will eventually seal 90% of the fistulae.[33] A fracture involving the sphenoid sinus occurs in about 15% of patients with rhinorrhea although in only one-half of these is the sphenoid fracture the sole site of dural tearing.[26] When studies indicates that the fracture is through the floor of the sella turcica or roof of the sphenoid sinus, a transsphenoidal approach is indicated and the dural tear is sealed with a muscle stamp and tissue adhesive. The sphenoid sinus is packed with fat. Although an intracranial approach to sella leaks has been described by Lewin and Cairns[26] and Ray and Bergland,[33] the transsphenoidal approach is safer and quite satisfactory for closure of the fistula.

Cerebrospinal Fluid Otorrhea and Fractures of the Petrous Bone

Drainage of cerebrospinal fluid from the ear occurs when three conditions are met: the petrous bone is fractured, the dura and arachnoid over the petrous bone are torn, and the tympanic membrane is perforated.

Fractures of the petrous bone are classified according to the relationship of the fracture to the long axis of the petrous pyramid[15] (see also Chapter 7). Longitudinal fractures occur following blows to the temporal or parietal skull. The fracture extends in an anterior-posterior direction starting in the temporal squama. The external auditory meatus and tympanic membrane are torn, and the middle ear ossicles are disrupted. Patients will present with conductive hearing loss, otorrhea, and bleeding from the external ear. In transverse fractures, the fracture originates in the occipital bone and is at right angles to the longitudinal axis of the petrous bone. The tympanic membrane generally remains intact, there is no bleeding from the external auditory canal, and sensorineural hearing loss occurs from damage to the labyrinth, cochlea, or the eighth cranial nerve within the auditory canal. Facial paresis is often present as well.

The diagnosis of cerebrospinal fluid otorrhea may be difficult as the initial discharge from the ear is usually bloody and the presence of cerebrospinal fluid may be difficult to ascertain. Probing, irrigating, or packing the external auditory canal adds nothing to the care of the patient and increases the risk of central nervous system infection. A non-tamponading sterile plastic bag may be placed over the ear to minimize the introduction of bacteria into the external auditory canal. The patient is placed in a position that minimizes the volume of fistulous drainage. In the overwhelming majority of patients, otorrhea ceases spontaneously. Raaf[32] reported only one persistent fistula in a series of 79 cases.

The incidence of meningitis in 156 patients with otorrhea compiled from the literature by MacGee et al.[28] was 4%, whereas the incidence in those with rhinorrhea was 17%. Leech and Paterson,[25] however, reported a higher incidence of meningitis with otorrhea than with rhinorrhea. Our own experience has been more consistent with the 4% figure of MacGee. Leech and Paterson[25] found that antibiotic prophylaxis resulted in a statistically significant decrease in the incidence of meningitis in their patients from 42 to 5%. It is not clear why the literature is so contradictory on this point. We do not treat patients prophylactically with antibiotics and we have noted a minimal incidence of meningitis.

In the unusual circumstance that cerebrospinal fluid ororrhea does not cease spontaneously within one week of the patient's injury, the fracture of the petrous bone may be localized with a Stenvers or Towne's view of the skull. More often, however, tomograms are necessary. Once the site of the fracture is localized, a bone flap is fashioned to expose the dura overlying the petrous bone in either the middle or posterior fossa. Exploration is begun intradurally and repair is carried out according to the principles outlined for anterior fossa dural tears.

Pneumocephalus

After a fracture of the base of the anterior fossa, plain films may show air within the subarachnoid space, or cerebral ventricles (Fig. 5.7). There are no statistics regarding the incidence of infection with pneumocephalus but the presence of air within the cerebral ventricles or subarachnoid space has the same implications as a cerebrospinal fluid fistula. Our policy is to repeat skull radiographs daily and if the amount of ventricular or subarachnoid air is increasing or has not begun to diminish in size within one week following injury, appropriate diagnostic studies are performed to localize the site of dural disruption and operative repair is

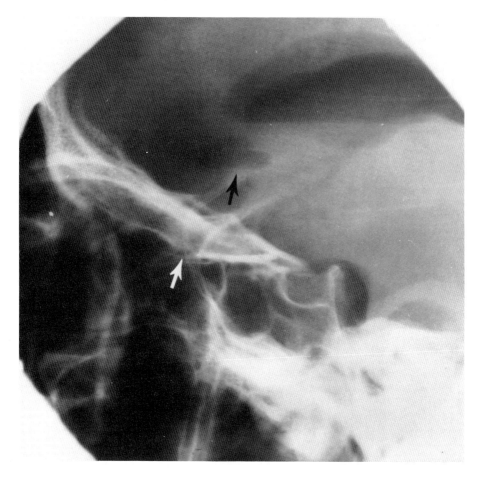

Figure 5.7.   Lateral roentgenogram of the skull in a patient with basal skull fracture (*white arrow*). Air is located within the cerebral parenchyma (*black arrow*), within the lateral ventricles and in the subarachnoid space anterior to the brain stem.

performed.

Air may also be seen within the substance of the brain. This generally occurs with larger defects of the frontal fossa when an increase in pressure in the paranasal sinuses forces air through the bony and dural defect into the brain. Operative therapy is the treatment of choice for this condition and conservative treatment is not justified. The floor of the frontal fossa and dura are repaired and the fistulous tract and air containing pocket of the frontal lobe are debrided.

SKULL FRACTURES INVOLVING THE FRONTAL SINUS

Correction of cosmetic deformity and prevention of central nervous system infec-

tion are the goals in the treatment of fractures of the frontal sinus. The majority of these fractures occur as a result of automobile trauma. Most patients will have external evidence of injury to the forehead and over one-half will have evidence of bony depression on the initial physical examination.[17] Almost one-half of all patients with fractures of the anterior wall of the sinus will have involvement of the posterior wall as well. Plain skull films will accurately delineate the fracture in about two-thirds of all patients (Fig. 5.8). If injury to the posterior wall is suspected but not confirmed, tomography should be obtained.

Closed, linear, non-displaced fractures of the frontal sinus need no operative therapy. However, the physician caring for these

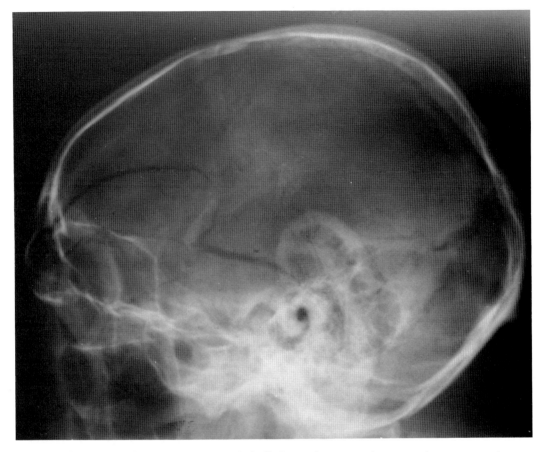

Figure 5.8.   Lateral roentgenogram of skull shows fracture of temporal squama and two frontal fractures with involvement of the posterior wall of the frontal sinus.

patients should be alert to the possibility of a cerebrospinal fluid fistula if the posterior wall of the sinus is fractured or if the fracture extends into the base of the frontal fossa.

In closed depressed fractures of the anterior wall of the frontal sinus with cosmetic deformity, a bicoronal scalp flap posterior to the hairline is fashioned. The fractured fragments are elevated and removed. To prevent the formation of a mucocele, the mucosa of the sinus is removed and the nasofrontal duct is plugged with a piece of muscle.[6] The anterior wall of the sinus is then reconstructed and the bone fragments wired in place as necessary. If the fracture is a compound one involving the anterior wall of the sinus, repair is generally not feasible without enlarging the overlying laceration of the forehead—a maneuver that

is not cosmetically acceptable. Therefore, the injury is approached through a scalp incision identical to that for closed fractures of the sinus. The frontal sinus fracture is treated in similar fashion to that employed for closed fractures.

Displaced fractures of the posterior wall are of particular significance because they may lacerate the dura and result in a cerebrospinal fluid leak via the frontal sinus. When there is X-ray evidence of a displaced fracture of the posterior wall of the frontal sinus, operative exploration and repair are indicated. The posterior wall of the frontal sinus is resected and the dura closed. The mucosa is exenterated and the sinus is plugged with muscle as previously described. The anterior wall of the sinus is replaced to minimize the cosmetic deformity.

References

1. Bell, R.S., Loop, J.W.: The utility and futility of radiographic skull examination for trauma. N. Engl. J. Med., 284:236–239, 1971.
2. Braakman, R.: Survey and follow-up of 225 consecutive patients with a depressed skull fracture. J. Neurol. Neurosurg. Psychiat., 34:106, 1971.
3. Braakman, R.: Depressed skull fracture: data, treatment, and follow-up in 225 consecutive cases. J. Neurol. Neurosurg. Psychiat., 35:395–402, 1972.
4. Brawley, B.W., Kelly, W.A.: Treatment of basal skull fractures with and without cerebrospinal fluid fistulae. J. Neurosurg., 26:57–61, 1967.
5. Calcaterra, T.C., Moseley, J.I., Rand, R.W.: Cerebrospinal rhinorrhea. Extracranial surgical repair. Western J. Med., 127:279–283, 1977.
6. Donald, P.J., Bernstein, L.: Compound frontal sinus injuries with intracranial penetration. Laryngoscope, 88:225–232, 1978.
7. Einhorn, A., Mizrahi, E.M.: Basilar skull fractures in children. The incidence of CNS infection and the use of antibiotics. Am. J. Dis. Child., 132:1121–1124, 1978.
8. Eyes, B., Evans, A.F.: Post-traumatic skull radiographs. Time for a reappraisal. Lancet, 2:85–86, 1978.
9. Fremstad, J.D., Martin, S.H.: Lethal complication from insertion of nasogastric tube after severe basilar skull fracture. J. Trauma, 18:820–824, 1978.
10. Galbraith, S.: Misdiagnosis and delayed diagnosis in traumatic intracranial haematoma. Br. Med. J., 1:1438–1439, 1976.
11. Galbraith, S., Smith, J.: Acute traumatic intracranial haematoma without skull fracture. Lancet, 1:501–503, 1976.
12. Glaser, M.A., Shafer, F.P.: Depressed fractures of the skull. Their surgery, sequelae and disability. J. Neurosurg., 2:140–153, 1945.
13. Harris, J.H. Jr.: High yield criteria and skull radiography. J. Am. Coll. Emerg. Physcians, 8:438–440, 1979.
14. Harwood-Nash, D.C., Hendrick, E.B., Hudson, A.R.: The significance of skull fractures in children. A study of 1,187 patients. Radiology, 101:151–155, 1971.
15. Henry, R.C., Taylor, P.H.: Cerebrospinal fluid otorrhea and otorhinorrhea following closed head injury. J. Laryngol. Otol., 92:743–756, 1978.
16. Hoff, J.T., Brewin, A., U, H.S.: Antibiotics for basilar skull fracture. J. Neurosurg., 44:649, 1976.
17. Hybels, R.L., Weimert, T.A.: Evaluation of frontal sinus fractures. Arch. Otolaryngol., 105:275–276, 1979.
18. Ingelzi, R.J., VanderArk, G.D.: Analysis of the treatment of basilar skull fractures with and without antibiotics. J. Neurosurg., 43:721–726, 1975.
19. Jamieson, K.G., Yelland, J.D.N.: Depressed skull fractures in Australia. J. Neurosurg., 37:150–155, 1972.
20. Jefferson, A., Reilly, G.: Fractures of the floor of the anterior cranial fossa. The selection of patients for dural repair. Br. J. Surg., 59:585–592, 1972.
21. Jennett, B.: Epilepsy After Non-Missile Head Injuries. London, A. William Heinemann Medical Books, 1975.
22. Jennett, B.: Some medicolegal aspects of the management of acute head injury. Br. Med. J., 1:1383–1385, 1976.
23. Jennett, B., Miller, J.D.: Infection after depressed fracture of skull. Implications for management of nonmissile injuries. J. Neurosurg., 36:333–339, 1972.
24. Jennett, B., Miller, J.D., Braakman, R.: Epilepsy after nonmissile depressed skull fracture. J. Neurosurg., 41:208–216, 1974.
25. Leech, P.J., Paterson, A.: Conservative and operative management for cerebrospinal-fluid leakage after closed head injury. Lancet, 1:1013–1016, 1973.
26. Lewin, W., Cairns, H.: Fractures of the sphenoidal sinus with cerebrospinal rhinorrhoea. Br. Med. J., 1:1–6, 1951.
27. Lewin, W.: Cerebrospinal fluid rhinorrhoea in closed head injuries. Br. J. Surg., 42:1–18, 1954.
28. MacGee, E.E., Cauthen, J.C., Brackett, C.E.: Meningitis following acute traumatic cerebrospinal fluid fistula. J. Neurosurg., 33:312–316, 1970.
29. Miller, J.D., Jennett, W.B.: Complications of depressed skull fracture. Lancet, 2:991–995, 1968.
30. Mincy, J.E.: Posttraumatic cerebrospinal fluid fistula of the frontal fossa. J. Trauma, 6:618–622, 1966.
31. Phillips, L.A.: Emergency services utilization of skull radiography. Neurosurgery, 4:580–582, 1979.
32. Raaf, J.: Posttraumatic cerebrospinal fluid leaks. Arch. Surg., 95:648–651, 1967.
33. Ray, B.S., Bergland, R.M.: Cerebrospinal fluid fistula: clinical aspects, techniques of localization and methods of closure. J. Neurosurg., 30:399–405, 1969.
34. Wyler, A.R., Reynolds, A.F.: An intracranial complication of nasogastric intubation. Case Report. J. Neurosurg., 47:297–298, 1977.

6

Cerebral Concussion and Diffuse Brain Injuries

THOMAS A. GENNARELLI

INTRODUCTION

Trauma to the brain can be classified into focal and diffuse injuries. *Focal brain injuries* are those in which a lesion large enough to be visualized with the naked eye has occurred and include cortical contusions, subdural hematoma, epidural hematoma, and intracerebral hematoma. These lesions cause neurological problems not only because of the local brain damage but, by causing masses within the cranium, they lead to brain shift, herniation and ultimately brainstem compression. *Diffuse brain injuries*, on the other hand, are associated with more widespread or global disruption of neurological function and are not usually associated with macroscopically visible brain lesions. Diffuse brain injuries are the consequence of the shaking effect of the brain within the skull and are thus lesions which are caused by the inertial or acceleration effects of the mechanical input to the head. Both theoretical[12] and experimental[10] evidence point to rotational acceleration as the primary mechanism for the production of diffuse brain injuries.

Since diffuse brain injuries, for the most part, are not associated with visible macroscopic lesions, they have historically been lumped together to mean all injuries not associated with focal lesions. Recently, however, diagnostic information has been gained from computerized tomographic scanning as well as from neurophysiological studies, which enables us to better define several categories within this broad group of diffuse brain injuries. These injuries will be discussed in detail. Four categories of diffuse brain injury are now recognized:

1) Mild concussion: several specific concussion syndromes exist which involve temporary disturbance of neurological function without loss of consciousness.

2) Classical cerebral concussion: classical cerebral concussion is a temporary, reversible neurological deficiency caused by trauma which results in temporary loss of consciousness.

3) Diffuse injury: diffuse injury is a traumatic brain injury with prolonged loss of consciousness (more than 24 hours). There are often residual neurological, psychological, or personality deficits which result.

4) Diffuse white matter shearing injury (shearing injury): shearing injuries are an extreme form of diffuse brain injury with considerable anatomical disruption of white matter fibers throughout both hemispheres. This lesion has been long recognized by neuropathologists and only recently diagnosed clinically.[2, 4, 18]

Nomenclature Problems

Considerable debate continues to confuse the nomenclature of the more severe categories of diffuse brain injury. Thus, there is no uniform consensus about the name of injuries more severe than classical concussion. The terms proposed here are designed to be clinically useful and to fit into current concepts of the mechanisms of diffuse brain injuries. Those who dislike the term "diffuse injury" argue that no proof exists that the injury is, in fact, diffuse and until this is established, prefer the term "severe head injury—unspecified." This term seems unnecessarily ambiguous and cumbersome and does not offer advantages to the commonly used term "diffuse injury." However, it should be recognized that, although clinically similar in presentation, this group of injuries is quite probably heterogeneous in terms of its pathophysiology.

The alternative to giving names to these injuries was provided by Ommaya and Gennarelli[17] who proposed a grading system of traumatic unconsciousness. Their grades I, II, and III are lumped together under the term "mild concussion" here and grade IV is called "classical cerebral concussion." "Diffuse injury" and "shearing injury" correspond roughly to grades V and VI.

Since traumatic unconsciousness may exist for varying periods of time, 24 hours is used to distinguish classical cerebral concussion from the more severe injuries. This cut off is arbitrary and others might argue for another time frame (6 or 12 hours) but 24 hours is a convenient and more easily determined time point.

Finally, the distinction between diffuse injury and shearing injury is difficult and as yet imprecise, but is important conceptually. It should also be noted that until widespread consensus occurs, the name "diffuse brain injuries" is a generic term which encompasses all four injury types, whereas the term "diffuse injury" is the name for a specific type of injury.

Mechanisms of Consciousness

Since most diffuse brain injuries involve a disturbance of consciousness, a brief review of the mechanisms which subserve the conscious state is in order. Consciousness, though difficult to define, is that easily recognized state in which a person can meaningfully interact with his environment. The neuroanatomical substrate of the awake state is a complex interaction involving the cerebral cortex, subcortical structures including the hypothalamus and numerous brainstem centers. The disconnection of one of these functions from the other two results in an altered state of consciousness. In general terms, the awake state requires the neural activity of the ascending reticular activating system of the brainstem to be projected to the cerebral cortex of both cerebral hemispheres. This projection may be either direct or indirect via hypothalamic-diencephalic centers. Similarly, feedback from the cerebral cortex of both hemispheres onto both the diencephalon and the reticular activating system of the brainstem is necessary for the conscious state.

In the most general terms then, unconsciousness can be produced either by dysfunction of the diencephalon-brainstem or by dysfunction of both cerebral hemispheres. In severe head injury, consciousness may be lost by compression or by hemorrhaging into the brainstem as a result of focal supratentorial mass lesions. Diffuse cerebral injuries, on the other hand, cause widespread dysfunction of both cerebral hemispheres and thereby alter consciousness by disconnecting the diencephalon or brainstem activating centers from hemispheric activity. Extremely severe diffuse brain injuries, such as that seen in the shearing injury, can cause bilateral cerebral hemisphere dysfunction as well as direct anatomical damage within the brainstem itself.

THE SPECTRUM OF DIFFUSE BRAIN INJURY

Diffuse brain injuries form a continuum (Table 6.1) of progressively severe brain dysfunction that is caused by increasing amounts of acceleration damage to the brain. Since normal brain function is a delicately balanced electrochemical series of events occurring in billions of cells at any one moment, it is easy to understand how mechanical forces can alter brain function. At low levels of input, this function can be

Table 6.1
Diffuse Brain Injuries

	Mild Concussion	Cerebral Concussion	Diffuse Injury	Shearing Injury
Loss of consciousness	None	Immediate	Immediate	Immediate
Length of unconsciousness	None	<24 hr	>24 hr	Days-weeks
Decerebrate posturing	None	None	Occas	Present
Posttraumatic amnesia	Min	Min-hrs	Days	Weeks
Memory deficit	None	Min	Mild-mod	Severe
Motor deficits	None	None	Mild	Severe
Outcome at 1 month				
Good recovery	100%	95%	21%	0
Moderate deficit	0	2%	21%	0
Severe deficit	0	2%	29%	9%
Vegetative	0	0	21%	36%
Death	0	0	7%	55%

disrupted, at least temporarily, without causing any structural disruption of the tissue. Thus, *physiological dysfunction can occur in the absence of structural or anatomical disruption*. This concept is the basis for our understanding of the concussion syndromes which, by definition, are transient, reversible events. It is also easy to imagine that if more profound mechanical input is delivered to the brain, structures within the brain can become physically or anatomically disrupted. In this instance, permanent sequelae in those structures anatomically disrupted would occur. Therefore, as the magnitude of mechanical input increases, function is first interrupted; later when anatomical disruption occurs, structure as well as function are disrupted. *The degree of functional disruption, since it precedes anatomical disruption, is always greater than the degree of anatomical disruption.*

To illustrate this concept one can envision a set of ten axons each of which participates to an equal degree in a particular neurological function. Each of the ten axons is, for the purpose of illustration, stronger and more resistant to mechanical strain than the one that comes before it. If a very mild mechanical stress is applied to the ten axons, none will be disrupted, but the first axon (the most sensitive one) will have a temporary loss of function. The overall result may not be noticeable because the other nine axons are still functioning perfectly normally. A more severe mechanical stress may cause dysfunction of the first five axons and at this point a decrease in the overall neurological function would be apparent. However, since none of the axons is structurally damaged, function will soon return. A still larger mechanical input now causes physical disruption (tearing) of the first three axons and physiological dysfunction of the remaining seven axons. Now all ten axons have had an anatomical or physical disruption so that neurological function is totally abolished. However, seven of the axons will recover their function so that little if any neurological deficit will be identified. If an even more severe mechanical input is delivered, seven axons could be torn and the remaining three could be physiologically disturbed. Again, the neurological function is totally abolished but after recovery of the three axons, severe neurological deficit is likely to result.

Mild Cerebral Concussion Syndromes

The syndromes of mild cerebral concussion are included in the continuum of diffuse brain injuries because they represent the mildest form of injury in this spectrum. Mild concussion syndromes are those in which consciousness is preserved but there is some degree of noticeable temporary neurological dysfunction. These injuries are exceedingly common and because of their mild degree are not often brought to medical attention.

The mildest form of head injury is that resulting in confusion and disorientation unaccompanied by amnesia. This temporary confusion without loss of consciousness lasts only momentarily after the injury and is so commonplace that it needs no further description. This syndrome is completely reversible and is associated with no sequelae.

Slightly more severe head injury causes confusion with amnesia that develops after 5 or 10 minutes. Again, this is an extremely frequent event, particularly in sports injuries. Football players may experience such an injury and, although confused, continue coordinated sensorimotor activities after the accident. If examined immediately after the accident, these players possess an intact recall of the events immediately prior to impact. However, retrograde amnesia then develops 5 or 10 minutes later and thereafter the player does not remember the impact or events immediately before impact. The amnesia usually extends for only several minutes before the injury and, although it may shrink somewhat, the player will always have some degree of permanent, though short, retrograde amnesia despite resumption of a completely normal consciousness. The confusion and disorientation completely resolve in a matter of seconds.

As the mechanical stresses to the brain increase, confusion and amnesia are present from the time of impact. Football players or boxers commonly can continue to play while having no recollection of prior events. By this stage some degree of post-traumatic amnesia (forgetting of events after the injury) also occurs in addition to retrograde amnesia (forgetting of events before the injury). The patient's length of confusion may last many minutes but then his level of consciousness returns to normal usually with some permanent degree of both retrograde and post-traumatic amnesia.

These three syndromes of mild cerebral concussion have been witnessed frequently and described in detail.[7, 20] Although consciousness is preserved, it is clear that some degree of cerebral dysfunction has occurred. The fact that memory mechanisms seem to be the most sensitive to trauma suggests that the cerebral hemispheres rather than the brainstem are the recipient of mild injury forces. The degree of cerebral cortical dysfunction, however, is not sufficient to disconnect the influence of the cerebral hemispheres from the brainstem activating system and therefore consciousness is preserved. No other cortical functions except memory seem at jeopardy and the only residual deficits that patients with mild concussion syndromes have is the brief retrograde or post-traumatic amnesia.

Classical Cerebral Concussion

Classical cerebral concussion is that posttraumatic state which results in loss of consciousness. This state is always accompanied by some degree of retrograde and posttraumatic amnesia and, in fact, the length of post-traumatic amnesia is a good measure of the severity of cerebral concussion. Inherent in the usual concept of classical cerebral concussion is the fact that the disturbance of consciousness is transient and reversible. In clinical terms this means that full consciousness has returned by 24 hours. Although it has also been frequently stated that classical cerebral concussion is associated with no pathological damage to the brain, this is not universally accepted.[19] Because of its transient and reversible state, patients with cerebral concussion do not have neuropathological examinations, but evidence from experimental cerebral concussion does suggest some mild degree of microscopic neuronal abnormalities.[3, 11] Although perhaps not strictly correct, *in practical terms* classical cerebral concussion can be viewed as a phenomenon of physiological neurological dysfunction without anatomical disruption.

In patients with classical cerebral concussion there is unconsciousness or coma from the moment of head impact. Although systemic changes such as bradycardia, hypertension, and apnea or neurological signs such as decerebrate posturing, pupillary dilatation or flaccidity may occur, they do so only fleetingly and disappear within several seconds. The patient then awakens and is temporarily confused before regaining full alertness and orientation. As in the mild concussion syndromes, classical cerebral concussion is always associated with both retrograde and post-traumatic amnesia. Although these states vary in length, they tend to be longer in cerebral concussion than in mild concussion syndromes.

It must be remembered that because the mechanisms which cause human head injury are so complex, classical cerebral concussion is often associated with other types of brain injury (Table 6.2). Thus, complicated concussion can arise if focal brain injuries are superimposed on a classical concussion. It is important for the clinician to distinguish the symptomatology resulting from the concussion from that arising as a result of focal injury. The most common lesion associated with concussion is cerebral contusion. Hemispheric contusion of course, does not alter consciousness (unless of massive size) but may cause lateralized or focal neurological deficit. Likewise, the initial loss of consciousness preceding the "lucid interval" in patients with extradural hematoma represents a classical cerebral concussion and has no relationship to the later loss of consciousness caused by brainstem compression. Thus, the clinical outcome of patients with concussion will often be dependent on associated brain injuries.

Insufficient attention has been placed on the precise sequence of recovery from uncomplicated classical cerebral concussion. Although by definition the loss of consciousness is transient and reversible, sequelae of concussion are commonplace. Certainly some sequelae such as headache or tinnitus may reflect injuries to the scalp, inner ear, or other non-cerebral structures. However, subtle changes in personality, and in psychological or memory functioning have been documented and must be of cerebral cortical origin.[13] Thus, although the great majority of patients with classical cerebral concussion have no sequelae other than amnesia for the events of impact, some patients may have more long-lasting though subtle, neurological deficiencies. Further investigations of these sequelae must be done.

Table 6.2
Lesions Associated with Classical Cerebral Concussion (N = 199)

	N	%
None	71	36
Cortical contusion	20	10
Vault fracture	19	10
Basilar fracture	13	7
Depressed fracture	5	3
Multiple lesions	71	36

The mechanisms which underlie classical cerebral concussion are but an extension of those of the mild concussion syndromes. With classical cerebral concussion, not only have the mechanical stresses and strains on the brain caused dysfunction of those cortical functions involving memory, but they have, in this instance, caused sufficient physiological disturbance so as to temporarily cause diffuse cerebral hemispheric disconnection from the brainstem reticular activating system. Since this dysfunction is physiological and not structural, when the electrochemical milieu of the brain returns to normal, the usual interaction between the cerebral hemispheres and brainstem is re-established and consciousness returns.

Diffuse Injury

Diffuse injury is the name given to a specific type of brain injury. Although this term is commonly used for all diffuse brain injuries more severe than classical cerebral concussion, it must be distinguished from shearing injury. Diffuse injury is evidenced by loss of consciousness from the time of injury and which continues beyond 24 hours. It is common for patients with diffuse injury to be unconscious for days or weeks before recovery begins. Diffuse injury is distinguished from shearing injury in that there are few signs of decerebrate posturing and no signs of increased sympathetic activity (hypertension, hyperhidrosis, hyperpyrexia). Thus, patients with diffuse injury are comatose with either purposeful movements to pain, or withdrawal to pain and only occasionally have brainstem reflexive decorticate or decerebrate posturing. Often these patients appear to be restless and may have an increased amount of random motor movements.

The longer length of unconsciousness in diffuse injury suggests a more profound disturbance of cerebral function than that which occurs in classical cerebral concussion. Since the length of unconsciousness may last for weeks, it is likely that diffuse injury represents a transition between pure physiological dysfunction and anatomic disruption. Therefore, it is not surprising that if some degree of anatomical disruption occurs, recovery will be incomplete. This indeed is the case with diffuse injury. As patients awaken from coma they are confused with long periods of post-traumatic and retrograde amnesia. Permanent deficits of intellectual, cognitive, memory, and personality functions may be mild to severe. Some patients, however, do make an adequate recovery and are capable of resuming all normal activities. Thus, the degree of presumed anatomical injury may vary greatly.

These patients present with Glasgow Coma Scores of 4 through 8 and thus fall into the group of severe head injuries. Because inappropriate movement, if present at all, disappears quickly, by 24 hours the Glasgow Coma Score improves to 6 to 8 but then remains there for a varying period before recovery. As indicated in Table 6.1, by one month after injury only one-fifth of the patients have attained a good recovery while another fifth have improved to a moderate disability status. By three months most of these patients will have improved enough to be considered good recoveries. At one month half of the patients with diffuse injury are either vegetative or have severe disability requiring continued hospitalization or intensive rehabilitative care. Seven percent of the patients succumb to the complications of prolonged coma.

Treatment of patients with diffuse injury requires intensive management to provide an environment which minimizes infectious and pulmonary complications, promotes adequate cerebral oxygenation, and prevents secondary complications due to intracranial hypertension. This management has been detailed elsewhere.[5] The role of intracranial pressure monitoring in this group of patients is still unsettled. The diffuse injury itself is not often associated with intracranial hypertension soon after the injury. However, acute diffuse brain swelling can frequently be present and, as discussed subsequently in this chapter, can be a factor in either early or delayed rises in intracranial pressure.

It is postulated that the diffuse injury results from the same types of mechanical strains on the brain that cause the mild concussion syndromes and classical cerebral concussion. Physiological function is impaired in a widespread area throughout the cerebral cortex and diencephalon and actual tearing (anatomical disruption) occurs in some weaker fibers in both hemispheres. The degree of recovery is then dependent on the amount and location of anatomical damage. Since the cerebral hemispheres are disconnected from the brainstem reticular activating system for a lengthy period, the resulting prolonged coma makes these patients prone to the numerous complications of the comatose state. Therefore, the recovery process can be curtailed by secondary complications which can result in death.

Diffuse White Matter Shearing Injury

The shearing injury, also called diffuse white matter shearing injury or diffuse axonal injury, is the most severe form of all the diffuse brain injuries. It is the next step in severity from diffuse injury and is associated with severe mechanical disruption of many axons in both cerebral hemispheres. Additionally, axonal disruption extends into the diencephalon and brainstem to a variable degree.

Patients with shearing injuries are immediately deeply unconscious and remain so for a prolonged period of time. They are differentiated from patients with diffuse injury by the presence and persistence of abnormal brainstem signs such as decorticate or decerebrate posturing. In addition, they usually exhibit evidence of immediate autonomic dysfunction such as hypertension, hyperhydrosis and hyperpyrexia. Although these patients were formerly diagnosed as having "primary brainstem injury" or brainstem contusion, there is now ample evidence that such injuries are exceedingly rare, and that shearing injury is present in most patients with this clinical picture.[15]

The abnormal brainstem signs of decortication and/or decerebration are often asymmetrical and, if the patient survives, will decrease after several weeks and eventually disappear. The same is true of the autonomic dysfunction. These events suggest that recovery of brainstem function is occurring. However, residual deficiencies are profound. Three types of recovery suggest that there is a continuum within this category of shearing injury. Patients with the least anatomic damage (*i.e.*, those with fewest axons torn) can recover to a greater or lesser degree. However, recovery rarely is good and rather severe intellectual or bilateral sensori-motor deficits occur (Table 6.1). Commonly, a second pattern of shearing injury occurs from which patients survive but do not recover. These patients remain in a vegetative state (36%), and although their eyes are open they have no cognitive connection or response to their environment. The most common pattern with the shearing injury is, however, death (55%). This indeed is the far end of the spectrum of all diffuse cerebral injuries and is associated with so much anatomical disruption as to be incompatible with life. Pathological evaluation of patients who die with shearing injury shows very little macroscopic change.[2, 4] Careful examination, however, does disclose two lesions which are regularly associated with shearing injury. These consist of hemorrhagic lesions in the superior cerebellar peduncle and corpus callosum. These may be the only visible findings, but disruption of the fornix or hemorrhages in the periventricular regions may also be seen.

The principal findings in shearing injury are seen only on microscopic examination of the brain. The lack of such examinations has caused an inadequate appreciation of the frequency of this severe lesion in the past. Careful microscopic examination will disclose evidence of axons which have been torn throughout the white matter of both cerebral hemispheres. The presence of axonal retraction balls or microglial clusters are a reflection of this and will be present if the length of time from injury to death has been sufficient. If survival has been many weeks, degeneration of long white matter tracts extending into the brainstem may be seen with special stains.

Thus, pathological information verifies the concept that at this end of the spectrum, anatomical disruption of innumerable axons has occurred. It is postulated that survivors who have recoverable or non-recoverable shearing injuries have slightly lesser amounts of anatomical damage.

Considerable difficulty exists in distinguishing the shearing lesion from diffuse injury on clinical grounds in the early post-traumatic period. It is important, however, to continue to improve our ability to make this differential diagnosis since the ultimate outcome from the two is so different. Because these two are not truly different lesions but rather part of a continuous spectrum of the same injury type there is no sharp cut-off which will unequivocally separate them. It should be possible, however, to distinguish the least severe diffuse injury from the most severe shearing injury.

In addition to the clinical differences cited above, two studies show promise of helping in making this distinction. In certain cases, high resolution CT scans done shortly after injury show findings compatible with the shearing injury.[21] These findings include small hemorrhages of the corpus callosum, superior cerebellar peduncle, or periventricular region in the absence of intracranial mass lesions. Since these lesions (especially the first two) are regularly associated with the shearing injury,[4] a shearing lesion can be assumed if these hemorrhages are seen on CT scan. If these hemorrhages are present on CT scan, and if the clinical status is as described, one can be confident of the presence of a shearing injury. Because these hemorrhages are quite small, it is possible to miss them on a CT scan. It is thus possible that a shearing lesion can be present with few, if any, CT abnormalities.

Far field brainstem auditory evoked responses (BAER) also show promise in the diagnosis and monitoring of the shearing

Table 6.3
Brain Stem Auditory Evoked Response (BAER)

	Initial BAER Latency (msec)						
	Wave						
	I	II	III	IV	V	VI	VII
Normal	1.74	2.78	3.82	4.71	5.48	7.03	9.12
SD	0.12	0.29	0.18	0.12	0.16	0.12	0.46
Diffuse injury	1.80	3.13	3.98	5.26[a]	5.80[a]	7.79[a]	10.20[a]
Shearing injury	1.77	3.09	4.23	5.43[a]	6.09[a]	7.78[a]	10.17[a]

Changes of BAER Latency (Wave 5) in Shearing Injury	
Day From Injury	Wave 5 Latency (msec)
Patient #1	
0	6.15[a]
19	5.73
142	5.31
Patient #2	
0	6.19[a]
1	6.92[a]
4	5.80[a]

[a] More than 2 SD from normal.

lesion. Comparing a series of patients with shearing lesions to other head-injured patients we have found significant prolongations of the transmission of impulses through the pontine-midbrain area (Table 6.3). Wave V latency reflects activity at the inferior colliculus and is significantly more delayed in patients with shearing injury than in other groups. In patients who survive to a vegetative state or who become severely disabled, this slowed conduction progressively normalizes.

Treatment for patients with shearing injury is similar to that for diffuse injury. Special attention must be paid to late rises in intracranial pressure (4–10 days after injury) and to prevention of pulmonary complications which are the primary causes of death in most patients. However, despite aggressive intensive management, the outcome in this group will probably never be satisfactory because of the amount of structural damage sustained at the time of impact.

Summary of the Spectrum of Diffuse Cerebral Injuries

The diffuse cerebral injuries form a spectrum of severity, beginning with the mild concussion syndromes on the one end and progressing to shearing injury which results in death on the other end (Fig. 6.1). It is postulated that as mechanical input increases, brain acceleration causes progressively more shear, tensile, and compression strains to the brain substance. At first, these strains are insufficient to cause any injury. As they increase, mild physiological disruption of cortical processing causes *the mild concussion syndromes*. More severe input increases the strains in the brain which, although insufficient to cause axonal disruption, is sufficient to cause temporary global dysfunction of cortical activity. This results in a temporary disconnection of the cerebral cortex from the reticular activation system and *classical cerebral concussion* with loss of consciousness results. As mechanical strains increase further, the structurally weakest axons fail, and anatomical disruption begins. In *diffuse injury*, physiological dysfunction is still more prominent than mechanical disruption, but as more and more axons are disrupted, the *shearing injury* is seen. By the time shearing injury occurs, sufficient physiological dysfunction of brainstem activity occurs, prolonged unconsciousness is produced, and depending on the amount of anatomical damage to

DIFFUSE BRAIN INJURIES

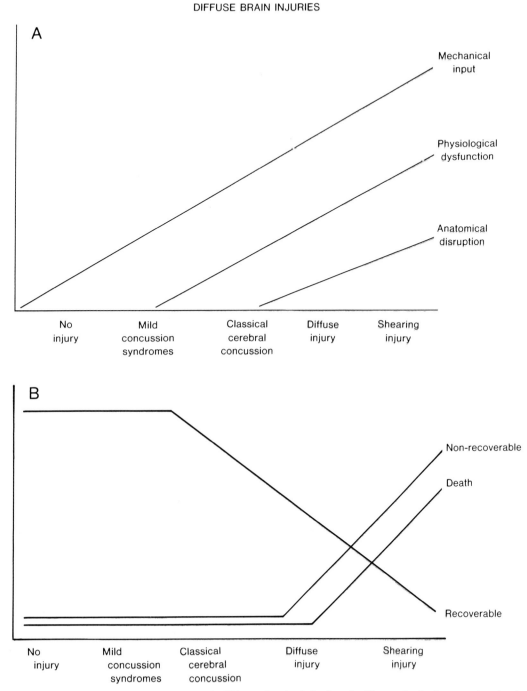

Figure 6.1. *A*, the continuum of diffuse brain injuries is illustrated. As mechanical strains increase, the mild concussion syndromes occur, followed by classical cerebral concussion, diffuse injury and shearing injury. Functional activity of the brain is always more disturbed than anatomic disruption. *B*, as diffuse brain injuries increase in severity, complete recovery is the rule until the diffuse injury is seen. Thereafter, the number of patients with non-recoverable injuries and death increases.

axons, either partial recovery, non-recovery, or death occurs. Thus, a shearing injury with death comprises that situation where the mechanical input forces cause such high strains that an overwhelming number of nerve fibers are destroyed.

PHENOMENA RELATED TO DIFFUSE BRAIN INJURIES

Several events are related to diffuse brain injuries which, because of different mechanisms of causation or because of different pathophysiological effects, must be differentiated from diffuse brain injuries. These events include vasovagal phenomena and brain swelling (see also Chapter 12).

Vasovagal Phenomena

Vasovagal syncope must be distinguished from the mild concussion syndromes and from classical cerebral concussion. This event is a fainting spell caused by a brief, intense, stimulation of the vagal parasympathetic nervous system. Activation of vagal centers occurs commonly from impacts or punches to the abdomen (the solar plexus punch of boxers), but may also be caused by head movements which stimulate the vagus nerve in or around the head. Blows to the face can cause sufficient head movements to activate the vagus. That this commonly occurs before the input forces are sufficient to cause classical cerebral concussion is well evidenced in experimental head injury.[1]

Whatever the cause, vagal hyperactivity results in profound bradycardia and hypotension. If mild, these may lead to lightheadedness or swooning sensations but if severe can decrease cerebral blood flow sufficiently to result in loss of consciousness. Thus, a mild vasovagal episode may mimic one of the mild concussion syndromes while a more severe event can cause fainting and loss of consciousness resembling a classical cerebral concussion. The true brain injury syndromes can usually be differentiated from vagal events by the lack of retrograde or post-traumatic amnesia and the presence of a slow, bounding pulse in the latter situation. Additionally, a momentary delay often occurs before the vasovagal syncope results in loss of consciousness and thus the patient may stagger for a few seconds before collapsing. Classical cerebral concussion, on the other hand, occurs exactly at the time of impact and is always due to head rather than body impact.

Brain Swelling

Brain swelling is a poorly understood phenomenon which can accompany any type of head injury. Swelling is not synonymous with cerebral edema, the latter term referring to a specific situation in which there is an increase in extravascular brain water. Such an increase in water content may, in fact, not be the case in brain swelling and current evidence favors the concept that brain swelling is due, at least in part, to increased intravascular blood within the brain. This is caused by a vascular reaction to head injury which disturbs the normal actions of the cerebral blood vessels and leads to vasodilatation and increased cerebral blood volume. If this condition of increased cerebral blood volume continues for long enough time, then vascular permeability may be increased and true edema may result.

Although brain swelling may occur in any type of head injury, the magnitude of the swelling does not correlate well with the severity of the injury. Thus, both severe and mild or moderate injuries may be complicated by the presence of brain swelling. The effects of brain swelling are additive to those of the primary brain injury, and may, in certain instances, be more severe than the primary injury itself.

Despite a lack of knowledge of the precise mechanism of causation of brain swelling, it can be conceptualized in two general forms (Table 6.4). It should be remembered that many different types of brain swelling may exist and that the following represents a phenomenological rather than a mechanistic approach to brain swelling.

Acute brain swelling occurs in several circumstances. That swelling which accompanies focal brain lesions tends to be localized, whereas diffuse brain injuries are associated with generalized swelling. Focal swelling is usually present beneath contusions but does not often contribute additional deleterious effects. On the other hand, the swelling which occurs with acute subdural hematomas though principally hemispheric in distribution may cause more mass effect than does the hematoma itself.

Table 6.4
Brain Swelling

I. Acute swelling
   A. Associated with focal lesions
      1. Acute SDH—hemispheric
      2. Contusions—focal
   B. Associated with diffuse lesions
      1. Diffuse injury—generalized
      2. Shearing injury—generalized
II. Delayed swelling
   A. Associated with lethargy
   B. Associated with light coma
   C. Associated with deep coma

In such circumstances, the small amount of blood in the subdural space may not be the sole reason for the patient's neurological state. If the hematoma is removed, the acute brain swelling may progress so rapidly that the brain protrudes through the craniotomy opening. Every neurosurgeon is all too familiar with this condition of external herniation of the brain which, when it occurs, is most difficult to treat. In an experimental model of acute subdural hematoma, this type of "malignant brain swelling" occurs regularly.[8] Shortly after the subdural blood is removed the brain swells so massively that it protrudes well beyond the outer table of the skull (Fig. 6.2). Measurement of tissue water content, studies

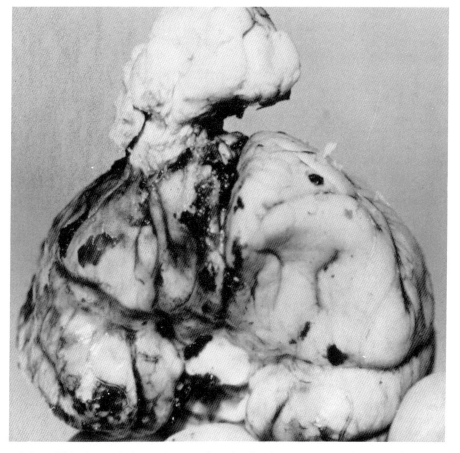

Figure 6.2. This frontal view of a monkey brain demonstrates the massive amount of acute brain swelling which can occur after the removal of an acute subdural hematoma. The "mushroom" over the frontal lobe (viewers left) is swollen brain which protruded through the craniotomy defect moments after a subdural hematoma was evacuated.

with labeled sucrose, and electron microscopic observations have failed to find evidence of cerebral edema in the swollen brain. This is indirect evidence that this variety of acute brain swelling is not due to cerebral edema but is a result of increased cerebral blood volume.

The more serious types of diffuse brain injuries are associated with generalized rather than focal acute brain swelling. Although not all patients with diffuse injury or shering injury have brain swelling, the incidence of swelling is higher than in patients with either classical cerebral concussion or one of the mild concussion syndromes. Because of the serious nature of the underlying injury, it is difficult to determine the relative importance of swelling in these patients. The swelling, though widespread throughout the brain, may not cause a rise in the intracranial pressure for several days. This late rise in pressure probably reflects the formation of true cerebral edema and it may be by the promotion of edema that diffuse swelling associated with the severe diffuse brain injuries is deleterious. In any event, this type of swelling is very different from the type of swelling associated with acute subdural hematomas.

Delayed brain swelling may occur minutes to hours after head injury. It is usually diffuse and is often associated with the less severe forms of diffuse brain injuries. Whether delayed swelling is the same or a different phenomenon than the acute swelling of the more serious diffuse injuries is unknown. The difference is that a distinct time interval exists before delayed swelling becomes manifest, thus allowing confirmation that the primary insult to the brain was not serious. Considering the high frequency of the mild concussion syndromes and of the classical cerebral concussion, the incidence of delayed swelling must be very low. However, when it occurs, delayed swelling can cause profound neurological changes or even death.

In its most severe form delayed swelling can cause deep coma. The usual history is that of an injury associated with a mild concussion or a classical cerebral concussion from which the patient recovers. Minutes to hours later the patient becomes lethargic, then stuporous, and lapses into a coma. The coma may be light, with appropriate motor responses to painful stimuli, or deep, associated with decorticate or decerebrate posturing. The key difference between these patients and those with diffuse injury or shearing injury is that in the latter cases the coma and abnormal motor signs are present from the moment of injury, whereas with delayed cerebral swelling there is a time interval when these signs are absent. This distinction is of major significance, since with diffuse or shearing injury a certain amount of primary structural damage has occurred at the moment of impact which is not present in delayed swelling. Therefore, the deleterious effects of delayed swelling should be potentially reversible and, if these effects are controlled, the outcome should be good. However, control of the effects of brain swelling may be difficult. Rigorous monitoring of intracranial pressure is necessary and prompt and aggressive treatment of brain swelling is required in order to control raised intracranial pressure. If this is successfully accomplished, the mortality rate from the increased intracranial pressure associated with diffuse brain swelling should be low.[6]

The severe form of delayed brain swelling often appears in a stereotyped fashion principally involving children between 4 and 10 years of age. The initial injury may occur from any variety of head trauma and is usually characterized by a more or less completely lucid interval immediately after injury. The children then become lethargic and lapse into coma often in association with an early post-traumatic seizure. Thereafter, a dynamic sequence of events occurs over the next several months. First, brain swelling is manifest on computerized tomographic scanning by the absence of cerebral ventricles and subarachnoid spaces. If adequate control of intracranial pressure is accomplished, a week or more after the injury brain swelling begins to diminish often to the point that extracerebral collections occur. By one month after injury these collections disappear spontaneously and the brain which had been swollen begins to shrink and the ventricular system is seen to be enlarged. This is often associated with enlargement of the sulci around the brain, giving a CT appearance of cerebral atrophy. By this time, some degree of neurological recovery from the deep coma has occurred. Still later, approximately six to nine months after injury, the CT appearance of cerebral atrophy disappears and the brain resumes its normal configuration. The exact mechanisms which cause this prolonged series of events to occur is unknown, but the final outcome in these patients if their intracranial pressure is controlled is good with no residual neurological deficit.

Less severe amounts of delayed cerebral swelling may also occur with the mild concussion syndromes and with classical cerebral concussion. These are not often diagnosed because they are associated only with early post-traumatic lethargy which soon disappears. However, these patients exhibit the same type of early clinical course as is seen in those patients with more severe delayed cerebral swelling. Again, after a mild concussion or classical cerebral concussion, the patient awakens and is normal for some moments to hours. Thereafter, a degree of lethargy occurs which lasts for hours to days. This state is reasonably common and probably represents a mild degree of delayed brain swelling.

Whether mild or severe, delayed brain swelling is an epiphenomenon associated with diffuse brain injuries which is poorly understood. Since it does not occur in all patients with diffuse brain injuries it can be viewed as a reaction to injury rather than as a primary injury itself. As with the immediate type of brain swelling it is likely that delayed brain swelling initially represents a vascular reaction to injury in which the cerebral blood vessels lose their normal vascular control mechanisms and widely vasodilate. This results in increased cerebral blood flow and increased cerebral blood volume.[16] True edema formation may subsequently occur and result in increased intracranial pressure. Thus, the effects of brain swelling, whether immediate or delayed, are added to the effects of the primary brain injury and, in the case of the milder forms of diffuse brain injury, may represent the most serious threat to survival.

The treatment of brain swelling is far from ideal but as a better understanding of this phenomenon develops more effective therapy will follow. It has been documented that brain swelling is often associated with increased cerebral blood flow and increased cerebral blood volume.[14, 16] In these patients, this hyperemia is always in excess of the metabolic needs of the brain and if cerebral blood flow (CBF) measurements are not available it can be adequately monitored by measuring the arterial-jugular venous difference of oxygen content ($AVDO_2$). Since the $AVDO_2$ represents the ratio of the cerebral metabolic rate of oxygen consumption to the CBF, instances of hyperemia (increased CBF) lead to a decrease of this ratio and thus the $AVDO_2$ is less than normal. In fact, this is the case and in all instances of significant hyperemia the $AVDO_2$ is low. Insertion of an internal jugular vein catheter and simultaneous measurement of jugular and arterial oxygen content can provide this useful clinical parameter in any intensive care unit. A low $AVDO_2$ (<3.5 vol.%) is diagnostic of the hyperemia associated with brain swelling and is best treated by hyperventilation to the degree necessary to increase the $AVDO_2$ to normal (3.5–7.5 vol.%). This is possible because vascular CO_2 responsivity is retained in spite of cerebral vasodilation which causes the hyperemia. In fact, this reactivity may be supra-sensitive to changes in arterial pCO_2. Thus, care should be taken to avoid such excessive hyperventilation that the $AVDO_2$ becomes higher than normal. This may result in a situation where the CBF becomes insufficient for the metabolic needs of the brain.

Hyperosmotic agents are not advisable as a primary treatment for brain swelling because they increase CBF and thus can potentially worsen an already hyperemic brain. They are, of course, useful in the treatment of increased ICP when brain swelling cannot otherwise be controlled.

SUMMARY

Diffuse brain injuries are consequences of shaking of the brain. They result from acceleration effects of head trauma and have little, if anything, to do with localized phenomena of the impact. Acceleration causes shear, tensile, and compression strains to be generated throughout the brain and these strains are the primary injurious factors. Since the brain is weakest in the shearing mode, rotational acceleration is more injurious than other types of acceleration because of the high shear strains it induces. The primary injuries to the brain caused by acceleration form a continuum of injury severity which increases as acceleration of the brain increases. Very low strains caused by low levels of acceleration may cause no injury whatsoever. As acceleration increases, the mild concussion syndromes result but these are not associated with loss of consciousness. Classical cerebral concussion is caused by a further increase in acceleration and is associated with transient reversible loss of consciousness.

If still further strains are induced in the brain by higher levels of acceleration, anatomic damage begins to occur and is associated with more severe functional changes of the brain. Diffuse injury is a primary injury associated with prolonged loss of consciousness and mild diffuse anatomical damage. Shearing injury is the most severe form of the diffuse brain injuries and is accompanied by deep coma, signs of decerebrate posturing, and autonomic dysfunction. It is associated with widespread disruption of axons throughout the white matter of both cerebral hemispheres. Though some patients with mild degrees of shearing may recover, most patients with shearing injury either die or remain in a vegetative state from which they do not recover.

The continuum of the diffuse brain injuries is associated with both physiological dysfunction and, at the most severe end of the spectrum, anatomical disruption. Although the individual primary diffuse brain injuries are distinct, they are a continuum and one syndrome may merge indistinguishably into the next. This can provide difficulty in making a precise diagnosis in certain cases. However, the end result of the primary injury is dependent on the amount of anatomical disruption which occurs at the moment of injury since the functional changes in themselves are reversible.

Brain swelling may be superimposed on the primary diffuse brain injuries. Although it does not occur in every case of diffuse brain injury, it can add deleterious effects to the primary injury by causing increased intracranial pressure. Rapidly occurring brain swelling is associated with severe diffuse brain injuries, whereas delayed brain swelling appears in conjunction with the less severe varieties of diffuse brain injuries.

Diffuse brain injuries and brain swelling form a distinct group of head injuries which have different mechanisms of causation, different pathophysiological influences on the brain, and different outcomes than do focal brain injuries.

References

1. Abel, J., Gennarelli, T.A., Segawa, H.: Incidence and severity of cerebral concussion in the rhesus monkey following sagittal plane angular acceleration. In: 22nd Stapp Car Crash Conference Proceedings, Soc. Auto. Engineers, New York, 1978, pp. 33–53.
2. Adams, J.H.: The neuropathology of head injuries. In: Handbook of Clinical Neurology, P.J. Vinken, G.W. Bruyn, R. Braakman, Eds. North-Holland Pub., Oxford, 23:35–65, 1975.
3. Adams, J.H., Graham, D.I., Gennarelli, T.A.: Acceleration induced head injury in the monkey. Acta Neuropath., Suppl. 7: 26–28, 1981.
4. Adams, J.H., Mitchell, D.E., Graham, D.I., Doyle, D.: Diffuse brain damage of immediate impact type. Its relationship to primary brain-stem damage in head injury. Brain, 100:489–502, 1977.
5. Bruce, D., Gennarelli, T.A., Langfitt, T.W.: Resuscitation from coma due to head injury. Crit. Care Med., 6:254–269, 1978.
6. Bruce, D.A., Schut, L., Bruno, L.A., Wood, J.H., Sutton, L.N.: Outcome following severe head injuries in children. J. Neurosurg., 48:679–688, 1978.
7. Fisher, C.M.: Concussion amnesia. Neurology, 16:826–830, 1966.
8. Gennarelli, T.A., Czernicki, A., Segawa, H.: Acute brain swelling in experimental head injury (in preparation).
9. Gennarelli, T.A., Obrist, W.D., Langfitt, T.W., Segawa, H.: Vascular and metabolic reactivity to changes in pCO_2 in head injured patients. In: Neural Trauma, Popp, A.J., Bourke, R.S., Nelson, L.R., Kimelberg, H.K., Eds. Raven Press, N.Y.,

1979, pp. 1–8.

10. Gennarelli, T.A., Thibault, L.E., Ommaya, A.K.: Pathophysiologic responses to rotational and translational acceleration of the head. 16th Stapp Car Crash Conference. New York, Society of Automotive Engineers, 1972, pp. 296–308.

11. Groat, R.A., Windle, W.F., and Magoun, H.W.: Functional and structural changes in the monkey's brain during and after concussion. J. Neurosurg., 2:26–35, 1945.

12. Holbourn, A.H.S.: Mechanics of head injury. Lancet, 2:438–441, 1943.

13. Jane, J., Rimmel R.: Mild head injury. In: Fourth Chicago Head Injury Symposium, Grossman, R., Gildenberg, P., Eds. Raven Press, New York (in press).

14. Kuhl, D.E., Alavi, A., Hoffman, E.J., Phelps, M.E., Zimmerman, R.A., Obrist, W.D., Bruce, D.A., Greenberg, J.H., Uzzell, B.: Local cerebral blood volume in head-injured patients. Determination by emission computed tomography of ^{99m} Tc-labeled red cells. J. Neurosurg., 52:309–320, 1980.

15. Mitchell, D.E., Adams, J.H.: Primary focal impact damage to the brainstem in blunt head injuries: does it exist? Lancet, 2:215–218, 1973.

16. Obrist, W.D., Gennarelli, T.A., Segawa, H., Dolinskas, D.A., Langfitt, T.W.: Relation of cerebral blood flow to neurological status and outcome in head-injured patients. J. Neurosurg., 51:292–300, 1979.

17. Ommaya, A.K., Gennarelli, T.A.: Cerebral concussion and traumatic unconsciousness. Correlation of experimental and clinical observations on blunt head injuries. Brain, 97:633–654, 1974.

18. Strich, S.J.: The pathology of brain damage due to blunt head injuries. In: The Late Effects of Head Injury, A.E. Walker, W.F. Caveness, M. Critchley, Eds. Charles C Thomas, Springfield, Ill., 1969, pp. 501–524.

19. Symonds, C.: Concussion and its sequellae. Lancet, 1:1–5, 1962.

20. Yarnell, P.R., Lynch, S.: The "ding": amnestic states in football trauma. Neurology, 23:196–197, 1973.

21. Zimmerman, R.A., Bilaniuk, L.T., Gennarelli, T.A.: Computed tomography of shearing injuries of the cerebral white matter. Radiology, 127:393–396, 1978.

7

Injuries of the Cranial Nerves

RICHARD L. ROVIT
RAJ MURALI

INJURIES TO THE OLFACTORY NERVES

Trauma is the most common cause of anosmia and is encountered in about 7% of all head injuries.[79] The incidence of post-traumatic anosmia may be even higher if one takes into account the obvious difficulties of testing olfaction in a seriously injured, unconscious patient. The detection of anosmia is rarely of diagnostic significance, but may be of medico-legal importance, especially if the victim's occupation has to do with the culinary arts. In about 50% of cases, anosmia is only of temporary duration. The reason for the return of olfaction is not entirely clear. However, recovery of the sense of smell can be expected at any time from a few days up to five years with a sharp increase in recovery being observed about 10 weeks after the injury. This may be related to clearing of edema and resolution of minor hemorrhages in the olfactory pathways.[79]

The exact site of injury in the olfactory pathway that produces anosmia is controversial. It had been thought that only serious injuries of the head with fractures of the anterior cranial fossa resulting in anatomical disruption of the olfactory filaments or tract caused permanent anosmia. However, Sumner[79] in his clinical thesis on this subject demonstrated that permanent anosmia could result from even trivial injuries to the brain. He observed further that the olfactory filaments are fairly well protected in the cribriform plate against the shearing stresses of the brain that often accompany even minor injuries to the head.

Two potential sources of error must be borne in mind when testing the sense of smell. The first is that the substance tested should be familiar to the patient. Second, the test substance should not stimulate the fibers of the trigeminal nerve in the nasal mucosa. The latter condition can be obviated by using pure stimulants such as floral odors and musk ketone instead of camphor, peppermint, or substances which irritate the nasal mucosa. One should also be sure that a local injury to the nose or nasal mucosa does not exist in conjunction with the head injury.

There are two objective tests of olfaction that are sometimes helpful in confirming the diagnosis of anosmia. These tests are also of value in differentiating true anosmia from malingering. The first is the *olfactory respiratory reflex*.[79] This test is based on the principle that sudden inhalation of an odor will cause a temporary arrest in the normal respiratory rhythm. The test is performed with the subject seated and blindfolded. The patient then breathes through a mask which in turn is connected to a spirometer. The respiratory excursions are recorded on graph paper. Once the normal respiratory pattern is established, a syringe containing a solution of pyridine is injected into the mask. If the subject is anosmic, the respiratory pattern remains unchanged. If, however, normal olfaction is present, there is a sudden transient arrest in the respiratory rhythm followed by a few small amplitude waves. This is a farily good test to detect malingering. The test may not, however, separate trigeminal and gustatory components from pure olfaction and this may be a limiting factor in its value. The other test of olfaction, *olfactory electroencephalography*[79] is an EEG performed with the eyes closed. Once the alpha rhythm is well established, an odoriferous substance is introduced. If olfaction is present, the alpha rhythm is abolished. This is a nonspecific response but is of value in identifying malingerers.

The investigation of a patient with posttraumatic anosmia should include careful ethmoidal tomography to disclose basal fractures. CSF rhinorrhea should be excluded and otolaryngological opinion should be obtained to evaluate any nasal trauma.

As there is no specific treatment, patients with post-traumatic anosmia can only be counseled with the known statistical information regarding their potential for recovery.

INJURIES TO THE OPTIC NERVE AND CHIASM

In this section discussion will be limited to direct and indirect trauma involving the optic nerve and chiasm. This represents a somewhat arbitrary decision. Trauma to the orbit, with or without significant craniocerebral trauma, is rarely neatly circumscribed and a severe injury to the eye may involve varying admixtures of optic nerve, extraocular muscles and nerves and optic globe insults. The subject of orbital trauma has been reviewed by Walsh and Hoyt.[93]

Anatomy

The optic nerve is not a true cranial nerve but rather a direct extension of the brain. Axons in the optic nerve do not regenerate after they have been injured. This lack of axonal regenerative capacity places a severe limitation on any therapeutic results that can be expected following severe optic nerve injury.

The optic nerve can be considered to have three components: intraorbital, intracanalicular, and intracranial. Isolated optic nerve injury occurs primarily within the tight bony optic canal, which measures from 4 to 9 mm in length and 4 to 6 mm in width. Each canal is directed posteriorly and medially from the posterior orbit. Within the canal, the optic nerve is surrounded by an extension of the dura mater, as well as the pia and arachnoid. The ophthalmic artery also traverses the canal, inferior and lateral to the nerve. Sympathetic fibers from the carotid plexus en route to the ciliary body of the pupil are also contained within the canal. The blood supply to the intracanalicular portion of the nerve is derived from small penetrating branches of the ophthalmic artery as well as a recurrent branch of the central retinal artery which arises within the orbit and extends back into the optic canal.

The orbital portion of the optic nerve measures 20–30 mm in length and extends from the anterior portion of the optic canal to the posterior portion of the globe. It lies rather loosely in a lazy-S shaped configuration covered by dura, pia, and arachnoid. The central retinal artery and vein penetrate the infero-medial portion of the nerve almost at right angles, entering it from 5–15 mm posterior to the globe.

The intracranial portion of each optic nerve is directed posteriorly and medially for a distance of 5–16 mm and ends where the optic chiasm is formed. The internal carotid artery lies lateral to the optic nerve, whereas the ophthalmic artery is usually lateral and inferior to the nerve. Inferiorly, the optic nerves have important relationships with the sphenoid sinus, posterior ethmoid cells, and the cavernous sinuses. The anterior cerebral arteries pass above the posterior portions of the optic chiasm where they generally form the anterior communicating artery.

Some Observations Regarding the Blood Supply to the Optic Nerve

Loss of vision following trauma may occur as a consequence of direct optic nerve injury or as a result of interference with the blood supply of the nerve. When loss of vision occurs immediately following the trauma, it is impossible to determine whether the optic nerve has been severed or the visual loss is secondary to ischemia of an intact nerve. If the loss of vision returns subsequently, it is obvious that the optic nerve is intact and the previous visual loss was secondary to transitory ischemia or nerve swelling with impaired axonal conduction. Delayed loss of vision following trauma always indicates that the optic nerve is intact, the late visual loss being secondary to infarction or less commonly to callus formation usually within the optic canal.

Certain ophthalmoscopic observations may provide clues regarding the site of optic nerve injury when blindness occurs after a cranial nerve insult. When division of the optic nerve occurs close to the globe, the central retinal vessels are also interrupted. The ophthalmoscopic picture is that of central retinal artery occlusion: immediate pallor of the optic disc, a gray retina with narrowed retinal vessels, and a cherry-red spot at the macula. Division of the optic nerve posterior to the point of entrance of the central retinal artery produces total blindness but funduscopic examination is initially normal. Pallor of the optic discs will develop in time, depending on the area of optic nerve disruption, and occurs most promptly with injuries closest to the globe. With an injury to the optic nerve within the optic canal, the ophthalmoscopic appearance of pallor of the fundus is usually evident three weeks after injury.

Incidence

Reliable statistics on the incidence of injuries to the optic nerve and chiasm are not available. Most reports on this subject come from single centers where retrospective analyses have been performed by individuals with a particular interest in a highly selected group of patients. From available data, however, injury to the optic nerve and chiasm occurs in 0.3–5.2% of patients with head injuries.

Trauma to the Intrabulbar Portion of the Optic Nerve

Injury to this part of the optic nerve invariably occurs in association with direct trauma to the globe as the nerve is pushed posteriorly and suffers a partial or complete avulsion at the back end of the globe.[18, 93] There is usually concomitant intraocular hemorrhage making funduscopic examination unrewarding, but Park et al.[57] have described cases where it has been possible to visualize a defect secondary to the nerve avulsion. Injuries to the globe extending into the optic nerve have been described by several authors.[34, 48] The ophthalmoscopic picture consists of a marginal hemorrhage extending to the disc. The hemorrhage soon disappears to be followed by a pigmented scar and on visual field examination there is a sector defect extending from the blind spot to the periphery.

Trauma to the Intraorbital Portion of the Optic Nerve

Although fractures of the orbit are common, isolated injury to the intraorbital portion of the optic nerve is rare.[15, 67] With severe trauma to the apex of the orbit, there may be a disruption of the sphenoidal fissure with loss of function of the third, fourth, sixth, and ophthalmic branches of the fifth nerve, accompanied by monocular blindness and proptosis secondary to hemorrhage into the muscle cone. Under these circumstances, a decompressive procedure through the maxillary antrum has been described to alleviate the proptosis.[95]

Trauma to the Intracanalicular Portion of the Optic Nerve

The most vulnerable component of the optic nerve in patients with head trauma is that portion of the nerve located within the optic canal (see anatomy). The literature on intracanalicular injuries of the optic nerve is extensive and has been compiled by Gjerris.[27] Although the intracanalicular portion of the nerve may be injured directly by penetrating foreign objects, such as missiles, the overwhelming majority of cases follow closed head injuries, primarily those involving frontal, temporal and orbital trauma.

Clinical Aspects. With a complete injury to the optic nerve within the canal, there is monocular blindness, a dilated pupil with an absent direct pupillary response, and a brisk consensual response to light. The funduscopic appearance is unremarkable initially but atrophy of the disc develops in several weeks. The pupil on the affected side is larger than the uninvolved one and there is some diminution in the pupillo-motor response to consensual stimulation. Although the clinical diagnosis should be established readily, optic nerve injuries may be overlooked initially in patients with severe concomitant head or eye injuries. In such instances, electroretinography (ERG) and visual evoked responses (VER) may be helpful. Although monocular blindness secondary to intracanalicular injuries is usually complete and permanent, immediate partial injuries may occur and these should be documented, if possible, since deterioration in vision may be the only clear indication for exploration and decompression. Partial visual defects may take the form of scotomas, sector defects, and upper or lower altitudinal hemianopsias.[1,8,34] The prognosis for restoration of vision in a patient with an optic nerve injury is poor. In a large review of the literature, 40–50% of patients remained blind and up to 75% showed no improvement in their reduced visual acuity or in a documented field defect.[27] If improvement is to take place spontaneously, it does so within the first several days and continues for four to six weeks at which time the condition becomes stationary.[65,73] The prognosis is said to be better in those patients whose visual acuity is diminished but who retain a good pupillary response to light.[73]

Bony Injury. In the vast majority of instances of injury of the intracanalicular portion of the optic nerve secondary to head injury, there are fractures of the base of the skull with extension into the optic canal. Whether the fracture of the optic canal is the primary cause of the nerve injury or constitutes an epiphenomenon associated with other insults (contusion, necrosis, ischemia, etc.) is a source of controversy. Most observers feel that the fracture represents an associated insult. The optic foramen is difficult to outline precisely radiographically, especially in a confused and/or restless patient and there are multiple sources of radiographic error.[44,82] Special views are usually required, including stereoscopic projections and polytomo-

grams. When these are performed, the most common fracture is seen to involve the roof of the optic canal with frequent extension into the roof of the orbit. Fractures of the lateral wall and floor of the canal are also seen but medial wall fractures are uncommon.[7,76]

Pathology of Optic Nerve Injury. The pathogenesis of optic nerve injuries is, in large part, inferential. Very few patients with well-documented clinical findings have had an operation with subsequent pathological confirmation of clinical deficits. In the majority of instances, the pathological findings have been derived from autopsy material on patients dying after severe cranial trauma where there was little information regarding visual function.[93,94] Pathological abnormalities are diverse and have been summarized by Gjerris[27]:

> The primary lesion is rarely a total section or laceration, but is usually a contusion necrosis, ischemic necrosis or interstitial hemorrhage due to the blow or shearing at the moment of injury. The pathogenesis of the immediate partial lesion is presumably the same but it is of lesser extent, and in both cases tearing or an injury to the pial vessels can lead to edema and infarction. This secondary edema occurs only sporadically, but it is of clinical importance if it develops two to six days after the injury and leads to a deterioration in a partial optic nerve lesion. Reaction to traumatic subarachnoid bleeding may lead to the late onset of arachnoiditis with secondary loss of vision.
>
> Formation of callus in the optic canal has been documented once.[46]

Treatment of Intracanalicular Injuries. Enthusiasm for operative treatment of optic nerve injury, with or without a demonstrable fracture of the optic canal, has waxed and waned over the years. Probably the only clear indication for operative treatment occurs in the special situation after head trauma where vision in the affected eye was documented to be quite good initially only to show progressive deterioration thereafter. This would be especially true when radiographs reveal a narrowed optic canal or a bone fragment dislocated into the canal. Under these admittedly unusual conditions, operations should be undertaken promptly, usually within the first 48 hours after injury. There are no compelling indications for operative treatment in patients who have a documented complete or partial visual loss immediately after trauma, patients with demonstrable fractures of the optic canal with or without visual loss, and patients with improving vision following a traumatic episode.

Traditionally, the operative approach to the optic canal has been via the transcranial route with unroofing of the canal and posterior orbit. An intracranial operation has obvious shortcomings in the acute stage following head injury where extensive retraction must be applied to swollen and contused frontal and temporal lobes. For this reason, there has been a recent resurgence of interest for acute decompression of the optic canal, using microsurgical techniques via the transethmoidal, transmaxillary and transorbital routes.[25, 28, 54, 77] Although technically feasible, there are no clear data indicating the advantages of early operative intervention in patients who have sustained an immediate post-traumatic optic nerve injury.

Steroids should probably be employed immediately following optic nerve injury to reduce secondary edema although their efficacy is not proved.[36, 93]

Trauma to the Intracranial Optic Nerve and Chiasm

Isolated injuries of the intracranial optic nerve and/or optic chiasm following head trauma are exceedingly rare. Only 0.7% of survivors of closed head injuries demonstrated clinical evidence of trauma to the optic nerve and chiasm.[7] In only 10% of these cases was there an isolated bitemporal hemianopsia.[93] Pure chiasmal injuries were present in only four cases compiled by Hughes[34] when he reviewed 90 instances of trauma to the anterior visual pathways. In closed head injuries, chiasmatic injury is most commonly associated with basal frontal fractures extending to the region of the sella turcica and pars petrosa. Probably the most common pathogenetic mechanism consists of a stretch injury to the chiasm followed by interstitial hemorrhages within the chiasm with associated contusions and

edema.[12, 93] Vascular insufficiency may also play a role in chiasmal injury,[87] but in view of the extensive vascular supply to this region, pure ischemic lesions are unlikely.

Clinically, patients with post-traumatic chiasmal lesions will, if conscious, demonstrate bitemporal hemianopsia with or without macular sparing depending on whether their macular fibers escape injury.[84] In the unconscious patient, Wernicke's hemianopic pupillary phenomenon may be helpful in diagnostic evaluation. Polytomography may also be of value in defining the precise area of injury.[41] It is expected that computed tomographic studies, especially with high resolution scanners, may be able to pinpoint precisely anatomic discontinuities, hemorrhages, and necrosis in the intracranial optic nerve and chiasm. There is general agreement that the early demonstration of a chiasmatic lesion *per se* is not an indication for exploration. Operative intervention may be indicated, however, for those rare cases where there is documented progressive visual deterioration, presumably secondary to adhesive arachnoiditis.[55]

INJURIES TO THE THIRD, FOURTH AND SIXTH CRANIAL NERVES

Injuries to the ocular motor system can result from trauma at multiple levels of the nervous system from the cerebral cortex to the muscles in the orbit. They can occur immediately as a result of direct mechanical trauma or secondarily due to cerebral herniation, cavernous sinus thrombosis, intracavernous carotid aneurysm formation, and carotid-cavernous fistulae. The section to follow will deal primarily with the direct injuries to the ocular motor system. Secondary insults, particularly those due to cerebral herniation, will be discussed elsewhere.

Incidence

The occurrence of pure ocular motor nerve palsies is often unclear due to difficulties of diagnosis in unconscious patients. Many reports do not clearly differentiate between immediate and delayed injuries. Orbital fractures with muscle entrapment, contusions and hemorrhage further compli-cate the issue. Partial trochlear nerve pal-sies and bilateral trochlear nerve palsies often escape attention. However, in spite of these limitations, the following large re-views are of interest: Turner[89] found 45 ocular palsies among 1,550 cases of cranio-cerebral trauma. Russell[69] disclosed a 3% incidence of ocular palsies among closed head injuries. Hughes[33] reported the follow-ing incidence of ocular palsy among pa-tients with closed head injuries: 2.6% third nerve palsy, 2.7% sixth nerve palsy, and 1.4% of combined third and sixth nerve palsies. There was only one case of fourth cranial nerve palsy. The sixth cranial nerve was the commonest to be involved bilat-erally. In a series of 1,000 ocular palsies from all causes Hughes[33] found 34 trau-matic third nerve palsies, 55 traumatic sixth nerve palsies, and 23 isolated fourth nerve palsies.

Traumatic Oculomotor Nerve Palsy

The third cranial nerve or oculomotor nerve projects from the anterior part of the midbrain to the tentorial incisura at the level of the posterior clinoid processes in an open "V" shaped fashion. The size of the opening in the tentorial incisura may play a part in determining whether the nerve is injured or not. A large tentorial opening may allow greater movement of the mid-brain without damage to the oculomotor nerves. The third nerve probably becomes damaged by a frontal blow to the acceler-ating head which results in stretching and contusion of the nerve. The exact site of damage has not been clearly defined but is believed to occur most commonly at the point where the nerve enters the dura at the posterior end of the cavernous sinus. Bilateral third nerve injuries are extremely uncommon. When the third nerve is injured at the superior orbital fissure or in the cavernous sinus, it is often accompanied by other cranial nerve injuries as they course through the fissure. Hughes[33] found a 56% incidence of associated optic nerve injuries, 25% incidence of associated trigeminal nerve injuries, and 25% incidence of facial nerve injuries when the oculomotor nerve was injured in the lateral wall of the cav-ernous sinus or in the superior orbital fis-sure.

The diagnosis of oculomotor nerve injury in conscious and cooperative persons is not difficult. In unconscious subjects, especially those with orbital bruising and hematoma, the diagnosis is more difficult and may es-cape detection if the pupil is not affected. Thus, in unconscious patients, a good his-tory with regard to previous oculomotor status and the findings of the immediate post-traumatic examination, when avail-able, are of great help in making an early diagnosis. Such information also helps in differentiating primary from delayed sec-ondary oculomotor nerve palsy.

The paralyzed nerve, if still in continuity, as it is in most cases, should begin to show signs of recovery in two to three months time. However, the "misdirection in regen-eration" phenomenon is often evident. The troublesome diplopia usually subsides but the paralyzed pupil rarely becomes normal. The pupil may not react to light but may constrict when any one of the muscles sup-plied by the third nerve contract. This amounts to a pseudo-Argyll Robertson pu-pil. Due to the misdirection of the growing axons, the levator muscle of the lid may receive fibers destined for other muscles. When such an individual attempts to look down, the lid becomes elevated rather than having the eyeball move down. This is re-ferred to as the pseudo-Graefe's sign.

Traumatic Trochlear Nerve Palsy

The fourth cranial nerve is the least fre-quently injured ocular motor nerve. When involved, the nerve is damaged by contu-sion or stretching as it exits the dorsal midbrain near the anterior medullary velum. Lindenberg[47] has shown that the dorso-lateral midbrain is particularly vul-nerable in severe frontal blows against the accelerating head. In this injury, the mid-brain is displaced against the posterolateral edge of the tentorial incisura causing con-tusion, hemorrhage, and damage to one or both fourth nerves. These injuries most commonly occur in automobile and motor-cycle accidents.

Lesions of the fourth nerve have to be

differentiated from a dislocation of the orbital pulley due to direct orbital trauma. This latter injury produces a vertical diplopia mimicking a trochlear nerve palsy but the symptom rarely persists beyond a few weeks.

The prognosis for recovery in fourth nerve palsy is not good as the nerve is so slender that it is often avulsed in the traumatic process.

Traumatic Abducens Nerve Palsy

The abducens or sixth cranial nerve is injured when the head is crushed in an antero-posterior plane with resultant lateral expansion and distortion of the skull. It may also be injured along with the seventh and eighth cranial nerves in fractures of the petrous bone. In such injuries, the sixth nerve is contused, stretched, or severed as it passes below the petroclinoid ligament. Vertical movement of the brain stem during trauma may severely stretch or avulse the sixth nerve as it leaves the pons before it enters the clival dura. Delayed secondary paralysis of the nerve due to increased intracranial pressure or herniation is considered elsewhere. The abducens nerve may also be injured at the superior orbital fissure and it is invariably accompanied by third and fourth cranial nerve palsies as well.

The diagnosis of abducens palsy in the unconscious patient can be made when the affected eye 1) fails to wander outward spontaneously; 2) fails to abduct when the head is passively turned away from the side of the sixth nerve paralysis; and 3) fails to abduct in response to ipsilateral cold caloric irrigation.

Many cases of abducens palsy recover spontaneously after about four months, a period of time consistent with axonal regeneration.

Treatment of Ocular Nerve Palsies

The treatment is initially symptomatic and consists of wearing a patch over the eye to prevent troublesome diplopia. It is customary to wait for four to six months for spontaneous regeneration to take place. If recovery does not occur, then local muscle shortening procedures may be carried out in the affected eye in certain situations. In oculomotor nerve palsy, even if recovery does take place, the "misdirection phenomenon" often occurs (see above) and may cause residual disability.

Ocular Motor Disturbances in Brain Injury

A brief description of certain ocular motor disturbances due to brain stem injury is mentioned here to enable one to differentiate these from more peripheral ocular nerve injuries. Rowbotham[66] noted that apart from restlessness and unconsciousness, disturbances of ocular posture and movements are the most distinctive neurologic manifestations of concussion. In concussion there is often some resistance as the examiner attempts to open the closed eye and the corneal reflex is intact. In deep coma, the eyelids can be opened easily and the corneal reflex is often absent. Abnormal, erratic wandering eye movements are present in midbrain injuries and usually disappear if the patient regains consciousness. Focal contusions of the midbrain may occur with or without alteration in the level of consciousness.

Various manifestations of nuclear and supranuclear oculomotor palsies can occur with or without pupillary involvement and the lesions may be unilateral or bilateral. Parinaud's syndrome has also been reported by Jefferson.[38] Occasionally, Weber's syndrome may occur from a primary contusional injury but this is much more common in transtentorial cerebral herniation. Bilateral internuclear ophthalmoplegia without any other evidence of brain stem injury has been reported by Baker.[2] Holmes[31] observed a peculiar form of gaze palsy ipsilateral to the side of cerebellar injury in gunshot wounds. This was ascribed to cerebellar atonia. Nystagmus is frequently seen after head injuries when either the labyrinth or the brain stem is involved. Vertical ocular and palatal myoclonus has also been reported following severe midbrain injury.

Contusion and laceration of the frontal cerebral cortex can become manifest as a supranuclear palsy of conjugate lateral gaze. During a focal seizure following cerebral injury, the eyes deviate away from the side of the lesion and in infarction of the cerebral hemispheres, the eyes deviate toward the side of the lesion. These conjugate lateral gaze palsies are often temporary unless accompanied by extensive cerebral infarction when they may last indefinitely.

Pupillary Changes in Head Injuries

Pupillary changes in head injuries as a result of cerebral herniation have been well described. However, changes in the pupillary size and shape occur from other mechanisms as well. Widely dilated pupils that are fixed to light are seen in deeply comatose patients with severe brain injury. If the patient improves, the light response returns before the pupils return to normal size. A unilateral pupillary dilation due to an epidural hematoma in an otherwise awake patient has been reported by DiTullio.[14] Blakeslee[6] has reported that a dilated pupil is occasionally seen on the side of contrecoup laceration of the brain. A unilateral fixation of the pupil to light may be due to optic nerve injury and this can be confirmed by the absence of both direct and consensual light reflexes.

Blakeslee[6] has also reported unequal, irregular pupils with sluggish light reflexes in acute head injuries, probably due to incompletely dilated or contracted pupils. Bilateral small pupils are often seen in severe head injuries usually as a result of pontine hemorrhage. Contracted pupils in these instances are probably the result of interruption of diencephalic and reticular inhibitory influences on the Edinger-Westphal nucleus. A unilateral contracted pupil with the retention of the light reflex may be due to interruption of the sympathetic system in the brain stem, cervical spinal cord, or the neck. Eccentric pupils have also been seen in midbrain injuries and are associated with a poor prognosis. The pupil may also be involved in direct injuries to the eye. This usually manifests as a dilated irregular pupil, reacting sluggishly to light.

A dilated pupil due to cerebral herniation often corrects itself quickly once the compression is relieved. However, a dilated pupil due to contusion of the oculomotor nerve may take a long time to recover and sometimes may never return to normal.

INJURIES TO THE TRIGEMINAL NERVE AND GANGLION

The most common form of trigeminal nerve injury following head trauma involves the supraorbital and supratrochlear nerves as they emerge from the supraorbital notch and superomedial aspect of the bony orbit. Branches of these nerves may be contused or divided resulting in anesthesia of a portion of the nose, eyebrow, and forehead extending as far back as the front of the ear. Russell[11] described 45 cases of this injury in a series of 1,000 head injured patients. Often sensation is only partially affected and some recovery may be expected. Patients with incomplete supraorbital and infraorbital nerve injuries (see below) often are left with a disagreeable hyperpathia of the involved portion of the face and/or scalp. On occasions we have administered carbamazepine to these patients for pain relief but the benefits are generally modest. In rare instances it may be justifiable to explore and section a contused, irritable supraorbital nerve if pain is not alleviated by conservative methods. We have performed selective percutaneous Gasserian ganglion thermocoagulation of the second division of the trigeminal nerve for intractable post-traumatic pain in the infraorbital region but have hesitated adopting this maneuver for supraorbital pain in the first division of the trigeminal nerve because of the risks of subsequent corneal anesthesia.

In rare instances, invariably associated with severe compound fractures of the frontal bone with disruption of the frontal and ethmoidal sinuses, the nasociliary nerve may be traumatized in the posterior-superior orbit. Six patients with this disorder were described by Jefferson and Schorstein,[39] one of whom had an isolated involvement of the ciliary nerve producing only numbness of the cornea, a situation first described by Lagrange.[45]

In facial trauma, especially with maxillary fractures, the infraorbital nerve may be injured resulting in variable sensory deficits of the ipsilateral cheek, upper lip, upper gum, upper teeth, and hard palate. The incidence of injury to the maxillary division in patients with head injury is not known precisely but it is undoubtedly more common than appreciated. Russell[70] observed eight cases of infraorbital nerve injury in 1,000 instances of cranial nerve trauma while Friedman and Merritt[24] described only one such case in 430 instances of severe head trauma. On the other hand, infraorbital nerve damage is seen frequently by surgeons involved in facial reparative surgery following maxillary-mandibular fractures. Ivy and Curtis[35] reported infraorbital nerve injuries in 9 of 10 patients with severe maxillary fractures and Ungley and Suggitt[91] described seven instances of similar injury in 14 cases of severe facial fractures. In their classic treatise on trigeminal nerve injuries, Jefferson and Schorstein[40] described 32 instances of post-traumatic maxillary nerve deficits, the vast majority of which involved the infraorbital nerve at its exit from the foramen.

Injuries of the mandibular nerve and its branches following cranial trauma are not common but have been described following fractures of the horizontal ramus of the mandible[35, 39, 66] or as a sequela, usually transitory, following tooth extraction.[5, 39]

The most informative discussion of intracranial injuries involving the trigeminal ganglion is that of Jefferson and Schorstein[39] in which these authors described seven cases of trigeminal ganglion injuries produced by penetrating head wounds and two cases where shell fragments traumatized only the maxillary division intracranially. An additional nine cases of Gasserian ganglion trauma following blunt head injuries with basal fractures are described by these authors along with two instances of intracranial ophthalmic nerve injury and one case each of closed head trauma involving the maxillary and mandibular divisions. Jefferson and Schorstein[39] also compiled and reviewed 25 additional cases from the literature in which blunt head trauma resulted in ganglionic injuries. Several additional cases have been reported since that time including an instance of bilateral tri-geminal and abducens neuropathies secondary to a crush injury in a young boy.[78] Although Jefferson and Schorstein's series of 66 personally observed cases of major injuries to the trigeminal ganglion and its divisions is remarkable in terms of sheer volume of material alone, it should be noted that these patients were derived primarily from injuries sustained during the two major world wars.

The pathophysiology of blunt head trauma to the Gasserian ganglion, often associated with adjacent cranial neuropathies (*e.g.*, oculomotor, abducens) and with occasional carotid-cavernous fistulas has been speculated upon. Most injuries of this type have not been subjected to operation and *postmortem* material is scarce. Skull fractures involving the base of the middle fossa are usually transverse and may run beneath the Gasserian ganglion. Only rarely (one out of 30 specimens) do these transverse fractures enter the foramen ovale.[64]

A more likely explanation of the pathogenesis of these injuries was provided by the experiments of Russell and Schiller[71] in which skulls were crushed in the *postmortem* room and the resultant fracturing was observed. In these studies there was a backward and medial rotation of the petrous tip, a fragment of which broke off, opening up the foramen lacerum, exposing the carotid artery and traumatizing the trigeminal root and ganglion. O'Connell[56] has suggested that the trigeminal nerve is especially vulnerable where the sensory root angulates as it passes through the dural foramen proximal to Meckel's cave.

INJURIES TO THE SEVENTH AND EIGHTH CRANIAL NERVES

Trauma to cranial nerves VII (facial nerves) and VIII (auditory and vestibular nerve) is commonly seen following head injuries. The literature on this field is voluminous and controversial especially when surgical therapy is discussed. A brief description of fractures of the temporal bone follows as these usually are the cause for injuries to either nerve.

Temporal Bone Fractures

Temporal bone fractures are said to account for 15–48% of all skull fractures.[60] The actual incidence is almost certainly higher as it has been clearly shown that many temporal fractures are missed on conventional X-rays and can only be demonstrated by tomography.[39] The petrous portion of the temporal bone is particularly vulnerable in traumatic situations due to its position at the base of the skull, its compactness and the presence of cavities within it. Fractures of the petrous portion of the temporal bone are classified as transverse or vertical, longitudinal or horizontal and oblique (see also Chapter 5).

Transverse fractures occur at right angles to the long axis of the petrous pyramid. They usually result from occipital blows and may be medial or lateral in position. Medial fractures involve the internal meatus and lateral fractures involve the bony labyrinth. These fractures are associated with seventh and eighth cranial nerve palsies about 50% of the time. A hemotympanum is common. Transverse fractures account for about 10–30% of all petrous bone fractures.[86]

Longitudinal fractures of the petrous pyramid are more common and account for 70–90% of temporal bone fractures[32] (Hough 1973). They occur parallel to the long axis of the petrous pyramid and the seventh and eighth cranial nerves are often spared as the nerves lie behind the fracture line. However, these fractures are associated with ossicular chain disruption.[32, 83] This was studied experimentally and the usual injury was found in the middle ear ossicular joints, the long process of the incus, the neck of the malleus and in the crura and the foot plate of the stapes.[17] Longitudinal fractures can also extend across the midline to the opposite side, can rupture the tegmen tympani and lacerate the tympanic membrane.

Oblique fractures are rare and occur as a combination of transverse and longitudinal fractures. These fractures often do not heal well due to the endochrondral development of this bone and are often associated with CSF otorrhea, otorrhagia, and occasionally spread of infection from the middle ear. Fractures of the mastoid process also occur causing facial paralysis and even fracture dislocation of the entire petrous pyramid has been reported.[13]

Injuries to the Facial Nerve

Trauma is the second most common cause of facial paralysis after Bell's palsy.[37] The nerve may be damaged anywhere along its course, although damage within the temporal bone is the most common site. Thirty to 50% of patients with a transverse petrous fracture and 10–25% of patients with a longitudinal fracture have an associated facial nerve injury. In transverse fractures, the nerve may be sectioned at the internal auditory meatus and more commonly in the horizontal portion of the fallopian canal on the medial wall of the tympanum. In longitudinal fractures, the nerve can be involved at the geniculate ganglion or immediately distal to it in the tympanic portion of the facial canal. Injury to the nerve before it enters the internal meatus is rare in head injuries and is more commonly associated with cerebello-pontine angle mass lesions. Lacerating injuries of the face can cause total or partial paralysis of the face depending on the branches involved.

Pathophysiology of Traumatic Facial Nerve Paralysis. Traumatic facial paralysis may be immediate, delayed, or mixed. The immediate type is probably due to an anatomical disruption of the nerve caused by splinters of bone or tearing of the nerve fascicles themselves from a fractured petrous bone. The delayed type of facial nerve trauma is seen an average of 2–3 days after injury but may occur as early as one day following injury or as late as two weeks after injury.[59] It is probably due to swelling of the nerve within its fibrous sheath or epineurium,[42] damage to the surrounding vasculature, or arterial spasm. External compression of the nerve by expanding hematoma fluid[38] or edema of loose fibrous tissue and periosteum between the nerve and the bony facial canal may also be responsible for the delayed onset. Although the nerve is structurally intact in these cases, prolonged compression of the nerve may result in incomplete recovery. In the mixed group an immediate incomplete paresis of the nerve is followed a few days later by complete paralysis.[59]

Methods of Diagnosis. A detailed systematic clinical examination of the facial nerve and its branches can be performed to pinpoint the location of damage to the nerve in the fallopian canal. The testing should include tear production by Schirmer test (greater superficial petrosal nerve), saliva secretion and taste in the anterior two-thirds of the tongue (chorda tympani), and the reflex reaction of the stapedius muscle. The methods of performing these tests and interpretation of the results have been summarized by Miehlke.[49]

Electrodiagnostic studies of the injured facial nerve should be done promptly in every case to serve as a baseline for subsequent follow-up examinations. Electromyography of the face, the transcutaneous nerve excitability test (NET), and evoked EMG are the methods favored at present. The NET test was found very useful by Miehlke[49] who could accurately predict irreversible nerve injury by noting the difference between the normal and injured side. When this difference is significant (3.5–4 mA) it is inferred that irreversible changes have begun in the nerve and operative intervention is offered. However, this opinion is not shared by others.[96] An ideal prognostic test for facial paralysis has not yet been found.

Radiologic studies should include polytomography of the petrous pyramid in at least two views to delineate the site of fracture.

Neurootologic tests of hearing and of labyrinthine function should be carried out in all cases of facial paralysis because of the high incidence of associated injury to these structures.

Management. The "watchful expectancy" approach in the management of facial paralysis has gained wide acceptance among neurologists and neurosurgeons. The vast majority of patients with traumatic facial paralyses in most series make a good spontaneous recovery.[59, 66, 88] Even where recovery is not complete, it is often

sufficient to satisfy many patients. The many types of peripheral supportive devices in the form of hooks and dental bars to support the sagging face do not achieve their goal and are not recommended, especially in the waiting period. Reassurance regarding the chances of recovery and active exercises in front of a mirror, in instances of partial paralysis, are helpful. Electrical stimulation of the muscles of the face ("galvanism") and massage are of no value except possibly for psychological purposes. The eye on the paralyzed side of the face must be carefully watched lest exposure keratitis develops.

The widespread use of the microscope and micro-techniques has attracted many surgeons (mostly otologists) to explore, decompress, or suture the nerve directly or with a cable graft as the situation demands. Before discussing briefly the timing and techniques available, it should be stated explicitly that the exact role of these direct surgical methods is far from settled and the question of whether a given surgical procedure is an "interesting technique" or an obligatory therapeutic maneuver is controversial.

In facial paralysis due to temporal fractures, Miehlke[49] prefers to wait for three or four days after the injury for the patient's condition to stabilize. From then on, depending on the results of the electrodiagnostic tests, operative intervention is carried out as soon as there is significantly diminished nerve conduction on the injured side. Harker and McCabe[29] carry out an exploration of the nerve three weeks after an immediate type of facial paralysis occurs and persists. In immediate types, exploration is not performed if there is no evidence of degeneration in EMG's. In the delayed type of paralysis, exploration is recommended soon after the onset of the paralysis.

The surgical methods employed include decompression of the nerve and nerve suturing either directly or with a cable graft to bridge the nerve defect. In delayed types of facial paralysis, only decompression is required. In immediate types with degeneration, if the nerve is found to be transected, meticulous microsuturing is carefully carried out to approximate the nerve fascicles. According to Millesi,[51] the suturing should be done without tension and the epineurium should be resected for 5 mm from the suture site.

Various grafting techniques have also been used. Fisch[21] has carried out 79 grafting procedures (32 extratemporal, 42 intratemporal and 5 intracranial) with good results. When the nerve is transected outside the stylomastoid foramen, grafting has been done with the sural or great auricular nerves.[11, 49, 61]

Hypoglossal-facial anastomosis[22] and a sural nerve graft from the pre-meatal facial nerve stump to the facial nerve distal to the stylomastoid foramen.[16] constitute other technical methods which are available. Plastic surgical procedures on the face in the form of "slings" and "face lift operations" can be performed in selected cases when the facial paralysis has been determined to be permanent or when neural repair is not feasible.

Injuries to Cranial Nerve VIII

Hearing and labyrinthine dysfunction occur in head injuries due to damage to the auditory and/or vestibular nerves (cranial nerve VIII), their end organs or trauma to the middle ear and conducting elements such as the ossicular chain. This discussion is limited to injuries of the nerve and end organs. A detailed discussion of trauma to the middle ear and ossicular chain is beyond the scope of this chapter.

Trauma to the Inner Ear. Transverse fractures of the temporal bone may cause disruption of the auditory and vestibular end organs or a concussion of these structures may produce transient eighth nerve dysfunction. The disabilities may be aggravated by associated injuries to the central auditory and vestibular pathways in the brain stem. In transverse fractures of the petrous bone, the anterior portion of the vestibule and the basilar turn of the cochlea are often damaged and many of these patients will have an accompanying facial paralysis. Patients with a fracture involving the otic capsule will often develop total degeneration of the cochlear and vestibular end organs.

It has been noted that a blow to the head creates a pressure wave which is transmitted through the petrous bone to the cochlea and that minor blows to the mastoid region resulted in temporary high tone hearing loss and tinnitus.[19] Schuknecht[74] described hair cell damage in the cochlea in head injured cats. As the severity of the blow increased, he noted histologic distortion of the outer hair cells, then loss of outer hair cells, finally loss of inner hair cells and degeneration of cochlear neurons.

Clinical Aspects. A simple neurootologic evaluation should be carried out in every patient with a head injury as soon as conditions permit. Unfortunately, in some seriously injured patients with systemic injuries such an evaluation may not be possible for a long time. However, even in minor head injuries, a baseline neurootological evaluation should be done for early detection of hearing loss and labyrinthine dysfunction. In conscious patients such an examination includes a good history, especially with regard to any previous otological problems, and a detailed analysis of the type of injury. Specific questions should be asked with regard to dizziness, vertigo, nausea, tinnitus, and impaired hearing. The bedside examination should include a search for CSF otorrhea, otorrhagia, and bruising over the mastoid (Battle's sign). At times CSF may accumulate behind an intact tympanic membrane and this condition is referred to as liquor tympanum. An otoscopic examination can be done if there is no obvious blood in the external canal obscuring vision. Tuning fork tests of hearing function and speech discrimination can also be carried out. If any abnormalities are detected, more thorough laboratory investigations of hearing and vestibular functions are in order. All patients should have their facial nerve function assessed at the same time.

Lacerations of the tympanic membrane and external auditory canal occur in about 58% of cases with longitudinal fractures.[86] Most will heal spontaneously. Ossicular chain disruptions occur for the most part in longitudinal fractures and these can be corrected surgically.[32, 86]

Vestibular symptoms are often not fully evaluated with caloric stimulation in the acute phase for fear of introducing infection in the presence of a perforated drum. If significant vestibular symptoms persist, these tests should be done once the patient is stable and has no perforation of the tympanic membrane. In a conscious individual the absence of nystagmus on caloric testing indicates damage to the vestibular nerve or end organ.

Auditory symptoms following head trauma are mainly those of tinnitus and impaired hearing. Tinnitus has been reported in 30–70% of patients with head injuries.[26, 40, 60]

Hearing loss of some degree following head trauma has been reported in over one-half of patients with serious head injuries. In the majority of cases, hearing loss is of a sensorineural type, the conductive variety accounting for only about 3% of cases.[3] A conductive hearing loss is usually temporary when caused by a hemotympanum and resolves as the hematoma is absorbed.

Laboratory Investigation. The main radiologic investigation in instances of serious head injury with eighth nerve dysfunction consists of X-rays of the skull followed by polytomography of the petrous bone in at least two views to show the otic capsule, ossicular chain, and the facial canal. CT of the posterior fossa with appropriate window levels to demonstrate the petrous bone may also be helpful.

Labyrinthine function is best assessed by caloric stimulation and electronystagmography. Auditory function is investigated further by audiometry, pure tone air conduction, pure tone bone conduction, speech discrimination and Bekesy audiometry. With these tests one can easily differentiate sensorineural hearing loss from conductive deafness.

Treatment and Prognosis. The prognosis for impaired hearing of the conductive type due to hemotympanum or ossicular chain disruption is usually good. Hemotympanum usually resolves spontaneously and ossicular chain disruption can be corrected surgically in most cases. The prognosis of sensorineural deafness is poor. Some improvement may occur with partial lesions. Tinnitus is usually self-limited, but occasionally becomes a disabling symptom.

Labyrinthine symptoms of dizziness, nausea, and vertigo usually subside in 6 to 12 weeks. If intractable vertigo persists along with sensorineural hearing loss, a tympanotomy may be done to rule out a perilymph fistula.[20] Labyrinthine sedatives, such as prochlorperazine, along with avoidance of sudden change of posture and firm reassurance, are the only means available for treatment of the minor types of dizziness, vertigo and nausea that are seen so frequently following trivial head injuries. These usually subside in time.

INJURIES TO THE GLOSSOPHARYNGEAL, VAGUS, SPINAL ACCESSORY AND HYPOGLOSSAL NERVES

The 9th, 10th, and 11th cranial nerves together with the internal jugular vein emerge through the jugular foramen at the base of the skull. The hypoglossal foramen, through which the 12th nerve passes, lies just medial to the jugular foramen. In this area at the skull base, the muscles attached to the styloid process and the parotid lie anteriorly and the carotid artery is in close proximity. An extracranial insult to the lower four cranial nerves, which may spare the major vessels, has been described most often as a consequence of gunshot wounds.[10, 52, 53, 58, 75, 92] Unilateral paralysis of the last four cranial nerves which may be traumatic, inflammatory or secondary to a neoplastic compression[4] is referred to as the Collet-Sicard syndrome.[23]

The symptomatology produced by an injury in this region can be inferred from the anatomy and function of the lower four cranial nerves. It consists of cardiac irregularities, excessive salivation, loss of sensation, and gag reflex of the ipsilateral palate, loss of taste sensation of the posterior third of the tongue, a hoarse voice with paralysis of the ipsilateral vocal cord, some dysphagia and hemiatrophy of the tongue with deviation to the side of the injury. Additional symptoms and signs may be present if neighboring structures (*e.g.*, the carotid artery, internal jugular vein, styloid process, facial nerve, etc.) are also involved in the traumatic process. Jefferson and Schorstein[39] have described one instance following a gunshot wound to the cheek which produced palsies of the ipsilateral 9th, 10th, 11th, and 12th nerves plus section of the lingual nerve. A suboccipital arteriovenous fistula was also present involving the vertebral artery and this was obliterated.

In instances of a pure Collet-Sicard syndrome, the treatment is usually expectant. Therapy consists of drainage of excess saliva by proper positioning, measures to control tachycardia if present and intravenous or nasogastric fluids and semi-solids in the days immediately following the injury.

References

1. Arseni, M.C., Lasco, F., Nicolesco, M.: Les lesions indirectes du nerf optique dans les traumatismes cranio-cérebraux fermés. Rev. Oto-Neuro-Ophthal., 32:321–335, 1960.
2. Baker, R.S.: Internuclear ophthalmoplegia following head injury. Case Report. J. Neurosurg., 51:552–555, 1979.
3. Barber, H.O.: Head injury. Audiological and vestibular findings. Ann. Otol. (St. Louis), 78:239–252, 1969.
4. Beck, J.C., Hassin, G.B.: A case of combined extracranial paralysis of cerebral nerves. Med. Rec. (N.Y.), 88:308, 1915.
5. Bell, C.: The nervous system of the human body. London, 1830.
6. Blakeslee, G.A.: Eye manifestations in fracture of the skull. Arch. Ophthal. (Chicago), 2:566–572, 1929.
7. Brändle, V.K.: Die posttraumatischen opticus-schädigungen (Insbeson-dere die opticusatrophie) Confin. Neurol. (Basel), 15:169–208, 1955.
8. Brihaye, J.: Lésions des nerfs optiques dans lés traumatismes fermés du crâne. Acta Chir. Belg., 53:891–912, 1954.
9. Byrnes, D.P.: Head injury and the dilated pupil. Am. Surg., 45:139–143, 1979.
10. Collet: Sur un nouveau syndrome paralytique pharyngo-larynge par blessure de guerre. (Hemiplégie glosso-laryngo-scapulo-pharyngée). Lyon. Med., 124:121–129, 1915.
11. Conley, J.J.: Facial nerve grafting. Arch. Otolaryng., 73:322–327, 1961.
12. Crompton, M.R.: Visual lesions in closed head injury. Brain, 93:785–792, 1970.
13. DeVilliers, J.C.: Fracture-dislocation of the petrous temporal bone. J. Neurol. Neurosurg. Psych., 34:105–106, 1971.
14. DiTullio, M.V. Jr.: Epidural hematoma with complete third nerve paralysis in an awake patient. Surg. Neurol., 7:193–194, 1977.
15. Dott, N.M.: Facial paralysis-restitution by extrapetrous nerve graft. Proc. Roy. Soc. Med., 51:900–902, 1958.
16. Dott, N.M.: Facial nerve reconstruction by graft bypassing the petrous bone. Arch. Otolaryng., 78:426–428, 1963.
17. Duerrer, J., Busek, J., Zemek, J.: Mechanical changes of the ossicular chain due to head injury. Pract. Oto-Rhino-Laryng. (Basel), 32:293–296, 1970.
18. Duke-Elder, S., Scott, G.I.: Neuropathology. In: System of Ophthalmology, 2nd Ed. Vol. 12, Duke-Elder, Ed., Henry Kimpton, London, 1971.
19. Escher, F.: Die otologische Beurteilung des Schädeltraumatikers. Basel, S. Karger, 1948.
20. Fee, G.A.: Traumatic perilymphatic fistulas. Arch. Otolaryng., 88:477–480, 1968.
21. Fisch, U.: Facial nerve grafting. Otolaryng. Clin. N. Amer., 7:517–529, 1974.
22. Fisch, U., Hof, E.: Die hypoglossus-fasialis-anastomose. Méd. et Hyg. (Genève), 31:450–452, 1973.
23. Fishbone, H.: Irreversible injury of the last four cranial nerves. (Collet Sicard syndrome). Handbook of Neurology, Chap. 8, P.G. Vinken, G.W. Bruyn, Eds., American Elsevier Publishing Co., New York, 1976, pp. 179–181.
24. Friedman, A.P., Merritt, H.H.: Damage to cranial nerves resulting from head injury. Bull. L.A. Neurol. Soc., 9:135–139, 1944.
25. Fukado, Y.: Diagnosis and surgical correction of optic canal fracture after head injury. Ophthalmologica. Additanent ad. 158:307–314, 1969.
26. Gaillard, L.: Les séquelles cochleo-vestibulaires des traumatismes crâniens fermés; étude clinique et médico-légale. Masson & Cie, Paris, 1961.
27. Gjerris, F.: Traumatic lesions of the visual pathways. In: Handbook of Neurology, Vol. 24, Chap. 2, P.J. Vinken, G.W. Bruyn, Eds., Am. Elsevier Pub. Co., 1976, New York, pp. 27–57.
28. Habal, M.B.: Clinical observations on the isolated optic nerve injury. Ann. Plast. Surg., 1:603–607, 1978.
29. Harker, L.A., McCabe, B.F.: Temporal bone fractures and facial nerve injury. Otolaryng. Clin. N. Am., 7:425–431, 1974.
30. Heinze, J.: Cranial nerve avulsion and other neural injuries in road accidents. Med. J. Aust., 2:1246–1249, 1969.
31. Holmes, G.: Symptoms of acute cerebellar injuries due to gunshot injuries. Brain, 40:461–535, 1917.
32. Hough, J.V.D., Stuart, W.D.: Middle ear injuries in skull trauma. Laryngoscope, 78:899–937, 1968.
33. Hughes, B.: Acute injuries of the head, their diagnosis, treatment, complications and sequels, 4th Ed. G.F. Rowbootham, Ed., Williams & Wilkins, Baltimore, 1964, pp. 408–433.
34. Hughes, B.: Indirect injury of the optic nerves and chiasma. Bull. Johns Hopkins Hosp., 111:98–126, 1962.
35. Ivy, R.H., Curtis, L.: Fractures of the Jaws, 3rd Ed. Lea, London, 1945.
36. Jampel, R.S.: Use of corticosteroids in neuroophthalmology. Int. Ophthal. Clin., 6:903–913, 1966.
37. Jaspen, O.: Thesis, Univ. of Aarhus, Denmark, 1955.
38. Jefferson, A.: Ocular complications of head injuries. Trans Ophthal. Soc. U.K., 81:595–612, 1961.
39. Jefferson, G., Schorstein, J.: Injuries of the trigeminal nerve, its ganglion and its divisions. Br. J. Surg., 42:561–581, 1955.

40. Jemmi, C.: Manifestazioni Auricolari dei Traumi Cranio-Cerebrali. A. Cordani, Milano, 1947.
41. Johnson, J.C., Lubow, M., Stears, J.: Polytomography of the optic chiasm and adjacent structures. Radiology, 114:629–634, 1975.
42. Jongkees, L.B.W.: On peripheral facial nerve paralysis. Arch. Otolaryng., 95:317–323, 1972.
43. Kalyanaraman, S., Ramamoorthy, K., Ramamurthi, B.: An analysis of two thousand cases of head injury. Neurology (Bombay), 18, Suppl., 1:3–11, 1970.
44. Kier, E.L.: Embryology of the normal optic canal and its anamolies. An anatomic and roentgenographic study. Invest. Radiol., 1:346–362, 1966.
45. Lagrange, F.: Fractures of the orbit and injuries to the eye in war. Military Medical Manuals, London, 1918.
46. Lillie, W.I., Adson, A.W.: Unilateral central and annular scotoma produced by callus from fracture extending into optic canal. Arch. Ophthal., 12:500–506, 1934.
47. Lindenberg, R.: Significance of the tentorium in head injuries from blunt forces. Clin. Neurosurg., 12:129–142, 1966.
48. Loewenstein, A.: Marginal hemorrhage on the disc. Partial cross-tearing of the optic nerve. Clinical and histological features. Br. J. Ophthal., 27:208–221, 1943.
49. Miehlke, A.: Recognition and management of facial nerve palsies of operative and traumatic origin. Proc. Roy. Soc. Med., 66:549–554, 1973.
50. Miller, G.R., Tenzel, R.R.: Ocular complications of midfacial fractures. Plast. Reconst. Surg., 39:37–42, 1967.
51. Millesi, H., Meissl, G., Berger, A.: The interfascicular nerve-grafting of the median and ulnar nerves. J. Bone Joint Surg., 54:727–750, 1972.
52. Mohanty, S.K., Barrios, M., Fishbone, H., Khatib, R.: Irreversible injury of cranial nerves 9 through 12. (Collet-Sicard Syndrome). Case report. J. Neurosurg., 38:86–88, 1973.
53. New, G.B.: Laryngeal paralysis associated with the jugular foramen syndrome and other syndromes. Am. J. Med. Sci., 165:727–737, 1923.
54. Niho, S., Niho, M., Niho, K.: Decompression of the optic canal by the transethmoidal route and decompression of the superior orbital fissure. Can. J. Ophthal., 5:22–40, 1970.
55. Obenchain, T.G., Killeffer, F.A., Stern, W.E.: Indirect injury of the optic nerves and chiasm with closed head injury. Bull. Los Angeles Neurol. Soc., 38:13–20, 1973.
56. O'Connell, J.E.A.: Trigeminal false localizing signs and their causation. Brain, 101:119–142, 1978.
57. Park, J.H., Frenkel, M., Dobbie, J.G., Choromokos, E.: Evulsion of the optic nerve. Am. J. Ophthal., 72:969–971, 1971.
58. Pollock, L.J.: Extracranial injuries of multiple cranial nerves. Arch. Neurol. Psychiat., 4:517–528, 1920.
59. Potter, J.M.: Facial palsy following head injury. J. Laryng. Otology, 78:654–657, 1964.
60. Proctor, B., Gurdjian, E.S., Webster, J.E.: The ear in head trauma. Laryngoscope, 66:16–59, 1956.
61. Pulec, J.L.: Total decompression of the facial nerve. Laryngoscope, 76:1015–1028, 1969.
62. Raja, I.A.: Aneurysm-induced third nerve palsy. J. Neurosurg., 36:548–551, 1972.
63. Rasquin, P.: Les anosmies traumatiques. Acta Oto-Rhino-Laryngologica Belg., 29:1159–1169, 1975.
64. Rawling, L.B.: The surgery of the skull and brain. Oxford Medical Publications, 1912.
65. Rodger, F.C.: Unilateral involvement of the optic nerve in head injuries. Br. J. Ophthal., 27:23–33, 1943.
66. Rowbotham, G.F.: Acute Injuries of the Head. 4th Ed. E&S Livingstone, London, 1964.
67. Rowe, N.L., Killey, H.C.: Fractures of the Facial Skeleton. 2nd Ed. E&S Livingstone, London, 1968.
68. Rucker, C.W.: The causes of paralysis of the third, fourth and sixth cranial nerves. Am. J. Ophthal., 61:1293–1298, 1966.
69. Russell, W.R.: In: Injuries of the Brain and Spinal Cord and their Coverings. 4th Ed., S. Brock, Ed., Springer-Verlag, New York, 1960.
70. Russell, W.R.: Injury to the cranial nerves and optic chiasm. In: Brock's Injuries of the Brain and Spinal Cord, 3rd Ed. Williams & Wilkins, Baltimore, 1960, p. 121.
71. Russell, W.R., Schiller, F.: Crushing injuries to the skull: clinical and experimental observations. J.Neurol., Neurosurg., Psych., 12:52–60, 1949.
72. Sarteschi, P., Ardito, R.: L'utilita dell olfattoelettroencefalografia nella obbiette-vazione delle anosmie. Riv. Neurol. (Nap), 30:555–557, 1960.
73. Scheschy, H., Benedikt, O.: Optikusatrophie durch indirekte traumen. Klin. Monatsbl. Augenheilkd., 161:309–315, 1972.
74. Schuknecht, H.F.: Mechanisms of inner ear injury from blows to the head. Ann. Otol., 78:253–262, 1969.
75. Sicard, J.A.: Syndrome du carrefour condylo-déchiŕe postérieur (type pur de paralysee laryngée associee). Marseille Med., 53:383, 1917.
76. Sollmann, H.: Die traumatische schadigurg des fasciculus opticus aus der sicht des neurochirurgen. Dtsch. Gesundh. - wes, 23:537–543, 1968.
77. Sugita, S., Sugita, Y., Yamada, J., Kawabe, Y.: Die sehstorung nach schadeltrauma und ihre operative behandlung. Klin. Monatsbl. Augenheilkd., 147:720–730, 1965.
78. Summers, C.G., Wirtschafter, J.D.: Bilateral trigeminal and abducens neuropathies following low-velocity, crushing head injury. J. Neurosurg., 50:508–511, 1979.
79. Sumner, D.: On testing the sense of smell. Lancet, 2:895–903, 1962.
80. Sumner, D.: Post-traumatic anosmia. Brain, 87:107–120, 1964.
81. Symonds, C.P.: Cranial nerve palsies in otitis media: the syndrome of the posterior fossa. J. Laryng., 52:656–664, 1927.
82. Taveras, J.M., Wood, E.G.: *Diagnostic Neuroradiology.* Williams & Wilkins, Baltimore, 1964.
83. Thorburn, I.B.: Post-traumatic conductive deafness. J. Laryng. Otol. 71:542–545, 1957.
84. Tibbs, P.A., Brooks, W.H.: Traumatic bitemporal hemianopsia: case report. J. Trauma, 19:129–131, 1979.
85. Toglia, J.U., Katinsky, S.: Neuro-otological as-

pects of closed head injury. In: Handbook of Clinical Neurology, Vol. 24, Am. Elsevier Publ., 1976, pp. 119–140.

86. Tos, M.: Fractures of the temporal bone. The course and sequele of 248 fractures of the petrous temporal bone. Ugeskr. Laeg., 133:1449–1456, 1971.

87. Traquair, H.M., Dott, N.M., Russell, W.R.: Traumatic lesions of the optic chiasma. Brain, 58:398–411, 1935.

88. Turner, J.W.A.: Facial palsy in closed head injuries. Lancet, 1:756–757, 1944.

89. Turner, J.W.A.: Indirect injuries of the optic nerve. Brain, 66:140–151, 1943.

90. Uetsuka, H.: Compression of the facial nerve. Arch. Otolaryng. 95:346–349, 1972.

91. Ungley, H.G., Suggit, S.C.: Fractures of the zygomatic tripod. Br. J. Surg., 32:287–299, 1944.

92. Vernet, M.: The syndrome of the foramen lacerum posterius. Paris Med., 7:78, 1917.

93. Walsh, F.B., Hoyt, W.F.: Clinical Neuro-Ophthalmology, Vol. 3, 3rd Ed., Williams & Wilkins, Baltimore, 1969.

94. Walsh, F.B., Lindenberg, R.: Die verauderungen des sehnerven bel indirekteim trauma. In: Entwicklung and Fortschritt in der Augnehellkunde. Ferdinand Enke, Stuttgard, 1963.

95. Watson, P.G., Holt-Wilson, A.D.: The traumatic orbital apex syndrome its differential diagnosis and treatment. Trans. Ophthal. Soc. U.K., 88:361–374, 1968.

96. Yanagihara, N., Kishimoto, M.: Electrodiagnosis in facial palsy. Arch. Otolaryng., 95:376–382, 1972.

8

Intracranial Pressure: Physiology and Pathophysiology

ANTHONY MARMAROU
KAMRAN TABADDOR

Under normal physiologic conditions, the pressure of the cerebrospinal fluid (CSF) that bathes the brain and circulates within the craniospinal axis is maintained below 15 mm Hg mean pressure. With trauma or disease, the normal homeostatic mechanisms controlling this pressure level may be disturbed and lead to a relentless increase of intracranial pressure (ICP) and eventual neurological death. Much has been written on the proposed mechanisms which govern this process; yet the exact sequence of events leading to pressure instability are poorly understood. It is the purpose of this chapter to review some of the more recent concepts underlying the physics of the intracranial cavity and attempt to explain how these principles are brought together in a unified theory which helps us to understand the dynamics of ICP.

THEORETICAL CONSIDERATIONS

Measurement of the ICP

The CSF pressure measured from a needle introduced into the CSF space may be defined, according to Davson,[3] as the pressure which must be exerted just to prevent the escape of fluid. Early studies used a glass manometer for measurement which in many cases smoothed the pulsatile variation of pressure. The introduction of low compliant strain gauge transducers enabled investigators to record pressure fluctuations with greater fidelity and the definition of ICP was extended to include these fluctuations. Thus, the normal ICP can be defined as a steady-state level reference to atmosphere upon which there is superimposed cardiac and respiratory components. Accurate specification of the ICP should include measurement of the baseline level as well as the amplitude of the rhythmic components (Fig. 8.1).

Classifications of ICP Dynamics into "Steady" and "Transient" State

If the ICP is observed for a long period of time and is unchanging, the system or combination of mechanisms governing the ICP is in equilibrium or "steady state." The ICP measured during this period of equilibrium may be defined as the "steady-state ICP." The abrupt change of ICP from a stable level, perhaps in response to a sudden change in volume, can be classified as the "transient ICP." It is necessary to distinguish between steady state and transient when we are discussing ICP, since it is conceivable that the mechanisms which govern the baseline or "steady-state ICP level" are different than those controlling the transient response of pressure.

Is there a form of ICP control? We know that if fluid is added or withdrawn from the CSF space, pressure will change transiently

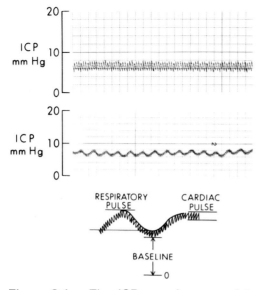

Figure 8.1. The ICP waveform consists of a respiratory and cardiac pulse superimposed upon a steady-state level which is above atmosphere. The upper panel displays the ICP at fast paper speed to accentuate the cardiac pulsation. Specification of ICP should include a measure of both baseline level and amplitude of pulsatile components.

from its initial value, followed by a gradual reduction to the pre-disturbance level. Ryder et al.[25] viewed this as a form of "dynamic control." They and other workers recognized that the magnitude of pressure change or "transient response" was somehow related to the elasticity of the intracranial contents and the persistent seepage of fluid into or out of the CSF space. However, the individual effects of these ongoing processes upon the ICP were difficult to isolate since formation, absorption, and elasticity seemed mutually interactive and their combined effects upon the ICP hydrodynamically complex.

One approach to a problem is to attempt a simulation or model of the system with the objective of isolating the mechanisms which control pressure. Theoretically, it is also possible using a modeling technique to uncover specific mechanisms or combinations of events which lead to instability and a relentless increase of pressure. The next

section will describe some of the progress made in the formulation of a theoretical pressure model of the CSF system.

A Theoretical Model of the ICP in the Steady State

In the condition of physiologic equilibrium, both the baseline ICP and the amplitude of the pulsatile component of ICP remain constant. This infers that the net intracranial volume is also in a state of dynamic equilibrium or steady state. If volume is removed or added to the system, the net seepage of fluid into or out of the CSF spaces will be in a direction which returns pressure to its steady-state value. Realizing that this must occur in a system where fluid is continually formed and absorbed, how does this volume interchange take place, and what factors govern the baseline level of ICP? These questions were addressed in a mathematical model of the cerebrospinal fluid system which subdivided the physical mechanisms into three major categories: mechanisms associated with *CSF formation*, the properties of the fluid storage or *compliance mechanism* and mechanisms dealing with *fluid absorption* (Fig. 8.2).

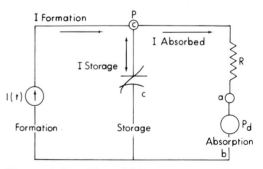

Figure 8.2. The CSF system was depicted by an equivalent electrical circuit that distributed the CSF parameters among three fundamental mechanisms: formation, represented by a constant current generator; storage, represented by a non-linear capacitance (*C*); and absorption represented by the resistance element (*R*). The venous outflow site (dural sinus) was represented by a constant pressure source P_D. The system equations were derived from this configuration.

Conceptually, the formation of CSF was depicted as a fluid pump which continuously introduces fluid into the CSF space of the neuraxis. The rate of formation of fluid was considered constant and independent of the pressure head seen by the pump mechanism, in accordance with observations that the rate of CSF formation is minimally, if at all, affected by changes in the ICP.

According to this model, the newly formed fluid entered a compliant storage space which could expand to accommodate the added volume or proceed *via* outflow pathways to be absorbed across the arachnoid villi into the venous sinuses.

The compliance mechanism was represented by an element (C) which decreased its contractibility with increasing volume, much like the increased resistance offered by a rubber balloon at maximum inflation. The resistance of both the CSF channels leading to the arachnoid villi and the resistance of the villi to fluid flow was combined into a single resistive element (R). This component represented the total resistance to outflow of CSF which, under normal conditions, was considered to remain fixed and independent of ICP.

The final element of this model was the representation of the dural sinus pressure as a pressure source positioned at the exit point of the absorptive pathway. Dural sinus pressure (P_D) was viewed as the exit pressure of the CSF system.

From this conceptual framework, a theory was developed to describe the interaction of the formation, storage, and absorptive elements in the steady state. First, with both pressure and volume in equilibrium there can be no net increase or decrease in the total volume of the CSF space. This implied that the amount of fluid formed passes through the absorptive element so that no fluid is stored and the total volume contained within the CSF space remains constant ($I_{\text{formation}} = I_{\text{absorbed}}$, $I_{\text{stored}} = 0$).

Since all fluid formed passes through the resistive element (R), a pressure gradient will be developed across the absorptive element which is equal to the product of fluid flow (CSF formation) and the fluidic resistance (R). The greater the magnitude of flow or resistance, the greater the pressure gradient ($I_a \times R$). As long as a condition of equilibrium is imposed upon the system, the pressure of the CSF space must be of sufficient magnitude to continuously force all newly formed fluid through the arachnoid villi and overcome the exit pressure. This requires that the CSF pressure (ICP) be equal to the sum of the pressure gradients developed by the absorptive element ($I_a \times R$) and the exit pressure (ICP $= I_a \times R + P_D$).

Thus, the steady-state ICP is proportional to three parameters: the rate of CSF formation, the resistance to CSF absorption, and the dural sinus pressure. When these parameters remain constant, the ICP level remains unchanged.

How is this dynamic equilibrium altered in cases of raised ICP? According to the model, a sustained elevation of pressure can develop with an increase in CSF formation, an increase of outflow resistance, or an increase in the venous pressure at the site of fluid absorption. Our computer studies show that the contribution of the product of outflow resistance and formation rate ($I_f \times R_0$) of the ICP is approximately 10%. The remainder is attributed to the magnitude of dural sinus pressure (P_D). With this distribution, the outflow resistance would have to increase markedly in order to effect a significant rise in the ICP. In contrast, elevations of sagittal sinus pressure by venous sinus obstruction would be transmitted directly to the CSF system, resulting in an increase of resting ICP level. Since the increase in P_D equals the change in ICP, the gradient across the arachnoid villi is not altered, CSF absorption remains constant, and the equilibrium shift to a higher ICP level is sustained. This concept is supported by the work of Johnston et al.,[8] who demonstrated normal CSF resistance in the presence of raised ICP induced by venous obstruction.

The resistance to outflow of CSF (R) is a function of both geometric and pressure factors. When outflow tracts of subarachnoid space and ventricular outflow tracts to subarachnoid space are patent, free flow of CSF can occur to either the spinal subarachnoid space or arachnoid villi, and rapid outflow with decrease in the ICP can occur. The outflow resistance will increase when occlusion of the CSF pathways occur either due to herniation of the brain, inflammation, subarachnoid hemorrhage, or ventricular obstructions. Under these conditions, it is postulated that the rise in ICP due to increased (R) will be proportional to the (formation × resistance) product of the steady state ICP equation.

Pressure/Volume Interactions; Intracranial Compliance

By definition, the steady-state analysis of ICP infers that the intracranial compartments which include blood, brain, and CSF remain in a condition of pressure and volume equilibrium. With homeostasis, a net increase or decrease of the volume within the storage element described in the model does not occur. However, pathologic settings are often associated with net changes in volume within the neuraxis. The Monroe-Kellie doctrine is the basis for understanding volume-pressure interaction and states that an increase in volume of one intracranial compartment (blood, brain, or CSF) must be compensated by a decrease in one or more of the other compartments so that total volume remains fixed. When this volume alteration involves the CSF space, the fluid pressure of the CSF is changed, and the magnitude of pressure change will depend on the amount of volume and the rate at which the interchange takes place. The change in CSF volume per unit change in pressure defines the "extensibility" of the CSF space and within the rigid skull this extensibility is provided by the resilient properties of the vasculature. In physical terms, the extensibility is quantified by a compliance ($\Delta V/\Delta P$) or the reciprocal term elastance ($\Delta V/\Delta P$) which can be derived from the slope of the CSF volume *vs.* pressure curve obtained by adding known amounts of fluid into the CSF space and recording the rise in pressure.

Many inanimate containers have "ideal" elastic properties. Such properties include a coefficient of compliance which does not vary with time and is constant for all degrees of expansion of the container. In such an "ideal" container, pressure varies linearly with volume and the slope of the volume pressure curve ($\Delta V/\Delta P$) or compliance is a constant. Pressure and volume in the CSF compartment are not linearly related. For equal volume increments the ($\Delta V/\Delta P$) ratio, or compliance decreases as pressure increases. This was first demonstrated by Ryder *et al.*,[25] who described the general form of the curve as "hyperbolic."

The relationship between neuraxis volume and ICP is hyperbolic up to an ICP of approximately 50 mm Hg. When pressure exceeds 50 mm Hg, the curve tends to flatten as the arterial blood pressure is approached and over the entire range of ICP the CSF pressure-volume curve may be described by a sigmoid shaped curve.[14]

Our studies have confirmed this non-linear relationship between pressure and volume. The analysis of the hydrodynamics involved in this process supports Ryder's concept of dynamic equilibrium. When volume is added or withdrawn from the CSF space, the reaction is completely reversible and both pressure and volume gradually return to their original resting level. Thus, the pressure-volume curve, in addition to providing an index of compliance, can be interpreted as a graphic representation of the trajectory that pressure must follow in response to transient changes in volume. For this reason, the P/V curve is of fundamental importance in the understanding of mechanisms leading to sustained elevations of the ICP. A stable ICP is analogous to a point (Q_1) of the exponential CSF pressure-volume curve which remains stable.[16] Small perturbations in volume such as those produced by vascular pulsation will cause the point to shift back and forth on the trajectory described by the P/V curve. The corresponding changes in pressure can be evaluated by projecting onto the pressure axis. A permanent increase of the ICP level represents a shift of the operating point to a new location of the curve (Q_2). The same perturbations in volume at raised ICP will result in an increase of the magnitude of pulsations due to the increased slope. Compliance then is not uniform throughout the range of pressure. As volume is measured, the slope tends toward the pressure axis which accounts for the increased pulse pressure observed at high levels of ICP. Because of the changing slope, the numerical value

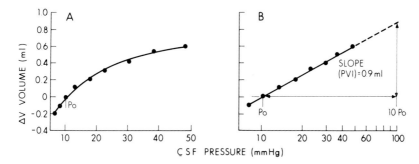

Figure 8.3.   The CSF volume-pressure curve plotted on a linear axis (*left*) was found to be exponential. The compliance given by the slope $\Delta V/\Delta P$ is not constant but decreases as pressure increases. The same data plotted on semilogarithmic axis can be approximated by a straight line (*right*). The slope of the straight-line segment is equal to the pressure-volume index (PVI), and can be defined as the amount of volume necessary to raise pressure by a factor of 10.

for compliance ($\Delta V/\Delta P$) or elastance ($\Delta P/\Delta V$) will depend upon the point of the curve for the pressure at which it is evaluated.

In pathological settings, the shape of the pressure-volume curve changes. The curve may become steeper, indicating a tight system, or flatter, as the system becomes slack. The slope of the curve reflects the ability of the neuraxis to accommodate or buffer additional increments of volume. Since the slope changes with pressure, compliance or elastance, which are derived from the slope, are pressure dependent. A compliance index that is not pressure dependent yet describes the overall steepness of the CSF pressure volume curve can be derived by plotting the pressure on a logarithmic axis against volume (Fig. 8.3). The logarithmic transformation of an exponential curve results in a straight line. The slope of this line is called the pressure-volume index (PVI).[18] A large PVI indicates a soft compliant system, whereas a small PVI indicates a tight system. In more practical terms, the PVI is numerically equal to the volume that must be added intracranially to increase pressure by a factor of 10.

Effect of Intracranial Compliance Upon the Dynamics of ICP—the Transient State

At equilibrium, it is proposed that the ICP is equal to the product of formation rate and outflow resistance added to the pressure of the dural sinus. The compliance parameter discussed in the previous section does not appear in the steady-state relationship. Theoretically, the intracranial compliance affects only the transient behavior and not the equilibrium level of the ICP. To describe the "transient response" or time course of pressure $P(t)$ which accompanies a volume change it is necessary to incorporate the compliance term into the theoretical model. This produced a complex differential equation which when solved for $P(t)$ yielded a formula which predicts both the transient response as well as the shifts in resting ICP level that would occur for any volume input (Eq. 1.0)

$$P(t) = \psi(t)/\{1/P_0 + (K/R)\int_0^t \psi(\tau)\,d\tau\} \quad (1.0)$$

where $\psi(t) = e^K \int_0^t I(\tau)d\tau$

and volume input is described by the term $I(\tau)$

Application of the General ICP Equation— Theoretical Estimates of Outflow Resistance (R_0)

It is possible to derive specific forms of the general equation by expressing the input volume function and solving for the corresponding time course of pressure in response to the volume change. For example, the time response of the ICP $P(t)$ to a bolus of volume (V) injected into the CSF system is given by

$$P(t) = \frac{P_0 e^{KV + KtP_0/R}}{1 + e^{KV} \{e^{KtP_0/R} - 1\}} \quad (2.0)$$

The time course of pressure to bolus injection is expressed in Eq. (2.0) as a function of the initial pressure (P_0), the compliance term ($K = 1/\text{PVI} \times \log e$), outflow resistance ($R$), input volume ($V$), and time ($t$). This expression defines the "output" for the special case of an "input" bolus injection.

One application of the modeling technique is to use the $P(t)$ equation to estimate the outflow resistance (R) and compliance index (PVI). The solution requires two steps. When the volume is injected into the system, the instantaneous rise in pressure is obtained by setting $t = 0$ in the $P(t)$ equation which yields $P(0) = P_{\text{peak}} = P_0 e^{KV}$.

The peak pressure (P_P), the initial pressure (P_0), and the volume injected (V) are known. It is then possible to solve for the PVI $= (\Delta V/\log P_p/P_0)$ and the parameter K. This is how the PVI can be determined from the instantaneous rise in pressure following bolus injection. Alternate techniques for compliance determination will be discussed in greater detail. Once the PVI is calculated using this method, it is possible to solve for the CSF outflow resistance R since all remaining parameters are known. This forms the basis of the bolus technique for estimates of R.

Infusion Technique for Estimate of Outflow Resistance (R)

Another method for estimating R can be derived by review of the ICP steady state equation (ICP $= I_f R + P_D$) where I_f is the rate of CSF production. According to the steady-state equation, if venous pressure (P_D) and resistance (R) were held constant, a linear increase in formation rate produces a linear or straight line increase of the ICP. The slope of the line equals the absorption resistance. Using this principle, the R can be estimated by infusing a known amount of fluid into the CSF space at a constant rate. Pressure will change from its initial value (P_0) and settle at a new steady state value (P_{ss}). The resistance to absorption (R) can be determined by dividing the infusion rate (ΔI) into the pressure difference ($P_{ss} - P_0$) or $R = (P_{ss} - P_0)/\Delta I$.

Withdrawal Technique for Estimation of Dural Sinus Pressure

The method for estimating the dural sinus pressure (P_D) is based on the structure of the steady-state ICP equation (ICP $= I_f \times R + (P_D)$). If fluid is withdrawn from the CSF space at a constant rate equal to the estimated formation rate, pressure will decrease gradually and plateau at a lower steady-state level. This new steady-state level will theoretically be equal to the dural sinus pressure. The reason for this is that removal of fluid at a rate of ($-I_f$) cancels the $I_f \times R$ product of the steady-state equation leaving the ICP equal to P_D. By this technique, it is possible to isolate the factor contributing most to the ICP level and is particularly useful in studying patients at high sustained ICP where volume addition is not clinically advisable.

Withdrawal Technique for Estimation of CSF Formation Rate (I_f)

In mathematical terms, a bolus withdrawal of fluid can be treated as a bolus injection of negative sign. This input to the general equation produces a specific solution for the predicted trajectory of ICP in response to a bolus removal of fluid. From this trajectory equation, it is possible to derive an expression which can be used to estimate the rate of CSF formation. The underlying assumption is that when fluid is removed so that pressure falls below a critical absorption threshold level, no fluid will be absorbed. The system will form new fluid and gradually increase in pressure until normal equilibrium pressure is reached. The rate of formation is calculated by noting the initial pressure (P_0), the pressure immediately following withdrawal (P_m), a pressure (P_1) extracted from the return curve at time t and inserting in the equation.

$$I_{\text{form}} = \frac{\text{PVI}}{t} (\log P_1/P_m) \quad (3.0)$$

Methods for Determining Intracranial Compliance/Elastance Parameters

As stated earlier, compliance (C) or its reciprocal elastance (e) can be derived from the slope of the pressure volume curve which can be obtained by CSF volume manipulation. However, because of the exponential nature of the PV curve, both these parameters are pressure-dependent and the compliance or elastance is ususally specified along with a baseline pressure. Miller et al.[19] studied the volume-pressure ratio (VPR) in head injured patients and examined the relationship of VPR to the resting level of the ICP. The VPR, introduced by Miller, is obtained by inserting a fixed increment of volume (1 ml) into the CSF space and computing the ratio of pressure to volume. ($\Delta P/\Delta V$) defines the magnitude of "elastance" (reciprocal of compliance) associated with the resting pressure at which it is measured.

The PVI is a compliance index which is not pressure-dependent and can be estimated by recording the baseline pressure (P_0), adding volume in a single bolus injection (ΔV), then recording the peak pressure (P_p) attained. The PVI is then calculated by dividing the volume (ΔV) by the logarithm of the ratio of P_p/P_0. With PVI determined, the compliance or PVR at any level of pressure (P) can be estimated by the relationship VPR = $P/0.4343$ PVI or C = 0.4343 PVI/P.

In certain clinical situations, it may be undesirable to inject fluid, particularly in patients with abnormally high ICP. In these cases, the PVI is estimated from bolus withdrawal data. The resting record is observed and average ICP determined. During a period of stable ICP, an aliquot of fluid is removed to reduce pressure by approximately 5 mm Hg. The PVI is estimated by inserting the initial pressure (P_0), the pressure immediately following withdrawal (P_{min}) and the volume removed (ΔV) into the equation PVI = $\Delta V/\log (P_0/P_{min})$. The withdrawal maneuver is incorporated into our clinical evaluation technique not only to estimate PVI and CSF formation but also to compute for subsequent R determination; the maximum injected volume corresponding to a pre-set pressure limit. For example, if it is desired to limit the pressure rise to bolus injection to 25 mm Hg, injected volume (V limit) can be estimated as V limit = (PVI) (log P_{limit}/P_0) where PVI is the value obtained from withdrawal data and P_0 is the resting pressure prior to the proposed bolus addition. Thus, the PVI obtained from withdrawal data allows us to compute the peak pressure that would result to bolus addition fluid and clinical judgment is used to determine the appropriate pressure limit.

Following the measurement of PVI and formation rate from withdrawal data, two or three bolus injections are conducted for repeated measurements of PVI and outflow resistance (R). The rate of injection does not exceed 1 ml/2 sec and sufficient time is allotted for pressure to return to equilibrium after each injection. When these tests are completed, fluid is removed at a fixed rate equal to the estimated CSF formation to circumvent the absorption mechanism and provide an estimate of venous exit pressure.

A summary table of ICP dynamics which describes the sequence of steps required to evaluate the parameters discussed in this chapter is presented in Table 8.1, along the physiologic range measured in normal adults.

Analysis of ICP Dynamics by Controlled Infusion

The linear relationship between ICP and CSF flow is described by the steady-state equation and forms the basis for the evaluation of CSF hydrodynamics using constant rate infusion techniques.

As fluid is added to the CSF space at a constant rate, ICP increases transiently and gradually plateaus at a new steady-state value. Higher steady-state pressures produced by increasing rates of infusion would result in a straight line relationship between pressure and infusion rate. The slope of this line equals the absorption resistance (R). The technique for calculation of R by this method was described earlier and is similar to the clinical test introduced by Katzman (11). An extensive review of the CSF phys-

Table 8.1
A Summary of the Methods Developed for Estimating CSF Parameters from Static and Dynamic Response of Intracranial Pressure to Known Volume Changes

Objective	Volume change	ICP Change	Data necessary	Equations	Normal values of adults
To estimate CSF formation and PVI using CSF bolus withdrawal	1. Remove CSF bolus of ΔV (ml)	2.	3. P_o, P_m, P_1, t_1	4. $PVI = \dfrac{\Delta V}{\log_{10} P_o/P_m}$ 5. $I_{form} = \dfrac{PVI}{t_1}(\log P_1/P_m)$	25-30 ml 0.3-0.4 ml/min
To estimate PVI, R_o, C or VPR using bolus injection	6. Inject bolus ΔV (ml)	7.	8. P_o, P_p, P_2, t_2	9. $PVI = \dfrac{\Delta V}{\log_{10} P_p/P_o}$ 10. $R_o = \dfrac{t_2 P_o}{(PVI)\log\left[\dfrac{P_2}{P_p}\cdot\dfrac{P_p - P_o}{P_2 - P_o}\right]}$ 11. $C = \dfrac{.4343\,PVI}{P_o}$ and $VPR = \dfrac{1}{C}$	25-30 ml 2-12 mm Hg/ml/min 0.25-1.5 ml/mm Hg
To estimate R_o using constant-rate infusion	12. Infuse fluid at rate I_{in}	13.	14. P_o, P_{ss}, I_n	15. $R_o = \dfrac{P_{ss} - P_o}{I_n}$	2-12 mm Hg/ml/min
To estimate PVI using constant rate infusion	16. Infuse fluid at rate I_{in}	17.	18. P_o, P_1, P_{ss}, R, I_n	19. $PVI = \dfrac{\Delta I\,P_{ss}t}{(P_o - P_{ss})\log\left[\dfrac{P_o(P_{ss} - P_1)}{P_1(P_{ss} - P_o)}\right]}$	25-30 ml
To estimate VPR from bolus injection (elastance) at pressure P_o	20. Inject bolus of 1.0 ml	21.	22. P_o, P_p	23. $VPR = \dfrac{\Delta P}{\Delta V} = P_p - P_o$ $VPR = \dfrac{1}{C}$	0-3 mm Hg/ml up to 30 mm Hg
To estimate P_d from constant-rate withdrawal	24. Remove fluid at a rate equal to estimated rate of formation from step 5	25.	26. P_d	27. Estimate of dural sinus pressure P_d equals ICP level after reaching equilibrium following withdrawal of fluid at rate estimated CSF formation (I_{form}).	

iology upon which these tests are based is provided by Welch.[34] In this method described by Ekstedt,[4] the infusion pressure is kept at a constant level, and the resulting CSF flow is recorded. In a modified version, the method has also been used by Portnoy and Croissant[24] and more recently by Sklar.[27] Special apparatus is required for evaluation of CSF parameters by these methods, particularly in the studies by Sklar, who has incorporated a servo-system for more precise control of the constant pressure source.

All of these methods, including the bolus and infusion technique described earlier, are based upon the rectilinear relationship between pressure and flow with the common assumption that pressure in the sagittal sinus remains unaffected when increasing the ICP. However, the infusion methods have a distinct advantage over the bolus techniques in that it is possible to determine R throughout a range of pressure. On the basis of the mathematical model, the measurement of R from both infusion and bolus techniques should be identical. However, Sullivan has reported differences between infusion and bolus R determinations in cats.[28] Resistance calculated by the bolus injection technique underestimated resistance calculations by the infusion method in animals with high R. Sullivan attributes these differences to pressure relaxation of the tissue. Further work is necessary to determine the extent to which viscoelastic properties of the brain affect measurements of R and compliance using these techniques.

Intracranial Pulse Pressure

The steady-state and dynamic properties of the ICP presented thus far have excluded the consideration of the pulsatile variation of the ICP. More recently, great interest has been shown in the analysis of the ICP pulse waveform and the changes in amplitude and frequency of the pulsatile components that accompany alterations in the level of the ICP and compliance of the neuraxis.

It is generally accepted that the pulsatile components derive from the transient changes in blood volume associated with the cardiac and respiratory cycle. These small volume changes may be considered to be superimposed upon a steady state volume level. The relationship of these volume changes to pressure is given by the pressure-volume curve of the craniospinal axis. It was stated earlier that the pressure-volume curve can be interpreted as a graphic representation of all possible steady and transient state changes of the CSF. This explains the increase in pulse amplitude with increasing pressure as illustrated in Figure 8.4. VanEijndhoven and Avezaat[32] have investigated the interrelationship of pulse pressure, ICP and compliance and view the pulse pressure as a continuous physiologic response which contains properties from which compliance parameters can be extracted. They point out that with an exponential P/V curve, the pulse component is proportional to the slope of the P-V curve which by definition is equivalent to the compliance. Since the volume is unknown, it is not possible to quantify the intracranial compliance solely from pulsa-

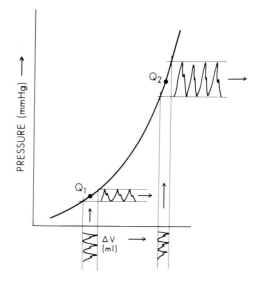

Figure 8.4. Under normal conditions, a stable ICP is analogous to a point Q, of the exponential CSF pressure volume curve. With increased ICP (Q_2) compliance is reduced and volume changes (horizontal axis) are reflected in pulsatile pressure components of greater magnitude.

tile amplitude measures. Conventional bolus techniques are still needed to identify the initial level of compliance and thereafter pulsatile amplitude parameters may be used to monitor compliance changes.

Other investigators have explored use of pulse pressure and waveform shape as possible indicators of neurologic deterioration and shifts in brain compliance. Portnoy and Chopp[23] utilized spectral analysis to determine characteristic changes of the ICP at different levels of pressure. Changes in spectral content in studies of cats were discernible with an expanding mass and raised ICP that were not detectable by conventional compliance testing.[2] The work of Avezaat et al.,[1] and Szewczykowski et al.,[29] concentrates on pulse amplitude correlates of compliance and provides further evidence that reliable techniques for compliance testing may be forthcoming which do not require manipulation of intracranial volume.

Summary—Theoretical Concepts of ICP

The nonlinear behavior of the ICP dynamics is primarily attributed to the sigmoid shaped pressure-volume curve. Within a range of pressure below 50 mm Hg, the curve is exponential and can be described mathematically. The incorporation of this exponential function into a theoretical model of the CSF system has led to the formulation of a general equation which defines the "static" and dynamic response of ICP. The analysis has shown that four parameters are necessary to adequately describe change of ICP: the rate of CSF production, intracranial compliance, the outflow resistance and the intradural sinus pressure. With knowledge of these parameters, the pressure response to a known volume change can be predicted. By reversing the process, methods for extracting the values of the parameters solely on the basis of pressure changes can be derived. These techniques have been condensed into a summary table (Table 8.1) and form the basis of continued investigation into the physiologic changes accompanying trauma.

Theoretical modeling efforts in this area

are continuing, and new approaches to noninvasive methods for compliance testing using pulse pressure data are promising. What is needed is a greater concentration in the high pressure portion of the pressure-volume relationship. When volume reserve is exhausted, the curve flattens and the monoexponential description of pressure and volume is not applicable. Under these conditions, new equations must be formulated to describe the dynamics of ICP.

CLINICAL CONSIDERATIONS

Although the clinical significance of ICP elevations in craniocerebral injuries has been questioned,[5] there is now general agreement that knowledge of the ICP and intracranial dynamics is useful in recognizing impending brain herniation, in guiding therapy, and in predicting the outcome of patients with severe head injuries.[9, 10, 15] In spite of this, however, the absolute value of the ICP is sometimes less important than the rate of increase of the ICP, the size, nature and location of the lesion and other extenuating factors such as the presence of herniation, cranial defects and CSF leaks. All these situations are the subject of the following discussion.

Brain Distortion

Expansion of the CSF compartment by obstruction of the CSF pathways or impaired absorption (as discussed in the theoretical section of this chapter) may lead to an increase in ICP. However, this elevation of ICP does not usually produce brain distortion and brain stem compression.[7] Introduction of a volume increment into the subarachnoid space produces an instantaneous pressure elevation uniformly transmitted across the entire neuraxis. Although injection of an equal volume into the epidural space raises epidural pressure, this is only partially transmitted to the subarachnoid space. Langfitt[13] has shown that the transmission of the pressure across the dural membrane is dependent on the adherence of the dura to the skull. If the dura is fully stripped from the skull the pressure gradient between the epidural and intradural space approaches zero. When the dura is adherent to the skull around the lesion, focal expansion of an epidural mass can distort and compress the brain stem before generating a significant rise in ICP. On the other hand, when the dura is stripped from the skull the pressure gradient between the epidural and intradural space approaches zero and the pressure of an expanding epidural mass is readily transmitted to the subarachnoid space, resulting in serious intracranial hypertension before brain stem distortion occurs. Similarly, in an expanding subdural hematoma, ICP elevation occurs prior to brain stem distortion; as long as the CSF pathways are patent, subdural pressure is virtually instantaneously transmitted to the subarachnoid space. This rapid transmission of pressure has also been shown in chronic subdural hematomas where simultaneous pressure fluctuations were recorded in the lumbar subarachnoid fluid and within the subdural capsule.[30]

Transmission of the pressure within the brain substance is more complex. When an expanding intracerebral lesion produces a focal increase in pressure within the brain parenchyma, only a portion of this increase is transmitted to the surface of the brain thus leading to a pressure gradient between the mass or adjacent brain and subarachnoid space.[13] This focal increase in pressure is not immediately propagated to all intracranial compartments; the direction of the pressure and the rate of transmission is dependent upon the relative distensibility or elastic properties of the brain tissue and vascular structures around the mass lesion.[22]

Location of the Mass

The location of an intracranial mass is associated with a variable risk of brain stem distortion and compression. For example, the bony boundaries of the temporal lobe laterally, anteriorly, and inferiorly, result in medial displacement of brain substance by a mass lesion.[7] Because of its proximity to the brain stem a relatively small amount of temporal lobe mass or distortion in a medial direction will cause midbrain compression and result in severe neurological dysfunction (see also Chapter 11). On the other

hand, occipital masses or those at the frontal pole need to be much larger before they can cause brain stem compression. In other words, the same size mass associated with an identical ICP value carries a higher risk of brain stem compression in the temporal lobe than lesions of the occipital or frontal regions.[33] This phenomenon must be taken into account when monitoring the ICP in patients with temporal lobe masses.

Rate of Expansion: Herniation

The rate of expansion of an intracranial mass is important in determining the degree of brain distortion and ICP elevation. In animal studies, Weinstein et al.,[33] have demonstrated that rapid introduction of a small volume into the intracranial cavity causes a significant rise of ICP and brain stem distortion, while slow injection of the same volume produces minimal ICP elevation and brain stem compression. Most clinicians have experienced this phenomenon in slow-growing tumors, and/or chronic subdural hematomas which can reach a considerable size with minimal clinical manifestations. Gradual growth of the mass without the production of symptoms occurs as a result of the utilization of compensatory mechanisms. When this intracranial buffering system is totally exhausted, any additional volume expansion precipitates a sharp rise in ICP and neurological decompensation. This condition is commonly referred to as a stiff or non-compliant brain.

Biomechanical characterization of brain elastance or compliance has been described in the theoretical section of this chapter and is readily determined from the pressure-volume curve. Since the compliance is not pressure-dependent, a critically low compliance may be observed in a patient with normal or only mildly elevated ICP. Therefore, it is useful to measure intracranial compliance in order to predict the risk of a sudden rise in ICP.

The normal values of PVI are dependent on the volume of buffering capacity within the neuraxis. This buffering capacity is provided by blood within the vascular compartment and CSF within the subarachnoid space and ventricles: as vascular structures are compressed there is a decrease in the intracranial blood volume. In infants and children with a smaller craniospinal volume, this buffering capacity is smaller and PVI values are proportionately less than that of adults.[26]

In both adults and children it has been estimated that 68% of the total buffering capacity is contained by the intracranial compartment and the remainder in the spinal compartment.[17] When cerebellar tissue herniates and obstructs the foramen magnum, the spinal compartment is isolated from the intracranial one and the buffering capacity of the former is no longer available. Intracranial compliance will, therefore, be reduced by about one third. Similarly, transtentorial herniation will reduce the compliance by about two thirds. In each case, decreased compliance shifts the pressure-volume curve to the left and makes it steeper than normal (*i.e.*, a given increase in volume will produce a larger increase in ICP). Therefore, detection of a markedly increased PVI in the absence of severe intracranial hypertension may be a reflection of an impending herniation and should be treated promptly.

Cranial Defects and CSF Leak

The characterization of the biomechanical properties of the neuraxis is made on the assumption that the craniospinal space is closed with a rigid covering. When the calvarium is removed because of trauma or decompressive surgery, compliance measurements and the relationship of compliance to ICP may not adhere to accepted models of intracranial dynamics. A bony defect in the presence of an intact dura does not influence these values significantly as the dura is virtually non-distensible and will maintain the properties of the craniospinal axis as a rigid container. However, a large cranial defect associated with a dural opening allows the intra-cranial contents to herniate into the bony defect with a low ICP reading. Therefore, ICP values, under these circumstances, are not useful in determining the course of treatment and outcome.

In normal circumstances, ICP in an upright position is less than atmospheric pressure.[12] But in the presence of a large defect, atmospheric pressure is directly transmitted to the intracranial contents. If ICP is greater than atmospheric pressure, the scalp becomes convex over the defect, and ICP elevation and compliance become dependent on the elastic properties of the scalp to compensate for the pressure gradient.[31] This conditiion is recognized clinically by the presence of a concave bony defect and may occasionally result in cortical compression.

The presence of a traumatic CSF fistula in association with severe head injury is not uncommon. As CSF finds its way to the extracranial space, one of the compensatory mechanisms of intracranial buffering system becomes prematurely exhausted resulting in an artifactually low ICP reading. The presence of pneumocephalus can further complicate the interpretation of CSF dynamic studies as the physical properties of air, which are different from other intracranial structures, can alter the compliance values. When a surgical decision is to be made using ICP information, the effect of these factors should be considered.

Knowledge of the ICP, when accompanied by studies of intracranial compliance, can be very useful in management of severely injured patients. As long as the clinician is aware of the limitations of ICP monitoring in specific conditions, knowledge of the ICP can be effectively used in conjunction with other clinical and diagnostic findings.

References

1. Avezaat, C.J.J., van Eijndhoven, J.H.M., Wyper, D.J.: Cerebrospinal fluid pulse pressure and intracranial volume-pressure relationships. J. Neurol. Neurosurg. Psych., 42:687–700, 1979.
2. Chopp, M., Portnoy, H.D.: Systems analysis of intracranial pressure. Comparison with volume-pressure test and CSF-pulse amplitude analysis. J. Neurosurg., 53:516–527, 1980.
3. Davson, H.: Physiology of the Cerebrospinal Fluid. Churchill Ltd., 1967, p. 337.
4. Ekstedt, J.: CSF hydrodynamic studies in man. 1. Method of constant pressure CSF infusion. J. Neurol. Neurosurg. Psych., 40:105–119, 1977.
5. Fleischer, A.S., Payne, N.S., Tindall, G.T.: Continuous monitoring of intracranial pressure in severe closed head injury without mass lesions. Surg. Neurol., 6:31–34, 1976.
6. Gudeman, S.K., Miller, J.D., Becker, D.P.: Failure of high-dose steroid therapy to influence intracra-

nial pressure in patients with severe head injury. J. Neurosurg., 51:301–306, 1979.

7. Johnson, R.T., Yates, P.O.: Clinico-pathological aspects of pressure changes at the tentorium. Acta Radiologica, 46:242–249, 1956.

8. Johnston, I., Gilday, D.L., Patterson, A., et al.: The definition of a reduced CSF absorption syndrome: Clinical and experimental studies, In: Intracranial Pressure II, Lundberg, N., Ponten, U., Brock, M., eds., Springer-Verlag, Berlin, 1975, pp. 61–66.

9. Johnston, I.H., Jennett, B.: The place of continuous intracranial pressure monitoring in neurosurgical practice. Acta Neurochir., 29:53–63, 1973.

10. Johnston, I.H., Johnston, J.A., Jennett, B.: Intracranial-pressure changes following head injury. Lancet, 2:433–436, 1970.

11. Katzman, R., Hussey, F.: A simple constant-infusion manometric test for measurement of CSF absorption. I. Rationale and method. Neurology, 20:534–544, 1970.

12. Langfitt, T.W.: Increased intracranial pressure. Clin. Neurosurg., 16:436–471, 1968.

13. Langfitt, T.W., Weinstein, J.O., Kassell, N.F., Gagliardi, L.J.: Transmission of increased intracranial pressure. II. Within the supratentorial space. J. Neurosurg., 21:998–1005, 1964.

14. Lofgren, J., von Essen C., Zwetnow, N.N.: The pressure-volume curve of the cerebrospinal fluid space in dogs. Acta Neurol. Scand., 49:557–574, 1973.

15. Lundberg, N., Troupp, H., Lorin, H.: Continuous recording and control of ventricular fluid pressure in neurosurgical practice. Acta Psychiatr. Neurol. Scand. (Suppl. 149), 36:1–193, 1960.

16. Marmarou, A.: A theoretical model and experimental evaluation of the cerebrospinal fluid system. Thesis, Drexel Univ., June, 1973.

17. Marmarou, A., Shulman, K., LaMorgese, J.: Compartmental analysis of compliance and outflow resistance of the cerebrospinal fluid system. J. Neurosurg., 43:523–534, 1976.

18. Marmarou, A., Shulman, K., Rosende, R.M.: A nonlinear analysis of the cerebrospinal fluid system and intracranial pressure dynamics. J. Neurosurg., 48:332–344, 1978.

19. Miller, J.D.: Clinical aspects of intracranial pressure-volume relationships. In: Head Injuries. McLaurin, R.L., Ed., Grune & Stratton, Inc., New York, 1976, pp. 239–245.

20. Miller, J.D., Becker, D.P., Ward, J.D., Sullivan, H.G., Adams, W.E., Rosner, M.: Significance of intracranial hypertension in severe head injury. J. Neurosurg., 47:503–516, 1977.

21. Miller, J.D., Leech, P.: Effects of mannitol and steroid therapy on intracranial volume-pressure relationships in patients. J. Neurosurg., 42:274–281, 1975.

22. Pollock, L. J., Boshes, B.: Cerebrospinal fluid pressure. Arch. Neurol. Psychiat., 36:931–974, 1936.

23. Portnoy, H.D., Chopp, M.: Spectral analysis of intracranial pressure. In: Intracranial Pressure IV. Shulman, K., Marmarou, A., Miller, J.H., Becker, D.P., Hochwald, G.M., Brock, M., Eds., Springer-Verlag, Berlin, 1980, pp. 167–172.

24. Portnoy, H.D., Croissant, P.D.: A practical method for measuring hydrodynamics of cerebrospinal fluid. Surg. Neurol., 5:273–277, 1976.

25. Ryder, H.W., Epsy, F.E., Kimbell, F.D., Penka, E.J., Rosenaver, A., Podolsky, B., Evans, J.P.: The mechanism of the change in cerebrospinal fluid pressure following an induced change in the volume of the fluid space. J. Lab. Clin. Med., 41:428–435, 1953.

26. Shapiro, K., Marmarou, A., Shulman, K.: Characterization of clinical CSF dynamics and neural axis compliance using the pressure-volume index. 1. The normal pressure-volume index. Ann. Neurol., 7:508–514, 1977.

27. Sklar, F.H. Non-steady state measurements of cerebrospinal fluid dynamics. In: Neurobiology of Cerebrospinal Fluid. Wood, J.H., Ed., Plenum Press, New York, 1980, pp. 365–379.

28. Sullivan, H.G., Miller, J.D., Griffith, R.L., Engr, D., Carter, W., Rucker, S.: Bolus versus steady-state infusion for determination of CSF outflow resistance. Ann. Neurol., 5:228–238, 1979.

29. Szewczykowski, J., Sliwka, S., Kunicki, A., Dytko, P., Korsak-Sliwka, J.: A fast method of estimating the elastance of the intracranial system. A practical application in neurosurgery. J. Neurosurg., 47:19–26, 1977.

30. Tabaddor, K.: ICP and compliance in chronic subdural hematoma. In: Intracranial Pressure IV. Shulman, K., Marmarou, A., Miller, J.H., Becker, D.P., Hochwald, G.M., Brock, M., Eds., Springer-Verlag, Berlin, 1980, pp. 358–361.

31. Tabaddor, K., LaMorgese, J.: Complication of a large cranial defect. A case report. J. Neurosurg., 44:506–508, 1976.

32. Van Eijndhoven, J.H.M., Avezaat, C.J.J.: The analogy between CSF pulse pressure and volume-pressure response. In: Intracranial Pressure IV. Shulman, K., Marmarou, A., Miller, J.H., Becker, D.P., Hochwald, G.M., Brock, M., Eds., Springer-Verlag, Berlin, 1980, pp. 173–176.

33. Weinstein, J.D., Langfitt, T.W., Bruno, L., Zaren, H.A., Jackson, J.L.F.: Experimental study of patterns of brain distortion and ischemia produced by an intracranial mass. J. Neurosurg., 28:513–521, 1968.

34. Welch, K.: The principles of physiology of the cerebrospinal fluid in relation to hydrocephalus including normal pressure hydrocephalus. Adv. Neurol., 13:247–332, 1975.

9

Medical Management of Intracranial Pressure

LAWRENCE F. MARSHALL
SHARON A. BOWERS

The ultimate outcome for the head-injured patient is dependent upon many factors, some of which are beyond the control of the treating physician. In our region, despite a sophisticated emergency medical services system, more than one-half of the deaths from head injury occur before the patient reaches the hospital.[34] This indicates that there may be such severe destruction of brain tissue that these injuries are irreversible.

If one extrapolates from the survivor statistics in San Diego County, nationally one can expect that approximately 60,000 severely head-injured patients per year will reach the hospital alive; and that approximately one-half of these patients will have intracranial hypertension some time during their post-injury course. Becker and Miller[2] found, as did Marshall and Smith,[46] that the single most frequent cause of death in aggressively managed head-injured patients is uncontrollable intracranial hypertension. Despite relatively systematized and well-organized approaches in these and other head injury centers, control of intracranial pressure (ICP) remains unsatisfactory in some patients. Nevertheless, it is apparent to neurosurgeons and critical care physicians that unless care is systematic and well organized, not only for the treatment of intracranial hypertension but also for the general maintenance of the patients, morbidity and mortality will rise exponentially.

The major thrust of this chapter is to review the treatment of increased ICP. It is appropriate to note that the treatment of intracranial hypertension must begin with the prevention of secondary insults to the brain (which lead to increases in ICP), and must go hand-in-hand with a systematic, relatively error-free approach to the entire management of the patient.

PREVENTION OF SECONDARY INSULTS LEADING TO INTRACRANIAL HYPERTENSION

The neuropathological studies of Graham and Adams[20] and, more recently, those of Clifton et al.,[9] have shown that severe generalized or focal disturbances, which result in irreversible neuropathologic changes, occur for one of two major reasons: because metabolic demands become too great or because cerebral blood flow (CBF) becomes inadequate. The former occurs in instances such as hyperthermia or status epilepticus where the brain's need for oxygen and glucose exceeds the ability of the cardiopulmonary system to deliver it. The latter occurs more frequently as a result of systemic hypotension and, in the head-injured population particularly, because of intracranial hypertension. Both of these conditions result in significant reductions in cerebral perfusion pressure (CPP); and the latter is responsible in large measure for the high incidence of ischemic brain damage that Graham and Adams found in their study of patients who died from their head injuries.[20]

One major objective then, in the treatment of the severely head-injured, is to maintain the patient in a milieu where the brain's metabolic demands can be met and where further insults to an already-damaged brain can either be prevented or obviated. It is imperative, therefore, that care of these patients begin from the moment of injury. Although neurosurgeons in the past have placed their focus in managing these patients in the operating room and/or the intensive care unit, it is now clear that they must take a more active role in both organizing and directing the initial care of these patients as well. No degree of surgical expertise on the part of the neurosurgeon can compensate for management errors made during the first minutes and hours after injury which subsequently may lead to uncontrollable intracranial hypertension.

Preliminary studies, both from our region and elsewhere, support the impression that early resuscitation, both in the field and during the emergency room phase of hospitalization has reduced the incidence of severe intracranial hypertension during the patients' subsequent course (see also Chapter 1).

In the initial 100 patients reported from San Diego, 25% had severe uncontrolled intracranial hypertension. This was defined as an ICP of greater than 40 mm Hg despite aggressive standard therapy.[46] In our latest series of patients, the incidence of uncontrolled intracranial hypertension has fallen to below 15%.[5] Considering that the incidence of surgical masses was identical in both groups (24%), and our policy regarding the management of contusion and non-extra-axial masses was unchanged, it appears that this difference might be explained by the expansion of the emergency medical services (EMS) in our region during the past several years. Both the City and County of San Diego are now covered by paramedic units capable of administering advanced life support with an average response time of ten minutes. Although response times and the adequacy of EMS systems will vary from region to region, our observation supports Miller's contention that the avoidance of "secondary insults to the brain"[51] may result in a reduced incidence of intracranial hypertension and, perhaps, an improved outcome.

CRITERIA FOR MONITORING INTRACRANIAL PRESSURE

It has been our policy to monitor ICP in all patients who have a Glasgow Coma Scale (GCS) of 7 or less following resuscitation. Recent evidence from Haar et al.[21] as well as our own experience, suggests the possibility that monitoring may not be necessary in certain patients with GCS scores of 6 or 7. That group includes patients who have initially normal computerized tomographic (CT) scans, and who have not suffered shock, hypoxia, hypercapnia, or a significant multiple injury. It is important to note, however, that a normal CT scan refers not only to the absence of shift and/or masses, but also to visualization of the brain stem cisterns and of the ventricular system. We have had several patients with markedly elevated ICP where the ventricular system was in the midline, and in whom the brain stem cisterns were not absent but compressed. Further experience is needed to determine whether or not such patients with "normal" scans can, in fact, be assumed not to have intracranial hypertension. As further information becomes available, it is possible that invasive monitoring may be more appropriately directed towards those patients in whom there is more significant likelihood of intracranial hypertension; and that the procedure might then be omitted in those patients in whom the probability yield is likely to be low or nil. One must recall, however, that in those patients who have suffered ischemic hypoxia or hypotensive insults prior to hospitalization, monitoring is mandatory. Late intracranial hypertension has often been observed in these patients.

INITIAL MANAGEMENT AND GENERAL INTENSIVE CARE OF THE PATIENT

Initial Management

The treatment of increased ICP is predicated upon the assumption that the care of the patient is well-organized, rapidly delivered, and that the treatment plan has enough flexibility to respond to changing circumstances. Our treatment scheme in San Diego is based on the post-resuscitation GCS score. Resuscitation in this context refers to non-surgical resuscitation and includes: endotracheal intubation, prophylactic anti-convulsant administration, hyperventilation to a PCO_2 of 25 to 30 torr, appropriate treatment of shock, if present; and in the absence of shock, the administration of at least one dose of an osmotic diuretic, preferably mannitol, 1 g/kg.

In patients who have a GCS score which remains 7 or less following the initial resuscitation, whether it has been carried out prior to arrival at the hospital or immediately upon admission to the emergency room, CT scanning should immediately follow the resuscitative effort. We routinely paralyze these patients with 10 mg of pancuronium bromide in order to allow for adequate and interpretable scans. Many patients, however, have already been paralyzed prior to or during the placement of the endotracheal tube. The exact techniques for the performance of the scan are discussed in Chapter 4.

Following the CT scan if no hematoma is found, the patient is transferred to the intensive care unit. If an intracranial mass is noted, the patient is taken directly to the operating room for evacuation of the clot or resection of contused brain and for placement of an intracranial pressure monitoring device. If the ICP exceeds 20 mm Hg in the first 24 hours after operation, the scan is repeated. It is also repeated in patients with non-operative lesions if control of ICP appears disproportionately difficult to that which would be predicted from the initial CT scan. Other authors advocate routine repetition of the CT scan following injury even if these criteria are not met (see Chapter 11).

Intensive Care Management

Table 9.1 summarizes the present method of management in our institution for patients with severe head injuries (GCS < 8) in whom no surgical mass has been demonstrated on the CT scan. It should be

Table 9.1

Management of Severely Head-injured Adult Patients with Intracranial Hypertension

1. Head up 30° and in neutral plane
2. Controlled ventilation to a pCO_2 of 25–30 torr with adequate paralysis and sedation
3. Maintain pO_2 >70 torr
4. Maintain SAP between 100 and 160 mm Hg systolic
5. Maintain normothermia
6. Use prophylactic anti-convulsants
7. Maintain fluid balance with 0.5 normal saline

For ICP Control

8. Ventricular drainage if possible
9. Dexamethasone 20 mg IV q 6 h
10. Mannitol 0.25 g–1 g/kg as needed
11. Avoid anesthetics and other drugs that are cerebral vasodilators

recalled that the basic goal in the treatment of intracranial hypertension is normalization of the cerebral perfusion pressure (CPP) which represents the difference between the mean arterial pressure and the ICP.[48] While we recognize that this measurement is only a crude guide to judging the adequacy of brain nutrition, it is one that is available to almost all neurosurgeons and is relatively reliable.

As stated previously, one must strive to create a milieu which permits recovery of those tissues not irreversibly damaged, and which avoids secondary injuries to an already damaged brain. We, as others, have learned that it is much easier to prevent intracranial hypertension than to treat it once high levels of pressure have been reached. It cannot be overemphasized that by instituting management early, and adhering to relatively standard protocols, the incidence of intracranial hypertension in brain-injured patients can be reduced from those high incidences reported initially by Miller and Becker,[50] and by Marshall and Smith.[46] Furthermore, the sequelae of repeated rises in ICP can be avoided if prehospital and emergency room treatment is instituted early and is successful.

Patient Position. Patient position is a significant factor in the prevention and treatment of increased ICP. It is important that all severely head-injured patients, with the exception of those who are in shock and those with spinal cord injuries, be managed in the head-up position, and that the head be kept in the neutral plane with respect to the body. Major rises in ICP can occur and sustained plateau waves can be precipitated if the head is turned to the side, particularly the left. This was demonstrated initially by Hulme and Cooper[24] in patients with brain tumors. Figure 9.1 demonstrates such changes in a patient in whom brain compliance had been reduced.

The head-up position is also advantageous in patients in whom positive end expiratory pressure (PEEP) is required to improve oxygen exchange. The increased venous volume which occurs in the superior portion of the body with the use of PEEP can be reduced if the patient is placed in the head-up position. This also reduces the probability of precipitating intracranial hypertension when PEEP is introduced into ventilatory management.

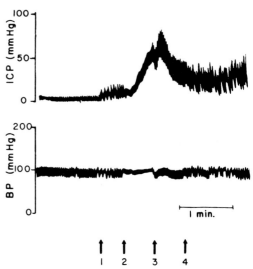

Figure 9.2.   Intracranial hypertension resulting from carbon dioxide retention during endotracheal suctioning. $PaCO_2$ during controlled ventilation immediately prior to suctioning was 21 torr. *Arrows*: 1) manual hyperventilation with anesthesia bag; 2) apnea followed by endotracheal suctioning; 3) return to mechanical ventilation; and 4) manual hyperventilation reinstituted. (With the kind permission of H.M. Shapiro, M.D.[58]).

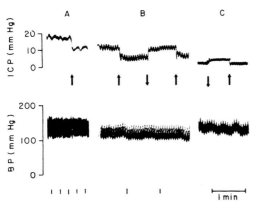

Figure 9.1.   Intracranial pressure effects of elevating the head of the bed to 30° (*Panel A*), and of rotating the patient's head from a lateral position (directed toward the ventilator hoses) to a midline position (*upward arrow*) and back to the laterally rotated position (*downward arrow*) at two different baseline intracranial pressures (*Panels B* and *C*). The lines at the bottom of the trace indicate 1-minute interval timing marks. (With the kind permission of H.M. Shapiro, M.D.[58]).

Airway Care and Chest Management. Coordination of the treatment of the respiratory tract with protection of the brain is critical, and not difficult to accomplish. However, the dangers inherent in the care of the chest must always be recognized. Figure 9.2 demonstrates the influence of endotracheal suctioning on ICP. As can be seen from the figure, difficulties with control of ICP during suctioning, chest physiotherapy, bronchoscopy, or other maneuvers to improve pulmonary function are common, but may be mitigated by small amounts of sedation and mild hyperventilation prior to performance of these procedures. The use of sedation and paralysis is described in the following section.

Intensive care unit monitoring equipment should be positioned and unit design should be such that personnel can look at the monitors while suctioning and while performing other maneuvers that may have a deleterious effect on ICP. Nursing and respiratory therapy personnel, as well as house staff, must be initially educated and continually reminded of the need for such vigilance. They should be instructed to immediately discontinue chest physiotherapy if the ICP exceeds 30 mm Hg unless specific orders to the contrary have been left to ignore such rises. Circumstances in which such rises might be ignored include those in patients who are emerging from high dose barbiturate therapy or other sedation and who are without midline shift on CT scan, or in those patients whose emergence from a narcotized state or other sedation has been deliberately planned prior to extubation. In patients in whom ventricular cannulas have been used for ICP monitoring, it is particularly useful to allow for ventricular drainage during respiratory care. Bronchoscopy is a particularly potent stimulant for the production of systemic arterial hypertension and intracranial hypertension. In brain-injured patients, it should always be performed using adequate sedation and occasionally under general anesthesia.

We utilize controlled ventilation to manage the airway in all patients who are severely head injured. The need to have an endotracheal tube in place for long periods of time makes it necessary to sedate or paralyze most of these patients. Any treatment modality which increases the incidence of noxious stimulation for the patient also carries with it the potential for increasing ICP. Endotracheal intubation is one such treatment modality. The use of paralyzing agents without sedation, which is not an uncommon practice, is not recommended. Agents such as pancuronium bromide, for example, have no analgesic effect and do not adequately protect patients from those reflex arcs which can occur from pain producing procedures; and most importantly from reflex arcs originating in the larynx.

As we have noted previously, autoregulation is often severely deranged in the head-injured patient.[52] In the absence of sedation, systemic arterial hypertension can often directly influence intracranial dynamics and precipitate catastrophic rises in ICP. Morphine sulfate in small doses, usually 2 to 3 mg per hour, administered intravenously will continue to permit assessment of the pupils while blunting the effects of noxious stimuli. Personal preference and experience should influence the choice of paralyzing agents and of sedative medication. We routinely use pancuronium bromide in an initial adult dose of 10 mg administered at the time of endotracheal tube placement and then a maintenance dose of 2 mg/hr. We prefer morphine as a sedative medication because it is reversible and in small doses has little effect on cardiac output. It does not interfere with pupillary dilatation in patients if tentorial herniation is about to occur. It does, however, carry considerable hazard under circumstances where severe dehydration is part of the management plan, or in patients in whom diazepam analogs have also been used for sedation. These drugs may interact synergistically and produce cardiovascular collapse.

Fluid Management. Fluid management is a source of continuing controversy in patients with the potential for developing intracranial hypertension. Some neurosurgeons continue to severely dehydrate their patients by restricting fluid intake to less than one liter per day. Others prefer more moderate dehydration, and still others simply replace urinary and insensible losses with half-normal saline solution.

The rationale for severe dehydration is to prevent intracranial hypertension by allowing for a hyperosmotic state to develop in the serum. While this approach appears to have some logic, it contains dangers which make it undesirable. Fluid losses can be severe in patients whose injuries are restricted to the head and can constitute even more of a problem in patients who are multiply injured. Intravascular fluid volume must be adequately maintained so that cardiac output remains satisfactory. Davis and Sundt have recently shown that CBF is, in fact, more dependent on cardiac output than it is on systemic arterial pressure (SAP) when intravascular volume is decreased.[14] SAP, therefore, is a relatively crude guide to cardiac performance.

Under circumstances where more aggressive therapies are needed to treat intracranial hypertension, severe dehydration often delays or makes these alternatives impossible. Hyperventilation is one such crucial alternative. When patients are severely dehydrated, the institution of hyperventilation can be extremely dangerous since cardiac output may drop precipitously, leading to irreversible ischemic brain damage. It appears desirable, therefore, to avoid severe dehydration. Mild dehydration, by limiting intravenous fluids to two liters of fluid per day, may be of some value in reducing ICP. The emphasis is on the word *mild*. In San Diego County the most frequent avoidable cause of death was fluid and electrolyte abnormalities which, at least in some instances, were iatrogenic.[5] Attention must be placed to fluid balance, and significant abnormalities in serum sodium and serum osmolality must be attended to immediately.

Trauma of any type is often accompanied by inappropriate ADH secretion. When this is present it should be treated with fluid restriction. The situation in head-injured patients, however, is often confused, because mannitol frequently has been given to these patients prior to their arrival at the hospital or during their intensive care unit stay. It becomes critical, therefore, to frequently measure the serum osmolality and to check the electrolytes. Unless this is done, the patient's management is often likely to result in severe electrolyte disturbances. One should always recall that there is a considerable amount of sodium in both the cerebrospinal fluid (CSF) and in the fluid obtained from nasogastric suctioning, two sources of sodium often ignored when sodium balance is being calculated.

Less frequently, diabetes insipidus may occur following severe head injury. In our experience, it has usually heralded the onset of more severe management problems in patients with intracranial hypertension. It also carries with it a very poor prognosis. The introduction of the new agent desmopressin acetate, which does not have the pressor or smooth muscle side effects of the natural hormone, may make the treatment and complications of the treatment of diabetes insipidus somewhat easier.[63] The administration of large fluid volumes, to replace urinary fluid losses, carries considerable hazard for the severely head-injured. When the natural hormone sodium vasopressin is used, significant sympathomimetic effects can be seen and they can result in rather dramatic rises in SAP which should be avoided, if possible, in such patients.

In patients with severe head injury, our general policy is to administer half-normal saline as the maintenance fluid in adults. Normal saline would be ideal, but its use often leads to sodium overload, and we have therefore selected the half-normal saline solutions. More hypotonic fluids, such as dextrose and water, not only have a deleterious effect on serum osmolality, but may also increase edema in the injured brain. Although significant brain edema is usually not present within the first 48 hours following head injury, it may occur later, and can be severely aggravated by fluid shifts caused by the inappropriate use of intravenous fluids.

Systemic Arterial Hypertension. SAP, though less well recognized than hypoxia or hypotension, is also a source of potential secondary injury. Patients with severe head injury are particularly sensitive to any changes in SAP because of the frequent failure of normal cerebral autoregulation.[36, 40, 52] CBF, therefore, either rises or falls passively with changes in SAP, rather than remaining within normal limits as occurs in healthy individuals. Lewelt and his colleagues[40] have shown that the more severe the head injury, the more severe is the impairment of autoregulation as well. Since increases in brain blood volume are the major cause of increased brain bulk and intracranial hypertension during the early phases of injury,[37, 38] it becomes as important in the severely head-injured to avoid systemic arterial hypertension as it is to avoid shock.

The philosophic basis for vigorous control of the SAP in patients with severe head injury is based not only on the fact that autoregulation is lost and that cerebral blood volume will increase as the blood pressure rises, but also on the observations made in animals by Johannson and co-workers,[21, 31, 32] and Forster *et al.*[18] They have shown that blood-brain barrier disruption following severe systemic arterial hypertension can lead to the extravasation of proteins, followed by the transudation of water.

We treat all sustained systolic blood pressure rises of greater than 160 mm Hg. Control of SAP may require nothing more than the administration of a sedative agent such as morphine. Small doses, given on a frequent basis, are often sufficient to blunt noxious stimuli, such as those that arise from an endotracheal tube, and prevent them from triggering rises in mean arterial pressure (MAP). In cases where sedation has proven inadequate in controlling SAP, it has been our preference to use intravenous trimethaphan (Arfonad) or hydralazine rather than sodium nitroprusside. Although the pupillary light response is usually preserved with the use of Arfonad, pupillary dilatation may occur, particularly if large doses are used, and this does represent a significant disadvantage.

Sodium nitroprusside often has a deleterious effect on cerebral perfusion because of the cerebrovascular dilatation that occurs following its administration.[13] This appears to be a direct effect of the drug on the cerebral vasculature. It has been shown in the laboratory by Marsh et al.,[43] and in patients by Cottrell *et al.*,[13] that intracranial hypertension can often occur in patients, even at a time when the blood pressure is falling, following the administration of sodium nitroprusside. Clubb *et al.*,[10] have shown in an experimental model of brain injury that this drug, while reducing the SAP, often causes dramatic rises in ICP, thus producing a profound decrease in CPP.

Under circumstances where agents such as trimethaphan or hydralazine are ineffective, sodium nitroprusside may be used in patients who are hypocarbic and hyperoxic if the dose is closely monitored and the infusion is delivered slowly. The ICP response to sodium nitroprusside is altered by hypocarbia and hyperoxia and the drug should be used only in closely controlled settings.[44] If ICP monitoring is not utilized, however, sodium nitroprusside and/or ni-troglycerin present real hazards and should not be used.

Fever. Temperatures in excess of 38°C should be treated while searching for the source of fever. The brain's metabolic demands, and CBF therefore, increase as body and brain temperature increase. Vigorous attempts should be made at maintaining normothermia, using antipyretic agents and/or cooling blankets.

TREATMENT CRITERIA AND STANDARD THERAPY FOR THE MANAGEMENT OF INTRACRANIAL HYPERTENSION

Treatment Criteria

It is generally accepted that failure to control intracranial hypertension almost invariably leads to a fatal outcome.[50] When ICP monitoring began in the United States, therapeutic attempts were relatively unsystematic and no definitive guidelines or goals were set. Over the past decade the major head injury centers in this country have begun to divide increases in ICP into two categories. The two categories generally define ICP's ranging between 20 and 40 mm Hg, and those pressures which exceed 40 mm Hg. This distinction is obviously arbitrary and should not lead one to conclude that pressure elevations above 20 mm Hg can be ignored.

In general, our policy is to treat any sustained ICP elevations above 20 mm Hg, if they persist for 15 minutes or more, in any patient with significant shift. We consider pressures above 15 mm Hg, when measured from the lateral ventricle, to be at the upper limit of normal or abnormal. It is often difficult to achieve ICP's below 15 mm Hg if the patient has significant brain swelling. A more realistic goal then is to reduce the ICP to below 20 mm Hg. Initial treatment should always consist of 1) maintaining the patient in the head-up position, 2) hyperventilation, 3) ventricular drainage if possible, 4) maintaining normothermia, and 5) preventing seizures.

If these measures are not successful, mannitol in a dose of 0.25–0.50 g/kg should be administered as a bolus infusion. If the addition of mannitol to the standard regimen outlined above is not effective in reducing the ICP to below 20 mm Hg, an additional dose of mannitol can be used and further attempts at ventricular drainage may also be useful. If the patient has been adequately sedated and paralyzed and the mean SAP is under control, and this regimen fails to control intracranial hypertension, the patient is in grave danger. It is under these circumstances that we have used high doses of barbiturates. High dose barbiturate therapy must still be considered investigational. It should be instituted only in centers with extensive experience in monitoring, and only when adhering to strict usage criteria which are described later in this chapter.

Standard Therapy

Respiratory Care. Hyperventilation continues to be the cornerstone of all attempts to acutely reduce ICP in the severely head-injured.[41] Increases in cerebral volume are the major cause of intracranial hypertension in the early phases of head injury and can often be satisfactorily treated by hyperventilation to a $PaCO_2$ of 25 to 30 torr. Although Overgaard has shown that the CO_2 responsiveness of the cerebral vasculature following severe head injury is reduced when compared to normals,[62] he also demonstrated that hyperventilation continues to be effective in such patients. The effectiveness of hyperventilation, however, does decrease over time. Nevertheless, we have shown that even small reductions in $PaCO_2$ can often lead to better control of the ICP on a chronic basis.[42] As the effect of PCO_2 on ICP control begins to diminish with a $PaCO_2$ between 28 and 31, further reduction to levels of 25 to 28 are often useful. A $PaCO_2$ of below 20 to 22 torr, however, must be avoided in adults because secondary brain ischemia has been reported in normals who were hyperventilated to these levels. Hyperventilation will reduce CBF to a point where secondary vasodilatation occurs because of ischemic hypoxia.[52] When the ICP shows no response to changes in $PaCO_2$, the outcome is invariably an unsatisfactory one with either death or vegetative survival.

An additional benefit of hyperventilation is the respiratory alkalosis that is induced which may be useful in combating brain tissue acidosis. Initial studies in the early '70's appeared to suggest that brain tissue acidosis did not interfere in any significant fashion with brain energy metabolism and other dynamic brain enzymatic systems. However, Siesjo has recently shown that severe brain tissue acidosis has a significant detrimental effect on brain energy metabolism and that the avoidance of such acidosis could conceivably be beneficial in the brain-injured patient.[59]

The Osmotic Agents. Osmotic agents have been shown to reduce ICP for more than 60 years. It was not until the introduction of urea by Javid in the late 50's and early '60's, however, that osmotic therapy had a rational base and came to be extensively used in neurology and neurosurgery clinics.[25-30]

Although urea remains a very satisfactory substance for the treatment of intracranial hypertension, it has been supplanted in most clinical centers in the United States by mannitol, which is the alcohol of the 6 carbon sugar mannose. The major reason behind the switch from urea to mannitol is the fact that unlike urea, mannitol is maintained almost entirely in the extracellular compartment. It is an excellent diuretic, and since its introduction into neurosurgery by Wise and Chater it has been the most widely used diuretic.[60, 61] Mannitol has been shown to have little, if any, rebound effect[60, 61]—a phenomenon that occurs when an osmotic diuretic is administered, and several hours following its administration the ICP returns to a higher level than that for which the drug has been initially given. Rebound has been attributed to influx into the brain of the hyperosmotic substance.

Mannitol is effective in lowering ICP because the serum which is presented to the brain is hyperosmotic. Water is removed from normal tissues rather than from foci of edematous brain. Kuhner and his colleagues[35] and Marshall *et al.*[45] have demonstrated that lower doses of mannitol can be effectively used in patients with intracranial hypertension. Table 9.2 demonstrates the response to varying doses of

Table 9.2
ICP Dose Responses for Mannitol in Patients with Intracranial Hypertension[a]

Mannitol Dose (g/kg)	Initial ICP	VPR	Time to Lowest ICP	Lowest ICP	ICP at 5 hr
	mm Hg		min	mm Hg	
0.25	41 ± 3.6	18 ± 3.6	14	16 ± 2.0	24 ± 1.8
0.5	48 ± 5.8	20 ± 3.4	13	17 ± 3.0	20 ± 3.0
1.0	44 ± 4.9	14 ± 2.7	17	18 ± 2.1	19 ± 3.0

[a] No differences ($p > 0.05$) existed among the required three dose ranges studied in the intracanial pressures (ICP's) or time required to achieve the lowest ICP. VPR, volume-pressure response.

mannitol and illustrates the fact that relatively good responses can be obtained even with 0.25 g/kg doses. It is true that at five hours there was a definite trend for the larger doses to remain effective; however, this offered no real advantage as a second smaller dose could be given in response to changes in monitored ICP. Miller and Leach have shown that mannitol not only reduces ICP but also favorably influences the volume-pressure curve.[49] Mannitol has also been shown, in both animals and man, to improve regional CBF. This may also account for its often dramatic long-term effectiveness in the absence of a sustained reduction in ICP.

Glycerol has also been recommended for use in the treatment of intracranial hypertension, but has not attained the popularity of mannitol in the United States. This is in part because mannitol has proven to be so satisfactory and so easy to use. The fact that glycerol can be given orally offers no real advantage in the severely brain-injured.

Non-Osmotic Diuretics. There has been considerable interest in the use of non-osmotic diuretics to treat intracranial hypertension. Bourke and his colleagues[40] have extensively studied furosemide and its cogeners in the laboratory. Cottrell reported that furosemide offered advantages over mannitol in the operating room setting.[12] However, the initial ICP's in the patients studied were not comparable, and the results, therefore, not as impressive as reported. Levin, in a study where patients served as their own controls, compared the effectiveness of the osmotic and non-osmotic diuretics.[39] He found that the non-osmotic agents were much less reliable in producing a reduction in ICP and that their use, although shown to be of value in acute laboratory experiments, appeared to be much more limited in man.

While mannitol continues to be the agent of choice, both for inital, acute, and chronic therapy, the search for agents to remove water from damaged brain, as well as from the brain as a whole, is a fruitful area of research. The development of analogs of furosemide in Bourke's laboratory may well often significant advantages if such agents can be shown to be effective in man.[4] Fluid and electrolyte problems that occur with the chronic administration of mannitol are real and could theoretically be avoided if an agent which had a specific effect on brain sodium and chloride could be developed.

Acetalzolamide is generally contraindicated in head-injured patients because of its cerebral vasodilator effect. Although the drug causes a significant reduction in CSF production, this effect in laboratory models of brain injury is less significant than the decreased compliance produced by the drug's cerebral vasodilator effect.[23]

Corticosteroids. Despite multiple attempts at controlled trials, the use of high doses of corticosteroids remains controversial. The initial enthusiasm for the use of high doses of dexamethasone emanated from Faupel et al.[17] and Gobiet.[19] When analyzing these two studies, the following must be kept in mind: The Gobiet study was not a randomized control trial, but rather a report of survivorship in patients in succeeding years, suggesting the possibility that other factors might have influenced outcome. If one combines the severely disabled survivors in Faupel's study with those who did not survive, there is not a significant difference in outcome in those patients who were treated with dexamethasone.

Pitts reported that the administration of high doses of corticosteroids did not influence survival. However, in those patients who did survive and had received corticosteroids, the quality of survival was significantly better.[53] Cooper noted no change and thus no benefit on outcome in patients with severe head injuries who received comparable doses.[11] As most patients who have had severe head injury do not initially have brain edema, but rather have brain swelling secondary to increased brain blood volume, this is not terribly surprising. Nevertheless, it is true that brain edema can occur later as areas of contusion resolve and osmotic pressure gradients develop within brain tissue. Figure 9.3 demonstrates two consecutive CT scans. The first shows an area of contusion and generalized hemispheric swelling. The second scan, 48 hours later, demonstrates edema around an area of hemorrhagic contusion. These findings were confirmed at the time of surgical intervention. It is possible that dexamethasone may prevent or at least ameliorate foci of edema in areas of already injured brain. This may be the only logical rationale for the use of this drug in acutely head-injured patients. As Becker has pointed out, only extremely large trials involving many hundreds of patients with very good patient matching is likely to give a definitive answer.

In our clinic, the use of dexamethasone has been based on the rationale described above. Our protocols call for the use of 80 mg a day during the first four days, with tapering of the drug so that the patient is no longer maintained on dexamethasone after 10 days.

HIGH DOSE BARBITURATE THERAPY FOR THE TREATMENT OF UNCONTROLLABLE INTRACRANIAL PRESSURE

Entry Criteria

It is our view that *high dose barbiturate therapy should only be used as an adjunc-* *tive therapy and only when other standard measures have failed.* Table 9.3 outlines the criteria for use of barbiturates in our institution. Despite the fact that we believe that the evidence is overwhelming that barbiturates do reduce ICP in patients who have become refractory to other treatments,[47, 54, 55] the absence of randomized control trials to demonstrate their influence on outcome makes their use investigational. It is therefore inappropriate to utilize these agents as the initial treatment tool.

Prior to instituting high dose barbiturate therapy, all efforts should be made to be certain the patient has been adequately hydrated and ventilated, that the airway is well established, and that all the standard methods to relieve elevated ICP have been attempted. A CT scan should be obtained prior to the administration of the drug to rule out the presence of a mass lesion as the cause of failure to control ICP. If pressure control continues to be a problem after administration of high doses of barbiturates, the neurosurgeon should have no hesitancy in re-scanning the patient. Absolute reliance on ICP monitoring is never advisable. Although pupillary dilatation will still occur with serum barbiturate levels of 3–4 mg% the clinical examination is partially lost once high serum levels of pentobarbital are reached.

Barbiturates have never been required in our center in patients with Glasgow Coma scores of 7 or more. It is our impression that the use of barbiturates in other centers in such instances probably reflects inadequate sedation and failure to use more standard measures appropriately. The use of the drug under these circumstances may only serve to prolong the level of the patient's intensive care unit hospitalization once this complex therapy is begun. Our sole deviation from an entry criteria pressure of 25 mm Hg or more, occurs in patients in whom a previous craniectomy has been performed and in whom the ICP exceeds 15 mm Hg and/or pupillary dilatation occurs. These patients deteriorate at much lower pressures because once a decompression has been performed the ICP becomes a much less accurate reflection of brain and brain stem distortion (see also Chapter 8).

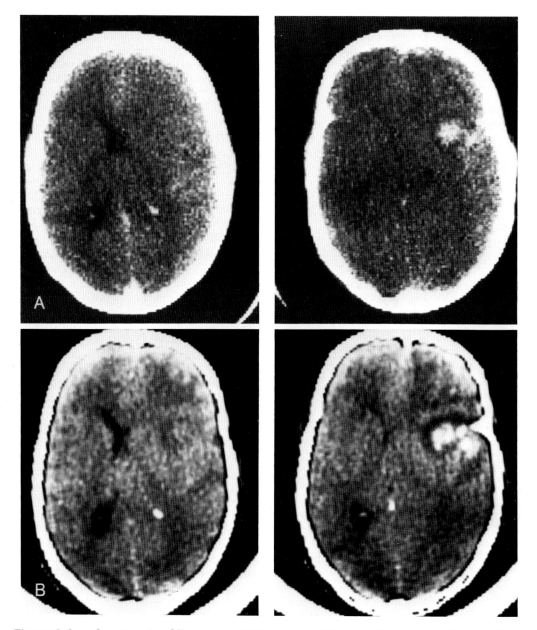

Figure 9.3.   Consecutive CT scans. (*A*) Initial scans (Glasgow Coma Score 13). Marked shift, hemorrhagic frontotemporal contusion. (*B*) Scans 48 hours later (Glasgow Coma Score 6). Note edema as manifested by decreased density about the area of contusion.

Monitoring Capabilities and Guidelines

The decision to begin high dose barbiturate therapy must not be made without the availability of strict pressure monitoring criteria and well-trained personnel. The clinical expertise and monitoring required of the intensive care unit personnel and of the hospital, if high dose barbiturate therapy is to be used, is defined in Table 9.4. All patients must have an ICP monitoring device in place as well as an intra-arterial

Table 9.3
Criteria for Patient Entry into High-dose Barbiturate Therapy Protocol

The patient has an ICP of >25 mm Hg[a] despite . . .

1. Appropriate positioning
2. Controlled hyperventilation with paralysis and adequate sedation
3. Normoxia
4. Normothermia
5. Adequate anti-convulsant therapy
6. Ventricular drainage if possible
7. Dexamethasone 20 mg IV q 6 h
8. Administering a total dose of 1 g/kg mannitol in the previous hour

and *does not* have

1. An inadequately treated surgical mass
2. A major continuing source of hemorrhage
3. Significant hypovolemia. Therefore,
   a. Mean pulmonary artery pressure is >8
   b. Mean SAP is >70 mm Hg
   c. Cardiac index is 2 or >

[a] 15 mm Hg in patients with craniectomy.

Table 9.4
Clinical Expertise, Monitoring, and Capabilities Necessary to Utilize High-dose Barbiturate Therapy

1. Experienced ICU team and a laboratory capable of measuring appropriate serum barbiturate levels rapidly
2. Continuous ICP monitoring
3. Continuous arterial pressure monitoring
4. Swan-Ganz catheter
5. In-house CT scanning capabilities

pressure line. The cerebral perfusion pressure should be maintained at a minimum of 50 mm Hg. Under most circumstances we have found that one can achieve an ICP of less than 20 mm Hg and preserve a CPP of 50 mm Hg. In adults, we have been reluctant to allow the mean SAP to fall below 65–70 mm Hg; and in children, we have chosen 55 mm Hg as a lower limit for the mean SAP. These recommendations may be somewhat conservative, but it is suggested that they be followed until we learn more about other methods for determining the adequacy of cerebral perfusion.

The placement of a Swan-Ganz catheter is also necessary to ensure that intravascular volume is maintained at a normal level and to allow measurement of cardiac output on a regular basis. In patients in whom multiple injuries are also present, a Swan-Ganz catheter is an absolute necessity. Pulmonary arterial wedge pressure should be normal prior to the institution of high dose barbiturate therapy so that the cardiac depressant effect of barbiturates are not exacerbated once the drug is administered.

The patient's temperature should be constantly measured by a rectal probe. We have not used deliberate hypothermia with barbiturates because the core temperature usually falls to 32–33°C when adequate serum barbiturate levels have been reached. This is an effect of the significant systemic metabolic depression that accompanies barbiturate administration. If hypothermia is superimposed on these already depressed body temperatures, life-threatening cardiac arrhythmias occur (particularly in younger patients with head injuries). Difficulties with gas exchange resulting in hypoxia have been observed by others when hypothermia has been added to high dose barbiturate therapy.

Brain stem auditory evoked responses have been extremely useful in monitoring patients who receive pentobarbital. Although small changes in latencies can occur when barbiturates are used, prolongations are not usually beyond those which occur normally. We have found the information derived from the serial examination of the brain stem, using the evoked response technique, to be useful in following the integrity of the brain stem in patients who have received high doses of barbiturates. When the brain stem evoked response deteriorates in the presence of satisfactory ICP control, the possibility of irreversible brain stem injury can often be demonstrated if adequate CT scanning is available (Fig. 9.4). We have also often seen improvement in brain stem auditory evoked responses as the ICP has come under better control, indicating that brain stem compression from tentorial herniation has been lessened and that the patient may therefore have an

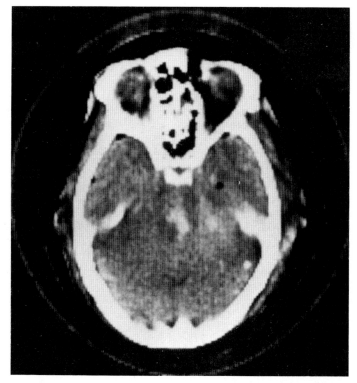

Figure 9.4. CT scan of brain stem hemorrhage seen 72 hours following intracranial hypertension from acute subdural hematoma. ICP well controlled but brain stem auditory evoked responses deteriorated. Initial scan did not demonstrate brain stem hemorrhage.

improved prognosis. Several centers are now investigating the utility of measuring other electrophysiologic parameters in patients who are receiving cerebral metabolic depressant agents. In the future, this type of monitoring is likely to occupy a more important place in the intensive care unit setting.

Barbiturate Dosage

Reduction in ICP is the major guiding factor in the administration of pentobarbital. In our initial series of patients, we began with relatively small doses of 3–5 mg/kg administered over several minutes.[47] We now feel that it is safe to begin with larger doses of 5–10 mg/kg provided that the patient is not hypovolemic. As a general guideline, we have administered pentobarbital until the ICP is reduced to 20 mm Hg and preferably until it is under 15 mm Hg and/or until the serum level exceeds 3 mg% but remains under 5 mg%. It has not been our experience that the ICP can be further reduced using barbiturates once a serum level exceeding 5 mg% has been achieved.

Kassell *et al.*,[33] have recently suggested that no further benefit secondary to a reduction of CBF or cerebral metabolism can be obtained if sufficient barbiturates have been administered to produce 60 second burst supression on the EEG. This laboratory finding, if confirmed, would at least partially eliminate the need for frequent determinations of serum pentobarbital level. Bruce, however, contends Kassell's laboratory observation is not consistent with his own observations in patients, and that he and his colleagues have seen further reductions in ICP if serum levels exceeding 5 mg% have been reached.[7]

It is critical to note that serum levels for each of the barbiturates presently being used to treat intracranial hypertension (thiopental, phenobarbital, and pentobarbital) are not equivalent. A serum level of 4 mg% from the administration of phenobarbital is compatible with a drowsy, but still partially wakeful state. A pentobarbital level of 4 mg% almost always results in an isoelectric EEG and respiratory arrest. If these drugs are used, it is important to know that the laboratory which determines barbiturate levels is actually measuring that barbiturate which is being administered.

We have no clinical experience with drugs other than pentobarbital and cannot comment on the relative efficacy of one agent versus another. The theoretical advantage of thiopental, as proposed by Demopoulos and Flamm, is based on their observation that free radical scavenging is much more efficacious with thiopental than pentobarbital.[15] However, there is recent evidence that free radical formation plays little, if any, role in the pathogenesis of brain injury. Moreover, the relatively brief effect of sodium thiopental on ICP tends to make its administration more difficult because the drug has to be given more frequently and serum sodium levels often rise because of the large volume of drug that needs to be given.

ICP Control; Discontinuance of the Drug

When satisfactory ICP control has been obtained using barbiturates and the ICP has been controlled in the normal range for 24 to 48 hours, one can consider reducing the dose of the drug. Barbiturates should never be stopped abruptly, as we have seen acute deterioration occur 8 to 10 hours following acute cessation of the medication despite the maintenance of adequate serum levels. This suggests that barbiturates act not only by causing metabolic depression but also by some direct effect of the bolus-administered dose on the cerebral vasculature.

The volume-pressure response, thought to be a reliable means of predicting when therapy could be stopped, has failed us in two instances and two deaths have resulted. Cerebral compliance testing is not reliable and we believe that slow reductions in the dose and increasing the time between each dose is a more satisfactory means of ensuring that no untoward rebound in ICP will occur.

On the first day, we maintain the patient on half the administered dose and on the second day, the time interval between doses is doubled. On the third day, the dose is halved again, and on the fourth day, the drug is discontinued. If intracranial hypertension develops while the drug is being tapered, but the ICP rises are relatively small, the reinstitution of mannitol therapy and/or ventricular drainage can usually ensure satisfactory reduction of ICP while the drug is being discontinued. If severe intracranial hypertension, defined as persistent pressures above 30 mm Hg, occurs while the drug is being tapered, resumption of therapy will often be effective. We have done this on several occasions with favorable outcomes. One must also be aware of the fact that as general metabolic suppression is reduced, $PaCO_2$ almost always rises and respiratory adjustments should be made to keep the $PaCO_2$ below 30 mm Hg. Bucking or straining on the endotracheal tube can also be blunted by the use of small doses of morphine or other sedative mediations.

When barbiturates are used in the manner described, and careful attention to detail is maintained, high dose barbiturate therapy, in our experience, is effective and safe. We must emphasize, however, that the complications of the administration of any potent drug can be disastrous unless a specific and organized plan is followed for its use.

Complications of High Dose Barbiturate Therapy

The avoidance of severe dehydration and an understanding of the problems which can occur if other therapies are superimposed on the use of these very potent agents, can prevent the occurrence of most potential complications. In a retrospective review of our experience, hypoxia has not occurred more frequently in patients who have been randomized to high dose barbiturate therapy than patients with equally severe head injury who have not received these drugs. If dehydration is used as the initial mode of therapy, and barbiturates are then superimposed on this setting, rather dramatic falls in cardiac output can be seen with subsequent poor peripheral and pulmonary perfusion and hypoxia.

When hypothermia is superimposed on the use of pentobarbital therapy, an increase in lung stiffness has been observed, leading to decreased compliance and subsequent hypoxia. If warming is instituted, this change is usually reversible. Therefore, extremely low body temperatures should be avoided when these drugs are employed.

Hypotension is another problem which often can be avoided in adults by assuring that the patient is adequately hydrated and that central pressures are continuously followed. We have had only minimal difficulty with systemic hypotension despite administration of initial doses of 10 mg/kg as long as we have taken care to support the intravascular volume. Dopamine, which is primarily an inotropic agent, can be used to support cardiac output if hypotension ensues. If hypotension disproportionate to that which one would expect from the administration of pentobarbital occurs, the possibility of an unrecognized intra-abdominal or pulmonary catastrophe should be suspected. Here, Swan-Ganz catheter monitoring can be very helpful and has enabled us to recognize intraperitoneal and other surgically treatable events which we had previously missed.

In patients receiving pentobarbital, it must not be assumed that all complications are secondary to barbiturate administration. Vigorous searches should be made for other possible causes of hypoxia, atelectasis, or pneumothorax. The inspired oxygen tension should always be increased in an attempt to maintain the $PaO_2 > 70$ torr, while vigorous efforts are made to find the source of the patient's problem.

When high dose barbiturate therapy has failed, and an inexorable rise in ICP has occurred, cerebral angiography can be used to determine whether the patient is brain dead (see Chapters 4 and 11). Barbiturates alone, no matter what the serum level, will not lead to an absolute cessation of blood flow in the absence of brain death. This is an important method to determine brain death, as the usual electroencephalographic techniques cannot be used in patients who have high serum levels of barbiturates.

CURRENT PHARMACOLOGICAL CLINICAL RESEARCH
Dimethyl Sulfoxide

Dimethyl sulfoxide (DMSO) has recently been introduced into clinical trials for the treatment of intracranial hypertension. It was initially postulated that DMSO had its major effect as a result of the tremendous diuresis that followed its administration. Recent experience in our clinic demonstrates that the diuresis occurs well after the abrupt fall in ICP. These changes in ICP are so rapid that it is tempting to postulate that the drug has some direct action on the cerebrovascular bed. This effect, however, must be produced by a different mechanism than that which causes the barbiturates to reduce ICP. Figure 9.5 demonstrates the effect of sequential administration of DMSO and pentobarbital. During previous episodes of intracranial hypertension, the ICP fell rapidly with DMSO. In this instance, there was no response to DMSO, but the administration of pentobarbital caused an immediate fall in ICP from 38 to 10 mm Hg.

DMSO has been dramatically effective in reducing ICP in several laboratory models of acute brain edema and the drug, therefore, deserves further investigation. Problems with its administration and potential complications are not well understood, and more work is needed before it can be used on more than an investigational basis. Difficulties include the large volume of fluid and salt needed to replace the naturesis and diuresis that follows DMSO administration. Electrolyte disturbances are much more se-

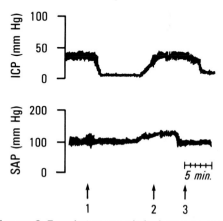

Figure 9.5. Intracranial hypertension treated with DMSO and then thiopental. *Arrows:* 1) first DMSO dose; 2) second DMSO dose; and 3) thiopental response following failure of DMSO to reduce ICP.

vere than those seen with mannitol, and the mild hemolysis which is seen with regularity when high concentrations of the drug are used, also presents problems. In addition, the mixture of the solutions and the care needed to administer the compound requires the use of glass IV bottles and glass syringes, and the odor is unpleasant for nursing personnel. However, because the drug appears to offer certain properties not available in agents currently in use, its efficacy should be investigated both in the laboratory and in man.

Lidocaine

Intravenous lidocaine is considered to be a promising agent for the treatment of intracranial hypertension. Initial reports from Donegan and his colleagues[16] demonstrated reductions in ICP in patients with head injury and other disturbances. However, many of these patients had little or no initial intracranial hypertension. The recent experience of Aidinis in some of our patients with severe intracranial hypertension demonstrated no decrease in ICP following the administration of lidocaine.[1] This brings into question whether the drug will be useful in the operating room or intensive care unit settings. A larger series of patients must be studied in a Phase II trial before we can be certain as to the efficacy of lidocaine.

PRESENT STATUS, NEEDS AND THE FUTURE

Significant advances appear to have been made in the treatment of brain-injured patients in the last decade. Perhaps the most important ones have not been those that have occurred in the intensive care unit setting, but rather the neurosurgical community's recognition that the prevention of secondary insults by rapid evacuation of mass lesions and early treatment of hypoxia, hypercapnea, and hypotension are prerequisites for the recovery of most brain-injured patients.[51] Our better understanding of the need for a systematic and rational well-organized approach to the treatment of these patients has also contributed to reduced mortality. The reduced mortality

reported initially by Becker et al.,[2] by Bruce et al.,[6] and more recently, by our own group,[46] strongly indicates that severely brain-injured patients can have improved outcomes with aggressive and systematic care. Although the regimens outlined by these three centers differ in detail, they all share a well-organized, systematic approach to managing these patients and the avoidance of management errors. If care is not well-organized and systematic, and all personnel do not understand what the goals are, management errors are common and often fatal.

The introduction of new therapeutic modalities such as high dose barbiturate therapy and aggressive pulmonary treatment also appear to have influenced mortality. These contributions must be viewed in the light of the well-organized and well-disciplined care team and not as panaceas for patients with acute, severe brain injury. Mortality rates of approximately 30% appear achievable if patients can be rapidly evacuated and rapidly studied in appropriate settings. One must recognize that a significant number of patients with severe brain injury, perhaps 25% or more who reach the hospital alive, have severe, irreversible structural injuries and that even optimal management will not yield useful survivors.[8, 9]

In the future, further research developments leading to the manipulation of CBF and cerebral metabolism are likely to come to the fore as methods for the treatment of severe brain injury. The flurry of research triggered by the initial application of metabolic suppression using barbiturates, as pioneered by Shapiro et al.,[56, 57] has led to renewed interest in the possibility of controlling brain metabolism in a beneficial manner for brain-injured patients with a variety of diseases. Other drugs with fewer cardiorespiratory depressant effects, such as long-acting diazepam analogs,[55] will be available in the next several years. We must be open in our search, and diligent and skeptical in our review of results when they are reported. We must keep in mind, however, as Clifton has recently shown, that even small reductions in mortality may be meaningful, given the fixed number of patients who suffer irreversible injuries and reach the hospital alive.[9] The future is not likely to hold any major surprises; rather, it will require consolidation of those gains already made and the careful application of potential new treatments.

References

1. Aidinis, S. Private communication.
2. Becker, D.P., Miller, J.D., Ward, J.D., Greenberg, R.P., Young, H.F., Sakalas, R.: The outcome from severe head injury with early diagnosis and inten sive management. J. Neurosurg., 47:491–502, 1977.
3. ecker, D.P. Commentary. Meeting of the American Association of Neurological Surgeons. Los Angeles, California, 1979.
4. Bourke, R.S., Kimelberg, H.K., Daze, M.A., Popp, A.J.: Studies on the formation of astroglial swelling and its inhibition by clinically useful agents. In: Neural Trauma, A.J. Popp, R.S. Bourke, L.R. Nelson, H.K., Eds. Raven Press, New York, 1979, pp. 95–112.
5. Bowers, S.A., Marshall, L.F.: The outcome in 200 consecutive cases of severe head injury treated in San Diego County: a prospective analysis. Neurosurgery, 6:237–242, 1980.
6. Bruce, D.A., Schut, L., Bruno, L.A., Wood, J.H., Sutton, L.N.: Outcome following severe head injury in children. J. Neurosurg., 48:679–688, 1978.
7. Bruce, D.A. Private communication.
8. Clifton, G.L., Grossman, R.G., Makela, M., Miner, M.E., Handel, S., Sadhu, V.: Neurologic course and correlated computed tomographic findings after severe closed head injury. J. Neurosurg., 52:611–624, 1980.
9. Clifton, G.L., McCormick, W.F., Grossman, R.G.: Neuropathology of early and late deaths after head injury. Neurosurgery, 1981 (in press).
10. Clubb, R.J., Maxwell, R.E., Chou, S.N.: Experimental brain injury in the dog. The pharmacological effects of pentobarbital and sodium nitroprusside. J. Neurosurg., 52:189–195, 1980.
11. Cooper, P.R., Moody, S., Clark, W.K., Kirkpatrick, J., Maravilla, K., Gould, A.L., Drane, W.: Dexamethasone and severe head injury. J. Neurosurg., 51:307–316, 1979.
12. Cottrell, J.E., Robustelli, A., Turndorf, H.: Furosemide- and mannitol-induced changes in intracranial pressure and serum osmolality and electrolytes. Anesthesiology, 47:28–30, 1977.
13. Cottrell, J.E., Patel, K., Turndorf, H., Ransohoff, J.: Intracranial pressure changes induced by sodium nitroprusside in patients with intracranial mass lesions. J. Neurosurg., 48:329–331, 1978.
14. Davis, D.H., Sundt, T.M.: Relationship of cerebral blood flow to cardiac output, mean arterial pressure, blood volume, and alpha and beta blockade in cats. J. Neurosurg., 52:745–754, 1980.
15. Demopoulos, H.B., Flamm, E.S., Seligman, M.L., Jorgensen, E., Ransohoff, J.: Antitoxidant effects of barbiturates in model membranes undergoing free radical damage. In: Cerebral Blood Flow. VIII. Cerebral Function, Metabolism and Circulation, D.H. Ingvar, and N.A. Lassen, Eds. Munksgaard, Copenhagen, 1977, pp. 152–153.
16. Donegan, M., Bedford, R.F., Dacey, R.: IV lidocaine for prevention of intracranial hypertension. Anesthesiology 51:S20, 1979.
17. Faupel, G., Reulen, H.J., Muller, D., Schurmann, K.: Double-blind study on the effects of steroids on severe closed head injury. In: Dynamics of Brain Edema, H.M. Pappius and W. Feindel, Eds. Springer-Verlag, Berlin, 1976, pp. 337–343.
18. Forster, A., VanHorn, K., Marshall, L.F., Shapiro, H.M.: Anesthetic effects on blood-brain barrier function during acute hypertension. Anesthesiology, 49:26–30, 1978.
19. Gobiet, W.: The influence of various doses of dexamethasone on intracranial pressure in patients with severe head injury. In: Dynamics of Brain Edema, H.M. Pappius, W. Feindel, Eds. Springer-Verlag, Berlin, 1976, pp. 351–355.
20. Graham, D.I., Adams, J.H., Doyle, D.: Ischemic brain damage in fatal non-missile head injuries. J. Neurol. Sci., 39:213–234, 1978.
21. Haar, FL., Sadhu, V.K., Sampson, J., Gildenberg, P.L., et al.: Can CT scan findings predict ICP in closed head injury patients? Transaction of Congress of Neurological Surgeons, Houston, 1980.
22. Haggendal, E., Johannson, B.: On the pathophysiology of the increased cerebrovascular permeability in acute arterial hypertension in cats. Acta Neurol. Scand., 48:265–270, 1979.
23. Harbaugh, R.D., James, H.E., Marshall, L.F., Shapiro, H.M., Laurin, R.: Acute therapeutic modalities in experimental vasogenic edema. Neurosurgery, 5:656–665, 1979.
24. Hulme, A., Cooper, R.: Cerebral blood flow during sleep in patients with raised intracranial pressure. Prog. Brain Res., 30:77–81, 1968.
25. Javid, M.: Urea—new use of an old agent. Reduction of intracranial and intraocular pressure. Surg. Clin. N. Am., 38:907–928, 1958.
26. Javid, M.: A valuable new method for the reduction of intracranial and intraocular pressure by the use of urea. Trans. Am. Neurol. Assn., pp. 113–116, 1958.
27. Javid, M.: Urea in intracranial surgery. A new method. J. Neurosurg., 18:51–57, 1961.
28. Javid, M., Anderson, J.: Observations on the use of urea in rhesus monkeys. Surg. Forum, 9:686–690, 1958.
29. Javid, M., Anderson, J.: The effect of urea on cerebrospinal fluid pressure in monkeys before and after bilateral nephrectomy. J. Lab. Clin. Med., 53:484–489, 1959.
30. Javid, M., Settlage, P.: Effect of urea on cerebrospinal fluid pressure in human subjects. Preliminary report. J.A.M.A., 160:943–949, 1956.
31. Johansson, B.: Blood-brain barrier dysfunction in acute arterial hypertension after papaverine-induced vasodilatation. Acta Neurol. Scand., 50: 573–580, 1974.
32. Johansson, B.B.: Water content of rat brain in acute hypertension. In: Dynamics of Brain Edema, H.M. Pappius, W. Feindel, Eds. Springer-Verlag, Berlin, 1976, pp. 28–31.
33. Kassell, N.F., Hitchon, P.W., Gerk, M.K., et al.: Alterations in cerebral blood flow, oxygen metab-

olism and electrical activity produced by high dose sodium thiopental. Neurosurgery, 7:598–603, 1980.

34. Klauber, M.H., Barrett-Connor, E., Marshall, L.F., Bowers, S.A.: Epidemiology of head injury: a prospective study of an entire community, San Diego, California, 1978. Am. J. Epidemiol., 113:500–509, 1981.

35. Kühner, A., Roquefeuil, B., Viguie, E., et al.: The influence of high and low dosages of mannitol 25% in the therapy of cerebral edema. In: Advances in Neurosurgery 1. Brain Edema, K. Schürmann, M. Brock, H.J. Reulen, Eds. Springer-Verlag, Berlin, 1973, pp. 81–91.

36. Langfitt, T.W., Weinstein, J.D., Kassell, N.F.: Cerebral vasomotor paralasis produced by intracranial hypertension. Neurology, 15:622–641, 1965.

37. Langfitt, T.W., Kassell, N.F., Weinstein, J.D.: Cerebral blood flow with intracranial hypertension. Neurology, 15:761–773, 1965.

38. Langfitt, T.W., Weinstein, J.D., Kassell, N.F.: Vascular factors in head injury: contribution to brain swelling and intracranial hypertension. In: Head Injury, W.F. Caveness, A.E. Walker, Eds. Conference Proceedings, Philadelphia J.F. Lippincott Co., 1966, pp. 172–194.

39. Levin, A.B. Treatment of increased intracranial pressure: a comparison of different hyperosmotic agents and the use of theiopental. In: Proceedings of the American Association of Neurological Surgeons Annual Meeting. New Orleans, Louisiana, 1978.

40. Lewelt, W., Jenkins, L.W., Miller, J.D.: Autoregulation of cerebral blood flow after experimental fluid percussion injury of the brain. J. Neurosurg., 4:500–511, 1980.

41. Lundberg, N., Kjallquist, A., Bien, C.: Reduction of increased intracranial pressure by hyperventilation. Acta Psychiat. Scand., 34:4–64, 1959.

42. Marsh, M.L., Marshall, L.F., Shapiro, H.M.: Neurosurgical intensive care. Anesthesiology, 47: 149–163, 1977.

43. Marsh, M.L., Shapiro, H.M., Smith, R.W., Marshall, L.F.: Changes in neurologic and intracranial pressure associated with sodium nitroprusside administration. Anesthesiology, 51:336–338, 1979.

44. Marsh, M.L., Aidinis, S.J., Naughton, K.V.H., Marshall, L.F., Shapiro, H.M.: Technique of nitroprusside administration modifies the intracranial pressure response. Anesthesiology, 59:538–541, 1979.

45. Marshall, L.F., Smith, R.W., Rauscher, L.A., Shapiro, H.M.: Mannitol dose requirements in brain-injured patients. J. Neurosurg., 48:169–172, 1978.

46. Marshall, L.F., Smith, R.W., Shapiro, H.M.: The outcome with aggressive treatment in severe head injuries. I. The significance of intracranial pressure monitoring. J. Neurosurg., 50:20–25, 1979.

47. Marshall, L.F., Smith, R.W., Shapiro, H.M.: Outcome with aggressive treatment in severe head injuries. II. Acute and chronic barbiturate administration in the management of head injury. J. Neurosurg., 50:26–30, 1979.

48. Miller, J.D., Stanek, A., Langfitt, T.W.: Concepts of cerebral perfusion pressure and vascular compression during intracranial hypertension. In: Progress in Brain Research: 35 Cerebral Blood Flow. Elsevier Pub., Amsterdam, 1971.

49. Miller, J.D., Leech, P.: Effects of mannitol and steroid therapy on intracranial volume-pressure relationships in patients. J. Neurosurg., 42: 274–281, 1975.

50. Miller, J.D., Becker, D.P., Ward, J.D., Sullivan, H.G., Adams, W.E., Rosner, M.J.: Significance of intracranial hypertension in severe head injury. J. Neurosurg., 47:503–516, 1977.

51. Miller, J.D., Sweet, R.C., Narayan, R., Becker, D.P.: Early insults to the injured brain. J.A.M.A., 240:439–442, 1978.

52. Overgaard, J., Tweed, W.A.: Cerebral circulation after head injury. I: Cerebral blood flow and its regulation after closed head injury with emphasis on clinical correlation. J. Neurosurg., 41:531–541, 1974.

53. Pitts, L.H., Kaktis, J.V.: Effects of megadose steroids on outcome following severe head injury. In: Proceedings of the American Association of Neurological Surgeons Annual Meeting. Los Angeles, California, 1979, pp. 90–91.

54. Rockoff, M.A., Marshall, L.F., Shapiro, H.M.: High dose barbiturate therapy in humans: a clinical review of 60 patients. Ann. Neurol., 3:83–84, 1979.

55. Rockoff, M.A., Naughton, K.V.H., Shapiro, H.M., Ingvar, M., Ray, K.F., Gagnon, R.L., Marshall, L.F.: Cerebral circulatory and metabolic responses to intravenously administered lorazepam. Anesthesiology 53:215–218, 1980.

56. Shapiro, H.M., Galindo, A., Wyte, S.R., Harris, A.B.: Rapid intraoperative reduction of intracranial pressure with thiopentone. Br. J. Anaesth., 45:1057–1061, 1973.

57. Shapiro, H.M., Wyte, S.R., Loeser, J. Barbiturate-augmented hypothermia for reduction of persistent intracranial hypertension. J. Neurosurg., 40:90–100, 1974.

58. Shapiro, H.M. Intracranial hypertension: therapeutic and anesthetic considerations. Anesthesiology, 43:445–471, 1975.

59. Siesjo, B. Influence of severe brain lactic acidosis on brain energy metabolism. Acta Neurol. Scand. (in press).

60. Wise, B.L., Chater, N.: Effect of mannitol on cerebrospinal fluid pressure. The actions of hypertonic mannitol solutions and of urea compared. Arch. Neurol., 4:200–202, 1961.

61. Wise, B.L., Chater, N.: The value of hypertonic mannitol solution in decreasing brain mass and lowering cerebrospinal-fluid pressure. J. Neurosurg., 19:1038–1043, 1962.

62. Wollman, H., Smith, T.C., Stephen, G.W., et al.: Effects of extremes of respiratory and metabolic alkalosis on cerebral blood flow in man. J. Appl. Physiol., 24:60–65, 1976.

63. Ziai, F., Walter, R., Rosenthal, I.M.: Treatment of central diabetes insipidus in adults and children with Desmopressin—a synthetic analogue of vasopressin. Arch. Intern. Med., 138:1382–1385, 1978.

10

Intracranial Pressure Monitoring: Techniques and Pitfalls

HAROLD A. WILKINSON

HISTORICAL

The first serious efforts to measure pressure in the central nervous system of human beings were spearheaded by Quincke,[87, 88] Queckenstedt,[86] Ayala,[3] and Ayer.[4] Using a lumbar puncture approach to the cerebrospinal fluid (CSF) space and measuring pressures manometrically the concept of intracranial pressure (ICP) and its potential significance came into clinical use even before arterial blood pressure monitoring had become generally accepted. These early pioneers delineated the normal range of CSF pressure, documented the influence of position (sitting *vs.* recumbent) on measured lumbar pressure, documented a respiratory effect (especially the Valsalva maneuver) on ICP, demonstrated the potential for compartmentalization or lack of communication of intracranial pressures below a spinal block, and described a method of demonstrating this compartmentalization (the Queckenstedt test). Ayala even anticipated our modern thinking about ICP "compliance" or "reserve." After extensive studies, largely in human volunteers, he formulated the once widely employed "Ayala Index" for estimating the degree of intracranial fluid volume and, therefore, indirectly measuring ventricular collapse caused by intracranial mass lesions—brain tumors, brain edema, etc.

One hundred years before Ayala's studies the Monroe-Kellie doctrine had been propounded.[53, 73] This doctrine conceptualizes the central nervous system as consisting of a closed and non-distensible box containing a mixture of liquid and solid structures. The doctrine specified that within this closed box a small increase in its contents would cause a dramatic increase in pressure, and *vice versa*. Although this doctrine has been modified in recent decades (see Chapter 8), the basic concept remains a valuable contribution and underlies much of our clinical thinking regarding intracranial hypertension.

Browder and Meyers[11, 12] used lumbar punctures extensively in head-injured patients and seriously questioned the reliability of clinical observations in predicting ICP. Even though they did not appreciate the potential significance of compartmentalization below a tonsillar herniation, the observations made by Browder and Meyers remain largely valid. They wrote:

> The 'classical pattern of signs,' consisting of steady rise above normal levels of blood pressure, steady fall in pulse pressure, decrease in respiratory rate, stupor, coma, vomiting, etc., which has been held to indicate that the intracranial pressure is on the increase, is not met in the present series of brain insults (and rarely in our general experience with head injuries). Therefore, it is of little help in determining whether a patient is improving or losing ground, in need

of operation, or if general supportive and symptomatic measures will suffice.

Whether singly or in combination, the blood pressure, pulse rate, respirations and the state of consciousness cannot be regarded as an index of the intracranial tension, whether high or low, rising, falling or on a plateau.

Guillaume and Janny[37] established the value of continuous direct ICP monitoring in human patients. They too pointed out the unreliability of neurological observation in estimating ICP, a conclusion amplified two years later by Ryder et al.[91] who stated:

There can be no syndrome specific for either high or low intracranial pressure . . . There is no valid physiological basis for two clinical inferences: first, fluid pressures within the range of normal indicate either the absence or the correction of a grave disorder of the central nervous system; second, the proper treatment of conditions associated with an abnormal fluid pressure consists of returning the pressure to normal.

Lundberg almost single-handedly began the "modern" era of direct ICP monitoring. His classic and scholarly monograph[63] is still required reading for all those seriously interested in the study of ICP monitoring and the pathophysiology of intracranial hypertension. He began by observing that:

. . . cerebral symptoms are often ascribed to variations in intracranial pressure without any conclusive evidence of the existence of such variations. In view of the fact that a major part of the neurosurgeon's time, skill and effort is devoted to combating intracranial hypertension and its consequences, it is a priori astonishing that more objective and exact methods for investigating this pressure have not found wider use.

He then reviewed his own experience and that of others with direct ICP monitoring in a series of 143 patients. He employed direct ventricular catheterization in all these patients and reported an amazingly low complication rate, with no intradural infections attributable to ICP monitoring.

Being acutely aware of the potential for compartmentalization, or lack of communication of pressures between the cerebral and spinal compartments, he demonstrated clearly the clinical value of direct ICP monitoring. Even more importantly, he observed and carefully described the ICP pressure waves which bear his name: the Lundberg "A" (or plateau) waves, "B" waves and "C" waves. The latter two waves he described as physiologic phenomena which become accentuated in pathologic states, the "B" waves reflecting respiration and the "C" waves reflecting arterial Traube-Hering waves.

The "A" waves, or plateau waves, are pathological and reflect a severe degree of decompensation of the brain's pressure controlling mechanisms. These waves are characterized by a steep rise in pressure to levels of 60–80 torr, with a usual duration of 2–5 minutes, and terminating in a prompt fall to pressures near the initial baseline value. Premorbidly, plateau waves may remain elevated for prolonged periods, or until they fall in concert with blood pressure as the animal dies. These plateau waves are ominous findings, heralding impending disaster. They occur with increasing amplitude, duration, and frequency as the animal approaches death. Their appearance does not denote an irreversible disturbance but should alert the clinician to a need for immediate and effective therapy.

By contrast, pathologic "B" waves, waves of greater than 10–20 torr magnitude with a frequency of one-half to two per minute, do not carry a similar ominous import. These pathologic "B" waves are seen more frequently with intracranial hypertension and with impaired intracranial compliance or reserve. On the other hand, they may occasionally be seen in patients with normal ICP and normal compliance or reserve and may fail to appear in patients with severely abnormal compliance or reserve or with intracranial hypertension. Nevertheless, they are clinically significant since they warn the clinician of an increased risk of intracranial hypertension or potentially dangerous impairment of intracranial compliance or reserve.

BASIC CONSIDERATIONS FOR CONTINUOUS ICP MONITORING

In his incisive and insightful way, Lundberg[63] stated what he considered to be six basic requirements for successful clinical application of ventricular ICP monitoring, requirements which remain equally valid two decades later. He stated:

(1) The procedure should cause as little trauma or irritation of intracranial structures as possible. (2) The risk of intracranial infection should be negligible. (3) It should be possible to establish and maintain the connection between the ventricle and recording apparatus without any leakage of fluid. (4) It should be possible to record pressure for long periods without disturbing the care and comfort of the patient. (5) It should be possible to continue recording the pressure during various diagnostic and therapeutic measures irrespective of changes in position of the patient, *e.g.*, during roentgen examination and general anesthesia. (6) The apparatus should be easy to handle, stable, reliable, and reasonably foolproof—so as not to require special training of nurses.

I would add to this list one additional requirement which I feel is essential if one is to realize the full potential of routine, continuous ICP monitoring: The capability for a continuous paper ("hard copy") printout of ICP recording at the patient's bedside or at the nursing station. With such a record, the neurosurgeon and neurosurgical nurse may rapidly review ICP events which occurred over the preceding hours and may thus assess increasing or decreasing trends in pressure, widening or narrowing of pulse width or the presence and frequency of "A" waves. All of these events give information which may be clinically useful, but which may be overlooked or not appreciated without a written record. To be practically useful a slow paper speed must be used so that the amount of record generated within a given day remains a manageable length—though it may be desirable to have short strips run at specified intervals at paper speeds rapid enough to permit assessment of waveform shapes.

An automatic alarm system to warn of persistent or brief elevations of ICP (the latter occurring during "A" waves) is a useful adjunct to a written "hard copy" record available at the bedside, and should be a minimum essential if a hard copy bedside record is *not* available. This is most important in warning of the presence of "A" or plateau waves. These ominous waves rarely last more than a few minutes, especially when they first begin to appear in a given patient's record. Even in a well-run intensive care unit it is impossible for a nurse to observe an ICP monitor at every minute of every day and night, so these early "A" waves may be missed without an alarm or hard copy record. The use of an alarm can be troublesome, however, since coughing, straining, or moving may trigger the alarm so frequently that its value is reduced as a result of personnel fatigue and inattention.

Electromagnetic tape recorders or electronic "trend" memories are useful, but do not provide as much immediately useful clinical information as a continuous hard copy record at the bedside. Trend memories may fail to record short duration, early "A" waves, are often incapable of recording "B" waves or changes in pulse width and do not permit a retrospective analysis of changes in waveform shape. Electromagnetic tape recorders are quite useful for research, permit sophisticated electronic analysis of slow or rapid features, and may also be tied into a bedside hard copy printer to increase their clinical usefulness.

ANATOMIC SITES OF MONITORING

Professor Bryan Jennett summarized the First International Conference on ICP Monitoring[48] with the caution that there is not, and never will be, a single ideal method for measuring ICP. Clinical indications for ICP monitoring vary widely and embrace a spectrum of disease entities which include acute head injuries, impending aneurysmal rupture, preoperative and postoperative brain tumor, and both acute and chronic hydrocephalus. Because of the clinical diversity of these diseases, the neurosurgeon must not be slavishly tied to a single method of ICP monitoring but must be prepared to apply to each clinical situation the form of ICP monitoring appropriate for that setting.

Cl-2 spinal puncture for long-term ICP monitoring has recently been suggested as an alternative to ventricular cannulation in head-injured patients with small ventricles and lumbar ICP monitoring may be valuable in situations where post-traumatic hydrocephalus is suspected as being clinically significant and treatable.[82] However, spinal monitoring becomes useless in the presence of compartmentalization of pressures which occurs not only with obstruction of the spinal canal but also with brain herniation and impaction of the cerebellar tonsils into the foramen magnum.[41, 45] In this condition, lumbar monitoring is potentially dangerous. Death or neurologic deterioration in patients with elevated ICP as a result of lumbar puncture has been a well-documented clinical phenomenon since the reports of Hirschberg[42] in 1894 and Nolke[75] in 1897, and was reviewed again by Duffy[28] in 1969. Puncturing the lumbar theca and not withdrawing fluid in the presence of demonstrated intracranial hypertension will not eliminate the potential for neurologic disaster.[45] Whether fluid is removed through the lumen of a monitoring system or through a leak in the violated theca following removal of the needle or catheter does not alter the result. Even removal of a small volume of fluid from the lumbar subarachnoid space causes a dramatic fall in pressure below a tonsillar herniation, leaving the elevated ICP relatively unopposed and therefore sharply aggravating the herniation.

ICP monitoring can be accomplished from any of several anatomic sites within the skull. The question of which site should be employed revolves around three major considerations: 1) the significance of ICP gradients, 2) the reliability of epidural pressures, and 3) the relative safety of monitoring at various intracranial sites.

Experimental studies have documented the existence of ICP gradients in a variety of pathologic situations,[9, 90, 95, 97, 99] but not in all models of experimental intracranial hypertension.[49] Edema fluid is released into brain tissue in subcortical areas, then distributes through white matter to be cleared at least partially transependymally.[90] As the wave of edema passes through brain tissue, local tissue pressures rise. In addition, mass lesions, whether focal brain edema or liquid or solid masses within or outside of the brain, cause a distortion of the brain. Because of the brain's high water content and fibrous construction, it distorts by plastic creep and pressures are not instantaneously transmitted as they would be through a pure fluid medium. In clinical practice, however, pressure gradients rarely are maintained for more than a few hours and gradients of more than a few torr almost never exist more than 24 hours after the initiation of the pathologic process.

The duration of existence of significant pressure gradients is also likely to be inversely proportional to the rapidity of enlargement of the pathologic process, so that rapid rises in ICP are likely to be transmitted throughout the cranial compartment relatively rapidly, at least in terms of clinically significant alterations in pressure. As a result, pressure gradients do exist but their clinical importance is probably relatively limited. If one were to be concerned enough about the existence of such gradients to seek an optimum site of pressure recording, this logically would mean direct pressure recordings from vital brain stem centers, an area where the risk of invasive monitoring is prohibitive. Consequently, measurements taken within the ventricle, the brain substance, or the subdural or subarachnoid spaces all provide information which is roughly equivalent in clinical usefulness. Compartmentalization of pressures certainly can occur between the intracranial cavity and the spinal space, but this is of little clinical significance when measurements are made from somewhere within the intracranial cavity. Compartmentalization of pressures can occur within the intracranial cavity in the presence of ventricular obstruction but this is rarely encountered. In these situations, measurement from a loculated ventricle with high pressure would yield a falsely high impression of ICP.

Monitoring ICP from the epidural space avoids the necessity of opening the dura but results in the interposition of the relatively tough and inelastic dura mater between the sensing device and the brain and subarachnoid space. Is epidural monitoring truly equivalent to subdural, subarachnoid, parenchymal, or intraventricular monitoring? Many clinical series suggest that, at least for clinical purposes, the pressures recorded are indeed equivalent and are extremely useful in patient care.[17, 22, 23, 27, 32, 33, 35, 36, 76, 92, 94, 99, 100] However, other experimental and clinical studies suggest that epidural pressure recording is subject to considerable artifact, which may be greater at higher levels of ICP[22, 23, 27, 32, 33, 64, 76, 89, 96, 99] (Fig. 10.1).

Because of the inelasticity of the dura mater, the design and application of pressure monitoring sensors used in the epidural space becomes critically important. Any device which employs a planar diaphragm which must be distorted to a concave shape in order to transmit pressure will function effectively only if it is applied in coplanar apposition to the dura. Even with careful placement at high pressures, the inelasticity of the dura mater limits the degree of concavity of the sensing membrane which can occur. As a result, monitoring devices with this mechanical configuration will exhibit increasingly severe artifact with increasing elevations of ICP. On the other hand, this

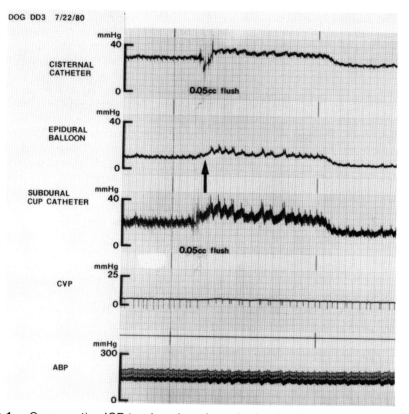

Figure 10.1.   Comparative ICP tracings in a dog, obtained using a cisternal catheter, an epidural recording balloon and a subdural ICP cup catheter. One milliliter injected into the contralateral "lesion" balloon (*arrow*) caused a rise in ICP which was much more evident in the subdural pressure tracing than in the epidural tracing. Balloon inflation also caused a slowing and irregularity of respiration as documented in the central venous pressure (CVP) tracing. Arterial blood pressure (ABP) failed to show any significant response and the classic "Cushing response" did not develop.

will be less of a problem with devices with convex surfaces or fluid coupled extradural systems (assuming, of course, that the devices do not suffer from specific design artifacts). If the inelasticity of the dura mater has been eliminated from the system as a potential for artifact, epidural pressure readings are found to be roughly parallel to intradural pressures. Even if the epidural pressures are somewhat higher or lower than those recorded from other intradural sites, the differences are generally reported to be within the acceptable range for clinical utility.

Safety and ease of insertion are the final considerations in an analysis of optimum anatomic siting for ICP monitoring. Monitoring from the epidural space with the dura mater intact provides a considerable safety advantage should sepsis intervene since infections in the epidural space are much less dangerous to the patient than are those located anywhere within the dura mater. Epidural monitoring also may offer greater safety from mechanical injury since the dura can protect the underlying brain during insertion of a monitor and from cortical irritation or injury during long-term pressure monitoring. Subarachnoid, subdural, parenchymal, and intraventricular monitoring all run the risk of introduction of infection into the meningeal spaces (meningitis), brain parenchyma (brain abscess), or ventricles (ventriculitis). Of these forms of infection, perhaps ventriculitis is most likely to be devastating and its occurrence is virtually limited to the use of intraventricular monitors.

Intraventricular fluid-coupled monitors do allow the possibility of daily withdrawal of CSF samples for culture and for white cell and differential counts. If an increasing number of white cells (especially polymorphonuclear cells) is discovered, ventricular infection can be suspected even before cultures are reported to be positive. At that point, a clinical decision must be made whether to terminate ventricular monitoring and/or whether to begin appropriate antibiotic therapy systematically or intraventricularly. Brain abscess is more likely to occur with monitoring from ventricles or brain parenchyma, but can occur with sub-

arachnoid or subdural monitoring if the pia and arachnoid have been violated mechanically at the time monitoring is begun or while the device remains in use. Most monitoring systems employing fluid coupling from the brain surface do not permit withdrawal of CSF for detection of incipient sepsis, but they do permit the introduction of antibiotic solutions for the prophylaxis of infection from cutaneous organisms. The author has even utilized an ICP monitoring cup catheter in patients operated upon for subdural empyema as the input arm of a through and through system for antibiotic irrigation.

The ease of insertion of all currently available ICP monitoring devices is limited chiefly by the protective coverings over the central nervous system. Spinal puncture, with or without catheter insertion, can be accomplished by insertion of a needle in the lumbar spine without the need for surgical incision. Catheters should be threaded cautiously into the lumbar subarachnoid space, especially in unconscious or anesthetized patients, for fear of having the catheter tip catch in a nerve root axilla with resultant neural injury. Although this rarely occurs, such a complication has been documented; it is safer to perform the puncture at a higher spinal level and to thread the catheter caudally within the subarachnoid space. Whenever rubber or plastic catheters are passed through a needle into the subarachnoid space, care should be taken never to withdraw the catheter into the needle once the needle has been inserted into the patient. This maneuver can amputate the catheter tip with remarkable ease if a sharp needle has been used.

If therapeutic catheterization of an obstructed ventricle has already been performed, ventricular monitoring can be added with little additional effort. Once a therapeutic burr hole or craniotomy has been done, ICP monitors of catheter configuration, or those not requiring precise seating into bone openings, can be easily placed into the epidural, subdural, or subarachnoid space. Devices which monitor pressure from the brain parenchyma or ventricle will still require penetration through the brain, adding the risk of brain injury or intracerebral hematoma formation from injury to parenchymal vessels. ICP monitoring devices whose design requires careful seating into a bone opening of precise size and shape will be equally difficult (or easy) to insert whether or not the patient has undergone concomitant surgery. Most of the devices designed to be used at the time of craniotomy can still be introduced through a burr hole made specifically to initiate ICP monitoring, but this introduction may be more difficult than that required for insertion of some of the devices which require only a twist drill opening for seating into the skull.

METHODS OF ICP MONITORING

The number of devices which have been described for monitoring ICP experimentally or clinically has expanded rapidly in the past few years. Many are being used at specific neurosurgical centers on a custom-made basis but only a relatively few devices are readily available commercially. I will attempt to review the spectrum of designs which have been described, but will emphasize particularly those devices which are readily available to the practicing neurosurgeon.

Intraspinal (Lumbar) Monitoring Devices

Long-term monitoring of ICP from the spinal subarachnoid space continues to be valuable clinically.[39, 40, 60] Papo and Caruselli[82] have suggested long-term ICP monitoring via lateral Cl-2 spinal puncture in head-injured patients with small ventricles as an alternative to ventricular catheterization. The equipment for performing simple spinal puncture is now readily available in nearly all hospitals. Simple lumbar puncture with a metal needle enables one to sample fluid for evidence of infection or hemorrhage but allows measurement of ICP only for a short period of time and then only in the absence of compartmentalization. "Ayala's Index" has now been largely discredited, but an extreme fall in measured pressure following removal of a small amount of CSF from a lumbar puncture strongly implies tonsillar herniation with pressure compartmentalization above and

below the foramen magnum. Diagnostic spinal puncture plays little useful role in the acute management of head injuries since: 1) the documentation of low pressure does not exclude the possibility of tonsillar herniation, while an elevated pressure confirms the presence of a head injury but also confirms that the puncture itself added to the patient's risk; and 2) the presence of blood in the CSF non-specifically confirms a head injury, yet the absence of blood does not exclude the possibility of hemorrhage confined to the subdural or epidural space or within the brain parenchyma. Spinal punctures performed more than 24 hours following head injury may be of clinical value, especially in patients who are clinically stable and only mildly neurologically impaired. In these patients, the presence of bloody spinal fluid documents an increased risk of cortical laceration and therefore predicts a somewhat greater risk of post-traumatic seizures. At this stage in management also, the documentation of intracranial hypertension in a symptomatic but minimally neurologically impaired patient may be a valuable guide to potential therapy.

Chronic monitoring (over hours, days, or even weeks) using intraspinal, implanted catheters requires more specialized equipment, but this is also readily available in most hospitals.[39, 60] Plastic catheters with rigid stylets may be used but many neurosurgeons prefer to employ a large caliber (generally a 14 gauge) side hole Touhey needle through which a flexible catheter is introduced. A variety of commercially available catheters, all of which will fit through the Touhey needle, have been used for chronic spinal monitoring of ICP. Devices should be equipped with multiple side holes near their indwelling tip to ensure free transmission of pressure by CSF and to permit reliable CSF withdrawal, which is valuable for fluid analysis to warn of impending infection. The soft silastic tubing available for pediatric shunting can be used with relatively less danger of damaging nerve roots but with greater difficulty in passing the catheter into the subarachnoid space. Polyethylene catheters may become water-logged with prolonged implantation and may lose their transmitting effectiveness. Tygon catheters provide a stiffer system, are easier but somewhat more risky to pass into the subarachnoid space, but are generally less readily available. Some neurosurgeons prefer commercial ureteral catheters (size 5 French) because of their molded tip and stiffness.

Lumbar ICP measurement by indwelling catheter adds an extra dimension to monitoring since it allows long-term monitoring over periods of days or even a few weeks. This form of monitoring may be valuable in assessing the symptomatic nature of documented post-traumatic hydrocephalus. It is also valuable in monitoring therapy of patients with diseases which cause acute intracranial hypertension of relatively short duration—*but should be used in these situations only if the risk of tonsillar herniation is felt to be small enough to justify the benefits of lumbar ICP monitoring*. In patients who have not had tonsillar herniation, especially those whose intracranial hypertension is directly related to disordered CSF circulation, lumbar catheter monitoring permits therapeutic withdrawal of CSF.

The major limitation of the use of intraspinal ICP monitoring is the risk of aggravation of brain herniation or loss of reliable pressure monitoring through compartmentalization separating spinal from intracranial spaces.

Extracranial, Non-invasive ICP Monitoring Devices

The ideal device for ICP monitoring is one which is totally non-invasive. Unfortunately, no such device has been successfully demonstrated for use in adults with intact skulls. Devices for recording a "fontagram" have been described for use in infants whose open fontanelle is capable of transmitting ICP to the cutaneous surface.[7, 29, 93, 104] Several versions of such devices have been described and variations of this basic concept have been used to measure ICP non-invasively at sites of cranial decompression.[65] None of these devices is currently being marketed in the United States. Although the Ladd ICP monitor (see subsequent section) has been used for extracranial, non-invasive monitoring, it

was not designed specifically for this application.

As is true of epidural monitoring, extracranial monitoring must take into account the potential for artifact introduced by the thickness, flexibility, and compressibility of those tissues which intervene between the monitoring device and the intracranial contents. These factors impose certain design restrictions, and recorded pressures may vary with changes in scalp edema or hematoma or with alterations in the manner and firmness with which the device is applied to the scalp.

Intraventricular Monitoring Devices

Intraventricular ICP monitoring can be carried out with a variety of devices which are currently clinically available. All of these devices must be inserted into a ventricular cavity, almost always into the lateral cerebral ventricle. Frontal, coronal-parasagittal, and occipital approaches to the ventricle are most commonly used, though occasionally the entry is made via Keene's point lateral to the trigone. Of the commercially available devices which are used for ventricular ICP monitoring only a few were designed specifically for pressure monitoring (*viz.*, the Holter company's "External Drain Unit" and the Pudenz-Schulte company's ICP monitoring system of "Becker design") (Fig. 10.2). Most of the devices used for ICP monitoring were designed for ventricular fluid sampling, introduction of diagnostic or therapeutic materials, or therapeutic drainage of fluid—thus reflecting the fact that ventricular ICP monitoring is often done in combination with other indications for ventricular entry (Fig. 10.3).

Two basic design configurations are used for ventricular ICP monitoring; both are fluid filled and fluid coupled to externalized pressure sensing and/or display devices. The first configuration is that of a catheter passing from the ventricle through the skin to an externalized component. The second configuration is that of a totally implantable device consisting of a catheter from the ventricular space to a subcutaneous reservoir either placed in a burr hole or

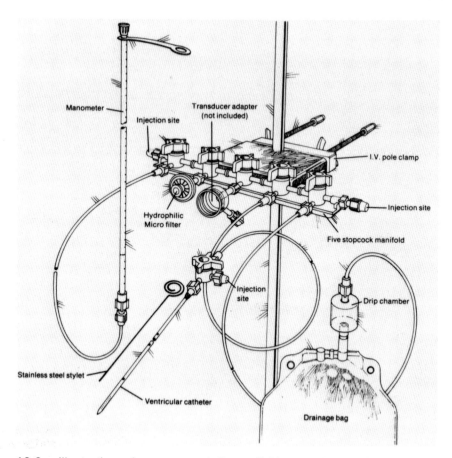

Figure 10.2. Illustration of a commercially available ventricular ICP monitoring and therapy set: the "Becker design" marketed by Heyer-Schulte Corporation. (Reproduced with permission of the manufacturer.)

subgaleally[31, 81, 105, 113]   (Fig. 10.4). Pressure monitoring with this design requires percutaneous needle entry into the reservoir with fluid coupling to an externalized pressure sensing and/or display component whenever monitoring is to be done.

Any form of catheter which is in clinical use for ventricular CSF drainage can be used for ventricular ICP monitoring. Depending in part on patient selection, but also on the individual neurosurgeon's preference, the device employed may consist of a red rubber catheter, an infant feeding tube, simple Silastic rubber tubing, or any of the commercially available Silastic rubber ventricular catheters designed for ventriculoperitoneal or ventriculovascular CSF

shunting. The tubing employed should have multiple holes near its end to permit better pressure transmission and to facilitate CSF withdrawal. The Ommaya or Rickham reservoir devices are most popular for the implanted configuration, although some surgeons prefer to use the Hakim reservoir (especially the reservoir containing a metal plate as a needle stop), with the outflow end of the reservoir occluded by a ligature of metal clip.

Fleischer *et al.*[31] have shown that an implanted system can be employed for acute and subacute ICP monitoring, but despite their expectations to the contrary the risk of infection remained quite high. Implantation of such a reservoir, with percuta-

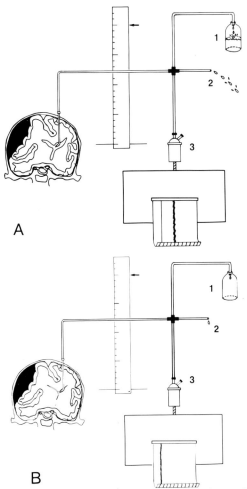

Figure 10.3. Advantage and limitations of ventricular monitoring. *A*, when ventricular system remains patent and filled with CSF, catheter drainage can be used *1*) to establish "automatic" CSF drainage against gradient whenever ICP rises sufficiently high, *2*) to drain CSF manually whenever deemed advisable by the surgeon, or *3*) to monitor ICP. ICP monitoring cannot be done simultaneously with CSF drainage since the release of pressure through the outflow valve will drop the recorded pressure to 0 or near 0 even though brain pressure remains elevated. *B*, when ventricular system collapses from excessive intracranial mass or fluid withdrawal, CSF can no longer be withdrawn and ICP recording capability is lost or seriously impaired.

neous needle coupling to the externalized pressure sensing and display components, is particularly useful in patients in whom long-term access to the ventricular system is felt to be useful (Fig. 10.4). Patients likely to require long-term intraventricular antibiotics or chemotherapy are particularly suitable for this technique So, too, are patients in whom long-term, periodic ICP monitoring is deemed likely to be an asset in patient care, such as patients with slow growing and incompletely resectable tumors or chronic hydrocephalus.

All forms of ICP monitoring have the potential for causing patient infections, but ventricular monitoring carries with it the greatest risk of ventricular infections. It also carries a significantly greater risk of brain abscess than that encountered with brain surface monitoring systems. A recent experimental study reports that the minimum number of staphylococcal bacteria necessary to induce infections by intradermal scalp injection is in the order of 10^5 organisms, while brain infection may result from injection of as few as 100 organisms.[70] By using meticulous aseptic technique and both topical and systemic antibiotics, Lundberg[63] was able to avoid significant central nervous system infection entirely in his large clinical series, but Fleischer *et al.*[31] showed that this enviable success may not always be achieved in routine clinical application.

Introducing a ventricular catheter necessitates passage of instruments through brain tissue into the ventricular system, placing the patient at a small but real risk of intracerebral hemorrhage from injury to parenchymal vessels. This risk is a cumulative one for each unsuccessful needle pass which the surgeon makes in attempting to catheterize the ventricle (Fig. 10.5). In a brain severely distorted by swelling or intracranial mass, the ventricle may be collapsed and shifted from its normal position so that ventricular catheterization may be quite difficult and require more than one passage of the needle or catheter.

Once a ventricle is catheterized, further collapse of the ventricle may seriously interfere with pressure recordings from the catheter.[63] This often results in a situation in which measured ICP rises sharply but

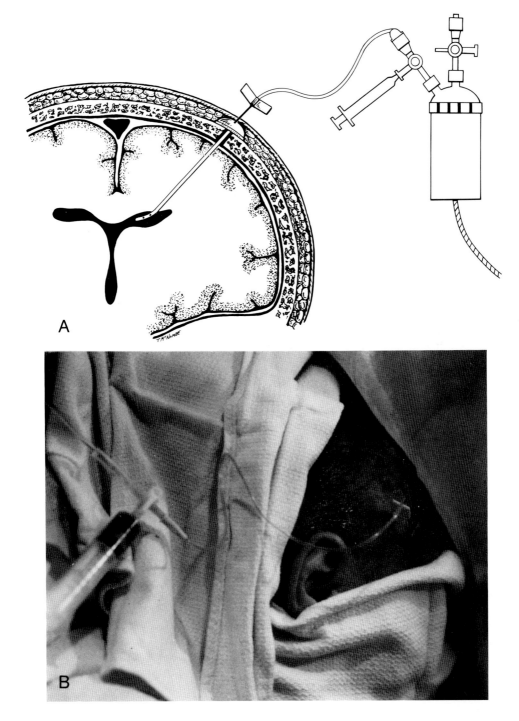

Figure 10.4. Implanted reservoir used for ICP monitoring and periodic ventricular drainage. *A*, drawing demonstrates ventricular catheter terminating in a reservoir device implanted beneath the scalp. *B*, photograph showing fluid withdrawal and ICP monitoring established via percutaneous puncture of the implanted reservoir.

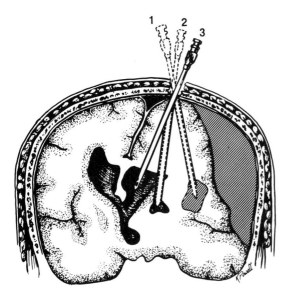

Figure 10.5. Graphic demonstration of some potential difficulties with attempted ventricular ICP monitoring. *1)* Passage of ventricular cannula (or catheter) may tear parenchymal vessels and cause intracerebral hemorrhage. *2)* Fluid injected intracerebrally when the catheter is not actually in the ventricular lumen can cause tissue damage and recording from such a placement can give seriously artifactual tracings. *3)* Ventricle may be severely shifted, even if not collapsed, and abnormal position may require multiple needle passes.

transiently following catheter flushing, then falls rapidly to zero or nearly so. A catheter left with its tip in brain parenchyma, rather than in the ventricle, may still transmit pressures, but these are likely to be artifactual. Even tiny fluid leaks may reduce the "coupling" fluid volume below that necessary for full and accurate transmission of pressure, resulting in artifactually low readings. Injection of small amounts of fluid into a loculated area within brain parenchyma may give artifactually high, but unsustained, pressures.

The major advantage of ICP monitoring via ventricular catheterization is that it offers the simultaneous opportunity for patient therapy by removal of ventricular fluid. One must be careful not to attempt

to record ICP at the same time that fluid drainage is being carried out since the pressure recorded will be no higher than the pressure of the fluid drainage, even though actual ICP may be much higher. Withdrawal of CSF, sometimes even withdrawal of volumes less than 10 ml, may be extremely effective in lowering ICP. On the other hand, withdrawal of fluid from a partially collapsed ventricle may cause further collapse of the ventricles and interfere with accurate ICP recording. If there is insufficient fluid to transmit pressures adequately, the recorded ICP will be artifactually lower than the actual ICP.

A second advantage of ventricular ICP monitoring is that it may be easy to introduce a catheter, especially if the ventricle is large. In patients with ventriculomegaly, ICP monitoring from a ventricular catheter would seem to be the method of choice. In patients with collapsed and distorted ventricles, the ease of insertion of a ventricular catheter, often requiring a simple twist drill opening through the skull, must be weighed against the potential difficulty in locating a collapsed and distorted ventricle. However, many neurosurgeons who deal extensively with severe head injuries feel that they have little difficulty locating the ventricle and that the ease of insertion of a ventricular catheter leads them to favor this method of ICP monitoring as their routine procedure.

Monitoring from Brain Parenchyma

ICP monitoring directly from the parenchyma of the brain has been described both experimentally and clinically but is not in widespread use.[10, 18, 19, 85, 95] As is true with all implantable systems, great care must be taken to avoid introducing infection into the implanted device. Devices designed specifically for measuring ICP from brain parenchyma often utilize a wick or filter at their open end to lessen the risk of herniation of brain into the lumen of the device.

It may well be that many instances of parenchymal ICP monitoring are actually carried out inadvertently when ventricular catheterization is attempted in a swollen brain and the catheter tip is located within the cerebral parenchyma rather than the ventricular cavity. Care must be taken in interpreting the data from such placements. Fluid flushed into such a device may well loculate about the catheter tip causing artifactually elevated local pressures. As the fluid then escapes along the catheter tract to the subarachnoid space, observed pressure will fall. Contrary to the expected situation with most fluid coupled systems, in this instance the more accurate pressure will be the lower one *not* the higher pressure seen immediately following flushing. No device is currently commercially available in the United States designed specifically for intraparenchymal monitoring.

Fluid Coupled, Surface Monitoring Devices

Balloon Devices. Monitoring ICP from the brain surface using fluid-coupled devices began with balloons implanted subdurally or epidurally.[43] Balloon devices continue to be used for short-term ICP monitoring in the experimental laboratory, but

their use in humans is restricted by an inherent technical problem: small balloons are quite sensitive to changes in their internal volume and larger balloons pose a threat to the patient because of the larger volume which must be inserted intracranially (Fig. 10.6). The loss of even a small volume from a small balloon will cause a drastic change in observed ICP. Although this may be corrected by periodic emptying and precise refilling of the balloon, this is cumbersome for clinical use and would have to be repeated any time an abnormal ICP was suspected. The greater danger would arise if ICP actually rose without being reflected in the measurement and if this elevated ICP were then not detected until some later time. Balloon rupture or leakage would also expose the intracranial cavity to the balloon's fluid contents.

Hollow Screw Device. Vries *et al.*[101] described and popularized the first commercially available device for surface, fluid coupled ICP monitoring: the so-called

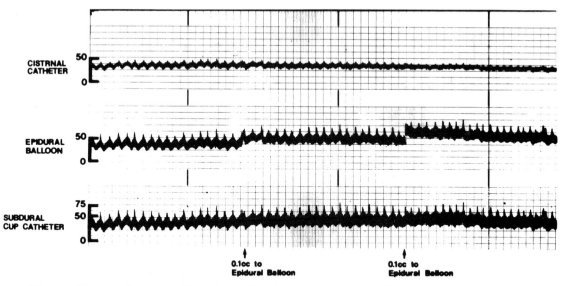

Figure 10.6. Influence of intraluminal volume changes on ICP recorded from an ICP monitoring balloon. 1.0 cc monitoring balloon chronically implanted into the epidural space of a dog recorded an epidural pressure equivalent to that recorded from a cisternal catheter and an ipsilateral subdural ICP monitoring cup catheter when the epidural monitoring balloon was filled with 0.2 cc of fluid. However, the addition of further small volume increments to the epidural monitoring balloon significantly altered the pressure which this system recorded even though it caused no significant change in the pressures recorded from the other two devices. (ICP measurements in torr.)

"Richmond screw" or "Becker bolt" (Fig. 10.7). This hollow bolt device circumvents the problem of a critical internal volume by using an open system which employs the pial or arachnoidal surface of the brain as its sensing membrane. The device was originally described for subarachnoid use but in actuality works best in subdural application with the arachnoid membrane left intact. The device does *not* work satisfactorily if the dura is *not* opened.[15] An optimum fluid volume within the device is insured by frequent infusions of small volumes of fluid (flushing the device). Excess fluid so introduced simply escapes into the subdural or subarachnoid space, leaving the device nicely fluid coupled to the externalized sensor and display apparatus. It does not require a free pool of fluid in the subdural or subarachnoid space and therefore it can be used in conjunction with subdural drains or close to a craniotomy defect—as long as the brain surface is in apposition to the open end of the device. To install the device, a 1-cm incision is made in the scalp and through this a one-quarter inch twist drill hole is made through the skull. For optimum functioning the dura should be curetted cleanly away, allowing the tip of the hollow bolt to seat firmly against the brain surface. The device is then screwed firmly into place in the bone to a measured depth

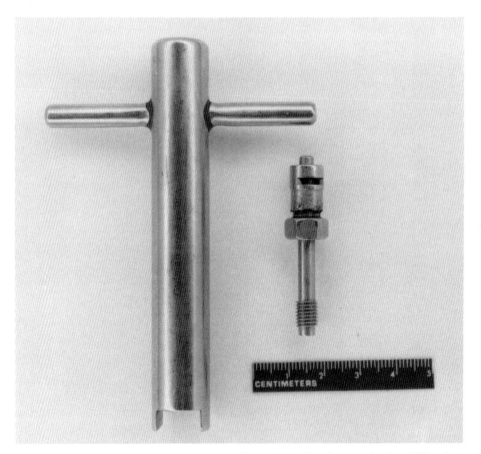

Figure 10.7.   "Becker Bolt" or "Richmond Screw" device for monitoring ICP subdurally via fluid coupling. The special screwdriver device on the left is used to seat the threaded end of the bolt device into a drill opening in the skull. For optimum use the dura must be cleanly curetted away so that the inner end of the device rests cleanly on the arachnoidal surface of the brain but does not penetrate into brain.

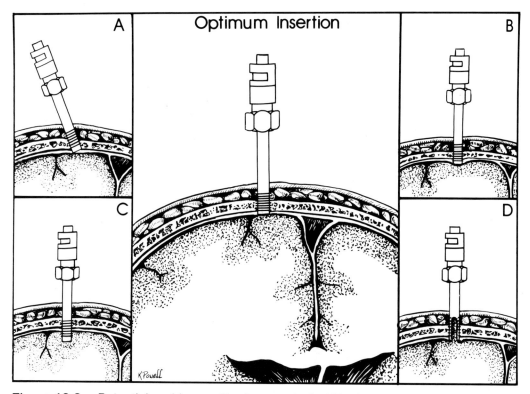

Figure 10.8. Potential problems with placement of a "Becker Bolt" for ICP monitoring: *A*, oblique penetration through the skull may prevent close approximation of the open end of the bolt to the arachnoid and may interfere with pressure recording. *B*, thin skulls may not provide sufficient thickness to hold the device firmly either initially or following several days of insertion. *C*, excessively deep insertion of the device can rupture through the arachnoidal surface into the brain causing local tissue damage. *D*, in the presence of intracranial hypertension brain tissue may herniate into the lumen of the device, causing local tissue injury and rendering the device nonoperational.

so that the open inner end protrudes a millimeter or so below the inner table and is occluded by the brain surface.

Perhaps the main attractiveness of the "Richmond screw" is its ease of application. Even so, precise introduction and apposition onto underlying brain through bleeding bone and a narrow drill opening requires some care (Fig. 10.8). If the dura is not cleanly curetted away, close apposition will be impeded and the device may fail to record pressures accurately. Proper depth of insertion is also important, since deep penetration will damage the brain surface and insufficiently deep penetration increases the likelihood of loss of pressure.

Application to the brain surface should also be made precisely coplanar to the surface of the brain as inadvertent tilting of the device can lead to improper functioning. Tearing of the arachnoid or of the pial surface can be a significant problem since it greatly increases the likelihood of herniation of brain into the hollow screw in the presence of elevated ICP—precisely those situations in which monitoring is most important (Fig. 10.9). The potential for herniation of brain tissue into the bolt is, in fact, one of the major drawbacks of the use of the device, both for fear of damaging the surface of the brain and because herniation of brain into the device often renders it

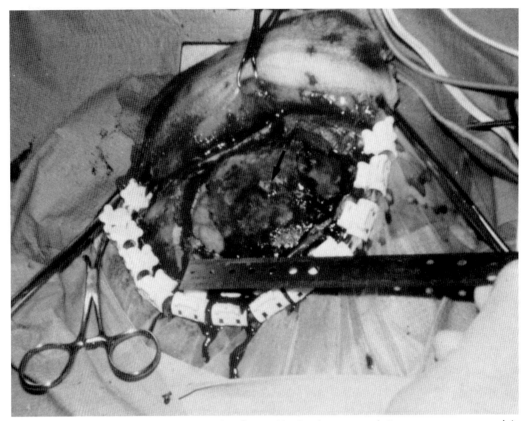

Figure 10.9. Operative photograph of a patient whose craniotomy was reopened to evacuate a postoperative hematoma one week following initial craniotomy and placement of a "Becker Bolt." The *arrow* points to brain tissue which herniated through the dura mater and which had completely filled the lumen of the bolt.

useless just when its functioning is most necessary. Frequent "flushing" with tiny volumes of fluid will help to prevent this complication but at high ICP's brain rupture may not be preventable.

The "Richmond screw" offers both advantages and disadvantages with respect to sepsis. Application of the device to the surface of the brain makes the possibility of ventricular infection or brain abscess considerably less likely, but the near approximation of the skin incision site to exposed brain offers some liability for infection, both during use and following removal of the device. Another potential problem may arise when CT scanning is needed. The older scanning units which require application of a fluid bag to the patient's head cannot be used when there is a prominent metal rod extending from the patient's skull. With the newer CT units severe artifact may be generated by the heavy metal object, but this can be avoided by placing the monitoring device near the parasagittal vertex or by altering the angle of CT scan cut to a plane tangential to the site of insertion.

Once the bolt is in use, either with or without a stopcock interposed between it and the pressure transmitting tubing, its length presents some minor awkwardness in patient positioning and presents the possibility of considerable leverage which can facilitate accidental dislodgement. The device does require firm seating in bone and may fail to stay seated or may fail to function if the drill hole is not cleanly made, if the bone is soft, if bone wears during prolonged insertion, or if the skull is thin—as is often encountered in children.

Other devices based on this same principle have been described and are in clinical use at various centers. A special pediatric version for use with thin skulls and hollow bolts similar to or more complex than the "Richmond screw" have been described.[16, 47, 64] Some neurosurgeons prefer to use a "homemade" version of the fluid-coupled, surface-monitoring design. This is accomplished simply by tightly wedging the male port of a disposable plastic stopcock or short IV tubing into a ⅛-inch hole drilled into the skull beneath a ½-inch scalp incision[34, 54] (Fig. 10.10). This simplified version is said to work nearly as well as the metal bolt. It has the advantage of even greater simplicity and ease of insertion as well as being radiolucent. Its shorter length minimizes the chance of dislodgement through leverage but it is held in place only by friction and its short length may be a problem in the presence of scalp swelling or edema.

Cup Catheter. The ICP monitoring cup catheter is a commercially available device which is a direct outgrowth of the bolt design and is also a fluid-coupled, surface-monitoring device[106, 112] (Fig. 10.11). Like the bolt it utilizes the arachnoid surface of the brain as its sensing membrane and functions better with periodic small volume flushing to insure optimum cup filling. Unlike the bolt, the cup catheter is ribbon-shaped and is designed to be passed through a subcutaneous tunnel beneath the scalp to exit from a remote scalp incision site. This design is intended to limit the risk of CSF leakage and bacterial ingress during use and following its removal. Since the sensing cup is on the flat surface of the ribbon-shaped device a larger sensing cup surface area can be applied to the brain than is possible with the open tip of a bolt configuration. This generally gives better transmission of pulsatile wave forms. This configuration of the sensing cup also presents a shallow wide cup to the brain surface so that herniation of brain into the device, with surface disruption of the brain, is less likely to occur.

Although the device is designed for insertion at the time of craniotomy, it can also be inserted through a burr hole when ICP monitoring is required in patients who do not need a craniotomy. In these patients, insertion is more difficult than is placement of a subarachnoid bolt and care must be taken to pass the catheter into the subdural space over a curved metal instrument such as a Penfield #3 dissector and to avoid plunging the rubber catheter into the brain substance. When the device is used in conjunction with craniotomy, the cup end can be placed over an area of brain where cortex is known to be intact. No additional bone openings are required, such as would be required for use with a bolt. Like the bolt, the catheter can be used simultaneously with a subdural drain, as long as the drain does not interfere with apposition of the cup end of the catheter to the brain. Problems may be encountered with the cup catheter if its cup end is positioned over the frontal poles in a patient who will be nursed predominantly in the supine position. Particularly if intracranial pressure is low, air may accumulate over the frontal poles following craniotomy and may interfere with good apposition of the cup end of the monitoring catheter to the brain surface.

Other Devices. Two devices have been described which employ the basic fluid-coupled bolt design, but which are intended specifically for epidural use. Even though the "Becker bolt" and the subdural cup catheter do *not* maintain accurate transmission of ICP for long when used epidurally, these other devices are said by their designers to function reliably. The rubber device described by deRougemont *et al.*[25, 26] must be applied to the dural surface, but the metal device described by Cheek *et al.*[17] is seated tightly in a hole drilled in the cranium and is not applied directly to the dura. Both require maintenance of precise volumes of fluid in the extradural space, and both are theoretically subject to the same potential errors inherent in other coplanar epidural sensing devices. Neither device has received an extensive clinical trial.

Another design configuration for a surface-monitoring, fluid-coupled system employs a metal pod or capsule which is inserted in the subdural or epidural space and

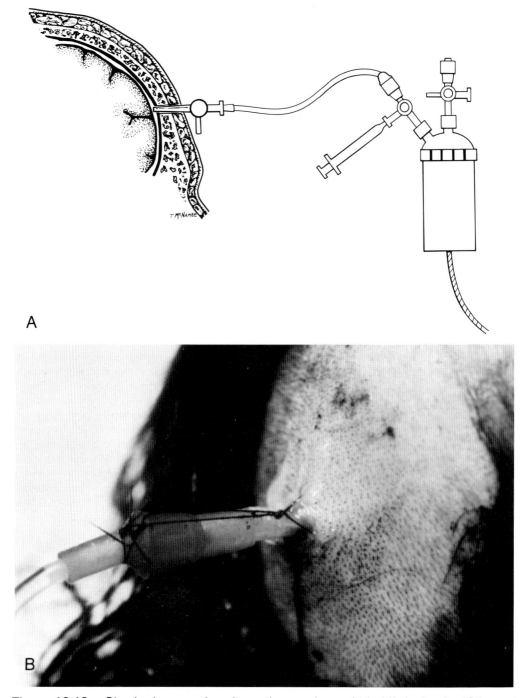

A

B

Figure 10.10. Simple, inexpensive alternative versions of ''bolt'' device for ICP monitoring. *A*, drawing of a disposable plastic stopcock used for this purpose, and *B*, photograph of a ''male'' intravenous tubing connector used in similar fashion. Both devices are anchored to bone by friction. Scalp edema may interfere with insertion of the stopcock device to an optimum depth.

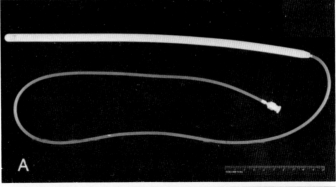

Figure 10.11. ICP monitoring cup catheter, a ribbon shaped, fluid coupled rubber device designed specifically for monitoring post-craniotomy. *A* and *B*, photographs of the device with a close up of the open cup end which is placed on the arachnoidal surface of the brain during monitoring. *C*, postoperative radiograph of an ICP cup catheter in use showing *1)* end of the device applied over intact brain, *2)* point of penetration of the device through dura, and *3)* point of skin exit, remote from dural entry point.

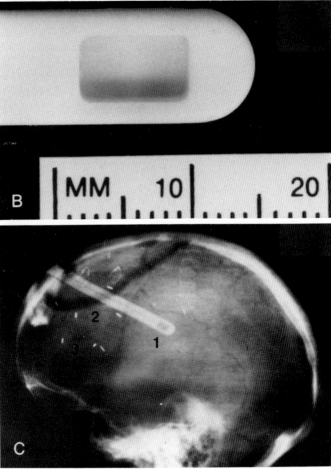

which transmits pressure from subdural fluid through lateral openings or ports in the device.[34, 35] This device, of course, requires fluid in the subdural space and may not operate properly near an opening in the skull. Care must be taken to insure that adequate fluid is available around the device to transmit accurate pressure. This device is not at present commercially available.

Non-fluid Coupled Devices for Surface ICP Monitoring—Mechanical or Optical Pressure Transmitters

Numoto was the first to describe a series of devices which measure ICP from the brain surface by means of extracranial application of measured pressures just sufficient to counterbalance the intracranial pressure.[77] The first of these was a small balloon containing electrical contacts fastened to the inner walls of the balloon. When intracranial pressure exceeded the applied pressure, the balloon flattened, bringing the electrodes into contact and closing a servo circuit. This circuit powered an infusion pump which raised the intraluminal pressure to a point where the electrical contacts separated, causing the servo circuit to open and the infusion pump to reverse. The result was an applied pressure which oscillated about the ICP and which was detected by the electronic and manometric devices outside of the patient. This device was appropriately given the name of

an "ICP pressure switch." A second device in this line of development was termed the "pressure indicating bag."[77, 78] This device employed the same mechanism but utilized a shifting meniscus between two differential fluids within the system to register the pressure outside of the patient. The culmination of this developmental sequence is the Ladd ICP monitoring device which uses optical switching transmitted through tiny fiber optic cables to detect the distortion by the applied ICP of a tiny mirror within a balloon system which is implanted in the patient's head[81, 82, 153] (Fig. 10.12). By eliminating the need for intracranial electrical circuitry, the risk of electrical excitation or injury of the brain has been eliminated. Each of these devices includes safeguards in case of balloon rupture to ensure against an unreversed infusion of excessive volumes or pressures intracranially. Because of this possibility, the sterility of the interior of the system must be maintained. This device is currently being marketed and is in use in a number of neurosurgical centers.

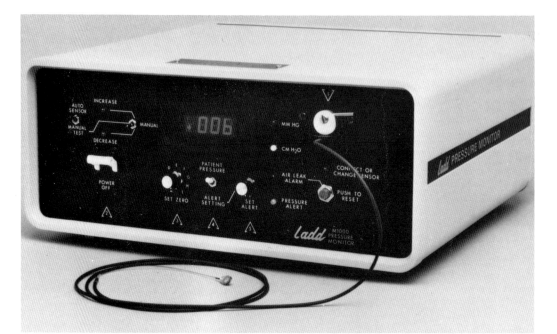

Figure 10.12. Ladd fiberoptic ICP monitoring device, a system wholly dedicated to ICP monitoring. This system does not display fine wave forms but can be used subdurally, epidurally and perhaps extracranially. (Illustration reproduced with permission of the manufacturer.)

The advantage of the Ladd ICP monitoring device is that it can be used subdurally or epidurally or even as a non-invasive extracutaneous device when it is applied over an open fontanelle or cranial decompression. Extracutaneous monitoring eliminates the risk of intracranial infection with ICP monitoring, but may be subject to artifact introduced by the intervening tissues and by different pressures used to hold the device in contact with the scalp. If the device is tightly strapped in place, an artifactually high pressure may be recorded—but no ICP will be recorded if the device is simply laid gently on the skin surface.

When used in the extradural space, the risk of dangerous intracranial infection is considerably less than when devices are used which penetrate the dura. Some artifact may be introduced by the thick and inelastic dura, though the design configuration of the Ladd device minimizes this problem to a sufficient degree that extradural usage should be quite valuable and reliable in clinical practice. The ribbon shape of the device is an asset since it allows the surgeon to interpose a subcutaneous tunnel between the site of skin entry and the point of penetration through the skull, thus minimizing the risk of extradural infection from skin contaminating organisms. This ribbon design does make it somewhat more difficult to insert than some of the other available devices when no cranial surgery is planned other than that necessary to initiate ICP monitoring. When used in conjunction with planned craniotomy or burr holes, however, the device is simpler to implant than other designs which require specially shaped or sized bony openings.

Two major drawbacks of the Ladd system have been encountered. The first of these is that the entire system, including the externalized electronic component, is solely dedicated to ICP monitoring. Whereas the fluid coupled systems can be linked to any existing external pressure monitoring device which records pressures over physiologic ranges (and most modern intensive care units are now equipped with such devices, often interconnected to a central station), the total dedication of the electronic components of this system (cost-ing several thousand dollars each) can increase the cost of setting up ICP monitoring capability in a neurosurgical unit and can cause problems if one wishes to couple the system to a central display panel.

Another problem encountered with this system is the cost and reliability of the implanted sensing catheters themselves. The catheters are relatively fragile and often do not hold up well to the rough treatment which most equipment receives in clinical use, so that they frequently must be replaced after use in a few patients. The catheters themselves are relatively expensive in comparison to disposable or reuseable ICP monitoring devices. A less serious drawback of these devices is that they are by design not capable of transmitting small and rapid fluctuations in the ICP wave. These small fluctuations generally are of limited clinical significance but this feature hampers the usefulness of this device in some research applications. Overall, many clinicians feel that the greater safety offered by the capability of extradural monitoring outweighs the drawbacks inherent in the Ladd ICP monitoring device.

Non-fluid Coupled Devices for Surface ICP Monitoring—Electronic Devices

A variety of devices has been described for experimental and clinical monitoring of ICP, all of which have in common a component which is placed inside the head to convert pressure to electrical impulses which are then transmitted via cables to external display or recording devices. Many devices have used a strain gauge for converting pressure to an electrical impulse.[6, 32, 33, 44, 64, 66, 76, 94, 100] Other devices have used measurement of capacitance changes or other electronic principles[20, 38, 112, 114]; the physical design of the devices has generally been either a ribbon[32, 33, 112] or a plug configuration for seating in a specially sized and shaped opening in the skull. All of these devices have suffered from problems with baseline drift. In general, the smaller the pressure-translating component has been made, the more serious the baseline drift problem has become. The larger devices, of course, have been limited to a plug configuration but this larger size has left an even greater area of potentially contaminated skin about the exposed dura or cortex following removal of the device.

Extradural pressure recording has often been troublesome in those designs employing flat sensing membranes for these membranes must be applied in an absolutely coplanar fashion to the dura. However, even when this is done, the stiffness and inelasticity of the dura has severely hampered the performance of these devices at higher ICP's. Thermal drift and drift with changes in atmospheric pressure have plagued some of the electronic devices, leading to development of compensating externalized circuitry. A few have been designed to permit re-zeroing *in situ*,[32, 112] although in practice this is often technically demanding and cumbersome for the average nursing staff. Some devices of this class remain in use in certain neurosurgical centers but none are being marketed in the United States for general neurosurgical use.

Fully Implantable Devices for ICP Monitoring

For long-term monitoring of ICP, a system ideally should be fully implantable with no external connections piercing the skin. Such devices would still act as foreign bodies but the elimination of skin penetration would sharply limit the risk of infection. Several such devices have been designed and their experimental and clinical use has been reported. The ingenious device designed by Meyer is unique in ICP monitoring in that it uses a radioactive source as a pressure indicator.[21] The radioisotope source is shielded but is moved from beneath the shield as a function of increasing pressure applied to the radioisotope-containing component from a compressible capsule implanted beneath the skull and fluid coupled to the isotope source. ICP can then be quantitated by a radiation detector probe which is positioned extracutaneously over the device.

Nakai *et al.*[74] reported the development of an indirect, purely mechanical method of ICP measurement which also employs an epidural tambour or balloon which is attached to a fully implanted subcutaneous cylinder. Pressure in the implanted cylinder is measured by the transcutaneous application of a second cylinder with matching, apposed diaphragms and then measuring the presence which must be applied to the external cylinder to bring the two diaphragms to a neutral position. The most obvious potential technical problem facing this design configuration is the constancy of the enclosed volume of the implanted portion of the device, since most fluids and gases slowly diffuse through plastics and rubber. Any swelling or distortion of the overlying skin will also introduce artifacts.

Other fully implantable ICP monitoring devices have utilized conversion of pressure to electrical signals, which have been detected transcutaneously by externally applied sensing antennae. The electronic principle employed has varied with the different devices, and has included battery-powered, frequency modulated (FM) radio transmitters,[103] passive FM radio transmitters powered by a transcutaneous power transmitter,[2, 5, 8, 92] frequency-tuned detectors,[36] detectors of capacitance alteration,[79, 80, 89, 115] and generation of an audible response to electromagnetic tuning of an oscillating magnet (Fig. 10.13).

These devices pose the potential risk of foreign body infection inherent in chronically implanted devices. Furthermore, they carry the potential for brain cortical surface injury through chronic pressure, since most of them depend on contact transmission of brain pressure and require continuous pressure on the brain surface. With chronic use there is also the potential for tissue reaction to the implanted material, which can potentially harm the underlying brain, or at least lead to formation of thickened membranes beneath the device, limiting its sensitivity and accuracy.

Long-term maintenance of accuracy and sensitivity are serious problems with many of these devices. Checking zero baseline pressure *in situ* is generally not possible, though Brock and Diefenthaler[8] accomplished this by incorporating a "snorkel" tube which passed through the skin to permit *in vivo* calibration by external application of a known negative pressure. Because they are chronically implanted, and thus

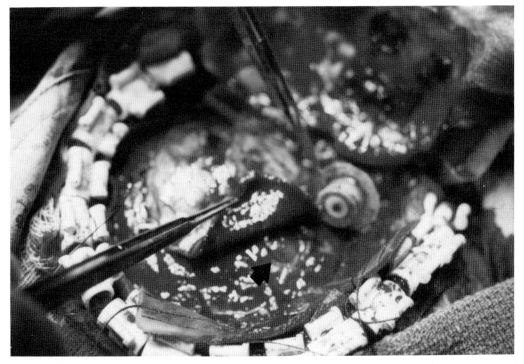

Figure 10.13. Fully implanted telemetric ICP monitor of Zervas-Cosman design removed three months following implantation at the time of repeat craniotomy for evacuation of recurrent tumor cyst. *Arrow* points to a circle of reactive arachnoidal thickening beneath epidural placement.

are generally usable only in a single patient, the cost of the device could become a consideration. A fully implantable device for ICP monitoring which was safe, accurate, and reliable for long-term use would be of little benefit to the large group of patients who require only short-term ICP monitoring of acute brain diseases but would be of potentially great benefit for that smaller group of patients who require long-term monitoring of ICP during therapy of their intracranial tumor, hydrocephalus, or other chronic brain diseases. At the present time, no device in this class has been marketed for general neurosurgical use.

BENEFITS OF ICP MONITORING

Some of the specific benefits of monitoring are discussed in Chapters 8, 9, and 20, and include the use of monitoring when clinical assessment is obscured by therapy, the use of monitoring to predict outcome, and the use of monitoring to guide therapy in the pre- and post-operative period. In this section, the use of ICP monitoring in predicting clinical changes and in documenting brain death will be discussed, as will the *clinical* application of the use of ICP monitoring for the quantitation of cerebral compliance or reserve.

Changes in ICP Precede Clinical Changes

Beginning well before Lundberg's classic treatise and continuing through every subsequently published clinical study, the lack of precise correlation between measured ICP and clinical status of the patient has been repeatedly demonstrated. In every case in which intracranial hypertension is the cause of a patient's deterioration, an elevation of ICP can be documented before changes in mental status or focal neurologic deficits can be detected. If intracranial hypertension develops slowly, clinical deterioration may be delayed by a day or more beyond the onset of intracranial hypertension. Rapid rises in ICP are followed more quickly by clinical deterioration, but early detection in these instances is even more valuable.

How much elevation of ICP is dangerous? In human volunteers, lumbar infusions can be continued without detectable clinical change until the ICP approximates systemic blood pressure.[3, 91] This experimental situation, of course, does not take into account the fourth dimension of time, so that over a longer period of time a modest elevation of ICP may be as dangerous as a higher pressure over a short period of time. When ICP exceeds 15 or 20 torr, capillary beds become compressed and microcirculation is compromised.[93] In areas of focal brain injury, an already compromised capillary circulation may decompensate as a result of the superimposition of relatively small degrees of intracranial hypertension resulting in focal brain dysfunction or shunting of blood away from these areas to other regions of the brain.[9] In areas of brain edema, oxygen and nutrients must diffuse over a greater distance before reaching local neurons so that blood flow of marginal volume may be insufficient to maintain normal cellular metabolism in these regions of the brain. As ICP exceeds 30 to 35 torr, venous drainage becomes compromised and brain edema can be aggravated. Once ICP approaches to within 40 or 50 torr of mean systemic blood pressure, cerebral perfusion begins to fall with resulting cerebral ischemia.[50-52, 71, 97] When the ICP approximates mean systemic blood pressure, the brain is deprived of perfusion and brain death rapidly ensues.

Early detection of changes in ICP is important since it permits therapy before clinical deterioration ensues, before edema accumulation progresses, and before CNS damage results.[24] The neurologic deterioration which results from a rise in ICP may be caused by microcirculatory impairment at localized areas of trauma, by shifts and herniations of brain or by generalized impairment of cerebral perfusion. The precise nature of the neurologic deterioration is significant since it sheds some light on the mechanism causing the deterioration, but the common element of importance is that neurologic deterioration represents a progressive deterioration of the intracranial status. If this deterioration results from increasing brain edema, cell membranes may be ruptured in areas of maximum edema or sufficient interruption of microcirculation may occur and cause local necrosis (Fig. 10.14). Brain shifts and herniations likewise may cause permanent changes in the brain if feeding arteries are overstretched to the point of rupture or if draining veins are distorted and compressed with resultant focal hemorrhagic congestion. All of these secondary complications are potentially preventable if intracranial hypertension is detected prior to neurologic deterioration, but permanent changes may have ensued before therapy can be instituted if one waits until neurologic deterioration is clinically apparent.

ICP Monitoring and the Detection of Brain Death

The diagnosis of "brain death" is probably best made by careful neurologic examination. However, it is often advisable, or at least reassuring, to have some supporting laboratory documentation. The "flat EEG" was the form of documentation called for in the original "Harvard Brain Death Criteria." Unfortunately, EEG documentation of brain death is not valid for patients who are being treated with high doses of barbiturates for intracranial hypertension until blood barbiturate levels have fallen to near zero. If ICP is being monitored continuously in these patients, this may offer sufficient proof of brain death if it confirms a lack of cerebral perfusion. If continuously monitored mean ICP approximates, equals, or exceeds mean systemic blood pressure, *and if the ICP loses its pulsatile character*, this confirms a cerebral perfusion pressure of zero or of approximately zero and consequently a severe impairment or termination of cerebral blood flow. If the brain is not perfused for a period of at least 5 minutes, brain death is confirmed. This criterion has been accepted by the United States Commission on Cerebral Death of the American College of Surgeons and is ac-

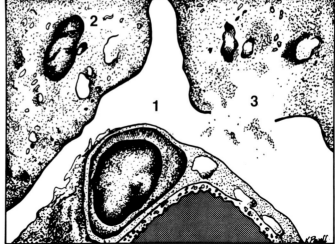

Figure 10.14. Drawing of electron photomicrograph of extracellular brain edema: extracellular edema (1), intracellular edema (2), and membrane rupture secondary to massive cellular swelling (3).

cepted by many hospitals, including my own hospital, the University of Massachusetts Medical Center.

ICP Monitoring Permits Quantitation of Cerebral "Compliance" or "Reserve"

Miller deserves credit for establishing the clinical significance of quantitative determinations of cerebral "compliance" in normal and pathological situations.[55–57, 72] He restudied the principle upon which Dr. Ayala had based his "Ayala Index" and which Lofgren had further delineated[61, 62] and found that the change in ICP which results from withdrawal or addition of aliquots of fluid intracranially is proportional to the initial ICP.[72] However, he also noted a wide variability in the ICP response to intracranial volumetric change and introduced into clinical usage his test for the quantitation of this pressure change in response to volume alteration, a pressure change which he termed cerebral "compliance." He was able to demonstrate that an increased compliance (*i.e.*, a greater rise in pressure in response to volumetric challenge with a given aliquot of fluid, usually 1.0 ml) was obtained from patients with intracranial mass lesions, brain shifts, or brain edema. Presumably, in these patients the brain's compensatory mechanisms are already partially compromised so that they have a reduced capacity to adapt to further increases in

pressure. This phenomenon is also conceptualized as a shift along the roughly exponential volume-pressure curve of ICP response to a rapid addition of added intracranial volume. The basic physiology behind this concept is discussed in greater detail in Chapter 8.

The clinical application of Miller's test for cerebral compliance consists of rapid intraventricular or subdural[67, 98] injection of a test volume of from 0.1 to 1.0 ml of fluid and quantitation of the immediate rise in ICP which this induces to give a measurement of cerebral compliance. In clinical use this test has been found generally to be quite safe but the small volume used sometimes makes it difficult to quantitate, especially in patients with fluctuating baseline ICP's or wide ICP pulse pressures (Fig. 10.15). The single injection employed in the test also increases the possibility of artifactual error (Fig. 10.16), so that several repetitions are advisable for increased accuracy.

An extension of the test for intracranial compliance has been described and is termed the "ICP Reserve Test."[107–111] This attempts to quantitate more than the brain's ability to react over a few seconds to a single volumetric challenge. Instead it attempts to reproduce in a safe and controlled fashion a situation more closely akin to the clinical situation in which the brain's pressure adapting response to a larger volume is quantitated over a longer period of

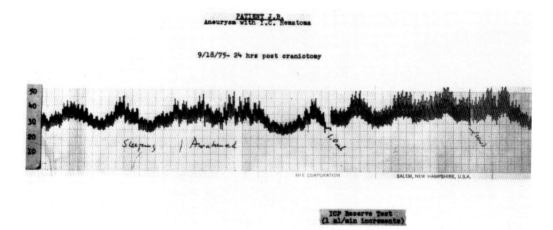

Figure 10.15. Test of cerebral "compliance" using Dr. Miller's technique in a patient with intracranial hypertension and fluctuating ICP. A 1 ml fluid injection subdurally caused minimal immediate rise in ICP but a sustained increase of greater than 5 torr was noted over the next 5 minutes.

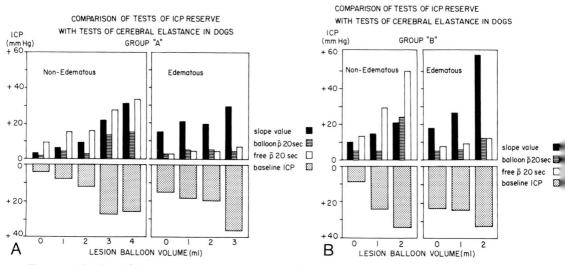

Figure 10.16. ICP, intracranial "compliance" and ICP "reserve" in dogs with large cranial vaults (group "A") and small cranial vaults (group "B"). Incremental inflation of "lesion" balloons at 40-minute intervals caused a rise in baseline ICP but an even more pronounced rise in "slope value" of ICP "reactivity," a measure of ICP "reserve." "Balloon p 20 sec." and "free p 20 sec." refer to two different tests of cerebral "compliance." (Reprinted from Arch. Neurol., 35:575, 1978, copyright 1978, American Medical Association.)

time. It has been nicely documented in the experimental laboratory that a sudden increase in intracranial volume will be slowly compensated over a period of 5–15 minutes, during which time other mechanisms come into play above and beyond those encountered in the first few seconds following rapid intracranial volumetric change (Fig. 10.17).

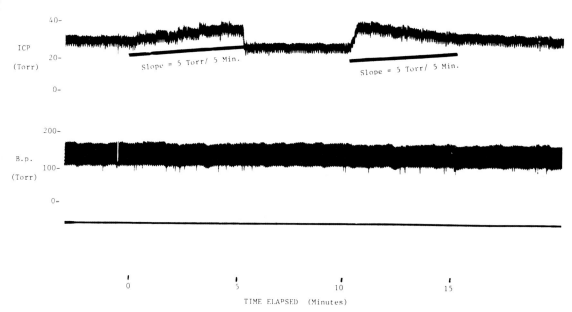

Figure 10.17. Theoretic basis for ICP "reserve" test. ICP remains elevated 5 torr above baseline following 5 incremental 1-ml injections over a 5-minute period and 5 minutes following a single incremental injection of 5 ml. The injection of a sequence of five 1-ml increments avoids the abrupt rise to extremely high ICP levels.

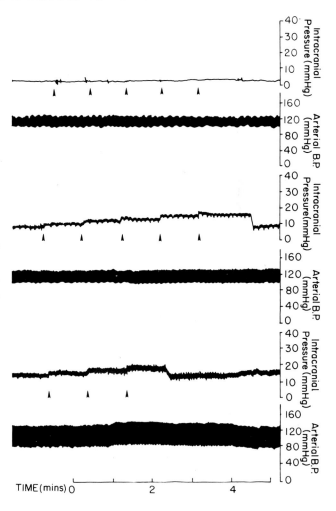

Figure 10.18. ICP "reserve" test in dogs showing: (*upper trace*) minimal ICP rise following 5 injections over 5 minutes in a dog with no mass lesion; (*middle trace*) moderate ICP rise following five injections over 5 minutes in a dog with a moderate intracranial mass lesion and (*lower trace*) sharp rise in ICP following only three injections over 3 minutes in a dog with a large intracranial mass lesion. At this point, the test was terminated and a "slope value" was calculated. (Reprinted from Arch. Neurol., 35:571, 1978, copyright 1978, American Medical Association.)

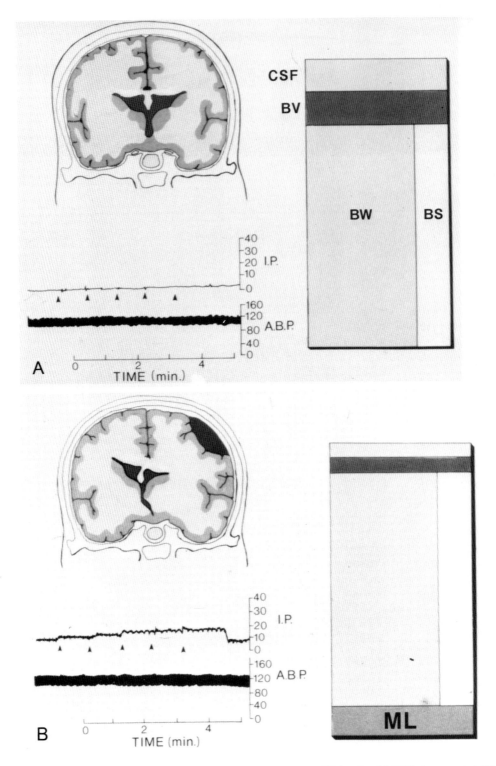

Figure 10.19. *A*, normal ICP ''reserve'' in a ''normal'' brain (*CSF*-intracranial CSF volume; *BV*-intracranial blood volume; *BW*-brain water; *BS*-brain solid). *B*, moderately impaired ICP ''reserve'' in a brain with intracranial volume partially replaced by a mass lesion (*ML* - mass lesion). *C*, severely abnormal ICP ''reserve'' in a brain in which compensatory mechanisms have been exhausted by the presence of a large mass lesion.

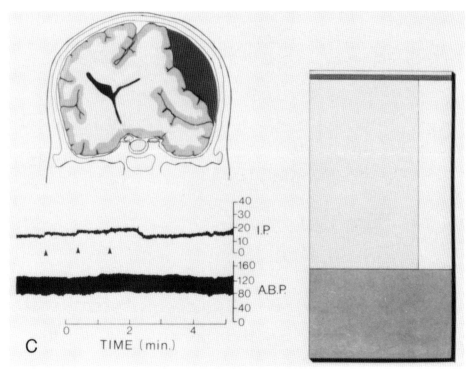

Figure 10.19. *C*

Since safety must be a prime consideration in patient management, the ICP Reserve Test involves challenging the brain with a series of up to five 1-ml aliquots of fluid injected intraventricularly or subdurally at one-minute intervals over a maximum five-minute duration (Fig. 10.18). The test is not done if baseline ICP already exceeds 30 torr, since intracranial decompensation can be assumed to have occurred without need of quantitation of the brain's reactivity to volumetric stress. The pressure rise which follows each test injection is recorded 60 seconds *following* each injection. If this rise is found to have exceeded 10 torr over baseline ICP, further injections of the planned series of 5 are omitted (Fig. 10.19). Instead the response which would have been observed is quantitated as a linear extrapolation using the following simple formula: observed rise in ICP divided by number of injections × 5 = "slope value" of the brain's "reactivity" to volumetric stress testing, a quantitative measurement of ICP "Reserve."

This test has been useful clinically in helping to determine when a normal ICP is a safe ICP. The presence of postoperative bleeding or severe brain edema may be detected as much as several days prior to clinical deterioration of the patient and often several days prior to an observed rise in ICP. In clinical use, most patients are unaware of any altered sensation during performance of the test. So far, with careful observance of the clinical safeguards built into the test, no incidence of neurologic deterioration or triggering of plateau "A" waves has been reported.

ICP reserve testing was initially described as a method for quantitating the brain's reactivity to subdural administration of a fluid volume challenge (Fig. 10.20). This test can be carried out by intraventricular fluid volume injections as well, but will be accurate *only* if the ventricular system is freely communicating with the subarachnoid space and if the presumed ventricular catheter is lying within the ventricular cavity and not within the brain paren-

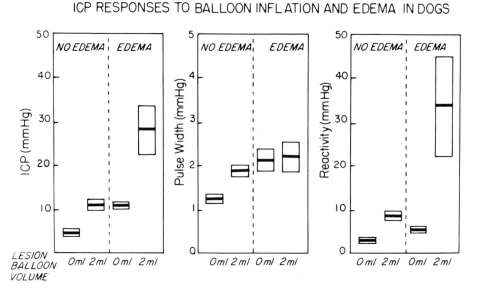

ICP RESPONSES TO BALLOON INFLATION AND EDEMA IN DOGS

Figure 10.20. Experimental mass lesions with and without brain edema in dogs showing response to lesion balloon inflation: Baseline ICP (*left*), ICP pulse width (*middle*) and quantitated ICP reactivity (*right*) show different responses with ICP "reserve test" best differentiating between the different brain states. (Reprinted from J. Neurosurg., 50:761, 1979.)

chyma.[109] Injections of even small volumes of fluid into an obstructed ventricle or directly into the parenchyma of the brain can cause severe local rises in pressure. This will result in an artifactual increase in observed reactivity of brain to volumetric challenge, will cause local tissue distortion, and may be dangerous to the patient. Intraventricular assessment of brain compliance or reserve should always be carried out initially with small fluid increments before proceeding to the full ICP reserve test or even before proceeding to a full test of intracranial compliance using a single milliliter of fluid.

Both of the above described volumetric tests of cerebral compliance or reserve involve introduction of added volume intracranially. Alternative methods of determining the brain's reactivity to volumetric stress have been sought by challenging the brain's ability to react volumetrically through manipulation of inspired gases,[30, 84] or through manipulation of positive end expiratory pressure.[1, 36] The former test has enjoyed some clinical popularity although

it is more difficult to quantitate precisely and may be unreliable in the presence of impaired cerebral autoregulation. It has been reported that this test can trigger plateau "A" waves, a pathologic change which can be demonstrated to be potentially dangerous to the patient.[52]

RISKS AND LIMITATIONS OF ICP MONITORING

The problems encountered with ICP monitoring fall into three categories: 1) problems which pose a risk to the patient; 2) technical problems resulting in failure to record accurate and reliable ICP; and 3) problems involving errors on the part of the clinician who utilizes the ICP data.

Problems Involving Risk to the Patient

The possibility of introducing intracranial infection is the most important single risk encountered with direct ICP monitoring. As discussed earlier, the type of monitoring device employed influences to a great degree the type of infection to which the patient is placed at risk. Intraventricular monitoring carries the potential of ventriculitis or brain abscess, complications which are often quite severe. Whereas epidural monitoring usually leaves the brain protected by the intact dura mater in the event of an epidural infection, subdural monitoring carries the risk of subdural empyema or brain abscess. Even continuous lumbar monitoring from an indwelling catheter can result in infection in the form of meningitis, epidural abscess, or occasionally subdural abscess.

The risk of infection is clearly proportional to the duration of monitoring with all systems currently employed. Reported incidences of infection have varied widely, with some authors reporting as much as 10% infection risk. On the other hand, most clinical series, as well as the present author's personal experience, have documented an infection rate of 0–6%.[13–15, 35, 63] Errors in sterile technique at the time of insertion of monitoring devices or during prolonged monitoring undoubtedly account for the major proportion of monitoring related infections. With fluid-coupled systems all potential portals of bacterial entry must be kept covered aseptically. Sterility of all solutions introduced into the system must be rigidly maintained and the number of entries into and changes in the system should be kept to an absolute minimum to avoid contamination. Nursing personnel must be impressed with the fact that during direct ICP monitoring, opening a stopcock, changing a syringe or reconnecting tubing are potentially *life-threatening* maneuvers, and must be done with rigid attention to sterile technique.

The design configuration of the ICP monitoring device may also influence the possibility of infection. Devices which penetrate the skin directly over the site of dural penetration present an increased risk of infection both during monitoring and following removal of the device because of the short distance interposed between the potentially contaminated skin opening and the point of penetration into the subdural or deeper spaces of the brain. In contrast, catheter-shaped devices which are tunneled beneath the scalp to a skin exit site remote from the point of dural penetration lessen the likelihood of bacterial ingress and CSF egress during use and following removal of the monitoring device.

An *extremely important* technical consideration for limiting infection with *any* form of ICP monitoring device which is at least partially externalized is the application of a large amount of occlusive antibiotic ointment at the skin site. In normal use, some movement of the skin around the penetrating portion of the monitoring device occurs and this adds to the risk of passive introduction of bacteria from the skin surface. Contamination by the roaming fingers of a confused patient can usually be avoided by vigilant nursing, patient restraints when necessary, and adequate head dressings. Even if fingers do manage to reach the skin exit site, an occlusive antibiotic ointment will provide a considerable safety factor. Administration of systemic prophylactic antibiotics throughout the entire period of ICP monitoring was recommended by Lundberg.[63] Some neurosurgeons still take this precaution, although this author does not; there is no convincing proof in the literature of the effectiveness of systemic antibiotic prophylaxis sufficient to outweigh the potential risks inherent in their use.

As is true with any neurosurgical operative procedure, the potential exists for harming the patient during placement of an ICP monitoring device. Ventricular catheterization is not always easy in a damaged and distorted brain and the need for multiple catheter passes before ventricular catheterization is accomplished compounds the risk. If cerebral engorgement and venous congestion are present, the risk of disruption of small parenchymal vessels during catheter passage is increased, with an increased risk of intracerebral hemorrhage. If the brain is severely distorted, vigorous attempts at ventricular catheterization can lead to inadvertent damage to basal ganglia or other deep brain structures.

Subdural catheter placement necessitates passing a catheter over the surface of the brain, often without benefit of direct vision. Bridging cortical veins may be encountered and may be torn or hematomas may be dislodged from the ends of previously torn brain surface blood vessels. If the brain is tense, swollen and softened great care must be taken during passage of these catheters to insure that they do not catch on the arachnoidal surface and tear through the arachnoid to plunge into the brain substance.

Bolt or plug type ICP monitoring devices which record pressure from the brain surface must be introduced to a depth sufficient to bring them in contact with the surface of the brain whose pressure they are to monitor, but excessively deep insertion may damage the brain surface at the time of insertion or subsequently as the brain moves about within the skull. The hollow bolt devices pose a particular problem in this regard since they carry the real potential for herniation of cortical tissue into the open lumen of the bolt. While the amount of tissue loss is usually not sufficient to cause a noticeable or persistent neurologic deficit, this local disruption may add to the problems of brain edema and may act as a focus for subsequent seizure activity. Devices which are left permanently or semi-permanently implanted also pose the risk of cortical brain injury through chronic pressure, irritation, or chemical reaction and likewise may generate seizure foci.

CSF leakage can be a problem both during and following ICP monitoring because it places the patient at increased risk of infection. Devices which exit from, communicate with, or traverse the subarachnoid space and which are in part externalized can provide a tract or passageway for CSF egress. This is true of lumbar subarachnoid catheters, ventricular catheters, devices left in brain cavities or brain parenchyma, and "subdural" monitoring devices (the latter often communicating with the subarachnoid space through tears in the arachnoid membrane). CSF leakage through the arachnoid and dura which does not reach the skin surface is rarely a problem with direct cerebral monitoring but may be a distinct risk to the patient with lumbar monitoring. Even an internal loss of lumbar CSF will produce a fall in lumbar CSF pressure, placing the patient at risk of brain herniation.

Another safety consideration concerns the volume of fluid injected intracranially through a fluid coupled device. Nearly all fluid-coupled devices function better with periodic "flushing" (usually done with an antibiotic solution) to clear the system and maintain an optimum volume within the system. Air bubbles introduced through these systems intracranially rarely if ever pose a risk to the patient, but attempts to clear air from the system by injecting large volumes of fluid pose a very real potential threat. The volume of fluid which the brain will tolerate under pathologic condition varies widely and when fluid coupled devices are in use, fluid "flushes" of the system should be kept to a minimum. Ideally, the effect of larger volume infusions on ICP should be quantitated in terms of compliance or ICP reserve at least daily. Certainly ICP reserve or compliance should be quantitated incrementally at any time larger volume infusions are felt to be necessary (*i.e.*, for clearing air bubbles from the system), especially when measurements have not previously been made. Because of the very real danger to the patient ICP monitoring systems should *never* be set up in such a way that the potential exists for accidental introduction of large volumes of fluid intracranially. Suspending a bag or bottle of fluid from a pole above an ICP monitoring system and having this container coupled into the system poses an unnecessary danger to the patient. In this situation, a stopcock may be accidentally opened by an inexperienced nurse or a confused patient. Occasionally, stopcocks have become entangled in bed clothes and have been opened "remotely" without this coming to the attention of a conscientious and attentive nurse (Fig. 10.21). It is useful to have attached to the system at least a sufficient volume of irrigating solution for 24-hour use to limit the necessity for frequent syringe changes. A sufficient volume can usually easily be stored in a large syringe. Remember Murphy's Law: "If things can go wrong, they will!"[68, 69]

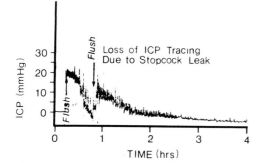

Figure 10.21. Decay of recorded ICP obtained with fluid coupled ICP monitor secondary to fluid leakage through a faulty stopcock. "Flush" denotes flushing the catheter system with 0.2 ml of fluid, sufficient to restore ICP tracings briefly. In this situation the most accurate ICP reading is the one obtained immediately *following* flushing.

Technical Problems: Failure to Obtain an Accurate and Reliable ICP Reading

Devices which pose a technical burden on personnel in the intensive care unit, recovery room, or operating room or on house officers or neurosurgeons will be fraught with considerable problems in routine use and daily application. The more technically demanding and functionally unique a device is, the more specialization will be required from personnel who operate and maintain the equipment. As a result, fewer people will be qualified for use of the device and failure of usefulness is more likely to occur when these key people are unavailable. It is well-known among instrument manufacturers that all forms of medical equipment receive considerable abuse during routine use and that this abuse potential increases dramatically if more than one or two people are involved and responsible. Experience further shows that apparatus which is difficult to operate and therefore which adds to the burden of personnel assigned to operate that equipment is more likely to receive abuse in operation and is more likely to give difficulty through equipment malfunction. If ICP monitoring can be accomplished at least in part with existing and familiar equipment, such as is true with most of the fluid coupled devices, personnel and maintenance problems are likely to be reduced.

Baseline drift and loss of accuracy are potential problems with electronic ICP monitoring devices. If accurate ICP monitoring is to be continued for more than a brief period it should be possible to check the accuracy and continued functioning of the pressure monitoring component of the device during use. For fluid-coupled devices this can usually be accomplished relatively easily by calibrating an electronic transducer located at the patient's bedside and fluid coupled to the ICP transmitting component. Some ICP monitoring devices which employ implanted electronic transducers have been designed to permit re-zeroing *in situ*, or by temporary removal of the plug shaped device, to permit determinations of continued accuracy. These maneuvers, however, have not always been technically easy to accomplish or totally devoid of risk to the patient. Some ICP devices which cannot be re-zeroed have depended instead on a reasonably accurate pre-implantation assessment of device stability, so that the neurosurgeon either relies on a knowledge of the expected change in function during use, must be content with an estimate of daily percent loss of accuracy[76] or must check the accuracy of the ICP monitor by lumbar puncture.[35, 36] My own experience with implantable devices which could be re-zeroed *in situ* has demonstrated that at times unexpected changes in device accuracy have occurred and have not been apparent through observation of the patient. This has the potential for being particularly harmful when a dangerous rise in actual ICP is counterbalanced by a downward drifting in machine performance and therefore goes undetected clinically.

Difficulties with ICP Monitoring Due to Physician Errors

The major source of physician error encountered with ICP monitoring is the reverse of that encountered when ICP monitoring is not used: an undue and uncritical dependence on ICP as displayed or recorded. Treatment decisions based on clinical assessment of the patient without the benefit of ICP recording may err since ICP may be abnormally elevated despite a normal or unchanged neurologic examination. Conversely, a recording of a normal ICP should not be allowed to induce a laxity in the clinical assessment and monitoring of the patient and should not be used as an excuse to withhold proper therapy when this is dictated by a clinical assessment of the patient.

A "normal" ICP reading may in fact be artifactual and this *technical* problem of ICP monitoring can easily be converted to a *patient management problem* if the neurosurgeon is not alert to the possibility of such an artifact and does not continue careful clinical monitoring of the patient. Frequently, a "normal" ICP is recorded *only* because the patient is receiving intensive medical therapy and fluid restriction. This patient, of course, does *not* have a normal intracranial status, and severe intracranial hypertension may develop rapidly if one is lulled into excessive therapeutic laxity, withdrawing medical management too rapidly, or beginning patient hydration too vigorously. It is obviously possible for a patient to suffer from severe disease of the central nervous system with *no* increase in ICP and treatment for these conditions should not be withheld or unduly delayed simply because of a lack of documented intracranial hypertension.

Tests of ICP reserve or brain compliance may be quite valuable if they give early warning of impending intracranial decompensation or intracranial disease of unexpected severity. However, these are only clinical tests and are therefore subject to potential artifact. As discussed earlier, unexpectedly severe rises in cerebral "reactivity" can occur if the volumetric challenge is administered into an obstructed ventricle or inadvertently into brain parenchyma instead of into the ventricle. On the other hand, the reactivity to intraventricular volumetric stress is characteristically reduced in patients with ventriculomegaly and will be reduced following subdural volumetric challenge if the subdurally injected fluid does not remain intracranially but escapes

extradurally through the catheter exit site. Certainly the demonstration of abnormal ICP reserve or brain compliance should alert the neurosurgeon to the possibility of serious intracranial abnormality, especially if the documented reserve or compliance becomes progressively more abnormal during the period of observation. However, the documentation of a normal compliance or reserve should be assessed cautiously as a decidedly optimistic but *potentially* misleading additional bit of clinical data in the course of patient management.

The other major source of physician error in ICP monitoring is the choice of a suboptimum method of ICP monitoring for a given patient. There is no single ideal method for measuring ICP. Because the indications for ICP monitoring vary widely, neurosurgeons should have available a variety of techniques for measuring ICP. The patient whose intracranial hypertension is caused by enlarged ventricles should undergo ventricular catheterization for ICP monitoring and for therapy of the ventriculomegaly. On the other hand, the patient with slit-like and compressed ventricles who is already undergoing craniotomy could best have his ICP monitored by a subdural or epidural catheter device. For the acutely head-injured patient some may prefer the relative ease of insertion of a bolt device, or stopcock or tubing used as a bolt device, for epidural or subdural monitoring.

SUMMARY

Direct ICP monitoring has now become an accepted and valuable part of the neurosurgeon's armamentarium. A variety of techniques for ICP monitoring have now been perfected so that they are safe and practical to use. Intracranial hypertension often develops well before clinical deterioration is apparent and clinical deterioration and CNS damage can often be prevented by the early warning which direct ICP monitoring gives.

The risks of ICP monitoring to the patient can be minimized by careful attention to surgical technique and asepsis. The limitations inherent in ICP monitoring can be minimized by careful personnel planning, device selection, and physician awareness of the continued need for clinical monitoring in addition to direct ICP measurement.

References:

1. Apuzzo, M.L.J., Weiss, M.H., Petersons, V., Small, R.B., Kurze, T., Heiden, J.S.: Effect of positive end expiratory pressure ventilation on intracranial pressure in man. J. Neurosurg., 46:227–232, 1977.
2. Atkinson, J.R., Shurtleff, D.B., Foltz, E.L.: Radio telemetry for the measurement of intracranial pressure. J. Neurosurg., 27:428–432, 1967.
3. Ayala, G.: Uber den diagnostischen wert des liquordruckes und einen apparat zu seiner messung. Ztschr. Neurol. Psychiat., 84:42–95, 1923.
4. Ayer, J.B.: Analysis of the lumbar cerebrospinal fluid in 67 cases of tumours and cysts of the brain. In: The Intracranial Pressure in Health and Disease, Assoc. Res. Nerv. Ment. Dis., 8:189–199, 1929.
5. Barbaro, V., Macellari, V.: Intracranial pressure monitoring by means of a passive radiosonde. Med. Biol. Eng. Conput., 17:81–86, 1979.
6. Beks, J.W.F., Albarda, S., Gieles, A.C.M., Kuypers, M.H., Flanderijn, H.: Extradural transducer for monitoring intracranial pressure. Acta Neurochir., 38:245–250, 1977.
7. Blaauw, G., Van der Bos, J.L., Mus, A.: On pulsation of the fontanelle. Dev. Med. Child Neurol., 16 (Suppl. 32):23–36, 1974.
8. Brock, M., Diefenthaler, K.: A modified equipment for the continuous telemetric monitoring of epidural or subdural pressure. In: Intracranial Pressure, Brock, M., Dietz, H., Eds., Springer-Verlag, Berlin, 1972, pp. 21–26.
9. Brock, M., Furuse, M., Weber, R., Dietz, H.: Changes in intracranial blood flow distribution following circumscribed hemispheric lesions as studied by the "single dye passage" technique. In: Pathology of Cerebral Microcirculation, Cervós-Navarro, Ed., Walder de Gruyter, New York, 1974, pp. 342–353.
10. Brock, M., Pöll, W., Furuse, M., Dietz, H.: Der Docht-Katheter—Ein neues verfahren zur postoperativen uberwachung des intrakraniellen druckes. Acta Neurochir., 28:201–212, 1973.
11. Browder, J., Meyers, R.: Observations on behavior of the systemic blood pressure, pulse and spinal fluid pressure following craniocerebral injury. Am. J. Surg., 31:403–426, 1936.
12. Browder, J., Meyers, R.: Behavior of the systemic blood pressure pulse rate and spinal fluid pressure associated with acute changes in intracranial pressure artificially produced. Arch. Surg., 36:1–19, 1938.
13. Bruce, D.A., Berman, W.A., Schut, L.: Cerebrospinal fluid pressure monitoring in children: physiology, pathology and clinical usefulness. Adv. Pediatr., 24:233–290, 1977.
14. Bruce, D.A., Goldberg, A., Schut, L.: ICP monitoring in critical care pediatrics. Intensive Care Med., 3:184–187, 1977.
15. Bruce, D.A.: The pathophysiology of increased intracranial pressure. The Upjohn Company Monograph, 1978.
16. Butler, A.B., Rosenthal, J.D., Bass, N.H., Johnson, R.N.: Multiport device for the assessment of cerebrospinal fluid dynamics under conditions of elevated intracranial pressure in man and experimental animals. Med. Bull. Eng. Comput., 16:601–602, 1978.
17. Cheek, W.R., Evans, A.F., Dennis, G.C., Stein, F.: Device for extradural monitoring of intracranial pressure: technical note. Neurosurgery 5:692–694, 1979.
18. Clark, R.M., Capra, N.F., Halsey, J.H. Jr.: Method for measuring brain tissue pressure: response to alteration in pCO_2, systemic blood pressure, and middle cerebral artery occlusion. J. Neurosurg., 43:1–8, 1975.
19. Clark, R.M., Capra, N.F., Halsey, J.H.: Methodology for measuring intracranial parenchymal pressure (ICPP). In: Intracranial Pressure II, Lundberg, N., Penten, U., Brock, M., Eds. Berlin, Springer-Verlag, 1974, pp. 209–210.
20. Cohadon, F., La Balme, M., Castel, J.P., Vandendriessche, M.: ICP microprobes series microfet. In: Intracranial Pressure II, Lundberg, N., Ponten, U., Brock, M., Eds. Springer-Verlag, Berlin, 1974, pp. 375–376.
21. Cooper, P.R., Moody, S., Sklar, F.: Chronic monitoring of intracranial pressure using an in vivo calibrating sensor: experience in patients with pseudotumor cerebri. Neurosurgery 5:666–670, 1979.
22. Coroneos, N.J., Turner, J.M., Gibson, R.M., McDowall, D.G., Pickerodt, V.W.A., Keaney, N.P.: Comparison of extradural with intraventricular pressure in patients after head injury. In: Intracranial Pressure, Brock, M., Dietz, H., Eds. Springer-Verlag, Berlin, 1972, pp. 51–58.
23. Coroneos, N.J., McDowall, D.G., Gibson, R.M., Pickerodt, V.W.A., Keaney, N.P.: Measurement of extradural pressure and its relationship to other intracranial pressures. J. Neurol. Neurosurg. Psych., 36:514–522, 1973.
24. Crockard, H.A.: Early intracranial pressure studies in gunshot wounds of the brain. J. Trauma, 15:339–347, 1975.
25. de Rougemont, J., Barge, M., Benabid, A.L.: Un nouveau capteur pour la mésure de la pression intra-crânienne. Neurochirurgie, 17:579–590, 1971.
26. de Rougemont, J., Benabid, A.L., Barge, M.: Intracranial pressure measurement by epidural technique—a simple solution. In: Intracranial pressure II, Lundberg, N., Ponten, U., Brock, M., Eds. Springer-Verlag, Berlin, 1974, pp. 384–385.
27. Dietrich, K., Gaab, M., Knoblich, O.E., Schupp, J., Ott, B.: A new miniaturized system for monitoring the epidural pressure in children and adults. Neuropaediatrie, 8:21–28, 1977.
28. Duffy, G.P.: Lumbar puncture in presence of raised intracranial pressure. Br. Med. J., 1:407–409, 1969.
29. Edwards, J.: An intracranial pressure tonometer for use in neonates: preliminary report. Dev.

Med. Child Neurol., 16 (Suppl. 32):38–39, 1974.

30. Fieschi, C., Battistini, N., Beduschi, A., Boselli, L., Rossanda, M.: Regional cerebral blood flow and intraventricular pressure in acute head injuries. J. Neurol. Neurosurg. Psych., 37:1378–1388, 1974.

31. Fleischer, A.S., Patton, J.M., Tindall, G.T.: Monitoring intraventricular pressure using an implanted reservoir in head injured patients. Surg. Neurol., 3:309–311, 1975.

32. Gobiet, W., Bock, W.J., Liesegang, J., Grote, W.: Experience with an intracranial pressure transducer readjustable *in vivo*. Technical note. J. Neurosurg., 40:272–276, 1974.

33. Gobiet, W., Brock, W.J., Liesegang, J., Grote, W.: Long-time monitoring of epidural pressure in man. In: Intracranial Pressure, Brock, M., Dietz, H., Eds., Springer-Verlag, Berlin, 1972, pp. 14–17.

34. Gosch, H.H., Kindt, G.W.: Subdural monitoring of acute increased intracranial pressure. Surg. Forum, 23:405–406, 1972.

35. Gücer, G., Viernstein, L.J., Chubbuck, J.G., Walker, A.E.: Clinical evaluation of long-term epidural monitoring of intracranial pressure. Surg. Neurol., 12:373–377, 1979.

36. Gucer, G., Viernstein, L., Walker, A.E.: Continuous intracranial pressure recording in adult hydrocephalus. Surg. Neurol., 13:323–328, 1980.

37. Guillaume, J., Janny, P.: Manométrie intracranienne continué. Intérêt de la méthode et premiers résultats. Révue Neurologique, 84:131–142, 1951.

38. Handa, H., Yoneda, S., Matsuda, M., Handa, J.: A miniature SFT transducer for continuous monitoring of intracranial pressure. In: Intracranial Pressure II, Lundberg, N., Pontén, U., Brock, M., Eds. Springer-Verlag, Berlin, 1974, pp. 378–379.

39. Hartmann, A., Alberti, E.: Differentiation of communicating hydrocephalus and presenile dementia by continuous recording of cerebrospinal fluid pressure. J. Neurol. Neurosurg. Psych., 40:630–640, 1977.

40. Hartmann, A., Alberti, E.: Eine einfache methode zur kontinuierlichen messung des liquordrucks. Acta Neurochir. (Wein) 36:201–214, 1977.

41. Hill, L.: The physiology and pathology of the cerebral circulation. An experimental research. London, 1896.

42. Hirschberg, R.: Traitment de la meningite tuberculeuse. In: Bulletin general du therapeutique medicale, chirurgicale, obstetricale et pharmaceutique. Paris, pp. 411–421, 1894.

43. Hoppenstein, R.: A device for measuring intracranial pressure. Lancet, 1:90–91, 1965.

44. Hulme, A., Cooper, R.: A technique for the investigation of intracranial pressure in man. J. Neurol. Neurosurg. Psych., 29:154–156, 1966.

45. Ingvar, S.: On the danger of leakage of the cerebrospinal fluid after lumbar puncture. Acta Med. Scand., 58:67–101, 1923.

46. Jacobson, S.A., Rothballer, A.B.: Prolonged measurement of experimental intracranial pressure using a subminiature absolute pressure transducer. J. Neurosurg., 26:603–608, 1967.

47. James, H.E., Bruno, L., Schut, L.: Intracranial subarachnoid pressure monitoring in children.

Surg. Neurol., 3:313–315, 1975.

48. Jennett, B.: Techniques for measuring intracranial pressure. In: Intracranial Pressure. Brock, M., Dietz, H., Eds., Springer-Verlag, Berlin, 1972, pp. 365–368.

49. Johnston, I.H., Rowan, J.O.: Raised intracranial pressure and cerebral blood flow 4. Intracranial pressure gradients and regional cerebral blood flow. J. Neurol. Neurosurg. Psych., 37:585–592.

50. Johnston, I.H., Rowan, J.O., Harper, A.M., Jennett, W.B.: Raised intracranial pressure and cerebral blood flow. 1. Cisterna magna infusion in primates. J. Neurol. Neurosurg. Psych., 35:285–296, 1972.

51. Johnston, I.H., Rowan, J.O., Harper, A.M., Jennett, W.B.: Raised intracranial pressure and cerebral blood flow. 2. Supratentorial and infratentorial mass lesions in primates. J. Neurol. Neurosurg. Psych., 36:161–170, 1973.

52. Johnston, I.H., Rowan, J.O., Park, D.M., Rennie, M.J.: Raised intracranial pressure and cerebral blood flow. 5. Effects of episodic intracranial pressure waves in primates. J. Neurol. Neurosurg., Psych., 38:1076–1082, 1975.

53. Kellie, G.: An account of the appearances observed in the dissection of two of the three individuals presumed to have perished in the storm of 3rd, and whose bodies were discovered in the vicinity of Leith on the morning of the 4th November 1821 with some reflections on the pathology of the brain. Trans. Med. Chir. Sci., Edinburgh, 1:84–169, 1824.

54. Kindt, G.W.: Simplification of intracranial pressure monitoring. In: Intracranial Pressure II, Lundberg, N., Pontén, U., Brock, M., Eds. Springer-Verlag, Berlin, 1974, p. 381.

55. Leech, P., Miller, J.D.: Intracranial volume-pressure relationships during experimental brain compression in primates. J. Neurol. Neurosurg., Psych., 37:1093–1098, 1974.

56. Leech, P., Miller, J.D.: Intracranial volume-pressure relationships during experimental brain compression in primates. 2. Effect of induced changes in systemic arterial pressure and cerebral blood flow. J. Neurol. Neurosurg. Psych., 37:1099–1104, 1974.

57. Leech, P., Miller, J.D.: Intracranial volume-pressure relationships during experimental brain compression in primates. 3. Effect of mannitol and hyperventilation. J. Neurol. Neurosurg. Psych., 37:1105–1111, 1974.

58. Levin, A.B.: The use of a fiber optic intracranial pressure transducer in the treatment of head injuries. J. Trauma, 17:567–574, 1977.

59. Levin, A.B.: The use of a fiber optic intracranial pressure monitor in clinical practice. Neurosurgery, 1:266–271, 1977.

60. Levinthal, R.: A simple method for continuous pressure recording. Bull. Los Angeles Neurol. Soc., 41:148–153, 1976.

61. Löfgren, J.: Effects of variations in arterial pressure and arterial carbon dioxide tension on the cerebrospinal fluid pressure-volume relationships. Acta Neurol. Scand., 49:586–598, 1973.

62. Löfgren, J., von Essen, C., Zwetnow, N.N.: The

pressure-volume curve of the cerebrospinal fluid space in dogs. Acta Neurol. Scand., 49:557–574, 1973.

63. Lundberg, N.: Continuous recording and control of ventricular fluid pressure in neurosurgical practice. Acta Psychiat et Neurol. Scand., 36 (Suppl. 149):1–193, 1960.

64. McGraw, C.P.: Epidural intracranial pressure monitoring. In: Intracranial Pressure II, Lundberg, N., Pontén, U., Brock, M., Eds., Springer-Verlag, Berlin, 1974, pp. 394–396.

65. McGraw, C.P., Alexander, E. Jr.: Durometer for measurement of intracranial pressure. Surg. Neurol., 7:293–295, 1977.

66. McKay, L.: Development of an intracranial pressure transducer. J. Audio Eng. Soc., 19:121–126, 1971.

67. Mann, J.D., Butler, A.B., Rosenthal, J.E., Maffeo, C.J., Johnson, R.N., Bass, N.H.: Regulation of intracranial pressure in rat, dog and man. Ann. Neurol., 3:156–165, 1978.

68. Matz, R.: Principles of medicine. N.Y. State J. Med., 77:99–101, 1977.

69. Matz, R.: More principles in medicine. N.Y. State J. Med., 77:1984–1985, 1977.

70. Mendes, M., Moore, P., Wheeler, C.B., Winn, H.R., Rodeheaver, G.: Susceptibility of brain and skin to bacterial challenge. J. Neurosurg., 52:772–775, 1980.

71. Miller, J.D., Garibi, J., North, J.B., Teasdale, G.M.: Effects of increased arterial pressure on blood flow in the damaged brain. J. Neurol. Neurosurg. Psych., 38:657–665, 1975.

72. Miller, J.D., Garibi, J., Pickard, J.D.: Induced changes of cerebrospinal fluid volume—effects during continuous monitoring of ventricular fluid pressure. Arch. Neurol., 28:265–269, 1973.

73. Monro, A.: Observations on the Structure and Function of the Nervous System. Creech and Johnson, Edinburgh, 1783.

74. Nakai, M., Togawa, T., Fujimoto, T., Inaba, Y.: Transcutaneous pressure measurement system for the intracranial pressure monitoring. Reports of the Institute for Medical & Dental Engineering, Tokyo, 8:75–80, 1974.

75. Nölke, O.: Beobachturgen zur pathologie des hindrucks. Deutsch Med. Wochenschr. 39:618–620, 1897.

76. Nornes, H., Serek-Hanssen, F.: Miniature transducer for intracranial pressure monitoring in man. Acta Neurol. Scand., 46:203–214, 1970.

77. Numoto, M.: Intracranial pressure monitoring methods by pressure balance technique. Brain Nerve, 228:365–370, 1976.

78. Numoto, M., Wallman, J.K., Donaghy, R.M.P.: Pressure indicating bag for monitoring intracranial pressure. J. Neurosurg., 39:784–787, 1973.

79. Olsen, E.R., Collins, C.C.: Passive radio telemetry for the measurement of intracranial pressure. In: Intracranial Pressure, Brock, M., Dietz, H., Eds. Springer-Verlag, Berlin, 1972, pp. 18–20.

80. Olsen, E.R., Collins, C.C., Loughborough, W.F., Richards, V., Adams, J.E., Pinto, D.W.: Intracranial pressure measurement with a miniature passive implanted pressure transensor. Am. J. Surg.,

113:727–729, 1967.

81. Ommaya, A.K.: Subcutaneous reservoir and pump for sterile access to ventricular cerebrospinal fluid. Lancet, 2:983–984, 1963.

82. Papo, I., Caruselli, G.: Long-term intracranial pressure monitoring in comatose patients suffering from head injuries. A critical survey. Acta Neurochir., 39:187–200, 1977.

83. Papo, I., Caruselli, G., Luongo, A., Scarpelli, M., Pasquini, U.: Traumatic cerebral mass lesions: correlations between clinical, intracranial pressure and computed tomographic data. Neurosurgery 7:337–346, 1980.

84. Paul, R.L., Polanco, O., Turney, S.Z., McAslan, T.C., Cowley, R.A.: Intracranial pressure responses to alterations in arterial carbon dioxide pressure in patients with head injuries. J. Neurosurg., 36:714–720, 1972.

85. Pöll, W., Brock, M., Markakis, E., Winkelmüller, W., Dietz, H.: Brain Tissue Pressure. In: Intracranial Pressure, Brock, M., Dietz, H., Eds., Springer-Verlag, Berlin, 1972, pp. 188–194.

86. Queckenstedt, H., Zur diagnose der ruckenmarkkompression. Deutch. Ztschr. Nerveh., 55: 325–333, 1916.

87. Quincke, H.: Die diagnostiche und therapeutische bedeutung der lumbalpunktion. Klinischer Vortrag. Deutsch. Med. Wochnschr. 31:1825–1928, 1869–1872, 1905.

88. Quincke, H.: Lumbar puncture. In: Modern Clinical Medicine, Diseases of the Nervous System. Church, A., Ed. Appleton, New York, 1911.

89. Ream, A.K., Silverberg, G.D., Corbin, S.D., Schmidt, E.V., Fryer, T.B.: Epidural measurement of intracranial pressure. Neurosurgery 5:36–43, 1979.

90. Reulen, H.J., Graham, R., Spatz, M., Klatzo, I.: Role of pressure gradients and bulk flow in dynamics of vasogenic brain edema. J. Neurosurg., 46:24–35, 1977.

91. Ryder, H.W., Rosenauer, A., Penka, E.J., Espey, F.F., Evans, J.P.: Failure of abnormal cerebrospinal fluid pressure to influence cerebral function. Arch. Neurol. Psych., 70:563–586, 1953.

92. Rylander, H.G., Taylor, H.L., Wissinger, J.P., Story, J.L.: Chronic measurement of epidural pressure with an induction-powered oscillator transducer. J. Neurosurg., 44:465–478, 1976.

93. Salmon, J.H., Hajjar, W., Bada, H.S.: The fontogram: a noninvasive intracranial pressure monitor. Pediatrics, 60:721–725, 1977.

94. Schettini, A., McKay, L., Majors, R., Mahig, J., Nevis, A.H.: Experimental approach for monitoring surface brain pressures. J. Neurosurg., 34:38–47, 1971.

95. Shulman, K., Marmarou, A., Weitz, S.: Gradients of brain interstitial fluid pressure in experimental brain infusion and compression. In: Intracranial Pressure II, Lundberg, N., Pontén, U., Brock, M., Eds. Springer-Verlag, Berlin, 1974, pp. 221–223.

96. Sundbarg, G., Nornes, H.: Simultaneous recording of the ventricular fluid pressure and the epidural pressures. Acta Neurol. Scand., 46:634–635, 1970.

97. Symon, L., Pasztor, E., Dorsch, N.W.C., Bran-

ston, N.M.: Physiological responses of local areas of the cerebral circulation in experimental primates determined by the method of hydrogen clearance. Stroke, 4:632–642, 1973.

98. Tabaddor, K., Shulman, K.: Comments following O.R. Hubschmann, "Twist drill craniostomy in the treatment of chronic and subacute subdural hematomas in severely ill and elderly patients." Neurosurgery, 6:233–236, 1980.

99. Turner, J.M., Gibson, R.M., McDowall, D.G., Nahhas, F.: Further experiences with extradural pressure monitoring. In: Intracranial Pressure II, Lundberg, N., Pontén, U., Brock, M., Eds. Springer-Verlag, Berlin, 1974, pp. 397–402.

100. Umlauf, B., Trappe, A.: Kontinuierlicke messung des hirndrucks mit cinem epiduralen druckaufnehmer A. EEG-EMG, 10–20–21, 1979.

101. Vries, J.K., Becker, D.P., Young, H.F.: A subarachnoid screw for monitoring intracranial pressure. Technical note. J. Neurosurg., 39:416–419, 1973.

102. Wald, A., Post, K., Ransohoff, J., Hass, W., Epstein, F.: A new technique for monitoring epidural intracranial pressure. Med. Instrum., 11:352–354, 1977.

103. Watson, B.W., Currie, J.C.M., Riddle, H.C., Meldrum, S.J.: The long term recording of intracranial pressure. Phys. Med. Biol., 19:86–95, 1974.

104. Wealthall, S.R., Smallwood, R.: Methods of measuring intracranial pressure via the fontanelle without puncture. J. Neurol. Neurosurg. Psych., 37:88–96, 1974.

105. White, R.J., Takaoka, Y.: Chronic monitoring of head injury with an implantable ventricular module. J. Trauma, 17:521–525, 1977.

106. Wilkinson, H.A.: The intracranial pressure-monitoring cup catheter. Technical note. Neurosurgery 1:139–141, 1977.

107. Wilkinson, H.A.: Intracranial pressure reserve testing. Initial clinical observations. Arch. Neurol., 35:661–667, 1978.

108. Wilkinson, H.A.: Intracranial pressure reserve testing. Initial clinical observations (abstract). Neurosurgery 2:161, 1978.

109. Wilkinson, H.A., Rosenfeld, S., Denherder, D.: The linearity of the volume/pressure response during intracranial pressure "reserve" testing. J. Neurol. Neurosurg. Psych., 44:23–28, 1981.

110. Wilkinson, H.A., Arredondo, D., Weems, S., Kaner, D.: Intracranial pressure reserve testing. A study in experimental animals. Arch. Neurol., 35:567–576, 1978.

111. Wilkinson, H.A., Schuman, N., Ruggiero, J.: Nonvolumetric methods of detecting impaired intracranial compliance or reactivity. Pulse width and wave form analysis. J. Neurosurg., 50:758–767, 1979.

112. Wilkinson, H.A., Weems, S.: Post-craniotomy intracranial pressure monitoring—two new devices emphasizing safety and ease of operation. 27th ACEMB, October, 1974.

113. Wood, J.H., Poplack, D.G., Flor, W.J., Gunby, E.N., Ommaya, A.K.: Chronic ventricular cerebrospinal fluid sampling, drug injections, and pressure monitoring using subcutaneous reservoirs in monkeys. Neurosurgery 1:132–135, 1977.

114. Yoneda, S., Matsuda, M., Shimizu, Y., Handa, J., Handa, H., Oda, F., Matsuo, K., Taguchi, N.: SFT—a new device for continuous measurements of intracranial pressure. Technical note. Surg. Neurol., 1:13–15, 1973.

115. Zervas, N.T., Cosman, E.R., Cosman, B.J.: A pressure-balance radio-telemetry system for the measurement of intracranial pressure. A preliminary design report. J. Neurosurg., 47:899–911, 1977.

11

Post-traumatic Intracranial Mass Lesions

PAUL R. COOPER

Subdural hematomas (SDH) have generally been divided into the acute variety and those which present in a chronic (or subacute) fashion. SDH, which are clinically manifest within 48–72 hours of injury, are considered to be acute.[78, 119, 124, 166, 181] Although all varieties have in common the presence of blood within the subdural space, they are dissimilar in most other respects—temporal course, signs and symptoms, pathogenesis, epidemiology, treatment, and outcome. It is therefore appropriate that they be discussed separately.

ACUTE SUBDURAL HEMATOMA
Epidemiology

The epidemiology of acute SDH is similar to that of other traumatic intracranial mass lesions. The patients are overwhelmingly male[32, 119, 162, 181] and most are in their middle years (the median age in most series is in the mid-forties).[48, 78, 93, 148] The predominant cause of injury varies from series to series but, for the most part, falls or motor vehicle accidents are the leading cause with lesser numbers of patients injured in sports mishaps, assaults and industrial accidents.[78, 93, 162] The frequency of the various causes of SDH is age-specific—traffic accidents being most common in patients in the first three decades and domestic accidents predominating in patients over the age of 50.

The exact frequency of occurrence of SDH is difficult to determine. Jamieson and Yelland[93] reported that acute SDH occurred in 5% of approximately 11,000 patients admitted with head trauma over an 11-year period. Echlin[43] stated that the incidence of SDH was 1% of all head injuries and 5% of serious injuries. Kennedy and Wortis[97] reported that acute SDH followed 9–13% of all severe head injuries.

Pathogenesis

Although acute SDH may, on occasion, occur without apparent head injury in patients who are receiving anti-coagulants or who have bleeding dyscrasias[67, 172] or as a result of rupture of cerebral aneurysms,[107] head injury is the usual cause.

Following impact injury, the brain is accelerated within the calvarium causing stretching of veins which drain from the surface of the hemisphere into the dural venous sinuses. When these veins which "bridge" the subdural space are sufficiently stretched, they rupture and venous blood escapes into the subdural space.

More commonly, however, following impact injury the brain may be contused as it is propelled over the rough edges of the sphenoid wing or the floor of the frontal fossa. Veins (or less commonly, arteries) on the cortical surface at the site of these contusions may rupture with resultant hemorrhage into the subdural space.[107, 124, 147] At operation it is often difficult to ascertain the etiology of the hemorrhage because active bleeding has ceased and removal of the clot exposes multiple bleeding points.

Frequently the impact that produces acute SDH also causes severe injury to the cerebral parenchyma. This co-existing severe brain injury is uncommon in chronic subdural and extradural hematoma (EDH) and explains, in large part, the superior outcome in these entities when compared to acute SDH. Indeed, in many cases of acute SDH, it is likely that the extra-axial collection is relatively unimportant in determining outcome.

Jamieson and Yelland[93] classified SDH into sub-groups based on the presence of associated brain injury. "Simple SDH" are those extra-axial collections not associated with any brain injury. "Complicated SDH" includes those cases where the extracerebral collection is associated with parenchymal laceration, intracerebral hematomas, or "exploded" temporal lobes. A third group consists of patients with contusions and acute SDH. Less than half of all patients had simple SDH and the mortality for this group in Jamieson and Yelland's series was 22%—a figure not very much higher than that reported in most recent series of patients with EDH. However, in the 40% of patients with complicated hematomas, the mortality was over 50%. For patients with contusions and SDH the mortality was 30%.

These figures would strongly suggest that mortality is influenced at least as much by the parenchymal injury as by the subdural hematoma. Indeed, it is likely that large numbers of patients with acute SDH sustain a diffuse brain injury at the time of impact with parenchymal damage that is not detectable by angiography or even by the CT scan. The mechanism of injury will, to a large extent, determine the location of parenchymal lesions which co-exist with the subdural hematoma.

Almost 70% of intracerebral hematomas, lacerations, and contusions associated with subdural hematoma result from contrecoup trauma.[93] As such, the majority are located in the temporal and frontal lobes. Although not all these lesions need operative treatment at the time of the evacuation of the SDH, 15–30% of patients with acute SDH will have intracerebral hematomas

that are large enough to require removal.[48, 78, 93] Between 7 and 15% will also have a co-existent EDH. The frequency with which these associated lesions are found is clearly a function of the type of pre-operative diagnostic study that is performed. Where pre-operative diagnostic studies were limited, for the most part, to skull films, less than 2% of patients were found to have co-existent EDH. Our own experience has been that the overwhelming majority of patients evaluated with the CT scan for acute SDH have associated intra- and extra-axial lesions—many of which would not be identified by other diagnostic techniques.

Clinical Course; Signs and Symptoms

The clinical course is determined by two factors: the severity of the injury sustained by the brain at the time of impact and the rapidity of the growth of the SDH. Patients with the most severe injuries may sustain diffuse irreversible brain damage which renders them immediately unconscious with brainstem signs.

Patients with less severe injury will regain consciousness in varying degrees, depending on the force of the initial impact. Their subsequent course will be determined by the rapidity with which an SDH accumulates and is treated. Those patients who sustain the least severe impact are not rendered unconscious at the time of their injury. SDH (or other enlarging mass lesion) should be suspected when the level of consciousness diminishes in the post-traumatic period. The relative frequency of the various clinical courses is seen in Table 11.1.

Clinical signs result from both the primary brain injury and external pressure on the brain from the SDH. The frequency of clinical findings noted by a number of authors has been compiled in Table 11.2. Anisocoria and motor deficit are the commonest clinical signs associated with SDH. Although these signs will not allow the clinician to distinguish SDH from other post-traumatic mass lesions, their presence may be an important clue as to the side of the lesion. Post-traumatic mass lesions will usually be located ipsilateral to the side of pupillary dilatation and contralateral to the side of motor deficit. Unfortunately, pupillary and motor signs are not consistently reliable indicators of the side of the hematoma. Motor signs may be falsely localizing because of multiple parenchymal injuries

unrelated to the side of the SDH or because of compression of the contralateral cerebral peduncle against the tentorial edge.[98] Direct trauma to the third nerve or midbrain at the time of impact may result in (falsely localizing) pupillary dilatation contralateral to the side of the hematoma.[22] For the most part, however, pupillary dilatation is a more reliable localizing sign than the motor deficit. The frequency with which falsely localizing motor and pupillary signs occur is seen in Table 11.3.

Diagnosis; Misdiagnosis

The diagnosis of acute SDH ought not to be difficult. External evidence of trauma or a history of a head injury is generally present. These findings, in the presence of a depressed or declining level of consciousness, should suggest an intracranial injury. Diagnosis may be a particular problem in

Table 11.1

Clinical Course of Patients with Acute Subdural Hematoma[a]

	% Patients with Finding
Unconscious throughout	17
Unconscious to lucid	12
Unconscious to lucid to unconscious	13
Conscious throughout	29
Lucid to unconscious	17

[a] (From data compiled by Jamieson, K.G., Yelland, J.D.N.: Surgically treated traumatic subdural hematomas. J. Neurosurg., 37:137–149, 1972.)

Table 11.2

Frequency of Clinical Findings in Acute Subdural Hematoma

	Jamieson and Yelland[93]	Browder[17a]	Laudig et al.[107]	Kennedy and Wortis[97]	McKissock et al.[119]	McLaurin and Tutor[124]
Anisocoria	28[b]	46	41		57	57
Papilledema			35	37	1	
Cranial nerve VI palsy				3		
Hemiparesis	40	55	43	68	44	44
Decerebration	16					7
Hypertension and/or bradycardia	21					
Aphasia	8			14	6	
Seizures	11		7		6	18

[a] Mixed series of acute and chronic SDH.
[b] Numbers represent percentage of patients with finding.

Table 11.3

Frequency of Falsely Localizing Signs in Acute Subdural Hematoma

	McLaurin and Tutor[124]	McKissock et al.[119]	Pevehouse et al.[152]	Talalla and Morin[181]	Mitsumoto et al.[136]	Browder[17]	Feldman et al.[47]
Pupillary dilatation contralateral to SDH	17[a]	11	9	22	19	29	44
Motor deficit ipsilateral to SDH	15	29		39		39	

[a] Figures represent percentage of patients with finding.

patients found unconscious or apparently intoxicated with no available history and without external evidence of head injury. It has been reported that as many as one-fifth of patients with subdural hematoma and other acute traumatic intracranial hematomas may die undiagnosed.[57] In 40% of patients, the initial diagnosis on admission did not include intracranial mass lesions.[47] In the overwhelming majority of patients

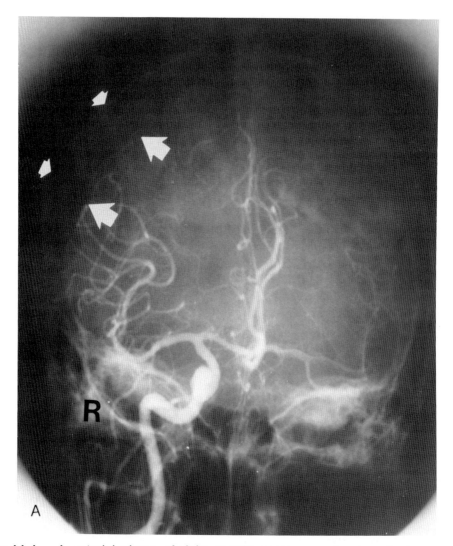

Figure 11.1.   *A*, arterial phase of right carotid angiogram showing displacement of middle cerebral artery branches (*large arrows*) away from the inner table (*small arrows*) by an acute subdural hematoma. The anterior cerebral arteries are shifted from right to left. *B*, venous phase of same angiogram as seen in *A*. *Arrows* delineate inner table of skull.

the sole cause of obtundation was mistakenly ascribed to acute alcoholism or to a cerebrovascular accident.[47, 57] Indeed, as many as one-third of patients with SDH may have acute alcoholism.[47]

The presence of focal neurological deficit or increasing obtundation should always suggest the presence of a traumatic intracranial mass lesion. Galbraith[57] states that in patients with blood alcohol levels of 200 mg% or less, coma is probably not due solely to alcoholism. In patients with suspected anterior circulation cerebrovascular occlusion, the resulting motor deficit may be profound but coma is rare in the period shortly after the accident. Massive hemispheric infarction may lead to obtundation and coma but this usually does not occur for several days.

The history and the initial clinical examination cannot, however, distinguish among the various types of intracranial masses. Moreover, in a patient who is unconscious when first examined, it may not be possible to distinguish between a mass lesion and diffuse brain injury. When a history of lucidity at some point after injury is available and the patient subsequently becomes unconscious, an expanding intracranial mass is the most likely diagnosis. In sum, the patient's clinical course and findings on examination can suggest the presence of a mass lesion. The confident diagnosis of the particular type of mass lesion depends on the specialized radiographic examinations discussed below.

Skull X-rays. Although skull X-rays are usually obtained in patients with head injury and a depressed level of consciousness, the usefulness of these studies in patients with suspected intracranial masses is questionable.[124] There is no consistent relation-

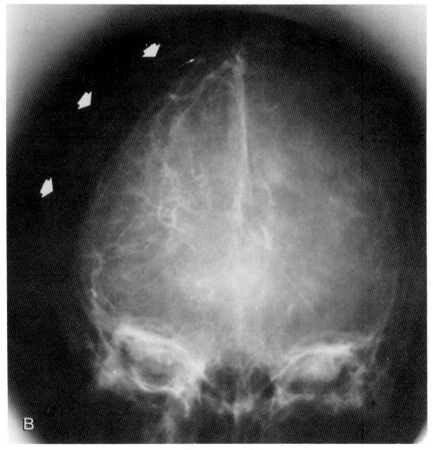

Figure 11.1 *B*

ship between skull fracture and the presence of an SDH—a fracture being visualized between 18 and 60% of the time.[47, 97, 107, 119, 124, 162] A fracture, when present, is as often as not contralateral to the side of the hematoma.[15, 97, 124] In the rapidly deteriorating patient without focal signs, skull X-rays in the frontal projection may be obtained to assess a pineal shift. Unfortunately, emergency skull films show a pineal shift less than 20% of the time in patients with acute SDH.[47, 97, 119, 124]

In summary, skull films have little to add to the diagnostic management of the patient with suspected SDH or other intracranial mass. They may, on occasion, show a pineal shift and may be helpful for delineating a depressed or basal skull fracture. In most circumstances they should not be done and the patient should be taken immediately for a CT scan or cerebral angiography.

Cerebral Angiography; CT Scanning. Until the advent of the CT scanner, cerebral angiography represented the diagnostic procedure of choice for delineation

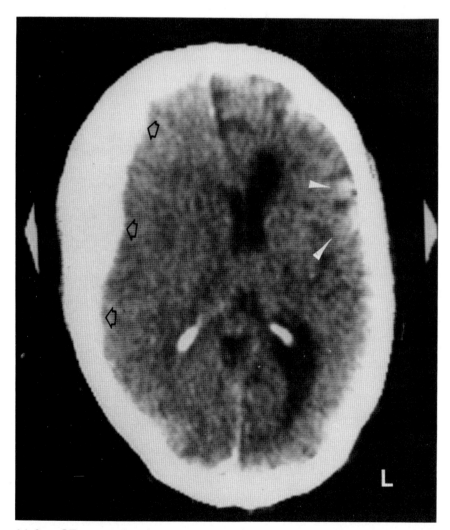

Figure 11.2. CT scan showing acute right subdural hematoma (*black arrows*) with compression and right to left shift of right lateral ventricle. *Arrowheads* identify left-sided cerebral contusion.

of acute SDH (Fig. 11.1). For the most part, angiography is quite adequate to delineate acute SDH. It is occasionally misleading[25]; and hematomas at the frontal or occipital poles may be missed unless appropriate oblique views are obtained.

The CT scan is now the diagnostic modality of choice when a post-traumatic mass lesion is suspected because it is rapid, visualizes the entire brain, and accurately distinguishes the extent and nature of intra- and extra-axial lesions (Fig. 11.2).

Lumbar Puncture. Lumbar puncture has no place in the diagnosis of acute SDH. The reasons are identical to that given in the subsequent section on EDH.

Treatment

In the pre-operative period, while diagnostic studies are being performed and the patient is being readied for operation, attention is directed toward lowering of intracranial pressure by medical means as outlined in Chapter 9.

In general, very thin subdural hematomas (less than 3 mm thick) usually do not require removal. Comatose patients with small hematomas most probably owe their obtundation to parenchymal injury. Adult patients who present flaccid, apneic, and without brain stem reflexes and who do not respond to initial resuscitative measures designed to lower ICP, with an improvement in their neurological status, will almost certainly have an unsatisfactory outcome and should not be considered operative candidates. In all other patients, however, operative evacuation remains the definitive treatment for acute SDH.

Operative treatment is directed toward evacuation of the entire SDH, control of the source of hemorrhage and evacuation of contused, non-viable brain and/or confluent intraparenchymal hemorrhage.

Trephines or burr holes have been advocated for the evacuation of acute SDH on the grounds that 1) the procedure may be performed rapidly and under local anesthesia, 2) that trephination is adequate for hematoma removal and may be enlarged to a craniotomy if necessary, and 3) that there is no difference in mortality when compared to more extensive proce-

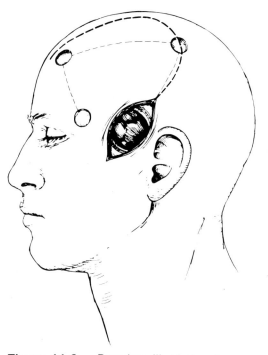

Figure 11.3. Drawing illustrates how a small subtemporal burr hole or craniectomy is converted to a large craniotomy to facilitate complete hematoma evacuation. (Reprinted with permission from Fell, D.A., *et al.*: Acute subdural hematomas. Review of 144 cases. J. Neurosurg., 42:37–42, 1975.)

dures.[42, 97, 166] In the patient who is deteriorating rapidly with clear-cut clinical signs indicating the side of the hematoma (and in whom angiography or CT scan cannot safely be performed) burr holes may be an appropriate diagnostic modality. However, once the hematoma is identified, burr holes are almost always inadequate for total evacuation and control of hemorrhage and the burr holes should be converted to a craniotomy (Fig. 11.3). Jamieson and Yelland[93] noted that satisfactory hematoma evacuation via burr holes could be accomplished in only 14 of 222 operations performed for SDH within the first 24 hours after injury. The inadequacy of burr hole evacuation is not surprising as the hematoma is usually solid and tenacious and ranges in volume up to 350 or 400 cc. Over one-fifth of patients have hematomas which exceed 200 cc in size.[107, 162]

Most authors prefer a large craniotomy.[15, 25, 48, 162] The size and location of the flap are determined by the extent of the hematoma and site of the parenchymal injury. The first burr hole is made over the area of maximal hematoma accumulation and the dura is opened and as much hematoma is aspirated as is possible. This maneuver results in an immediate decrease in an elevated ICP. The remainder of the burr holes are made and a free bone flap is removed. The dura is widely opened and the remaining hematoma is removed from the surface of the brain. A catheter is passed into the subdural space in all directions and any additional hematoma is irrigated. Contused brain and intracerebral hematomas are resected. A drain is generally left in the subdural space, the dura is tightly closed and the remainder of the wound is closed in routine fashion.

In an attempt to improve outcome from acute SDH, Ransohoff et al.[159] recommended that a large decompressive craniectomy be performed to facilitate complete clot removal, hemostasis, and external decompression of the swollen brain in the post-operative period. Post-operative angiographic examination of patients who underwent this procedure showed that the incidence of residual and recurrent post-operative hematoma was minimal and that midline structures returned to their normal anatomical position faster than in patients who did not have this operation.[137] Others[173] have also advocated this procedure and have claimed that ICP is decreased and that intracranial elastance is beneficially affected. None, however, has shown a convincing improvement in outcome. Indeed, a subsequent study by Ransohoff's group showed only 10% survival in patients who had massive surgical decompression.[32] The reasons for the failure of large, external decompression to improve outcome probably relates to the diffuse parenchymal injury sustained at the time of impact and the inability of decompression to reverse this injury. Experimental evidence also shows that large decompressions may actually increase edema.[30] It is possible that

enhanced swelling contributes to strangulation of cortical veins at the edge of the craniectomy and results in venous infarction.

Complications of Treatment. Dangerous elevations of ICP from cerebral swelling in the post-operative period may occur in one-half of all patients,[135] and must be anticipated and treated according to the principles outlined in Chapter 9. Recurrent (or residual) hematoma is not an infrequent complication[82, 162] and one that may be easily and non-invasively identified by the *routine* use of CT scanning in the post-operative period. Similarly, delayed intracerebral hemorrhage may occur following hematoma evacuation.[119] Recent CT studies have shown that this complication is more frequent than had heretofore been thought.[31]

Late post-operative seizures will occur in over one-third of all patients.[95] This high incidence mandates that all patients be started on anti-convulsant prophylaxis in the pre-operative period. Infectious and systemic complications are discussed in Chapters 17 and 18.

Outcome

Outcome from acute SDH has been very poor. There is no large series where the mortality is less than 35% and 13 of the 15 series listed in Table 11.4 show a mortality of 50% or more. Moreover, when the quality of survival is examined, a large proportion of survivors are disabled. Nevertheless, there are subgroups of patients who do considerably better or worse than overall outcome figures for any one series indicate. The factors which influence mortality are examined in the remainder of this section (see also Chapter 20).

Outcome and Age. Younger patients have a generally better outcome from acute SDH than older ones. Richards and Hoff[62] reported that the average age of survivors was 36 as compared to 51 for non-survivors. The age at which the reported mortality rate increases varies. McKissock et al.[119] noted a mortality of less than 20% for patients under 40 years and 65% for those over that age. Jamieson and Yelland[93] found an essentially constant mortality until the age of 70 at which point it increased

Table 11.4
Outcome from Acute Subdural Hepatoma

	McKissock et al.[152]	Hoff et al.[82]	Rosenørn and Gjerris[166]	Cooper et al.[32]	Laudig et al.[107]	Ransohoff et al.[159]	Hernes-niemi[78]	Becker et al.[10]	Fell et al.[48]	Talalla and Morin[181]
Dead	54[a]	55	73	90	83	60	70	42	50	68
Good recovery				4		20	7	23		
Moderately disabled						8	12.5	27		
Severely disabled						6	9.5	4		
Vegetative				6		6	1	4		

[a] Figures represent percentage of patients with finding.

from 30 or 35% to over 50%. Hernesniemi[78] found that mortality increased after 60 and Tallala and Morin[181] after age 50. When Fell et al.[38] compared outcome in patients under 40 and those over 40, they found a very similar mortality (42 vs. 49%). Outcome differed significantly only when patients under 10 years and those over 60 were compared (a mortality of 33 vs. 69%).

Outcome and Clinical Examination. The level of consciousness at the time of operation is the single most important determinant of outcome. Jamieson and Yelland[93] reported that patients who were conscious at the time of operation had a mortality of 9%, whereas those who were unconscious had a mortality of 40–65%. Similar findings have been noted by others.[78, 119, 166, 181] On the other hand, Richards and Hoff[162] could find no relationship between the level of consciousness and outcome. Pupillary abnormalities are associated with a higher mortality,[124, 162, 166] the difference being most pronounced when patients with bilaterally fixed dilated pupils are compared to those who do not have this finding. The influence of motor deficit on survival has not been extensively commented on but does not appear to affect survival.[124, 162]

Outcome and Operative Findings. Although Richards and Hoff[162] found that larger hematomas are associated with a higher mortality than smaller ones, other authors[107, 181] have found no consistent relationship between outcome and hematoma size. There does, however, seem to be a statistically significant decrease in survival when patients have bilateral hematomas.[162] As discussed in the section on pathogenesis, the severity of the associated brain injury seems to be more important in determining outcome than the size of the extra-axial hematoma.

CHRONIC SUBDURAL HEMATOMA

The term chronic SDH applies to those hematomas which present over 20 days following injury. Hematomas are considered "subacute" when symptoms develop between 3 and 20 days following trauma[119, 166] (Fig. 11.4). Those subacute hematomas presenting 3–4 days following injury have much in common with acute SDH and those presenting in the third week are, in their manner of presentation, little different from chronic SDH. For this reason subacute SDH will not be discussed separately.

Epidemiology

It has been estimated that the incidence of chronic SDH is 1–2/100,000/year.[51, 107, 191] The overwhelming majority of patients are elderly or in late middle age. Svien and Gellety[177] reported that over three-quarters were over 50 years of age with an average age of 63. Cameron[23] reported an average age of 56. The median age in other series has also been the late fifties or early sixties.[51, 116, 119] The age-specific incidence increases sharply with advancing age and is 7.4/100,000/year for a population in their

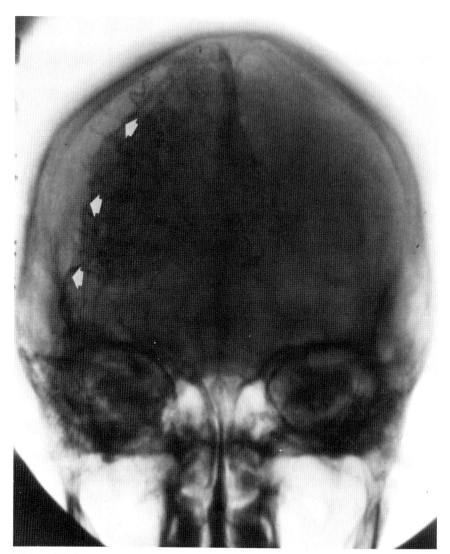

Figure 11.4.   Right carotid angiogram showing subacute subdural hematoma (*arrows*). The shape of the hematoma is midway between the lentiform shape of the chronic subdural hematoma and the appearance of an acute subdural hematoma (see Fig. 11.1).

seventies, whereas the incidence is only 0.13/100,000/year for those in the third decade of life.

Between 25 and 48% of patients have no history of head injury.[51, 116, 119, 177] Even when remembered, the injury is often mild.[119, 177] As many as one-half of all patients[51] are said to have a history of chronic alcoholism and this may account for the failure to obtain a history of head injury. Other precipitating factors are epilepsy, shunting procedures, and anti-coagulation.[116]

Pathogenesis

At the time of trauma, hemorrhage into the subdural space may not produce symptoms. The initial hemorrhage may be quite small and fails to compress the underlying brain. In elderly patients with a decrease in cerebral volume as a result of atrophy, a relatively large initial accumulation of hemorrhage may occur without cerebral compression or clinical symptoms. Regardless of the initial size of the hemorrhage, within 24 hours the hematoma is invaded by fibroblasts from the undersurface of the dura. After one week, these fibroblasts have organized into an outer membrane which is grossly visible. In the third week an inner membrane forms. Thus, the hematoma comes to be encapsulated by a thin inner and a thick outer membrane.[141]

Although there is general agreement regarding the sequence of membrane formation, there has been considerable controversy over the pathogenesis of the subsequent enlargement of the hematoma. In 1932, Gardner[60] postulated that the capsule of a chronic SDH acted as an osmotic membrane and that fluid was drawn into the hematoma from the cerebrospinal fluid. Gardner felt that the progressive decrease in the protein concentration of the subdural fluid occurred as a result of dilution of cerebrospinal fluid (CSF) entering the encapsulated hematoma. He dialyzed a cellophane bag filled with SDH fluid against CSF and found that the volume within the bag increased markedly. However, when he used a SDH capsule as the dialyzing membrane, there was only a minimal increase in

volume. Zollinger and Gross[201] provided an additional explanation for Gardner's hypothesis. In an experimental model, they induced hemolysis of blood in a cellophane membrane and found an increase in osmotic pressure within the sac when compared with non-hemolyzed blood. They felt that hemolysis caused an increase in the number of osmotically active particles in human chronic SDH and accounted for the enlargement of the hematoma. Ingraham[86] also subscribed to this theory.

Recent observations have discredited the osmotic theory of hematoma formation. Gitlin[61] found that the albumin/gamma globulin and albumin/total protein ratios were higher in subdural fluid than in serum samples suggesting that effusion of albumin must be taking place through the walls of capillaries of the hematoma membrane. Because albumin is not found within red blood cells, an increase in concentration of this substance cannot be attributed to red blood cell lysis. Weir[66] measured the osmolality of chronic SDH of varying ages. He could find no change in osmolality with increasing age of the hematoma and no significant difference in osmolality when blood and hematoma were compared. Rabe et al.[156] found that I^{131}-tagged albumin given intravenously rapidly appeared within SDH fluid. This supports Gitlin's concept[61] of effusion through the capillary walls. Sato and Suzuki[168] presented ultrastructural morphologic evidence that the capillary endothelial cells of the chronic SDH capsule had cytoplasmic protrusions and fenestrations which are known to be associated with high permeability and which could permit passage of protein moieties into the hematoma. In an experimental study, Glover and Labadie[64] proposed that corticosteroids inhibited formation of this protein-permeable membrane and thus decreased the size of the hematoma.

However, effusion of protein is not the only mechanism for enlargement of chronic SDH. It is likely that hematoma enlargement may occur by recurrent hemorrhage into the hematoma capsule. Clinically during evacuation of chronic SDH it is not uncommon to see hematomas of varying age and consistency co-existing within the capsule suggesting that recurrent hemorrhage has occurred. Ito *et al.*[87] proposed that there were fibronolytic enzymes in the hematoma membrane which enhanced the chances of recurrent hemorrhage into the cavity. In a series of patients with chronic SDH who were given ^{51}Cr-labeled red cells prior to hematoma evacuation, the appearance of tagged red cells confirmed recent hemorrhage into the hematoma. In fact, mean daily hemorrhage into the hematoma in 18 patients studied amounted to over 10% of the hematoma volume.

Thus, escape of protein through leaky vessels and recurrent hemorrhage (and not osmotic effect) probably account for hematoma enlargement. Why some hematomas enlarge and others resolve is not clear. It is possible that at some point a critical size of the hematoma is reached at which re-absorptive processes are overwhelmed by the fresh hemorrhage and protein exudation. This may explain why twist-drill aspiration and subtotal removal of a large hematoma will lead to recovery and ultimate resorption of the hematoma in most patients.

Signs and Symptoms

The diagnosis of chronic SDH is often not considered and therefore overlooked. The head injury is often minor or has taken place many weeks or even months before. The patient or his family may not remember it and the clinician may not suspect the diagnosis or try to elicit a history of head injury. Because the signs and symptoms are often insidious in onset in patients who are in their sixth to eighth decade, it is not surprising that chronic SDH is frequently misdiagnosed as dementia. Trotter[186] noted that "a slight degree of sleepiness, a loss of initiative, absentmindedness and forgetfulness are the symptoms most commonly noted . . . The whole picture suggests a very slight reduction of functional capacity of a large area of the cerebral cortex."

What makes the diagnosis even more complex is the fact that there are multiple patterns of presentation[7]: 1) The pseudotumoral form—which is characterized by a slow progression of focal neurological signs;

2) a course characterized by symptoms of increased ICP with headache and vomiting but without focal neurological signs; 3) mental disturbance consisting of dementia or inappropriate behavior; 4) a meningeal syndrome with neck stiffness and photophobia but without focal signs; 5) a picture mimicking generalized cerebral atherosclerosis with headaches, apathy, amnesia and gait disturbance; 6) a course mimicking cerebrovascular accident with a sudden onset of focal neurological deficit; 7) a syndrome similar to that of cerebral circulatory insufficiency or symptoms consistent with transient ischemic attacks with focal motor or sensory disturbances with a fluctuating course sometimes with total clearing of the symptoms; 8) seizures without other neurological signs or symptoms. Other authors have also emphasized the variable presentation of patients with chronic SDH.[23, 40, 116, 130, 160]

In most series, less than half of all patients present with impaired consciousness.[96, 143, 154] The frequency with which various signs have been elicited is seen in Table 11.5. The *symptoms* reflect the patient's perception of some of the clinical signs listed in Table 11.5. Headache is a cardinal symptom and is frequently found in patients without other signs or symptoms of elevated ICP. Other common symptoms include confusion, mental changes, nausea, vomiting and seizures.

Because the signs and symptoms of chronic SDH are non-specific and a history of head injury may not be obtained, the admission diagnosis is in error as often as 40% of the time.[160] In over one-third of all patients with chronic SDH, the diagnosis is not made until autopsy is performed.[40, 51] Common misdiagnoses include stroke or transient ischemic attacks, brain tumor, senile dementia and encephalitis.[40, 47, 51, 130, 150, 154]

Specialized Diagnostic Examinations

Skull X-rays. Skull radiographs are of little use in making the diagnosis of chronic subdural hematoma. A fracture is found less than 10% of the time.[23, 40, 116, 119] Other non-specific abnormalities include erosion

Table 11.5
Frequency of Various Clinical Signs in Patients with Chronic Subdural Hematoma

	Luxon and Harrison	Feldman et al.[47]	Dronfield et al.[40]	McKissock[119]	Kaste et al.[96]	Pevehouse et al.[152]
Hemiparesis	58[b]	40	62	41	24	
Papilledema	34		14	22	41	22
Dysphasia	20	10		11		
Meningismus	14					
Hemianopia	11		10	3		3
Sensory changes	9					
Cranial nerve III abnormality	10	10	10			15
Impaired consciousness		50	100	59	28	
Personality change		30				
Ataxia		10				
Dementia				27	38	

[a] Patients all over age 50.
[b] Figures represent percentage of patients in each series with finding.

of the sella turcica or shift of the calcified pineal gland. In at least one-half of all patients no abnormalities are found. No single finding on skull roentgenography is diagnostic of a chronic SDH and additional examinations are always indicated.

Isotope Brain Scans. The diagnosis of chronic SDH by radioisotope brain scan is dependent on the uptake of the isotope by the membranes of the chronic SDH.[129] Chronic SDH of more recent origin without well-developed membranes will therefore be less likely to result in a positive scan. Cowan et al.[35] were able to detect only 50% of hematomas less than 10 days from the time of injury, whereas the scan was positive in 91% of lesions of greater duration. The overall accuracy of the brain scan in detecting chronic SDH has been reported to range from 50–100%.[23, 40, 85, 114, 160] A false-negative scan will result when bilateral hematomas cause symmetrical peripheral uptake of isotope. A false positive scan may occur in the presence of scalp trauma, previous craniotomy, infection, or peripherally located metastatic tumors. The isotope scan may remain positive even after most of the hematoma has been resorbed in patients who did not receive operation. Although isotope scans can identify chronic SDH its use has been superceded by cerebral angiography and the CT scan both of which are more accurate.

Echoencephalography. Before the advent of the CT scan, echoencephalography was frequently used as a screening procedure for the evaluation of chronic SDH or acute traumatic lesions that might produce a midline shift. The accuracy of this procedure in detecting a shift of midline structures has been reported to range between 44 and 57%.[85, 116] Because it is so unreliable, it is now little used and has been replaced by more definitive studies such as CT or angiography.

Electroencephalography (EEG). The EEG is usually abnormal in patients with chronic SDH. Dysfunction may be diffuse or unilateral and manifest by voltage suppression, delta activity, or depression of alpha rhythm.[47, 114, 116] These findings are non-specific and cannot reliably be used to diagnose a chronic SDH. Moreover, a normal EEG does not rule out a mass lesion.

Lumbar Puncture. The results of CSF examination in patients with chronic SDH are variable. The fluid is xanthochromic or blood-stained in only a minority of cases. The protein content is usually normal. The lumbar puncture pressure is elevated in less than half of all cases.[23, 40, 116, 119, 154, 164] Therefore, normal findings on lumbar puncture cannot be accepted as evidence that a chronic SDH is absent. Even if there is xanthochromia or elevations of protein content or CSF pressure, the findings are not specific for a chronic SDH. Although deterioration following lumbar puncture was not observed in one large series,[23] most authors stress the dangers inherent in performing this procedure in the presence of a mass lesion.[119, 154, 165]

Cerebral Angiography. Before the advent of the CT scan, cerebral angiography was the diagnostic procedure of choice for detecting chronic SDH. It is accurate in 99% of patients studied.[23] The hematoma appears as an avascular area between the cortical surface and the inner table of the skull in the frontal projection. With increasing age the hematoma assumes more of a lenticular pattern on this view (Fig. 11.5). On the lateral projection there is usually distortion of the vessels of the sylvian triangle.

Most authors report that between 15 and 20% of hematomas are bilateral, although in some series bilateral hematomas are said to occur up to 50% of the time.[47, 116, 119, 164, 177] The signs and symptoms are not dissimilar

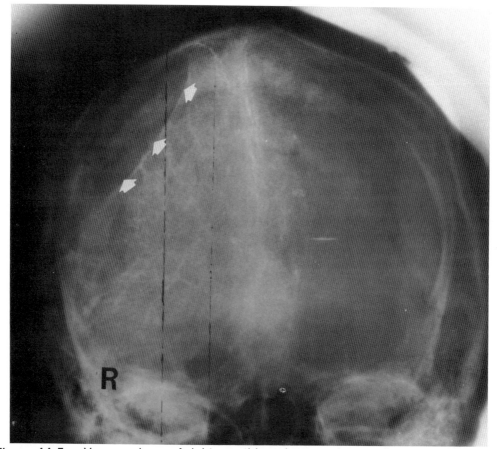

Figure 11.5. Venous phase of right carotid angiogram. *Arrows* show cortical vessels which have been displaced from the inner table of the skull. Lenticular shaped avascular area is typical of a chronic subdural hematoma.

from unilateral hematoma and the diagnosis cannot be made on clinical grounds alone.[96] Therefore, bilateral carotid angiography should always be performed. When angiography is carried out via the transfemoral route it is generally easy to catheterize the contralateral carotid artery. When angiography is performed by direct carotid puncture, compression of the opposite carotid artery during injection of contrast material will often result in visualization of both the ipsilateral and contralateral intracranial vessels and facilitate diagnosis of bilateral hematomas. If visualization of both the left and right sided circulations cannot be achieved because of technical factors or time constraints, exploratory burr holes should be placed on the opposite side of the skull at the time of operation. Bilateral visualization of cere-

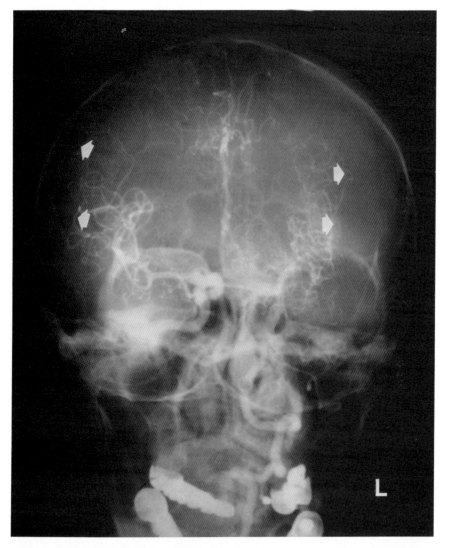

Figure 11.6. Cerebral angiogram with bilateral filling of anterior cerebral circulation. *Arrows* show bilateral displacement of cerebral vessels away from the inner table as a result of bilateral subdural hematoma. Note absence of shift of anterior cerebral artery as a result of these counterbalancing hematomas.

bral vessels is particularly important where the patient's signs and symptoms are not appropriate to the side of the hematoma or the size of the shift is not proportional to the size of the hematoma (Fig. 11.6). Unilateral operation in the presence of bilateral hematoma has been suspected of enhancing brain stem distortion and hastening an unsatisfactory outcome.[96]

CT Scan. The CT scan is now the preferred method for the evaluation of patients with suspected chronic SDH because it is rapid, accurate, non-invasive, and permits the evaluation of all intracranial structures in a single study. In the first week following injury, all hematomas are hyperdense compared to brain. In the second and third weeks the majority are isodense and a few are hypo- or hyperdense (Fig. 11.7). After the third week, however, over three-quarters are hypodense.[171] With increasing time the hematoma assumes a lenticular pattern like that seen on angiography,[72] although Radcliffe[157] feels that the shape of the hematoma is more a function of the age of the patient than the age of the hematoma. The

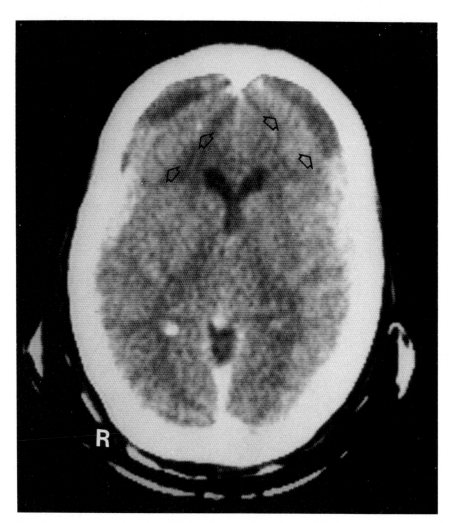

Figure 11.7.   CT scan showing bilateral chronic subdural hematomas two weeks after trauma. *Arrows* delineate cortical surface. Note that there is layering in the hematoma with both hyperdense and hypodense material.

diagnosis of chronic SDH by CT scan is usually not difficult. The typical CT appearance is seen in Figure 11.8.

Misdiagnosis is most likely to occur when the hematoma visualized on the CT scan is isodense in relation to the brain (Fig. 11.9). Although a hematoma may not be visualized, a shift or compression of the cerebral ventricles or obliteration and shift of the cortical sulci should alert the clinician or radiologist to the possibility of an occult isodense hematoma. When bilateral isodense hematomas are present, a midline shift may be minimal or absent and ventricular compression will be symmetrical.[69, 120] If an isodense SDH is suspected, the intravenous injection of contrast material (300 cc of 30% diatrizoate meglumine over 15–30 minutes) will permit enhancement of the inner membrane of the subdural hematoma, cerebral cortex, and cortical vessels[75, 126, 181] (Fig. 11.10) (see also Chapter 4).

Treatment

The treatment of chronic SDH has been a subject of controversy. Although patients

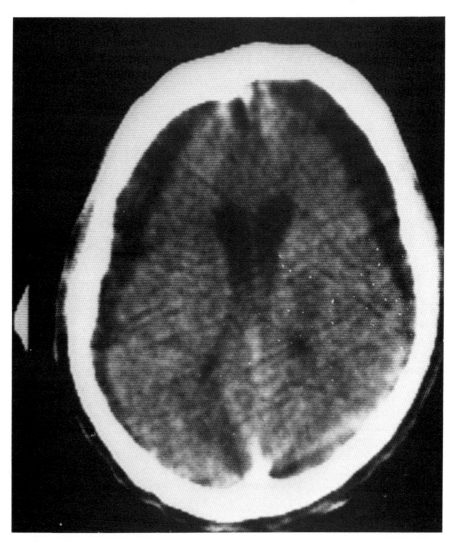

Figure 11.8.   CT scan of a patient with bilateral chronic subdural hematomas. Although there is no midline shift, the hypodense appearance of these hematomas is characteristic.

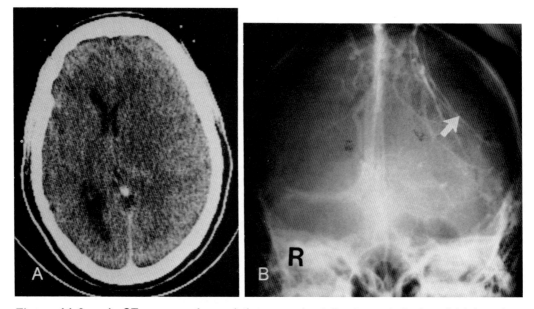

Figure 11.9. *A,* CT scan performed three weeks following relatively mild injury in a patient with signs and symptoms of increased ICP. There is a left-to-right shift of the lateral ventricles but no definite subdural hematoma is seen. *B,* left carotid angiogram of patient whose CT scan is seen in Figure 9A. *Arrow* marks displacement of cortical veins from inner table typical of a chronic subdural hematoma.

have been managed successfully without operative therapy using regimens of diuretics, bed rest, or corticosteroids, the prevailing neurosurgical opinion is that symptomatic patients are best managed with operation. However, there is no unanimity on the choice of procedure and a number of operations have been proposed: craniotomy (with or without excision of membranes), burr holes, or twist-drill evacuation of the hematoma.

Non-operative Treatment. It is likely that some patients with chronic SDH remain asymptomatic and have spontaneous regression of their lesions. The finding of thick membranes of a resorbed chronic SDH at post-mortem examination of patients dying of other causes would support this concept. Gannon *et al.*[59] reported resolution of chronic SDH in four patients who received no treatment.

Ambrosetto[3] and Bender and Christoff[12] proposed that in selected patients spontaneous (or medically assisted) resolution of chronic SDH might take place and that

non-operative therapy might be preferable to surgical treatment. Treatment consisted of bed rest alone or in combination with corticosteroids. In a few patients, this treatment was combined with mannitol. For the most part the patients chosen for medical treatment were neurologically intact or had mild depression of their level of consciousness. The more depressed the patient's level of consciousness, the more likely it was that operative treatment was the primary treatment modality. Of 97 patients selected for medical treatment, 22 eventually needed operation. The average duration of treatment was three weeks. More recently, Suzuki and Takaku[76] reported success in 22 of 23 patients treated with mannitol. The mean treatment length was 41 days and the total dose of mannitol averaged 30 liters. On the other hand, Gjerris and Schmidt[62] reported failure in all seven patients with chronic SDH in whom mannitol treatment was tried.

In carefully selected patients, a combination of diuretic therapy and corticoste-

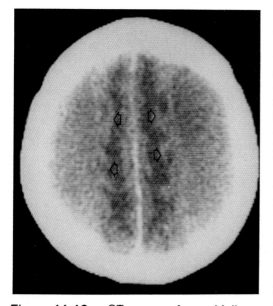

Figure 11.10. CT scan performed following intravenous injection of contrast. Bilateral isodense chronic subdural hematomas are present. The contrast enhanced cortex (*arrows*) is displaced from the inner table by bilateral high vertex chronic subdural hematomas. Lower cuts failed to show ventricular displacement or evidence of hematoma.

roids may result in the resolution of chronic SDH. In certain patients with a small chronic SDH found incidentally, no therapy may be necessary. In the vast majority of patients, however, non-operative treatment offers several disadvantages: the length of hospitalization is prolonged and patients require an extensive course of steroids and/or potent diuretics both of which may be associated with adverse reactions. Most importantly, patients remain at continued and prolonged risk of deterioration from a mass lesion.

Craniotomy. Putnam and Cushing[155] noted that recovery from chronic SDH "followed even the simplest procedure." However, they recommended craniotomy for the access it provided to solid components of the SDH. They also recommended sub-temporal decompression for those cases where postoperative brain edema was expected. Although a craniotomy flap is sometimes needed for adequate evacuation of solid hematoma, the usual chronic SDH is liquefied and easily evacuated through smaller openings. Another reason given for craniotomy is to facilitate the removal of membranes surrounding the subdural hematoma. However, Svien and Gelety[177] could find no difference in outcome when patients with and without membranectomy were compared.

Burr Holes. A burr hole at the site of the angiographically demonstrated maximal thickness of the hematoma has been the commonest mode of treatment for chronic SDH.[23, 119, 164, 177] The procedure may be performed under local anesthesia in cooperative patients. A single burr hole usually provides adequate exposure for removal of the liquid hematoma. If there are solid bits of clot, it is sometimes helpful to place two burr holes to irrigate hematoma out of the subdural space by flushing saline solution in one hole and out the second. A drain is placed in the subdural space and left in place postoperatively for 24 hours for drainage of the residual hematoma. We formerly placed clips on the dura and subjacent inner membrane to follow the progress of re-expansion of the brain on skull roentgenograms. Clips are no longer used as the progress of cerebral re-expansion and the recurrence of hematoma can be followed by the CT scan.

Some authors[23, 106, 184] have emphasized the importance of the failure of the brain to immediately re-expand following evacuation of the hematoma. They believe that this intracranial "hypotension" may produce signs similar to those of *increased* ICP and treat patients whose brains fail to expand with lumbar puncture and intrathecal infusion of saline or Ringer's lactate solution. There is no evidence that "intracranial hypotension" retards recovery from operative evacuation of hematomas. Moreover, there is no evidence whatsoever that lumbar infusion improves the post-operative course of these patients. The course of recovery in the post-operative period is variable and is a function of the patient's pre-operative level of consciousness, neurological deficit, age, and other factors which will be discussed subsequently.

Twist-drill Craniostomy. Because most chronic subdural hematomas are composed of homogeneous liquefied material they may be evacuated by a needle or twist drill craniostomy as described by Negron *et al.*,[145] Burton,[21] and most recently by Tabbador and Shulman[180] (Fig. 11.11). The advantage of this procedure is that it can be rapidly performed at the bedside using local anesthesia and involves minimal operative trauma. A 1 cm incision is made in the scalp at the site of maximum thickness of the hematoma as determined angiographically or by CT scan. A hole is made with a twist drill at a 45° angle to the skull. The dura mater and outer membrane are perforated with a #16 needle and a Scott Cannula or small gauge red rubber catheter is passed into the subdural space. The catheter is connected to a sterile, closed collection apparatus (we use a bile bag or empty plasma bag). The bag is initially kept slightly below head level for the first few hours and then placed 8–10 cm below head level so that the fluid siphons off. After 24 hours, the catheter is removed and the patient allowed out of bed. The outcome of patients treated by this technique is superior to that obtained by craniotomy or burr hole. For hypodense hematomas without a solid component, twist drill craniostomy is the treatment of choice. The procedure must only be performed, however, when the clot is liquid and of sufficient thickness to preclude injury to the cortex when the dura is penetrated.

Complications of Operative Treatment for Chronic Subdural hematoma. When a residual collection of hematoma is discovered after operation it is often difficult to ascertain whether there has been incomplete removal or recurrence of the hematoma. Before the widespread use of the CT scan it was common to find a space between the cortical surface and the inner table of the skull when "clip" films or angiography was obtained in the post-operative period. Experience with the CT scan

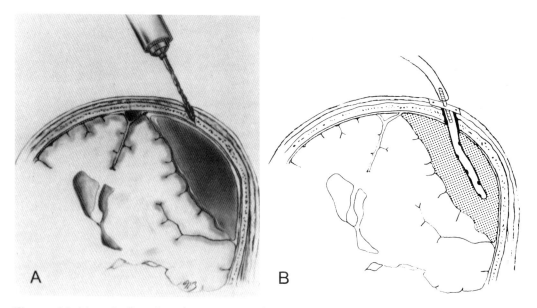

Figure 11.11. *A,* Drawing demonstrates how a twist drill hole is made at an oblique angle to the skull over the site of maximum thickness of a chronic subdural hematoma. *B,* a rubber catheter is passed into the subdural space through the twist drill hole for evacuation of liquefied chronic subdural hematoma. (Reproduced with permission from Tabaddor, K., Shulman, K.: Definitive treatment of chronic subdural hematoma by twist-drill craniostomy and closed-system drainage. J. Neurosurg., 46:220–226, 1977.)

shows that residual collections of subdural hematoma fluid are remarkably common. For the most part, however, evacuation of only a portion of the hematoma will produce amelioration of symptoms and will tip the balance in favor of eventual hematoma resorption.

True re-accumulation of the hematoma has been reported to occur between 8 and 45% of the time.[184] The possibility of re-accumulation should be considered in those patients who deteriorate or who do not improve following operation. A CT scan should be done when recurrence is suspected and, if present, it will show hematoma of mixed or greater density than was seen on the pre-operative scan.

The commonest cause of re-accumulation of a chronic SDH is bleeding from the vascular outer membrane. This is more likely to occur if this membrane is widely incised. Data[177] would indicate that recurrence is almost twice as common (37 vs. 20%) in patients who have craniotomy when compared with patients who have evacuation of the hematoma performed via burr holes. Although we routinely insert subdural drains for 24 hours after operation, it is not clear that this reduces the incidence of recurrent hematoma.

Following rapid evacuation of large chronic subdural hematomas, a small group of patients deteriorate and go on to die. In most, diagnostic studies show a decrease in the size of the shift and no recurrence of the hematoma. The deterioration may occur quite suddenly; McKissock et al.[119] described a patient who had rapid evacuation of 100 ml of fluid under local anesthesia with sudden loss of consciousness and death. Autopsy showed a large brain stem hemorrhage probably induced by rapid evacuation of this large lesion. Slow evacuation of chronic SDH with twist drill craniotomy as described by Tabaddor and Shulman[180] may prevent this occurrence.

Although it is possible that compression of the brain substance by a hematoma may result in brain edema, CT scans in patients with unevacuated chronic SDH usually show surprisingly little edema. In a small group of patients, neurological deterioration with signs of elevated ICP occurred 1 to 3 days following operation.[155] Cerebral swelling may result from rapid relief of brain compression. Treatment with mannitol and steroids may result in clinical improvement.

Infection after chronic SDH is uncommon. Cameron[23] reported only one infection in a review of 114 cases, Svien and Gelety[177] three infections out of 69 cases, and Raskind et al.[160] only two infections in 52 patients. The common infectious complications include subdural empyema, brain abscess, bone flap infection, and meningitis. Patients with infectious complications are treated according to the principles outlined in Chapter 18.

Seizures in the post-operative period occur 11% of the time[23] and all patients should be treated prophylactically with anti-convulsants.

Outcome

The outcome of patients with chronic SDH is variable. The reported mortality ranges from zero[160] to 38%[40]. Most larger series report a mortality rate of about 10% or less.[23, 96, 116, 119] There is little data on morbidity. Luxon and Harrison[116] report a 14% incidence of minor morbidity and a 17% incidence of serious disability. Raskind et al.[160] reported that three-quarters of all patients were returned to normal function.

In most series, outcome is most closely related to the patient's neurological function at the time of operation. In the patients reported by McKissock et al.,[119] a 13% mortality occurred in patients who had operation when stuporous or comatose, whereas only 5% of those who were alert or drowsy went on to die. Cameron, however, states that the patient's neurological status had no bearing on outcome and that 13 of 15 patients in coma at the time of operation in their series made a complete recovery.

There is no consensus on the influence of age on outcome: Munro[139] found no relationship between age and outcome, whereas McKissock et al.[119] found that patients over 50 had a three-fold increase in mortality when compared to those in younger age groups.

The size of the hematoma does not appear to influence outcome.[119] The reported mortality of patients with bilateral hematomas[96] is approximately the same (about 11%) as that reported for unilateral hematoma.

SUBDURAL HYGROMA

Subdural hygromas are collections of clear, xanthochromic, or blood-tinged fluid collections located within the subdural space after head injury. Because many collections are associated with parenchymal injury, they are often composed of a mixture of cerebrospinal fluid and varying amounts of blood.[81] Stone et al.[174] have classified patients with subdural hygromas into two groups: complex hygromas associated with extracerebral hematomas or intraparenchymal injury, and simple hygromas where associated injuries were absent or minor.

Pathogenesis

The pathogenesis of traumatic subdural hygroma has not been established with certainty. In 1924, Noffziger[144] speculated that a tear in the arachnoid allows the escape of cerebrospinal fluid into the subdural space. Others[81, 149, 174] have accepted this as an explanation of hygroma formation. The hygroma enlarges because cerebrospinal fluid becomes trapped in the subdural space as a result of a flap-valve effect.[36] Hoff et al.[81] performed isotope cisternography using RISA on 99 mTc albumin in three patients. In one patient, isotope passed from the lumbar subarachnoid space into the subdural space overlying the hemisphere. A hygroma was found at operation. This would appear to support the hypothesis that the hygroma may result from passage of cerebrospinal fluid into the subdural space.

Stone et al.[174] suggest that hygromas may also originate as a result of effusions into the subdural space from injured capillaries in the underlying brain. The fact that the protein content of the hygroma fluid is frequently higher than could be expected from red blood cell breakdown alone would support this theory.

Although membrane formation surrounding the hygroma has been reported[149] most authors[81, 174] have failed to observe this phenomenon. The presence of a membrane would suggest that the patient has a chronic subdural *hematoma* rather than a subdural hygroma.

Epidemiology

The incidence of subdural hygroma has been reported to represent 7%[149] and 12%[174] of all traumatic intracranial mass lesions. The severity of the head injury as judged by the duration of the loss of consciousness varies widely, and hygromas appear in patients who have never lost consciousness as well as in those with prolonged episodes of coma.[149] The reported age of patients ranges from two months to over 70 years.[81, 149, 174]

Signs and Symptoms

An altered level of consciousness is the commonest sign in patients with hygroma. Symptoms of increased ICP are frequently present as well, and include headache, nausea, and vomiting. Focal motor deficit, and symmetrical or unreactive pupils may be present and seizures have also been reported in one-third of patients.[149, 174]

The temporal course (*i.e.*, the interval from injury to operation) is variable and ranges from less than 24 hours to over 3 weeks.[81, 149, 174] The presence of a complex hygroma with co-existing parenchymal injury or an extraparenchymal hematoma results in the early appearance and rapid progression of symptoms. Patients with simple hygromas generally had operation much later. Their course was characterized by neurological deterioration after a period of improvement or stabilization. A second group of patients never fully recovered following their initial injury.

Diagnosis

The signs and symptoms of patients with subdural hygroma are not pathognomonic and there is no way, on clinical grounds alone, to distinguish subdural hygroma from intracranial hematomas. In particular the signs and symptoms of patients who experience neurologic deterioration weeks after head injury from a hygroma are indistinguishable from chronic subdural hematoma.

The diagnosis of subdural hygroma may be made by cerebral angiography or CT scanning. Angiography characteristically reveals a crescentic extracerebral space which, on A.P. views, is quite similar in appearance to an acute SDH. The midline shift commonly seen with SDH is absent or minimal.

CT scanning is the preferred diagnostic modality if a hygroma is suspected. The hygroma will appear as an extra-axial collection of similar density to cerebrospinal fluid. The collections may be unilateral but are bilateral in over 50% of cases.[174]

Treatment

Patients with asymptomatic subdural hygromas do not need treatment. However, all patients with subdural hygroma who deteriorate in the post-traumatic period or whose neurological status plateaus short of full recovery, should have operation. Midline shift is usually absent even in unilateral hygromas but absence of shift should not be misconstrued to mean that the hygroma is of no clinical significance.

Patients with simple hygroma may be adequately treated with evacuation, *via* burr holes or small trephines. In spite of the absence of midline shift, the fluid is generally under increased pressure. In patients with intracranial hematomas in addition to hygromas, the operation must be adapted so that the hematoma as well as the hygroma may be fully evacuated.

Outcome

Mortality has been reported as 12%[149] and as 25%.[81, 174] Outcome would appear to be most closely related to the associated cerebral injury. Stone et al.[174] reported a mortality of 20% in patients with simple hygroma and 43% for those with complex hygroma. Advanced age also appears to have an adverse effect on outcome with 17 of 19 deaths occurring in patients over the age of 50.

EXTRADURAL HEMATOMA

Epidemiology

Extradural hematoma (EDH) is an infrequent sequel to head trauma. Jamieson and Yelland[92] reported an incidence of only 1.5% in 11,000 patients admitted to hospital with head injury. Galbraith[56] reported a 0.2% incidence, Kvarnes and Trumpy,[104] 1.4%, Phonprasert et al.,[153] 2.8%, Heiskanen, 4.6%[76] and Weinman and Muttucumaru, 6%.[192] The reason for the large variation and the frequency of EDH from one series to another is unclear. The incidence of EDH is greatly influenced by the threshold for admission of patients with relatively minor injuries. Thus, in centers where few minor injuries are admitted, the incidence of EDH will be high.

The type of trauma that causes EDH is diverse but in most series traffic accidents and falls predominate.[58, 76, 83, 92, 153] The age distribution of patients with EDH is similar to that of patients with other traumatic intracranial lesions. However, EDH is unusual in elderly patients and in two large series only 2–4% of the total number of patients with EDH were over the age of 60.[92, 153] This is a lower percentage of elderly patients than that seen in series of SDH, for example, and is probably a result of the increased adherence of the dura to the inner table that occurs with advancing age.[58] In most series, the peak incidence is in the second and third decades.[92, 84, 153] EDH occurs less frequently in the first decade of life and most series report between 5 and 10% of the total patients in this age group.[58, 83, 92, 153] EDH is, however, most unusual in the first two years of life. Hooper[83] reported that only two of 83 patients were in this age group and Phonprasert et al.,[153] none in 138 cases. It has been postulated that EDH in this very young group of patients is infrequent because the dura is stripped from the inner table only with difficulty—a situation analogous to that seen in the elderly.[121]

Pathogenesis

Jamieson and Yelland[92] have emphasized that the acceleration-deceleration stress which plays a large part in producing the brain injury seen following motor vehicle accidents or falls, has nothing to do with the production of EDH. Indeed, an EDH occurs as a result of trauma to the skull and the underlying meningeal vessels and not to brain injury. Impact to the head causes an inward bending of the calvarium resulting in dural detachment from the inner table of the skull, and is essential for the subsequent formation of an EDH.[52] As a result of this inbending and dural detachment, meningeal vessels may be torn (Fig. 11.12). Although a fracture is usually found (at autopsy, operation of or on X-rays), tearing of meningeal vessels and subsequent formation of EDH may occur in the absence of a fracture.[121]

Ford and McLaurin[52] presented experimental evidence showing that a "hydraulic press" effect is created following separation of the dura from the skull. The amount of hydraulic force is the product of the pressure at which blood escapes from a torn vessel and the area of the initial dural separation. If the pocket of dural separation is large enough (6–8 mm in diameter), then the dura can be progressively stripped from the inner table by blood escaping from a torn meningeal artery. As the hematoma accumulates, the hydraulic force increases resulting in further dural stripping and growth of the hematoma. Hematomas of venous origin clearly occur from laceration of middle meningeal veins or dural sinuses (Fig. 11.13). Because venous pressure cannot exert sufficient hydraulic force it is probable that venous bleeding occurs only into a preformed space created by a large area of primary dural separation.[192]

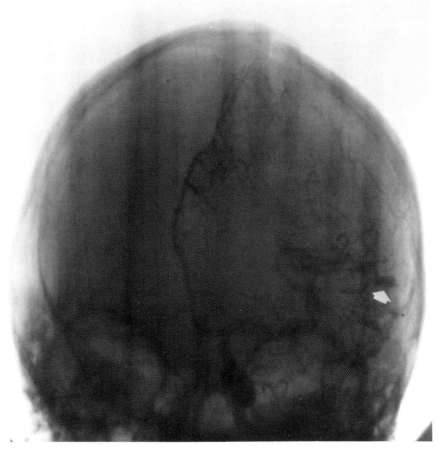

Figure 11.12. Left carotid angiogram showing extravasation of contrast (*arrow*) from middle meningeal artery in patient with an extradural hematoma and large midline shift of anterior cerebral artery.

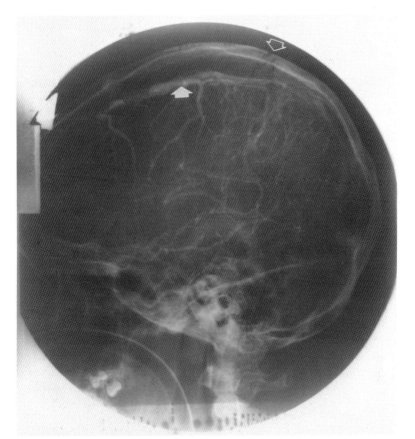

Figure 11.13. Venous phase of carotid angiogram. Sagittal sinus (*solid arrow*) is displaced from inner table of skull by an extradural hematoma. Midline fracture (*open arrow*) resulted in laceration of sagittal sinus with formation of extradural hematoma of venous origin.

Occurrence of Fracture. Under experimental conditions an EDH can form without a skull fracture. In clinical situations, a fracture is usually (but not invariably) present. Treil *et al.*[185] documented traumatic rupture of the midline meningeal artery in 30 patients—20% of whom had no evidence of skull fracture. Gallagher and Browder[58] could not demonstrate skull fracture by skull roentgenography, operation, or autopsy in 9% of 152 patients. Freytag[54] found skull fractures in all but 3% of patients with EDH who came to *postmortem* examination. Munro and Maltby[140] reported a skull fracture in each of 44 patients with EDH. McKenzie[118] reported a skull fracture in 19 of 20 patients with EDH. More recently, Jamieson and Yelland[92] reported the presence of a skull fracture in about two-thirds of their patients, Kvarnes and Trumpy[104] in

72% and Phonprasert *et al.*[153] in 75%. The frequency with which a fracture is associated with EDH is age-related. Children are less likely to have a skull fracture than adults. Mealey[127] reported that 5 of 12 patients below the age of 15 in his series of patients did not have a skull fracture. Galbraith[56] confirmed these findings. Of 46 patients with epidural hematoma without skull fracture, 42 were under the age of 30 and 30 were under the age of 20. Campbell and Cohen[24] attributed the lower incidence to the increased elasticity of the skull in children with a lesser tendency to fracture when deformed.

Although most patients with EDH have a skull fracture and the skull roentgenogram has been used as a screening procedure to identify those patients at risk for developing EDH, patients without roentgenographic evidence of skull fracture clearly develop EDH and the use of this screening procedure as a determinant of hospital admission must be questioned.

Source of Bleeding; Site of Hematoma. Supratentorial EDH may occur from injury to the middle meningeal artery, the middle meningeal veins, diploic veins, or the dural sinuses.[58, 192] Laceration of the carotid artery before it enters the intracranial dura has also been reported to result in EDH.[194] At operation, active bleeding may be seen where the fracture line crosses the middle meningeal artery or veins or venous sinuses. In over one-half of all cases, the middle meningeal artery gives rise to the hematoma. In one-third, the hemorrhage originates from a tear in a meningeal vein. In less than 10%, hemorrhage results from a tear of one of the venous sinuses (Fig. 11.13).[192]

The hematomas are almost always unilateral, although bilateral ones have been reported.[58, 117] The commonest location of EDH is in the temporal region. At least one-half of all hematomas are located here, although extension to the frontal, parietal, or occipital areas is common.[58, 83, 92, 153]

Associated Intracranial Injury. Fifty to sixty-eight percent of patients with EDH have no significant intracranial pathology.[58, 104, 121, 153] In the minority of patients who do have associated injuries, subdural hematoma and cerebral contusion predominate. The presence of these associated lesions has an important influence on outcome and will be discussed in a subsequent section of this chapter.

Clinical Manifestations

Temporal Course. There are five basic variations in the clinical course of patients with EDH: 1) No loss of consciousness at any time; 2) unconscious at all times; 3) initially lucid and subsequently unconscious; 4) initially unconscious and subsequently lucid; and 5) initially unconscious followed by a period of lucidity with subsequent unconsciousness. The relative incidence of each of these clinical courses varies widely when a number of large series are compared (Table 11.6).

In the minds of many physicians (neurosurgical specialists and non-specialists alike), the term "lucid interval" conjures up a picture of a patient with an EDH. The initial transient loss of consciousness results from a concussion after which the patient recovers consciousness and remains alert until an expanding hematoma results in a second period of unconsciousness. The actual sequence of changes in consciousness will vary as a function of the severity of the initial blow and the rapidity of the development of the hematoma.

Although a lucid interval is often a feature of the course in patients with EDH, in most series the lucid interval occurs less frequently than has been generally assumed. Expeditious management of patients whose level of consciousness is deteriorating will decrease the incidence of the lucid interval. Moreover, it must be emphasized that the lucid interval is not pathognomonic for EDH and a secondary loss of consciousness after a period of lucidity may

Table 11.6
Clinical Course of Patients with Extradural Hematoma

	Weinman and Muttucumaru[192]	Heiskanen[76]	Jamieson and Yelland[92]	Kvarnes and Trumpy[104]	Phonprasert et al.[153]
Unconscious-lucid-unconscious	67[a]	32	12	11	37
Unconscious throughout	19	26	23	56	14
Unconscious-lucid		26	20	15	22
Lucid-unconscious			21	18	16
Conscious throughout	9	16	25		11
Unknown	5				

[a] Figures represent percentage of patients in each series with finding.

also occur with other intracranial mass lesions.

The rate of development of signs and symptoms in patients with EDH is variable. About one-third come to operation within 12 hours, 60% within the first 3–4 hours, and between 60 and 75% within 48 hours. The remainder develop signs and symptoms at some later time in the first week or even during the second week following injury.[92, 121, 192] Iwakuma and Brunngraber[89] report operating on a total of 21 chronic extradural hematomas 13 days or longer following trauma. This represents almost one-third of their series of 69 patients. This high incidence of chronic lesions is unusual. Twelve of these 21 patients were alert, and indeed it was not clear why operation was performed. The venous origin of the hemorrhage in these chronic lesions has been noted before.[58]

Clinical Signs. The clinical signs will depend on the amount of time which has elapsed since the injury, the rapidity of hematoma growth, and the presence of concomitant intradural lesions. Pupillary dilatation, hemiparesis, and decerebration are commonly associated with EDH. Although these signs may be helpful in diagnosing the side of the lesion, they are not useful in distinguishing EDH from other traumatically induced mass lesions. The frequency with which these signs have been reported is presented in Table 11.7.

Papilledema has also been reported in patients with EDH[192] but its presence is not important in the diagnosis of this entity. Indeed, in the vast majority of patients, signs and symptoms of elevated ICP develop quickly before papilledema has a chance to appear. When present, a more useful sign of increased ICP is the presence of retinal hemorrhages. Bradycardia has been frequently noted[58, 192] but while it

sometimes occurs with increased ICP its presence is not specific for EDH.

Diagnosis

CT scanning is the preferred diagnostic procedure of choice for patients with suspected EDH and other post-traumatic intracranial masses[53, 200] (Fig. 11.14). If a CT scanner is unavailable, angiography will accurately delineate the presence of an EDH[185] (Fig. 11.15). Carotid angiography is performed ipsilateral to the site of pupillary dilatation and contralateral to the side of the patient's motor deficit.

Treatment

A major issue in the management of patients suspected of having EDH is how to manage the patient whose level of unconsciousness or focal neurological deficit is worsening while waiting for diagnostic studies to be completed. The condition of most patients can be stabilized with endotracheal intubation, hyperventilation, and diuretics. When this is not possible, diagnostic studies should be cancelled and operation performed immediately.[131] In this situation, a burr hole should be placed ipsilateral to the side of the pupillary dilatation or contralateral to the side of motor deficit. If, on the basis of clinical signs, the side of the suspected lesion is not clear, the presence of a skull fracture on plain film examination may provide clues to the side and site of the hematoma. In over 85% of patients, the hematoma is found beneath the fracture.[104, 121, 153]

In patients who are experiencing rapid deterioration, the operation can be begun with local anesthesia and is completed using general anesthesia. A linear scalp incision is made over the site of the fracture. A

Table 11.7
Motor and Pupillary Signs in Extradural Hematoma

	Jamieson and Yelland[92]	Phonprasert et al.[153]	Weinman and Muttucumaru[192]	Heiskanen[76]	Gallagher and Browder[58]
Pupillary dilatation, unilateral	38[a]	28	42	31	63
Pupillary dilatation, bilateral	9	17	5		10
Decerebration	21	28	24		43
Hemiparesis	27		79	45	67

[a] Figures represent percentage of patients with this finding in each series.

burr hole is placed over the fracture line. Hematoma is aspirated from beneath the burr hole and adjacent area using flexible catheters or angled instruments. This will result in an immediate decrease in the level of ICP. The burr hole is then enlarged for removal of the entire hematoma. Hematoma removal may release a tamponade over a lacerated middle meningeal artery but the site of the bleeding which ensues may be easily controlled when it is directly beneath the burr hole. When this is not the case, rapid craniectomy may have to be performed to control blood loss from the lacerated vessel.

After evacuation of the hematoma, the dura is tented up against the bone edges, and a drain is placed in the epidural space. When craniectomy is performed beneath the temporalis muscle a cranioplasty is usually unnecessary. For craniectomies in other locations a wire mesh and/or acrylic cranioplasty minimizes cosmetic deformity and provides protection for the brain.

If an EDH or SDH is not found when the initial burr holes are placed, additional holes should be made in the ipsilateral frontal and parietal regions. If the hematoma is still not found, three holes should be made in similar locations on the opposite side. In all patients who have not had a definitive pre-operative radiographic study to localize the site of the hematoma, a CT scan or angiogram should be performed as early in the post-operative period as is practicable. This is of obvious importance in those cases where hematoma is not found through burr hole exploration.

In patients who are stable, or are deteriorating less rapidly, it is generally more convenient to perform a craniotomy with a free bone flap. The scalp incision is tailored to the location of the hematoma as determined by diagnostic studies. The general strategy is the same as outlined above. In patients with temporal hematomas, the temporal squama should be removed to the floor of the middle fossa to gain access to the more proximal portions of the middle meningeal artery.

Management Errors; Complications

Outcome is related to the patient's pre-operative state and failure to recognize clinical deterioration when it occurs will result in increased morbidity and mortality.[121, 192] Delay in diagnosis has been reported to be the commonest avoidable cause of morbidity and mortality in patients with EDH.[76, 118, 153, 192] Mendelow et al.[131] examined the relationship of outcome to delayed treatment in 83 patients with EDH without intradural lesions. The mean delay in evacuation of the hematoma in patients who died was over 15 hours, whereas the delay in those who made a good recovery was less than 2 hours.

In the rapidly deteriorating patient, the placement of burr holes to diagnose and treat a suspected EDH is an appropriate and accepted form of management. However, the limited visualization of the intracranial space this technique provides may result in failure to locate an EDH.[153, 192]

Recurrent hematoma formation after initial satisfactory operative evacuation will result in increased morbidity and mortality [121, 153] and can be minimized by accurately identifying and controlling bleeding from the lacerated section of the middle menin-

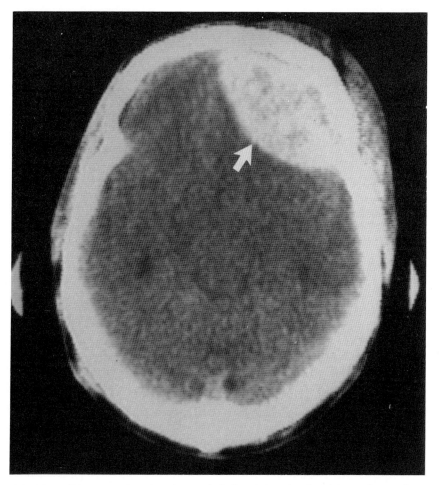

Figure 11.14.   CT scan showing large left frontal extradural hematoma (*arrow*) with typical lentiform appearance.

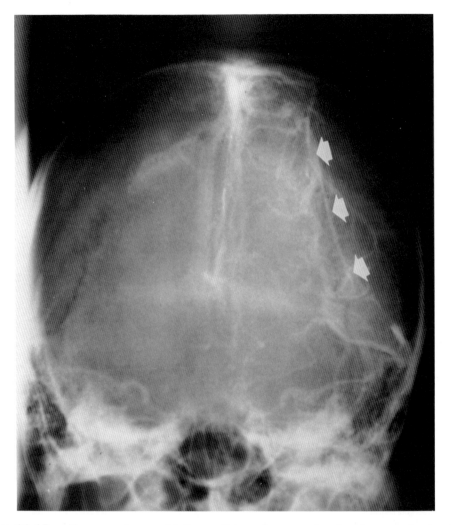

Figure 11.15. Venous phase of left carotid angiogram showing large extradural hematoma. *Arrows* mark cortical vessel displaced from inner table by hematoma. Lenticular shape of hematoma is similar to that seen with chronic subdural hematoma.

geal artery as well as multiple small dural bleeders which are often found.

Although lumbar puncture has been advocated in the investigation of patients with suspected EDH,[104] it should not be performed as death has been reported as a direct consequence of this procedure.[121, 192]

Outcome

The reported mortality of patients with EDH varies from a low of 15 or 16%[92, 153] to a high of 43%.[103] The factors which influence outcome will be discussed separately and include: age of the patient, presence of intradural lesions, the time from injury to the appearance of symptoms, level of consciousness, and neurological deficit at the time of operation.

Age. As with other types of head injury, mortality appears to increase with age. Campbell and Cohen[24] reported a good outcome in 90% of a series of pediatric patients. Jamieson and Yelland[92] reported a mortality of less than 5% for patients under the age of 10. McLaurin and Ford[121] reported an unsatisfactory outcome in 18% of patients below the age of 20 and in 52% of patients over the age of 20. Phonprasert et al.[153] reported a mortality rate of 13% in patients under 40 and 33% in those over that age.

Presence of Associated Intracranial Lesions. The presence of intradural mass lesions (SDH, intracerebral hematoma, cerebral contusion or laceration) results in a mortality rate at least four times that of patients with EDH without these lesions (5–8% vs. 26–32%).[92, 153] McLaurin and Ford[121] reported a 12% mortality in patients with uncomplicated EDH and a 60% mortality with EDH and associated cerebral contusions.

Site of Epidural Hematoma. The data on the relationship between the site of the EDH and mortality is somewhat contradictory. Kvarnes and Trumpy[104] reported that the site of EDH has no influence on mortality. In other series, hematomas in the temporal region were associated with the worst outcome.[58, 121] Frontal and vertex hematomas would seem to have the most favorable prognosis.[92] It has been postulated that mortality is more closely related to the speed of formation of the hematoma rather than to location; temporal hematomas form most rapidly and those in other locations accumulate more slowly.[58, 92]

Rate of Development. Mortality is highest (20–60%) in patients who develop symptoms early after head trauma.[92, 104, 121, 153] This is true for two reasons: patients symptomatic from the time of injury often have intradural mass lesions and diffuse parenchymal injury that adversely affect outcome[92] and hematomas which expand very rapidly may produce irreversible injury before therapy may be instituted. Operation performed after the third day (in patients with slowly expanding lesions) is generally associated with a mortality of less than 10%.

Neurological Examination. Unconsciousness, pupillary abnormalities, and decerebration are all associated with an outcome that is less favorable than when these clinical signs are not present. The deleterious effect of these clinical findings on outcome may be seen in Table 11.8.

Table 11.8
Mortality of Patients with Extradural Hematoma Related to Neurological Findings at Time of Operation

	Gallagher and Browder[58]	Jamieson and Yelland[92]	McLaurin and Ford[121]	Phonprasert et al.[153]	Weinman and Muttucumaru[192]
Conscious	18[a]	1	20	3	
Unconscious	55	26	64	28	82
Pupillary Abnormalities		23	62	28	
Pupils Reactive		11	29	5	7
Decerebration Present	49		62	39	
Decerebration Absent	31		29	4	

[a] Figures represent percentage of patients with this finding in each series.

CEREBRAL CONTUSION

Cerebral contusion is a brain injury which consists of heterogeneous areas of necrosis, pulping, infarction, hemorrhage, and edema.[170] The gyral crest is maximally involved and the subjacent white matter is affected to a more variable extent.[112]

Incidence

Cerebral contusion is the most frequently encountered lesion following head injury.[54] In a study of 1,000 brains examined at *post-mortem* examination contusion was absent in only 11%. However, under the age of one year it was seen in less than half of all brains examined. In these instances, the usual hemorrhagic contusions were replaced by contusions consisting of non-hemorrhagic tears of the white matter.[112]

Cerebral contusion is also the commonest traumatic lesion visualized on CT scan. Dublin *et al.*[41] reported a 40% incidence, Sweet *et al.*, 23%,[178] and Zimmerman *et al.*, 21%.[200] The reason for the lower incidence of CT-visualized contusions probably relates to the inability of the CT to resolve very small lesions that are readily seen at autopsy. In addition, patients studied with the CT scan had less severe injuries than those examined at *postmortem*, as only a minority of patients who had CT scans went on to die.

Pathogenesis

Following head injury, contusions may occur at the site of impact or at distant points.[33] Contusions occurring at points of impact are known as "coup" lesions and are produced by the deformation and inbending of bone at the point of impact. The brain is transiently compressed by this inbending and the severity of the contusion is a function of the amount of energy transmitted by the skull to the underlying brain. With a given impact energy, the smaller the area of contact, the greater the severity of the contusion, and the more likely it is that the contusion will expand into deeper areas of the white matter.[70]

For the most part, however, cerebral contusions at the site of impact are minor.[111]

The most significant lesions are found at a distance from the impact site. These injuries occur when the stationary head is free to move at the time of impact or when the moving head is suddenly decelerated.[70] These injuries, distant from the site of impact, are known as "contre-coup" contusions and occur predominantly at the frontal and temporal poles which are impacted against the irregular bony floor of the frontal and middle fossa. They are classically produced by forward acceleration of the brain within the calvarium when the occiput is struck (Fig. 11.16). Interestingly, frontal blows only rarely produce occipital contre-coup contusions—probably because of the smoothness of the bone against which the occipital lobe is impacted.[70] Contusions may also occur on the medial surfaces of the cerebral hemispheres as a result of acceleration of the brain against the falx. Small hemorrhagic contusions also occur in the deep white and gray matter. These "intermediate" lesions probably occur as a result of shearing with rapid acceleration or deceleration of the brain at the time of

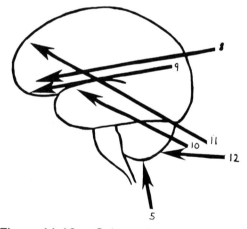

Figure 11.16. Schematic drawing of brain showing variability of impact direction in six cases of falls on the occiput. The *arrows* connect areas of impact with the corresponding area of contrecoup contusion. (Reproduced with permission from Lindenberg, R., Freytag, E.: The mechanism of cerebral contusions. Arch. Pathol., 69:440–469, 1960.)

impact. In an autopsy study, 27% of brains examined had contusions of the corpus collosum and basal ganglia.[54] The location of contusions found in 191 autopsy cases is seen in Fig. 11.17. The frontal and temporal lobes (and particularly their undersurfaces) are the commonest sites in virtually all series.[70, 170] The parietal lobe only occasionally is affected and the occipital lobe least frequently. It should be emphasized that contusions are most often multiple and are frequently associated with other lesions, both within and external to the cerebral parenchyma (cerebral hemorrhage, SDH, EDH). Almost one-half of all patients are reported to have more than one focal mass lesion.[170, 199]

Skull fracture is a frequent finding in patients with contusion and has been reported to be present in 60–80% of patients.[122, 199] Adams *et al.*[2] found that the contusion tends to be worse on the side of the fracture and much more severe when a fracture is present than when it is absent. However, McLaurin and Helmer[122] could find no correlation between the side of the fracture and the intracranial pathology.

Signs and Symptoms; Temporal Course

The signs and symptoms of cerebral contusions are related to the location of the contusion, the severity of the injury, and the presence of associated lesions. Patients with isolated, localized contusions of the

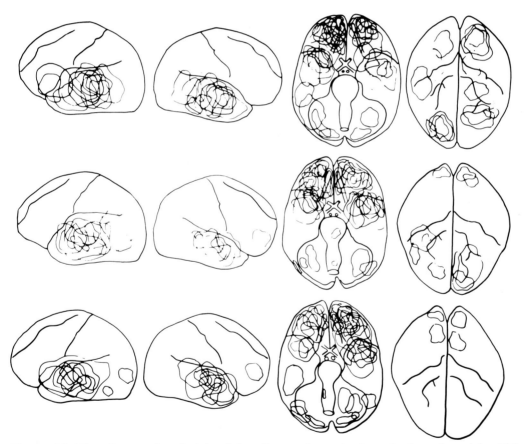

Figure 11.17. Composite sketch of locations of cerebral contusions found in 191 autopsied cases. (Reprinted with permission from Gurdjian, E.S., Gurdjian, E.S.: Cerebral contusions: re-evaluation of the mechanism of their development. J. Trauma, 16:35–51, 1976.)

motor or speech areas will have focal deficits related to dysfunction of these areas. Initial loss of consciousness at the time of impact is generally not related to a local contusion but to cerebral concussion or diffuse brain injury. The severity of the diffuse brain injury varies and the patient may have but a brief period of unconsciousness or diffuse white matter shearing and irreversible anatomical destruction of deep structures. In other patients, the symptoms of contusion are obscured by the presence of parenchymal or extraparenchymal hematomas.

Small focal contusions most often resolve spontaneously although the patient may be left with a motor or speech deficit. Larger contusions, especially those in the temporal lobe and those involving multiple areas (*e.g.*, tetrapolar injuries with bilateral contusions of the frontal and temporal lobes) often act as a mass lesion and threaten the patient with dangerous elevations of ICP. In the days following injury, the contusion becomes necrotic and heterogeneously hemorrhagic. The patient is not immediately at risk unless the lesion is quite large. The mass effect at this time is proportional to the size of the contusion.[199] By the latter part of the first week after injury, the hemorrhage begins to resolve but the mass effect may be very much increased because of the appearance of edema. The ICP may rise, focal neurological deficits may increase, and the patient's level of consciousness may deteriorate.

Because of the proximity of the incisura and midbrain, temporal lobe contusions are a particularly treacherous entity. Initially, the patient may be relatively intact or may have varying degrees of dysphasia if the lesion involves the dominant hemisphere. McLaurin and Helmer[122] have emphasized that "temporal contusion is most frequently a part of more generalized intracranial injury, and the syndrome may, therefore, be masked by the effects of other neurological damage." Deterioration may occur quite rapidly with little or no warning as a result of increasing mass effect from edema. The ICP is often deceptively low even in the period immediately prior to deterioration

and diagnostic studies may show little shift of midline structures.

Diagnosis

The diagnosis of cerebral contusion is best established by the CT scan. Angiography cannot identify the small contusion with minimal or no mass effect and cannot reliably distinguish between contusion and hematoma. Following trauma, the CT appearance of a cerebral contusion is that of a heterogeneous area of increased density which is a reflection of multiple small hemorrhages intermixed with edema and necrotic brain tissue[199] (Fig. 11.18).

Treatment

The management of patients with cerebral contusion is often not clear-cut. Patients with small, multiple and/or deep lesions may not need operation and can be followed with frequent assessments of their medical status. The ICP should be monitored and elevations treated according to the principles described in Chapter 9. Patients with larger contusions and considerable mass effect should have craniotomy at the time of presentation.

There is sometimes hesitation in recommending operative removal when contusion involves a dominant temporal lobe. Medical therapy can be employed in an attempt to see if the patient can be tided over during the period of maximum edema without operation. Our experience with this policy has not been wholly satisfactory. It is not uncommon to find patients with normal ICP and a relatively stable neurological condition who suddenly herniate as long as seven or nine days after injury.

It has been our policy to remove large contusions at the time of injury. Resection of contused brain results in immediate reduction of mass effect and precludes or minimizes the subsequent development of edema through damaged capillaries in the region of the contusion. When multiple contusions are present, they most often involve the frontal and temporal lobes and a frontotemporal flap on the side of maximal involvement and resection of contused brain is the treatment of choice. Large decom-

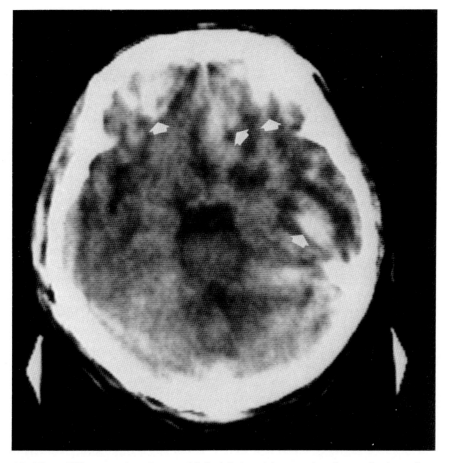

Figure 11.18. CT scan showing multiple bilateral hemorrhagic contusions (*arrows*) of the frontal and temporal lobes.

pressive craniectomy with opening of the dura without resection of injured brain has been recommended as a treatment for cerebral contusion.[197] However, when the outcome of patients treated in this fashion is compared to those who receive more conventional resection of contused areas, there is no clear-cut improvement in survival.

Outcome

Mortality from contusions is reported to range from 25–60%.[77, 170, 197] The factors that adversely affect outcome are similar to those for other post-traumatic mass lesions: adults (particularly those over age 50) fare worse than children and patients in coma at the time of operation have a generally poor outcome.[170]

INTRACEREBRAL HEMATOMA

Intracerebral hematomas are composed of hemorrhagic areas within the cerebral parenchyma that may be as small as 1 mm in size or large enough to involve several lobes of the brain. Although the differentiation between an intracerebral hematoma and hemorrhagic contusion is sometimes difficult, intracerebral hematomas are well-defined, homogeneous collections of blood. Hemorrhagic contusions are mixtures of blood and contused and edematous cerebral parenchyma. The distinction between the two is easily made by the CT scan but cannot be made with any degree of certainty by angiography as the vessel displacement caused by a confluent intracerebral hematoma and hemorrhagic contusions is indistinguishable.

Incidence

The actual incidence of intracerebral hematoma has undoubtedly been underestimated in the past because of the failure of angiography to resolve small lesions and to distinguish hematoma from contusion. In a review of 11,000 head-injured patients prior to the advent of the CT scan, Jamieson and Yelland[94] reported the incidence of intracerebral hematoma to be 0.6%. Similarly, Levinthal and Stern[110] reported only 12 cases in a six-year period. Recent series utilizing CT scans report an incidence of 4 to 23%.[118, 200]

Pathogenesis

The mechanisms by which traumatic intracerebral hematoma and cerebral contusions are produced is similar. Courville[34] defined three circumstances which will result in the production of intracerebral hematoma: 1) blows to the head causing depressed fractures beneath which there forms an intracerebral hematoma; 2) penetrating wounds (missiles, knives, pointed implements); 3) when the moving head strikes a fixed object. Levinthal and Stern[110] confirmed the second and third mechanisms in their small series. McLaurin and McBride[123] reported that all their cases of intracerebral hematoma resulted from sudden acceleration or deceleration of the head.

The last mechanism described by Courville is almost certainly the commonest manner by which intracerebral hematomas are produced. A blow (generally to the posterior part of the vault) causes the brain to be propelled forward in the cranium. Confluent hemorrhages are found originating at the undersurface and anterior tips of the frontal lobe where the brain is traumatized by the irregular surface of the floor of the anterior fossa.

The mechanism of production of temporal lobe hematomas is similar to that noted for frontal lobe hemorrhages. The temporal lobe is injured as it slides over the rough surface of the sphenoid wing. The hemorrhage generally begins superficially and extends deeply into the white matter as far as the lateral ventricle in one-third of the cases.[200]

Hemorrhages are seen in other structures as well. Bleeding into the corpus callosum probably results from shear stresses induced in the structure by acceleration-deceleration type injuries[34] (Fig. 11.19). Small hemorrhages involving the centrum semiovale and deep gray matter as well as the brain stem probably originate in similar fashion. The use of the CT scan has revealed that intraventricular hemorrhages are more frequent than had previously been thought and may occur without any evidence of parenchymal hematoma or other injury.[37, 150]

Eighty to ninety percent of intracerebral hematomas are located in the white matter of the temporal or frontal lobes.[9, 18, 69, 94, 198] The parietal or occipital lobes are less commonly involved.[9] Primary hemorrhages also occur within the brain stem, but these are unusual. Multiple hemorrhagic lesions occur 20% of the time,[41] although one lesion is usually consideraly larger than the others and 60% are associated with extracerebral hematomas.[18, 41]

Clinical Course; Signs and Symptoms

Over one-half of all patients are rendered unconscious by the initial impact.[94] Their subsequent state of consciousness is a function of the severity of the immediate impact injury and the size and subsequent growth of the intra-parenchymal hematoma and any extra-parenchymal hematomas which may be present. One-third of all patients remain lucid throughout their course. Jamieson and Yelland[92] noted that 19% have a classic lucid interval—a figure higher than the one reported by the same authors for patients with EDH.

The signs and symptoms of patients with traumatically induced intracerebral hematomas are similar to those which occur as a result of extracerebral collections and cerebral contusions. Moreover, because of the frequency with which these lesions coexist with extracerebral hematomas, this entity cannot be reliably distinguished from

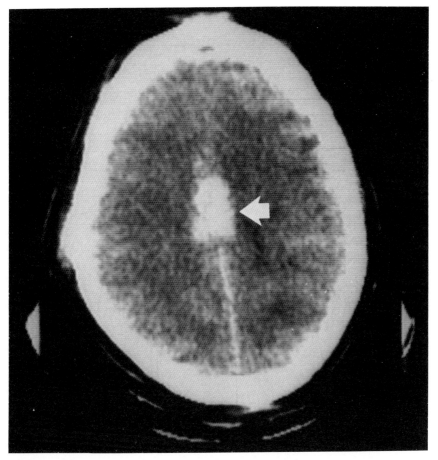

Figure 11.19.   CT scan of a patient with a corpus callosum hemorrhage sustained in a high speed motor vehicle accident. Hemorrhage probably originated as a result of shear stress and was associated with a clinical picture of diffuse brain injury.

other post-traumatic intracranial mass lesions. The type of focal neurological dificit depends upon the location and size of the hematoma. Anterior frontal hematomas, particularly on the non-dominant side, may fail to produce any symptoms. More posteriorly placed hematomas or large anteriorly located hematomas will produce focal motor deficit or speech dysfunction when located in the dominant hemisphere. Patients with temporal lobe lesions of the dominant hemisphere will present with speech dysfunction. Enlargement of the hematoma or an increase in edema surrounding the hematoma will produce additional mass effect with further depression of the patient's level of consciousness, increase in

motor or speech deficit and eventually ipsilateral compression of the third nerve and midbrain. The length of time from trauma to neurological deterioration is variable. It may occur within minutes after injury, or as long as 7–10 days following trauma.

Delayed Hemorrhage. Occasionally patients with head injury have no evidence of intracerebral hemorrhage on their initial CT scan, and one or more days after their trauma they develop a hemorrhage with associated neurologic deficit and depressed level of consciousness. This occurrence is referred to as delayed traumatic intracerebral hemorrhage (DTICH). Patients with this entity must be distinguished from those in whom edema around a *pre-existing* hemorrhage causes an increase in mass effect and results in neurological deterioration. DTICH was originally described 90 years ago by Bollinger[16] and multiple reports of this phenomenon have subsequently appeared.[38, 91, 138, 179] It is only since the advent of the CT scanner that there has been absolute confirmation of the *de novo* genesis of hemorrhages in areas shown to be normal on the initial CT study.[19, 20, 39, 113] The fact that delayed hemorrhage occurs in patients who have had unequivocally normal scans or patients with focal contusions makes it imperative that all patients who experience clinical deterioration be restudied even if the initial CT scan was normal. The overall incidence of DTICH in a large series of patients with closed head injuries has been reported as 1.5%.[39] In another series, as many as 10% of all patients with traumatic intracerebral hematomas had normal initial scans.[113] The reason for the occurrence of delayed hemorrhage has been the subject of considerable speculation. Brain injury is thought to result in a decrease in vascular resistance allowing an increased head of arterial pressure and increased blood flow to be transmitted to an already traumatized capillary-vascular bed with resultant hemorrhage into the cerebral parenchyma.[39, 69, 113, 138]

Diagnosis

Definitive diagnosis of traumatic intracerebral hemorrhage is made with the CT scan (Fig. 11.20). Because the CT scan can resolve differences in density, intracerebral hematomas are reliably distinguished from cerebral contusion or post-traumatic edema. Isotope brain scans have been used in the past for the diagnosis of intracerebral hematomas[110] but they are of limited usefulness as they do not become positive until at least 3–4 days have passed from the time of trauma and cannot reliably distinguish cerebral contusions from hematomas.

Treatment

The treatment of patients with large intracranial hematomas with a depressed level of consciousness, focal neurological deficit, and shift of midline structures is straightforward and consists of operative evacuation. It has been our policy to fashion large bone flaps centered over the site of the hematoma to provide adequate visualization for hematoma evacuation, resection of adjacent contused brain, and removal of any extra-parenchymal hematomas that may also be present. Although intracerebral hematomas may be removed through burr holes[123] the exposure is generally inadequate for hematoma evacuation, resection of damaged brain, and control of hemorrhage.

When hematomas involve the frontal lobe, we do not hesitate to perform a frontal lobectomy to provide room for cerebral swelling in the post-operative period. We are also aggressive in the resection of the non-dominant temporal lobe surrounding the hematoma. In the dominant temporal lobe only the hematoma and obviously contused brain are removed.

Patients with hematomas involving the deep white matter or basal ganglia without superficial extension are not operative candidates and should have medical management for the control of elevated ICP. Patients with small hematomas who are neurologically intact and those who have minimal deficit may also be managed without operation. They must be followed closely with ICP monitoring and serial CT scans at 2–4 day intervals for at least 7–10 days. Operation is performed if neurological deficit appears or increases, if the size of the mass increases as a result of swelling around the hematoma, or if the ICP cannot be controlled by medical means. The initial levels of ICP may also be helpful in deciding which patients need operation. Teasdale *et al.*[183] report that the majority of patients with ICP levels of greater than 20 mm Hg upon admission needed operation within 1–3 days following trauma, whereas those admitted with ICP levels below 20 mm Hg usually did not.

The management of the patient who is neurologically stable with fixed motor or speech deficit and a relatively small hematoma is sometimes difficult. For the most part we have chosen not to operate on these patients, although one series[110] reports con-

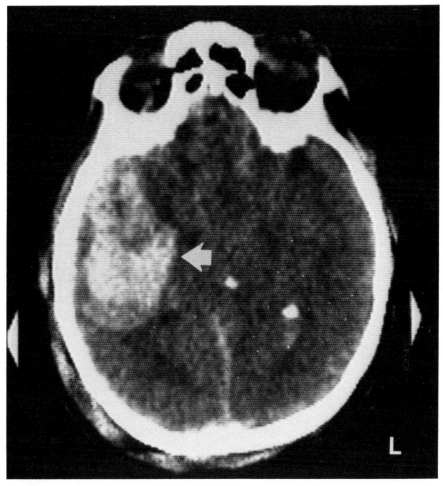

Figure 11.20. CT scan showing large right temporal intracerebral hematoma (*arrow*).

siderable resolution of deficit in patients who had hematoma evacuation.

The management of patients with temporal lobe hematomas is similar to that for temporal lobe contusions. The midline shift is often deceptively small and the ICP may be normal or only minimally elevated, even when patients show incipient signs of cerebral herniation. Because sudden deterioration is not an uncommon phenomenon in patients with temporal lobe hematomas our threshhold for operation is lower than it is for lesions in other locations.

Outcome

The mortality for traumatic intracerebral hematoma reported by Browder and Turney[18] was 72%. More recently, Jamieson and Yelland[94] documented a 25% mortality in 63 patients. In this latter series, mortality was closely related to the patient's level of consciousness following injury; patients who were unconscious at the time of operation had a mortality of 45% whereas those lucid just prior to operation had a mortality of only 6%.

MASS LESIONS OF THE POSTERIOR CRANIAL FOSSA

Incidence

Traumatically induced mass lesions of the posterior fossa are unusual. In a 10-year period Wright[196] was able to identify only

17 cases of traumatic infratentorial hematomas. During the same period of time 344 cases of supratentorial hematomas were seen. In particular, traumatic intracerebellar hemorrhage is infrequently encountered.[169, 196]

EDH is the most frequently reported mass lesion of the posterior fossa but it represents but a small fraction of the total number of EDH seen.[196] Gallagher and Browder[58] make no mention of the occurrence of posterior fossa EDH in their large series. Hooper noted only seven posterior fossa collections in a series of 47 EDH, and McLaurin and Ford[121] reported one case in a series of identical size. Jamieson and Yelland[92] collected 12 cases in a series of 167 EDH.

SDH of the posterior fossa is a rare lesion and represents less than 1% of the total number of SDH. Estridge and Smith[45] could find only 15 cases in a review of the literature.

Epidural Hematoma of the Posterior Fossa

Mechanism of Injury. Infratentorial EDH usually occurs as a result of a blow to the back of the head.[84, 196] External signs of injury (scalp hematomas, abrasions, lacerations or open skull fracture) are often present.[11] A skull fracture of the occipital bone is seen on X-rays in two-thirds of the cases and, when present, will usually be seen to cross a venous sinus.[11, 84, 102] The frequency with which fractures are visualized at operation is usually higher than this and in one series a fracture was seen in each of ten patients with an EDH of the posterior fossa.[14] On occasion, however, a fracture is absent.[8, 102] In the majority of patients, bleeding into the epidural space occurs from a tear of the outer wall of the transverse or sigmoid sinus or torcular directly under the site of the fracture.[14, 84]

Signs and Symptoms. The signs and symptoms of a posterior fossa EDH are variable[202] and no one sign or symptom is pathognomonic. Initial loss of consciousness with a lucid interval followed by progressive deterioration of the level of consciousness is inconstantly present. Beller and Peyser[11] reported that half of their patients did not lose consciousness immediately after the trauma and one-third had no secondary depression of their level of consciousness. Kosary et al.[102] reported the classic lucid interval in only 7 of 13 patients. However, Hooper[84] found the lucid interval to be the usual course in all patients except those with rapidly progressive hemorrhage or a co-existing supratentorial mass.

The rate of progression of signs and symptoms is also variable.[1, 83, 202] Hooper[84] has emphasized three clinical courses: 1) acute (signs of medullary compression within 24 hours); 2) subacute (symptoms and signs within 2–7 days of injury); and 3) chronic (symptoms one week or later following injury). Although these hematomas are unusual and the experience at any one institution is limited, at least one other series confirms the variability of the temporal course[196]. Of 100 cases collected by Besson et al.[14] from the literature, 52 had a subacute course, 42 an acute course, and 4 had a chronic course.

Headache and stiff neck are the commonest symptoms seen in patients with infratentorial extradural hematomas.[84, 196] Signs referable to dysfunction of posterior fossa structures are variable. Cranial nerve deficits have been noted but are not reliably present.[84, 196]

Papilledema occurs only in the subacute or chronic forms. Cerebellar signs are reported in less than one-half of all patients.[11, 102] Indeed, Besson et al.[14] have emphasized that in patients with an acute clinical course, 95% did not have cerebellar signs. Corticospinal tract findings (pathological reflexes, hemiparesis have been frequently reported,[11, 102] and present a particular problem because they tend to draw suspicion away from a posterior fossa hematoma. In the latter stages of hematoma expansion corticospinal tract signs may be a reflection of direct medullary compression. However, when seen early after the injury they probably result from a co-existing supratentorial injury. Indeed, contrecoup frontal or temporal contusions and hematomas are frequently present as a result of a blow to the occipital skull.[202]

The diagnosis of posterior fossa EDH is difficult for a number of reasons: it is often not suspected, the signs and symptoms are non-specific, posterior fossa EDH is rare, and co-existing supratentorial injury confuses the clinical picture. Eighty-five percent of patients with the acute syndrome and one-half of all patients with a subacute course have no localizing findings.[14] As many as one-half of all patients with this condition die without a correct diagnosis.[196] A posterior fossa EDH should be considered "whenever stupor follows upon an occipital injury."[102]

Specialized Diagnostic Studies. A CT scan is the diagnostic procedure of choice for patients with suspected posterior fossa EDH. More often than not, the lesion is not suspected and is discovered when a scan is performed for a suspected supratentorial mass. When the CT scan is used for the diagnosis of head injury with a paucity of localizing signs, it is important that appropriate cuts be obtained to delineate posterior fossa structures. The radiologist should be instructed to angle the plane of scanning steeper and to perform cuts at more frequent intervals than is usual for supratentorial structures. The configuration of the hematoma is similar to those located above the tentorium.

Ventriculography and angiography have been used in the past for the diagnosis of this lesion but are now indicated only when the CT scan is unavailable. Ventriculography will demonstrate displacement of the fourth ventricle by a mass lesion but the nature of the lesion (whether intra- or extra-axial) is usually difficult to determine. Carotid angiography performed for the diagnosis of a supratentorial traumatic mass lesion may show large ventricles, or displacement of the transverse sinus away from the inner table.[14] When hematoma extends above the tentorium, the sagittal sinus may be seen to be displaced. If radiographic signs are equivocal, or no supratentorial mass lesion is found, vertebral angiography is indicated. The basilar artery will be seen to be displaced anteriorly as will the posterior inferior cerebellar artery. An avascular area corresponding to the site

of the hematoma will also be seen on the venous phase. Anterior displacement of the precentral cerebellar vein will further serve to localize the lesion in the posterior part of the infratentorial space.

Ideally, operative treatment for symptomatic infratentorial EDH is undertaken after precise localization of the hematoma utilizing the CT scan. In patients with a subacute or chronic course, the slow progression of signs should allow the diagnostic evaluation to be completed. The diagnosis of *any* traumatic posterior fossa mass lesion on clinical signs alone is so difficult that radiologic evaluation should be omitted only if there is exceedingly rapid deterioration without localizing signs in a patient with occipital trauma or an occipital fracture on plain skull roentgenograms.

Treatment. In patients who experience rapid neurological deterioration and in whom angiography or CT scan shows large ventricles, the frontal horn of the right lateral ventricle is cannulated and enough CSF is removed to reduce the ICP to normal. While there is the theoretical possibility of upward tentorial herniation as a result of this procedure, this is more than outweighed by the benefits of decompression of an obstructed ventricular system.

In cases of suspected or proven EDH, a linear paramedian incision is made in the suboccipital region. A burr hole is centered over the point where the skull fracture crosses the torcula, transverse, or sigmoid sinus. As much hematoma as possible is removed through the burr hole. Hemostasis at the site of the sinus tear is obtained by using muscle or thrombin-soaked gelfoam. The burr hole is enlarged to a craniectomy. In a significant number of cases the hematoma extends above the transverse sinus to the region of the occipital lobe and bone removal may have to be extended superiorly for complete visualization of the hematoma.[14] After hematoma removal is completed, dural bleeders are cauterized, dural tenting sutures are placed and th wound is closed without drainage.

Outcome. Outcome correlates with the patient's neurological status at the time of operation. In a series of 10 patients, Besson *et al.*[14] reported a 40% mortality. Beller and Peyser[11] and Kosary *et al.*[102] reported mortality rates of 37 and 69%, respectively, in cases collected from the literature.

Subdural Hematoma of the Posterior Fossa

In most instances, infratentorial SDH results from injury to the occipital area. There are no signs or symptoms pathognomonic of this entity and it cannot be distinguished from EDH of the posterior fossa or traumatic cerebellar hematoma on clinical grounds alone.[29] Disturbance of consciousness, headache, and vomiting are the most common findings.[29, 45] Cranial nerve palsies, nucchal rigidity, cerebellar signs and symptoms, and papilledema are each seen in less than one-half of all patients. The course is variable: trauma may result in an immediate loss of consciousness with progression of neurological signs or a prolonged lucid interval of greater than 24 hours.[29, 196] A quarter or more of all patients will also have supratentorial subdural hematomas with signs of cerebral hemispheric dysfunction.[45, 50] The presence of an occipital skull fracture is variable and is reported from 20–80% of the time.[45, 196]

The pathogenesis of posterior fossa SDH has been attributed to tearing of bridging veins, injury to the venous sinuses, or cerebellar contusion.[29, 45] The favored diagnostic procedure is a CT scan, although angiography will also delineate the presence of the hematoma. The hematomas are usually unilateral and operative removal is accomplished via a unilateral suboccipital craniectomy. The outcome is not good and only one-half of patients treated survive.[29, 50, 196]

Traumatic Intracerebellar Hematoma

Traumatic intracerebellar hematomas are caused by blows to the occiput. Suture line separations or occipital fractures are often seen.[169, 196] The contusion or hematoma is usually located directly under the area of occipital trauma. A co-existing posterior fossa SDH is sometimes present and the occipital blow causing the brain to be propelled forward in the calvarium commonly results in contre-coup contusions and hematomas of the frontal and temporal poles.

The signs and symptoms are similar to those seen with extra-axial posterior fossa hematomas. Depression of the level of consciousness may occur quite rapidly in patients who are intact or apparently stable.[169]

Unilateral suboccipital craniectomy *via* a paramedian incision and resection of contused and hemorrhagic cerebellum is the treatment of choice. If a co-existing supratentorial mass exists attention should be directed first toward the lesion that is clinically and radiographically most significant. There is little data on outcome in the literature but it is probably not different from that reported for extra-axial lesions of the posterior fossa.

References

1. Achslogh, J.: Hématome sous-dural chronique de la fosse cérébrale postérieure. Acta Neurol. Psych. Belg., 52:790–794, 1952.
2. Adams, J.H., Scott, G., Parker, L.S., Graham, D.I., Doyle, D.: The contusion index: a quantitative approach to cerebral contusions in head injury. Neuropath. Appl. Neurobiol., 6:319–324, 1980.
3. Ambrosetto, C.: Post-traumatic subdural hematoma. Further observations on nonsurgical treatment. Arch. Neurol., 6:287–292, 1962.
4. Apfelbaum, R.I., Guthkelch, A.N., Shulman, K.: Experimental production of subdural hematomas. J. Neurosurg., 40:336–346, 1974.
5. Arkins, T.J., McLennan, J.E., Winston, K.R., Strand, R.D., Suzuki, Y.: Acute posterior fossa epidural hematomas in children. Am. J. Dis. Child, 131:690–692, 1977.
6. Aronson, S.M., Okazaki, H.: A study of some factors modifying response of cerebral tissue to subdural hematomata. J. Neurosurg., 20:89–93, 1963.
7. Arseni, C., Stanciu, M.: Particular clinical aspects of chronic subdural haematoma in adults. Eur. Neurol., 2:109–122, 1969.
8. Bacon, A.: Cerebellar extradural hematoma. Report of a case. J. Neurosurg., 6:78–81, 1949.
9. Baratham, G., Dennyson, W.G.: Delayed traumatic intracerebral haemorrhage. J. Neurol. Neurosurg. Psych., 35:698–706, 1972.
10. Becker, D.P., Miller, J.D., Ward, J.D., Greenberg, R.P., Young, H.F., Sakalas, R.: The outcome from severe head injury with early diagnosis and intensive management. J. Neurosurg., 47:491–502, 1977.
11. Beller, A.J., Peyser, E.: Extradural cerebellar hematoma. Report of three cases with review of the literature. J. Neurosurg., 9:291–298, 1952.

12. Bender, M.B., Christoff, N.: Nonsurgical treatment of subdural hematomas. Arch. Neurol., 31:73–79, 1974.
13. Bergström, M., Ericson, K., Levander, B., Svendsen, P.: Computed tomography of cranial subdural and epidural hematomas: Variation of attenuation related to time and clinical events such as rebleeding. J. Comp. Asst. Tomogr., 1:449–455, 1977.
14. Besson, G., Leguyader, J., Bagot D'Arc, M., Garré, H.: L'Hématome extra-dural de la fosse postérieure. Problèmes diagnostiques (10 observations). Neurochirurgie, 24:53–63, 1978.
15. Bisgaard-Frantzen, C.F., Dalby, M.: Acute subdural hematoma. Acta Psych. Neurol. Scand., 32:117–124, 1957.
16. Bollinger, O.: Über traumatische spät-apoplexie. Ein beitrag zur lehre von der hirnerschütterung. Internationale beiträge zur wissenschaftlichen medicin. Festschrift. Rudolph Virchow. Berlin: Hirschwald. 2:457–470, 1891.
17. Browder, J.: A resumé of the principal diagnostic features of subdural hematoma. Bull. N.Y. Acad. Med., 19:168–176, 1943.
18. Browder, J., Turney, M.F.: Intracerebral hemorrhage of traumatic origin. Its surgical treatment. N.Y.S. J. Med., 42:2230–2235, 1942.
19. Brown, F.D., Mullan, S., Duda, E.E.: Delayed traumatic intracerebral hematomas. Report of three cases. J. Neurosurg., 48:1019–1022, 1978.
20. Brunetti, J., Zingesser, L., Dunn, J., Rovit, R.L.: Delayed intracerebral hemorrhage as demonstrated by CT scanning. Neuroradiology, 18: 43–46, 1979.
21. Burton, C.: The management of chronic subdural hematoma using a compact hand twist drill. Military Med., 133:891–895, 1968.
22. Byrnes, D.P.: Head injury and the dilated pupil. Am. Surg. 45:139–143, 1979.
23. Cameron, M.M.: Chronic Subdural Haematoma: A review of 114 cases. J. Neurol. Neurosurg. Psych., 41:834–839, 1978.
24. Campbell, J.B., Cohen, J.: Epidural hemorrhage and the skull of children. Surg. Gynecol. Obstet., 92:257–280, 1951.
25. Cantore, G.P., Delfini, R., Neri, L.: Contribution to the surgical treatment of acute supratentorial subdural haematomas. Acta Neurochir., 41: 349–353, 1978.
26. Caplan, L.R., Zervas, N.T.: Survival with permanent midbrain dysfunction after surgical treatment of traumatic subdural hematoma: The clinical picture of a Duret hemorrhage? Ann. Neurol., 1:587–589, 1977.
27. Carcassonne, M., Choux, M., Grisoli, F.: Extradural hematomas in infants. J. Pediat. Surg., 12:69–73, 1977.
28. Chambers, J.W.: Acute subdural hematoma. J. Neurosurg., 8:263–268, 1951.
29. Ciembroniewicz, J.E.: Subdural hematoma of the posterior fossa. Review of the literature with addition of three cases. J. Neurosurg., 22:465–473, 1965.
30. Cooper, P.R., Hagler, H., Clark, W.K., Barnett, P.: Enhancement of experimental cerebral edema following decompressive craniectomy: Implications for the management of the severely head injured. Neurosurgery 4:296–300, 1979.
31. Cooper, P.R., Maravilla, K., Moody, S., Clark, W.K.: Serial computerized tomographic scanning and the prognosis of head injury. Neurosurgery, 5:566–569, 1979.
32. Cooper, P.R., Rovit, R.L., Ransohoff, J.: Hemicraniectomy in the treatment of acute subdural hematoma: a reappraisal. Surg. Neurol., 5:25–28, 1976.
33. Courville, C.B.: Coup coutre-coup mechanism of craniocerebral injuries. Arch. Surg., 45:19–43, 1942.
34. Courville, C.B.: Traumatic intracerebral hemorrhages. With special reference to the mechanisms of their production. Bull. Los Angeles Neurol. Soc., 27:22–38, 1962.
35. Cowan, R.J., Maynard, C.D., Lassiter, K.R.: Technetium-99m pertechnetate brain scans in the detection of subdural hematomas: A study of the age of the lesion as related to the development of a positive scan. J. Neurosurg., 32:30–34, 1970.
36. Da Costa, D.G., Adson, A.W.: Subdural hydroma. Arch. Surg., 43:559–567, 1941.
37. Danziger, A., Price, H.: The evaluation of head trauma by computed tomography. J. Trauma, 19:1–5, 1979.
38. De Jong, R.N.: Delayed traumatic intracerebral hemorrhage. Arch. Neurol. Psych., 48:257–266, 1942.
39. Diaz, F.G., Yock, D.H., Larson, D., Rockswold, G.L.: Early diagnosis of delayed post traumatic intracerebral hematomas. J. Neurosurg., 50: 217–223, 1979.
40. Dronfield, M.W., Mead, G.M., Langman, M.J.S.: Survival and death from subdural haematoma on medical wards. Postgrad. Med. J., 53:57–60, 1977.
41. Dublin, A.B., French, B.N., Rennick, J.M.: Computed tomography in head trauma. Radiology, 122:365–369, 1977.
42. Echlin, F.: Traumatic subdural hematoma—acute, subacute, and chronic. An analysis of seventy operated cases. J. Neurosurg., 6:294–303, 1949.
43. Echlin, F.A., Sordillo, S.V.R., Garvey, T.Q. Jr.: Acute, subacute and chronic subdural hematoma. J.A.M.A., 161:1345–1350, 1956.
44. El Gindi, S., Salama, M., Tawfik, E., Aboul Nasr, H., El Nadi, F.: A review of 2,000 patients with craniocerebral injuries with regard to intracranial haematomas and other vascular complications. Acta Neurochir., 48:237–244, 1979.
45. Estridge, M.N., Smith, R.A.: Acute subdural hemorrhage of posterior fossa. Report of a case with review of the literature. J. Neurosurg., 18:248–249, 1961.
46. Evans, J.P., Scheinker, I.M.: Histological studies of the brain following head trauma. II. Post-traumatic petechial and massive intracerebral hemorrhage. J. Neurosurg., 3:101–113, 1946.
47. Feldman, R.G., Pincus, J.H., McEntee, W.J.: Cer-

ebrovascular accident or subdural fluid collection? Arch. Intern. Med., 112:966–976, 1963.

48. Fell, D.A., Fitzgerald, S., Moiel, R.H., Caram, P.: Acute subdural hematomas. Review of 144 cases. J. Neurosurg., 42:37–42, 1975.

49. Ferguson, G.G., Barton, W.B., Drake, C.G.: Subdural hematoma in hemophilia: Successful treatment with cryoprecipitate. Case report. J. Neurosurg., 29:524–528, 1968.

50. Fisher, R.G., Kim, J.K., Sachs, E., Jr.: Complications in posterior fossa due to occipital trauma—their operability. J.A.M.A., 167:176–182, 1958.

51. Fogelholm, R., Waltimo, O.: Epidemiology of chronic subdural haematoma. Acta Neurochir., 32:247–250, 1975.

52. Ford, L.E., McLaurin, R.L.: Mechanisms of extradural hematomas. J. Neurosurg., 20:760–769, 1963.

53. French, B.N., Dublin, A.B.: The value of computerized tomography in the management of 1000 consecutive head injuries. Surg. Neurol., 7: 171–183, 1977.

54. Freytag, E.: Autopsy findings in head injuries from blunt forces. Statistical evaluation of 1367 cases. Arch. Path., 75:402–413, 1963.

55. Gaab, M., Knoblich, O.E., Fuhrmeister, U., Pflughaupt, K.W., Dietrich, K.: Comparison of the effects of surgical decompression and resection of local edema in the therapy of experimental brain trauma. Investigation of ICP, EEG and cerebral metabolism in cats. Child's Brain, 5:484–498, 1979.

56. Galbraith, S.L.: Age-distribution of extradural hemorrhage without skull fracture. Lancet, 1:1217–1218, 1973.

57. Galbraith, S.: Misdiagnosis and delayed diagnosis in traumatic intracranial haematoma. Br. Med. J., 1:1438–1439, 1976.

58. Gallagher, J.P., Browder, E.J.: Extradural hematoma. Experience with 167 patients. J. Neurosurg., 29:1–12, 1968.

59. Gannon, W.E., Cook, A.W., Browder, E.J.: Resolving subdural collections. J. Neurosurg., 19:865–869, 1962.

60. Gardner, W.J.: Traumatic subdural hematoma with particular reference to the latent interval. Arch. Neurol. Psych., 27:847–858, 1932.

61. Gitlin, D.: Pathogenesis of subdural collections of fluid. Pediatrics, 16:345–352, 1955.

62. Gjerris, F., Schmidt, K.: Chronic subdural hematoma. Surgery or mannitol treatment. J. Neurosurg., 40:639–642, 1974.

63. Glista, G.G., Reichman, O.H., Brumlik, J., Fine, M.: Interhemispheric subdural hematoma. Surg. Neurol., 10:119–122, 1978.

64. Glover, D., Labadie, E.L.: Physiopathogenesis of subdural hematomas. Part 2: Inhibition of growth of experimental hematomas with dexamethasone. J. Neurosurg., 45:393–397, 1976.

65. Goodell, C.L., Mealey, J. Jr.: Pathogenesis of chronic subdural hematoma. Experimental studies. Arch. Neurol., 8:429–437, 1963.

66. Gordy, P.D.: Extradural hemorrhage of the anterior and posterior fossae. J. Neurosurg., 5:294–298, 1948.

67. Grayson, M.J.: Chronic subdural haematomata associated with anticoagulant treatment. Proc. Roy. Soc. Med., 55:804–805, 1962.

68. Greenhouse, A.H., Barr, J.W.: The bilateral isodense subdural hematoma on computerized tomographic scan. Arch. Neurol., 36:305–307, 1979.

69. Gudeman, S.K., Kishore, P.R.S., Miller, J.D., Girevendulis, A.K., Lipper, M.H., Becker, D.P.: The genesis and significance of delayed traumatic intracerebral hematoma. Neurosurgery, 5:309–313, 1979.

70. Gurdjian, E.S., Gurdjian, E.S.: Cerebral contusions: re-evaluation of the mechanism of their development. J. Trauma, 16:35–51, 1976.

71. Guthkelch, A.N.: Extradural hemorrhage as a cause of cortical blindness. J. Neurosurg., 6:180–182, 1949.

72. Haar, F.L., Lott, T.M., Nichols, P. Jr.: The usefulness of CT scanning for subdural hematomas. Neurosurgery, 1:272–275, 1977.

73. Handa, J., Handa, H., Nakano, Y.: Rim enhancement in computed tomography with chronic epidural hematoma. Surg. Neurol., 11:217–220, 1979.

74. Hase, U., Reulen, H.-J., Meinig, G., Schürmann, K.: The influence of the decompressive operation on the intracranial pressure and the pressure-volume relation in patients with severe head injuries. Acta Neurochir., 45:1–13, 1978.

75. Hayman, L.A., Evans, R.A., Hinck, V.C.: Rapid-high-dose contrast computed tomography of isodense subdural hematoma and cerebral swelling. Radiology, 131:381–383, 1979.

76. Heiskanen, O.: Epidural hematoma. Surg. Neurol., 4:23–26, 1975.

77. Heiskanen, O., Vapalahti, M.: Temporal lobe contusion and haematoma. Acta Neurochir., 27:29–35, 1972.

78. Hernesniemi, J.: Outcome following acute subdural haematoma. Acta Neurochir., 49:191–198, 1979.

79. Hill, T.R.: Subdural hematoma. Proc. Roy. Soc. Med., 52:1043, 1959.

80. Hoessly, G.F.: Intracranial hemorrhage in the seventeenth century. A reappraisal of Johann Jacob Wepfer's contribution regarding subdural hematoma. J. Neurosurg., 24:493–496, 1966.

81. Hoff, J., Bates, E., Barnes, B., Glickman, M., Margolis, T.: Traumatic subdural hygroma. J. Trauma, 13:870–876, 1973.

82. Hoff, J., Grollmus, J., Barnes, B., Margolis, M.T.: Clinical, arteriographic, and cisternographic observations after removal of acute subdural hematoma. J. Neurosurg., 43:27–31, 1975.

83. Hooper, R.: Observations on extradural hemorrhage. Br. J. Surg., 47:71–87, 1959.

84. Hooper, R.S.: Extradural haemorrhages of the posterior fossa. Br. J. Surg., 42:19–26, 1954.

85. Hurwitz, S.R., Halpern, S.E., Leopold, G.: Brain scans and echoencephalography in the diagnosis of chronic subdural hematoma. J. Neurosurg., 40:347–350, 1974.

86. Ingraham, F.D., Matson, D.D.: Subdural hematoma in infancy. J. Pediatr., 24:1–37, 1944.

87. Ito, H., Komai, T., Yamamoto, S.: Fibrinolytic enzyme in the lining walls of chronic subdural

hematoma. J. Neurosurg., 48:197–200, 1978.

88. Ito, H., Yamamoto, S., Komai, T., Mizukoshi, H.: Role of local hyperfibrinolysis in the etiology of chronic subdural hematoma. J. Neurosurg., 45:26–31, 1976.

89. Iwakuma, T., Brunngraber, C.V.: Chronic extradural hematomas. A study of 21 cases. J. Neurosurg., 38:488–493, 1973.

90. Jackson, I.J., Speakman, T.J.: Chronic extradural hematoma. J. Neurosurg., 7:444–447, 1950.

91. Jamieson, K.G.: Delayed traumatic intracerebral hemorrhage. (Traumatische spätapoplexie). Aust. New Zeal. J. Surg., 23:300–307, 1954.

92. Jamieson, K.G., Yelland, J.D.N.: Extradural hematoma. Report of 167 cases. J. Neurosurg., 29:13–23, 1968.

93. Jamieson, K.G., Yelland, J.D.N.: Surgically treated traumatic subdural hematomas. J. Neurosurg., 37:137–149, 1972.

94. Jamieson, K.G., Yelland, J.D.N.: Traumatic intracerebral hematoma. Report of 63 surgically treated cases. J. Neurosurg., 37:528–532, 1972.

95. Jennett, B.: Epilepsy After Non-Missile Head Injuries, 2nd ed. Chicago, Year Book Medical Publishers, 1975.

96. Kaste, M., Waltimo, O., Heiskanen, O.: Chronic bilateral subdural haematoma in adults. Acta Neurochir., 48:231–236, 1979.

97. Kennedy, F., Wortis, H.: "Acute" subdural hematoma and acute epidural hemorrhage. A study of seventy-two cases of hematoma and seventeen cases of hemorrhage. Surg., Gyn. and Obstet., 63:732–742, 1936.

98. Kernohan, J.W., Woltman, H.W.: Incisura of the crus due to contralateral brain tumor. Arch. Neurol. Psych., 21:274–287, 1929.

99. Kim, K.S., Hemmati, M., Weinberg, P.E.: Computed tomography in isodense subdural hematoma. Radiology, 128:71–74, 1978.

100. Klug, W., Loew, F., Wüstner, S.: Zur frage der häufigkeit chronischer subduraler hämatome nach schädelverletzungen. Zentralbl. Neurochir. 21:51–56, 1961.

101. Koo, A. H., La Roque, R.L.: Evaluation of head trauma by computed tomography. Radiology, 123:345–350, 1977.

102. Kosary, I.Z., Goldhammer, Y., Lerner, M.A.: Acute extradural hematoma of the posterior fossa. J. Neurosurg., 24:1007–1012, 1966.

103. Kristransen, K., Tandon, P.: Diagnosis and surgical treatment of severe cranio-cerebral injuries. J. Oslo City Hosp., 10:105–213, 1960.

104. Kvarnes, T.L., Trumpy, J.H.: Extradural hematoma. Report of 132 cases. Acta Neurochir., 41:223–231, 1978.

105. Labadie, E.L., Glover, D.: Physiopathogenesis of subdural hematomas. Part 1: Histological and biochemical comparisons of subcutaneous hematoma in rats with subdural hematoma in man. J. Neurosurg., 45:382–392, 1976.

106. LaLonde, A.A., Gardner, W.J.: Chronic subdural hematoma. Expansion of compressed cerebral hemisphere and relief of hypotension by spinal injection of physiologic saline solution. N. Engl. J. Med., 239:493–496, 1948.

107. Laudig, G.H., Browder, E.J., Watson, R.A.: Subdural hematoma. A study of one hundred forty-three cases encountered during a five-year period. Ann. Surg., 113:170–191, 1941.

108. Leeds, N.E., Reid, N.D., Rosen, L.M.: Angiographic changes in cerebral contusions and intracerebral hematomas. Acta Radiol. Diagnosis, 5:320–327, 1966.

109. Levander, B., Stattin, S., Svendsen, P.: Computer tomography of traumatic intra- and extracerebral lesions. Acta Radiol., 346:107–118, 1975.

110. Levinthal, R., Stein, W.E.: Traumatic intracerebral hematoma with stable neurological deficit. Surg. Neurol., 7:269–273, 1977.

111. Lindenberg, R., Freytag, E.: The mechanism of cerebral contusions. A pathologic-anatomic study. Arch. Path., 69:440–469, 1960.

112. Lindenberg, R., Freytag, E.: Morphology of cortical contusions. Arch. Path., 63:23–42, 1957.

113. Lipper, M.H., Kishore, P.R.S., Girevendulis, A.K., Miller, J.D., Becker, D.P.: Delayed intracranial hematoma in patients with severe head injury. Radiology, 133:645–649, 1979.

114. Lusins, J., Jaffe, R., Bender, M.B.: Unoperated subdural hematomas. Long-term follow-up by brain scan and electroencephalography. J. Neurosurg., 44:601–607, 1976.

115. Lusins, J., Katz, J.H.: The natural history of nonsurgically treated subdural hematoma as studied by rapid-sequence scintiphotography. J. Nucl. Med., 15:1084–1088, 1974.

116. Luxon, L.M., Harrison, M.J.G.: Chronic subdural haematoma. Quart. J. Med., 189:43–53, 1979.

117. MacCarty, C.S., Horning, E.D., Weaver, E.N.: Bilateral extradural hematoma. Report of a case. J. Neurosurg., 5:88–90, 1948.

118. McKenzie, K.G.: Extradural haemorrhage. Br. J. Surg., 26:346–365, 1938.

119. McKissock, W., Richardson, A., Bloom, W.H.: Subdural haematoma. A review of 389 cases. Lancet, 1:1365–1369, 1960.

120. McLaurin, R.L.: Contributions of angiography to the pathophysiology of subdural hematomas. Neurology, 15:866–873, 1965.

121. McLaurin, R.L., Ford, L.E.: Extradural hematoma. Statistical survey of 47 cases. J. Neurosurg., 21:364–371, 1964.

122. McLaurin, R.L., Helmer, F.: The syndrome of temporal-lobe contusion. J. Neurosurg., 23:296–304, 1965.

123. McLaurin, R.L., McBride, B.H.: Traumatic intracerebral hematoma. Review of 16 surgically treated cases. Ann. Surg., 143:294–305, 1956.

124. McLaurin, R.L., Tutor, F.T.: Acute subdural hematoma. Review of ninety cases. J. Neurosurg., 18:61–67, 1961.

125. Makino, H., Yamaura, A.: Assessment of outcome following large decompressive craniectomy in management of serious cerebral contusion. A review of 207 cases. Acta Neurochirurg. Suppl., 28:193–194, 1979.

126. Marcu, H., Becker, H.: Computed-tomography of bilateral isodense chronic subdural hematomas. Neuroradiology, 14:81–83, 1977.

127. Mealey, J.: Acute extradural hematomas without

demonstrable skull fracture. J. Neurosurg., 17:27–34, 1960.

128. Mealey, J. Jr.: Gamma-ray image of subdural effusions. Scanning after injection of radio-iodinated serum albumin into subdural space and its clinical application. J. Neurosurg., 19:934–942, 1962.

129. Mealey, J. Jr.: Radioisotopic localization in subdural hematomas. An experimental study with arsenic-74 and radioiodinated human serum albumin in dogs. J. Neurosurg., 20:770–776, 1963.

130. Melamed, E., Lavy, S., Reches, A., Sahar, A.: Chronic subdural hematoma simulating transient cerebral ischemic attacks. Case report. J. Neurosurg., 42:101–103, 1975.

131. Mendelow, A.D., Karmi, M.Z., Paul, K.S., Fuller, G.A.G., Gillingham, F.J.: Extradural haematoma: effect of delayed treatment. Br. Med. J., 1:1240–1242, 1979.

132. Meredith, J.M.: Chronic or subacute subdural hematoma due to indirect head trauma. Report of two cases. J. Neurosurg., 8:444–447, 1951.

133. Merry, G.S., Stuart, G.: Extradural hematoma in the neonate—case report. J. Neurosurg., 51:713–714, 1979.

134. Messina, A.V.: Computed tomography: Contrast media within subdural hematomas. A preliminary report. Radiology, 119:725–726, 1976.

135. Miller, J.D., Becker, D.P., Ward, J.D., Sullivan, H.G., Adams, W.E., Rosner, M.J.: Significance of intracranial hypertension in severe head injury. J. Neurosurg., 47:503–516, 1977.

136. Mitsumoto, H., Conomy, J.P., Regula, G.: Ophthalmologic aspects of subdural hematoma. Cleve. Clin. Quart., 44:101–105, 1977.

137. Morantz, R.A., Abad, R.M., George, A.E., Rovit, R.L.: Hemicraniectomy for acute extra-cerebral hematoma: an analysis of clinical and radiographic findings. J. Neurosurg., 39:622–628, 1973.

138. Morin, M.A., Pitts, F.W.: Delayed apoplexy following head injury ("Traumatische spät-apoplexie"). J. Neurosurg., 33:542–547, 1970.

139. Munro, D.: Cerebral subdural hematomas. A study of three hundred and ten verified cases. N. Engl. J. Med., 227:87–95, 1942.

140. Munro, D., Maltby, G.L.: Extradural hemorrhage, a study of 44 cases. Ann. Surg., 113:192–203, 1941.

141. Munro, D., Merritt, H.H.: Surgical pathology of subdural hematoma. Based on a study of one hundred and five cases. Arch. Neurol. Psych., 35:64–78, 1936.

142. Munro, D., Sisson, W.R.: Hernia through the incisura of the tentorium cerebelli in connection with craniocerebral trauma. N. Engl. J. Med., 247:699–708, 1952.

143. Murthy, J.M.K., Chopra, J.S., Gulati, D.R.: Subdural hematoma in an adult following a blast injury. Case report. J. Neurosurg., 50:260–261, 1979.

144. Naffziger, H.C.: Subdural fluid accumulations following head injury. J.A.M.A., 82:1751–1752, 1924.

145. Negron, R.A., Tirado, G., Zapater, C.: Simple bedside technique for evacuating chronic subdural hematomas. Technical note. J. Neurosurg., 42:609–611, 1975.

146. Nelson, T.Y.: Acute subdural haematoma in the posterior fossa. Med. J. Australia, 2:792–794, 1959.

147. O'Brien, P.K., Norris, J.W., Tator, C.H.: Acute subdural hematomas of arterial origin. J. Neurosurg., 41:435–439, 1974.

148. Ogsbury, J.S., Schneck, S.A., Lehman, R.A.W.: Aspects of interhemispheric subdural haematoma, including the falx syndrome. J. Neurol. Neurosurg. Psych., 41:72–75, 1978.

149. Oka, H., Motomochi, M., Suzuki, Y., Ando, K.: Subdural hygroma after head injury. Acta. Neurochir., 26:265–273, 1972.

150. Oliff, M., Fried, A.M., Young, A.B.: Intraventricular hemorrhage in blunt head trauma. J. Comput. Asst. Tomogr., 2:625–629, 1978.

151. Parkinson, D., Chochinov, H.: Subdural hematomas—some observations on their post-operative course. J. Neurosurg., 17:901–904, 1960.

152. Pevehouse, B.C., Bloom, W.H., McKissock, W.: Ophthalmologic aspects of diagnosis and localization of subdural hematoma. An analysis of 389 cases and review of the literature. Neurology, 10:1037–1041, 1960.

153. Phonprasert, C., Suwanwela, C., Hongsaprabhas, C., Prichayudh, P., O'Charoen, S.: Extradural hematoma: analysis of 138 cases. J. Trauma, 20:679–683, 1980.

154. Potter, J.F., Fruin, A.H.: Chronic subdural hematoma—the "great imitator." Geriatrics, 32:61–66, 1977.

155. Putnam, T.J., Cushing, H.: Chronic subdural hematoma. Its pathology, its relation to pachymeningitis hemorrhagica and its surgical treatment. Arch. Surg., 11:329–393, 1925.

156. Rabe, E.F., Flynn, R.E., Dodge, P.R.: A study of subdural effusions in an infant, with particular reference to the mechanisms of their persistence. Neurology, 12:79–92, 1962.

157. Radcliffe, W.B., Guinto, E.C. Jr., Adcock, D.F.: Subdural hematoma shape. A new look at an old concept. Am. J. Roentgenol. Rad. Ther. Nucl. Med., 115:72–77, 1972.

158. Rand, B.O., Ward, A.A. Jr., White, L.E. Jr.: The use of the twist drill to evaluate head trauma. J. Neurosurg., 25:410–415, 1966.

159. Ransohoff, J., Benjamin, M.V., Gage, E.L. Jr., Epstein, F.: Hemicraniectomy in the management of acute subdural hematoma. J. Neurosurg., 34:70–76, 1971.

160. Raskind, R., Glover, M.B., Weiss, S.R.: Chronic subdural hematoma in the elderly: a challenge in diagnosis and treatment. J. A. Geriatr. Soc., 20:330–334, 1972.

161. Reigh, E.E., Nelson, M.: Posterior-fossa subdural hematoma with secondary hydrocephalus. Report of case and review of the literature. J. Neurosurg., 19:346–348, 1962.

162. Richards, T., Hoff, J.: Factors affecting survival from acute subdural hematoma. Surgery, 75:253–258, 1974.

163. Rieth, K.G., Schwartz, F.T., Davis, D.O.: Acute

isodense epidural hematoma on computed tomography. Case report. J. Comp. Asst. Tomog., 3:691–693, 1979.

164. Robinson, R.G.: The treatment of subacute and chronic subdural haematomas. Br. Med. J., 1:21–22, 1955.

165. Rosenbluth, P.R., Arias, B., Quartetti, E.V., Carney, A.L.: Current management of subdural hematoma. Analysis of 100 consecutive cases. J.A.M.A., 179:759–762, 1962.

166. Rosenørn, J., Gjerris, F.: Long-term follow-up review of patients with acute and subacute subdural hematomas. J. Neurosurg., 48:345–349, 1978.

167. Samiy, E.: Chronic subdural hematoma presenting a Parkinsonian syndrome. J. Neurosurg., 20:903, 1963.

168. Sato, S., Suzuki, J.: Ultrastructural observations of the capsule of chronic subdural hematoma in various clinical stages. J. Neurosurg., 43:569–578, 1975.

169. Schneider, R.C., Lemmen, L.J., Bagchi, B.K.: The syndrome of traumatic intracerebellar hematoma. With contrecoup supratentorial complications. J. Neurosurg., 10:122–137, 1953.

170. Schonauer, M., Schisano, G., Cimino, R., Viola, L.: Space occupying contusions of cerebral lobes after closed brain injury. Considerations about 51 cases. J. Neurosurg. Sci., 23:279–288, 1979.

171. Scotti, G., Terbrugge, K., Melancon, D., Belanger, G.: Evaluation of the age of subdural hematomas by computerized tomography. J. Neurosurg., 47:311–315, 1977.

172. Seeler, R.A., Imana, R.B.: Intracranial hemorrhage in patients with hemophilia. J. Neurosurg., 39:181–185, 1973.

173. Shigemori, M., Syojima, K., Nakayama, K., Kojima, T., Watanabe, M., Kuramoto, S.: Outcome of acute subdural haematoma following decompressive hemicraniectomy. Acta Neurochir. Suppl., 28:195–198, 1979.

174. Stone, J.L., Lang, R.G.R., Sugar, O., Moody, R.A.: Traumatic subdural hygroma. Neurosurgery, 8:542–550, 1981.

175. Strang, P.R., Tovi, D.: Subdural haematomas complicating anticoagulant therapy. Br. Med. J., 1:845–846, 1962.

176. Suzuki, J., Takaku, A.: Nonsurgical treatment of chronic subdural hematoma. J. Neurosurg., 33:548–553, 1970.

177. Svien, H.J., Gelety, J.E.: On the surgical management of encapsulated subdural hematoma. A comparison of the results of membranectomy and simple evacuation. J. Neurosurg., 21:172–177, 1964.

178. Sweet, R.C., Miller, J.D., Lipper, M., Kishore, P.R.S., Becker, D.P.: Significance of bilateral abnormalities on the CT scan in patients with severe head injury. Neurosurgery, 3:16–20, 1978.

179. Symonds, C.P.: Delayed traumatic intracerebral haemorrhage. Br. Med. J., 1:1048–1051, 1940.

180. Tabaddor, K., Shulman, K.: Definitive treatment of chronic subdural hematoma by twist-drill craniostomy and closed-system drainage. J. Neurosurg., 46:220–226, 1977.

181. Talalla, A., Morin, M.A.: Acute traumatic subdural hematoma: a review of one hundred consecutive cases. J. Trauma, 11:771–777, 1971.

182. Teasdale, G., Galbraith, S.: Extradural hematoma: effect of delayed treatment. Br. Med. J., 1:1793, 1979.

183. Teasdale, G., Galbraith, S., Jennett, B.: Operate or observe? ICP and the management of the "silent" traumatic intracranial hematoma. Intracranial Pressure IV. Shulman, K., Marmarou, A., Miller, J.D., Becker, D.P., Hochwald, G.M., Brock, M. Eds., Springer-Verlag, Berlin, 1980, pp. 36–38.

184. Tindall, G.T., Payne, N.S. II, O'Brien, M.S.: Complications of surgery for subdural hematoma. Clin. Neurosurg., 23:465–482, 1976.

185. Treil, J., Morel, C., Bonafe, A., Manelfe, C.: Traumatic rupture of the middle meningeal artery. Angiographic appearances—a review of 30 cases. J. Neuroradiol., 4:399–414, 1977.

186. Trotter, W.: Chronic subdural haemorrhage of traumatic origin and its relation to pachymeningitis haemorrhagica interna. Br. J. Surg., 2:271–291, 1914.

187. Tsai, F.Y., Huprich, J.E., Segall, H.D., Teal, J.S.: The contrast-enhanced CT scan in the diagnosis of isodense subdural hematoma. J. Neurosurg., 50:64–69, 1979.

188. Turnbull, F.: Extradural cerebellar hematoma. A case report. J. Neurosurg., 1:321–324, 1944.

189. Ugrumov, V.M., Zotov, Yu.V., Shchedryonok, V.V.: Early surgical treatment of traumatic intracranial haematomas and laceration foci as the main factor for favourable prognosis. Acta Neurochir. Suppl., 28:199–200, 1979.

190. Watanabe, S., Shimada, H., Ishii, S.: Production of clinical form of chronic subdural hematoma in experimental animals. J. Neurosurg., 37:552–561, 1972.

191. Webber, G.: Das chronische subduralhämatom. Schweiz Med Wochenschr 99:1483–1488, 1969.

192. Weinman, D., Muttucumaru, B.: Extradural hematoma. Ceylon Med. J., 14:60–71, 1969.

193. Weir, B.: The osmolality of subdural hematoma fluid. J. Neurosurg., 34:528–533, 1971.

194. Whitehurst, W.R., Christensen, F.K.: Epidural hemorrhage from traumatic laceration of internal carotid artery. J. Neurosurg., 31:352–354, 1969.

195. Williams, R.S.: Chronic subdural hematoma simulating transient ischemic attacks. Ann. Neurol., 5:597, 1979.

196. Wright, R.L.: Traumatic hematomas of the posterior cranial fossa. J. Neurosurg., 25:402–409, 1966.

197. Yamaura, A., Uemura, K., Makino, H.: Large decompressive craniectomy in management of severe cerebral contusion. A review of 207 cases. Neurol. Med. Chir. (Tokyo), 19:717–728, 1979.

198. Zimmerman, R.A., Bilaniuk, L.T.: Computer tomography of traumatic intracerebral hemorrhagic lesions: the change in density and mass effect with time. Neuroradiology, 16:320–321, 1978.

199. Zimmerman, R.A., Bilaniuk, L.T., Dolinskas, C., Gennarelli, T., Bruce, D., Uzzell, B.: Computed tomography of acute intracerebral hemorrhagic contusions. Comp. Axial Tomogr., 1:271–280, 1977.

200. Zimmerman, R.A., Bilaniuk, L.T., Gennarelli, T., Bruce, D., Dolinskas, C., Uzzell, B.: Cranial computed tomography in diagnosis and management of acute head trauma. Am. J. Roentgenol.,

131:27–34, 1978.

201. Zollinger, R., Gross, R.E.: Traumatic subdural hematoma. An explanation of the late onset of pressure symptoms. J.A.M.A., 103:245–249, 1934.

202. Zuccarello, M., Pardatscher, K., Andrioli, G.C., Fiore, D.L., Iavicali, R., Cervellini, P.: Epidural hematomas of the posterior cranial fossa. Neurosurgery, 8:434–437, 1981.

12

Traumatic Brain Swelling and Edema

RICHARD D. PENN
RAYMOND A. CLASEN

Many of the most perplexing clinical and experimental problems in trauma are related to the role of cerebral edema. Gross evidence of brain swelling after head injury is a familiar sight in both the operating room and at the autopsy table, but the histologic basis for this has remained elusive.[40] Fortunately, a number of new techniques are available to study human traumatic cerebral edema in much greater detail than was previously possible. The most notable is computerized tomography (CT) which, for the first time, allows visualization and quantification of cerebral edema in the living patient. The correlation of the CT image with histologic studies of brains obtained at autopsy should provide a clarification of the histologic basis of brain swelling. Other techniques, such as positron emission tomography will provide measurements of cerebral blood volume and metabolism in the brain-injured patient.[78] It is hoped that these tools will provide information which will soon lead to more appropriate therapy.

In this chapter, the various forms of cerebral edema will be reviewed briefly. The CT characteristics of cerebral swelling in brain trauma will be presented. To empha-size the importance of correlating the CT image with corresponding pathological changes in the brain, a histologic study of a case of acute brain trauma in which a CT scan was obtained shortly before death will be described in detail. Since experimental models of cerebral edema have been so important in the development of current therapeutic approaches, various models will be evaluated. Finally, the thorny problems of the treatment of cerebral edema will be discussed.

The definitions of brain swelling and edema have changed as knowledge of their causes has evolved. Current usage in the United States is often confusing because swelling and edema are used interchangeably by some authors. Cerebral edema is a specialized form of swelling in which the brain substance is expanded because of an increase in tissue fluid.[47]

Brain swelling may also result from an increase in the cerebral intravascular blood volume (hyperemia).[55] This distinction is of more than academic importance; for if this type of swelling is present, the treatment would be quite different from that for cerebral edema. In fact, mannitol, commonly employed to decrease brain volume in patients with cerebral edema, might be contraindicated for patients with hyperemia or vascular congestion. For these reasons we will distinguish between the general term cerebral swelling and the specialized type of swelling, *e.g.*, edema, that occurs when fluid is added to the brain substance.

Acknowledgements: Support for this work was provided by grants from the National Institute of Neurological and Communicative Disorders and Stroke #NS15522 (Richard D. Penn, M.D.) and Grant #NS=03677 (Raymond Clasen, M.D.).

VARIETIES OF EDEMA

Five different types of cerebral edema have been recognized from laboratory and clinical studies; vasogenic, cytotoxic, hydrocephalic, osmotic, and ischemic (Table 12.1). Vasogenic edema involves primarily white matter, is extracellular, and the edema fluid contains plasma proteins. Cytotoxic edema is intracellular, involves either white or gray matter, and the edema fluid contains only electrolytes.[49] In hydrocephalic edema, the edema fluid is cerebrospinal fluid.[60] Osmotic edema is intracellular in gray matter and extracellular in white matter.[101] The edema fluid is a hypotonic ultrafiltrate of plasma.[102] This form of edema is often classified with the cytotoxic form.[26] While ischemic edema has some of the characteristics of cytotoxic edema, there are sufficient differences to use separate terms.

Vasogenic edema is relatively easy to identify in routine histologic sections because the protein containing edema fluid may be stained red with the periodic acid-Schiff (PAS) technique and the nerve fibers a contrasting blue with luxol fast blue. The red staining of the edema fluid is a reflection of its globulin content.[12] Cytotoxic edema shows vacuolation of tissue without histologic evidence of cellular necrosis. Hydrocephalic and osmotic edema show a similar histologic picture. In ischemic edema, there is vacuolation with accompanying neuronal necrosis. The white matter stains poorly with myelin stains and there is enlargement of the extracellular space.[31]

CT SCANNING AND EDEMA

The visualization of the brain and intracranial pathology by CT scanning is so striking an advance that one frequently forgets the physical basis for the image. The basic data of the CT scanner are a series of numbers, representing X-ray absorption of tissue, displayed in a matrix. To understand how these numbers are found, the concept of attenuation must be considered. Attenuation is the reduction in the intensity of an X-ray beam as it traverses matter by either the absorption or deflection of photons.[8]

The CT scanner offers great promise for measuring cerebral edema in the human brain. If tissue water increases without changes in chemical composition, its absorption values will fall. The actual value of the edematous tissue reflects its relative dry weight, or conversely the percentage increase in water. In vasogenic edema, water, electrolytes, and varying amounts of plasma protein enter the tissue together. Complete replacement by an edema fluid low in protein would result in spinal fluid density. The displayed image composed of these absorption values therefore shows edema as a darker region than normal white matter but lighter than CSF. If it can be

Table 12.1

Type of Edema	Vasogenic	Cytotoxic	Hydrocephalic	Ischemic	Osmotic
Pathogenesis	Increased capillary permeability	Disturbed intracellular metabolism	Increased ventricular pressure	Diminished oxygen supply	Hypo-osmolarity of plasma
Fluid	Plasma filtrate	Plasma ultrafiltrate	Cerebrospinal fluid	?	Hypotonic plasma ultrafiltrate
Location	White matter extracellular	White or gray matter intracellular	White matter extracellular	White and gray matter	Gray matter intracellular; white matter extracellular
Blood-Brain Barrier	Disrupted	Intact	Intact	Variable	Intact
CT	White matter hypodensity	?	White matter hypodensity	White and gray matter hypodensity	?
Clinical or experimental example	Head injury brain tumor	Triethyl tin poisoning	Hydrocephalus	Cerebral infarction	Water intoxication

assumed that edematous tissue contains no significant neutral lipid, the water content may be determined from the magnitude of decrease of the attenuation number.[74]

All regions which are darker than normal on the CT scan are not regions of edema. Edema implies swelling so there must be an associated mass effect. Hypodensity reflecting a relative increase in water due to a decrease in tissue dry mass may be seen in the cystic atrophy of infarction. This is of great importance in interpreting CT pictures of trauma, especially several weeks or months after the initial injury when such a condition might occur. While vasogenic edema is readily identified, cytotoxic swelling which involves gray matter may not be obvious. The water shifts are less, and gray matter may be difficult to visualize on the scan. Ischemic edema has been studied in detail in stroke patients, and is a much more complex process because of the biochemical changes which occur. The usual course of an ischemic region is to be of normal density for hours to days and then to become hypodense whether or not mass effect develops.[10] Hydrocephalic edema, which may occur in the aftermath of trauma with the blockage of CSF flow, is hypodense on the CT scan.

Although enhancement by intravascular infusion of contrast agents is not frequently used in trauma, a few points should be made about the technique. Normally, the contrast material remains within the vascular space. The falx enhances because it is outside the blood-brain barrier and the glomus of the choroid plexus appears because of its high blood volume. To the eye, the normal brain does not seem to increase in density, but measurements show that in fact, it does go up reflecting the blood volume, which is approximately 3% of the brain parenchyma.[76]

If the blood-brain barrier is disrupted in traumatized brain, the contrast material will extravasate into the tissue and will be visualized as a whiter region because of increased absorption. The edema fluid does not enhance. Indeed, as the fluid in an area of vasogenic edema increases, the blood volume decreases. For this reason, enhancement in these areas is *less* than normal.[75]

Cerebral Swelling in Trauma as Revealed by the CT Scan

Primary traumatic cerebral swelling usually involves both hemispheres. This diffuse form has been reported to occur in 4%,[19] 7%,[56] and 16%[111] of all patients and in 28%[110] of head-injured patients in the pediatric age group. Some authors, however, do not recognize the entity,[21, 28, 53] and those who do admit that the diagnosis is difficult and may require serial scans.[103] The swelling is characterized by obliteration of ventricles and cisterns by homogeneous tissue which, in the adult, has normal density.[56] In children, there is a measurable increase in the attenuation number of white matter and a subsequent decrease in attenuation back to normal levels as the condition resolves over a one week period.[110] In adults, the mortality rate has been reported as 33 and 50%, but in children it is only 6%. The difference in mortality and in the density on scan implies that these are different conditions.

When diffuse swelling is associated with small parenchymal hemorrhages (especially in the region of the corpus callosum) and subarachnoid hemorrhage, the condition has been designated as shearing injury of the white matter.[109, 112] Typically, patients with this injury are in deep coma and generally have decerebrate posturing. In another similar report, patients showing immediate decerebration after trauma were found to have swollen white matter with decreased attenuation.[15] The prognosis for recovery in these patients is poor, but some do survive. After six months, the few survivors had marked atrophic changes in the white matter.

Occasionally, cerebral swelling may be confined to one hemisphere and has been described as occurring as early as 20–30 minutes after trauma.[52, 100] Beginning resolution is demonstrable in six hours and is complete by two weeks. The initial clinical picture has been variable. Of two patients reported with this condition and no other demonstrable lesions, one was comatose on admission but the other never lost consciousness. The latter made a complete recovery and the former showed only a persistent Babinski sign on discharge. Swelling confined to one hemisphere is rare and was not mentioned in several large series of hospitalized patients.[19, 28, 56, 110, 111] One reason may be related to its transient nature, and to the fact that if this swelling were associated with other conditions, such as hemorrhage, it could not be diagnosed.

The presence of diffuse traumatic swelling on scan does not necessarily imply increased intracranial pressure (ICP).[110] In fact, quite the opposite is found. In one series in which ICP monitoring was done, 27 out of 29 had ICP less than 15 mm Hg. This relatively low pressure was associated with good functional recovery.[91]

Diffuse traumatic swelling of both the general and hemispheric form has been attributed to vascular congestion. Initial studies utilizing the xenon washout method reported an increased blood flow in these patients.[68, 111] The investigators recognized that increased flow alone could not quantitatively account for the rise in attenuation number.[110] Furthermore, vascular congestion could not provide a sufficient increase in volume to collapse the cerebral ventricles. Even a doubling of the cerebral blood volume would increase the brain volume by only 45 cc. Recent studies using technetium-labeled red blood cells and emission computed tomography in several patients have shown that diffuse traumatic swelling may occur in the face of a measured *decrease* in cerebral blood volume.[54] If this is confirmed in a large number of patients, a blood volume increase would be eliminated as an explanation for the swelling. An alternative theory has not yet been proposed to account for this important clinical and CT phenomenon (see Chapter 16).

A second form of primary traumatic ·swelling appears as focal areas of hypodensity on the CT scan. This has been variously described as Type I (non-hemorrhagic) contusion[56] or focal cerebral edema.[112] It occurs in 14% of patients.[63] Increased ICP is seen in approximately one-third of these patients. Mortality rates of 7%[56] and 35%[63] have been reported. The lesions resolved in 2–3 weeks[56] or earlier.[77] There is also a form of hypodense cerebral swelling which may involve one entire hem-

isphere.[53, 99] This lesion may be responsible for neurologic deterioration in the first week after trauma.[13] Whether holohemispheric edema should be considered an extensive Type I contusion or diffuse edema cannot be determined since the histopathology of neither has been defined. One group has expressed the opinion that the focal hypodense lesions in trauma are due to anoxia,[63] but again, histological proof is lacking.

Type II contusions contain areas of hemorrhage in the hypodense foci producing a mottled or salt and pepper appearance.[56] The mortality rate for Type II contusion is 41%. Contusions plus perifocal edema occur in 27% of patients, and the mortality rate is 43%. Increased ICP occurred in 58% of these patients. From the CT scan alone, one cannot determine if the perifocal edema involves only the necrotic tissue of the contusion or if there is also involvement of the adjacent viable white matter.

In any correlative study of CT scans and pathology, timing is important. In a recent study of traumatized patients, a correlation of only 72% was reported for CT findings and neuropathology.[86] This could well be related to the time intervals between the scan and the autopsy which were not stated in the paper.

In the absence of a clinical history, a hypodense area on the CT scan which does not show mass effect may not be confidently labeled as edema. For example, to attribute a low density lesion seen 25 days after trauma to edema is inappropriate.[66] At this time, the edema has subsided and there is active phagocytosis with transformation of compound lipids into neutral lipids.[58] This is yet another factor in producing hypodensity on the CT scan,[47] small contusions generally resolve within two weeks[109] but larger lesions may persist on the CT scan as cystic areas. This point is illustrated in Figures 12.1 through 12.3. The specimen was obtained from an epileptic patient with a history of old head trauma. The cystic areas on the base of the frontal lobes are not infarcts. They do not have a vascular distribution and their histopathology differs from old infarction.[58] It is not appropriate to call hypodense areas which persist on the CT scans of patients with head trauma infarcts[77] unless it can be proven that they are not old contusions.

CT and Histopathology of Trauma— Case Study

Pathologic changes seen in acute head trauma are illustrated in the following case report: the patient, a 31-year-old white male, was admitted to an outlying hospital in coma a short time after an automobile accident. He had a right temporal hematoma, proptosis of the right eye, periorbital hemorrhage and bilateral hemotympanum. The right pupil measured 2 mm and the left 5 mm. Both were nonreactive. Doll's eye movements were absent, and no caloric response could be obtained. The extremities were flaccid and a Babinski sign was present bilaterally. Skull X-rays revealed an extensive depressed fracture of the right

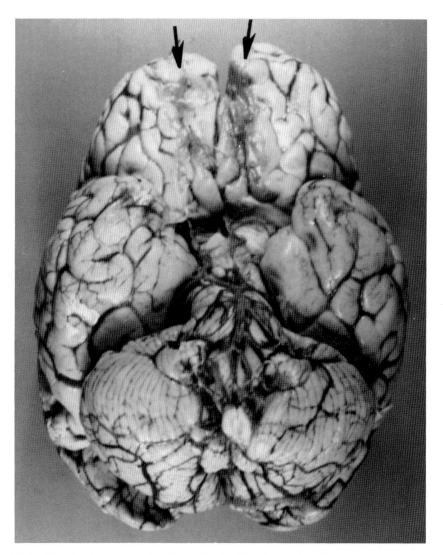

Figure 12.1 The brain of an epileptic patient with a long-standing history of head trauma showing bifrontal contusions (*arrows*).

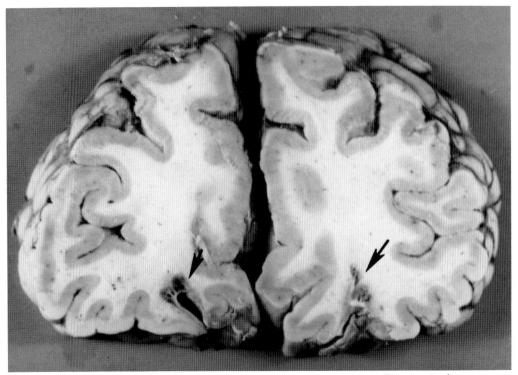

Figure 12.2 Coronal section of the brain shown in Figure 12.1. The contusions appear as cystic areas (*arrows*) but are not infarcts.

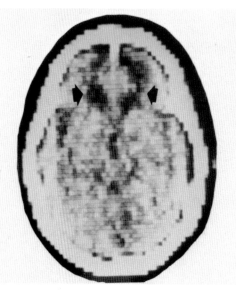

Figure 12.3 CT scan of the patient whose brain was shown in Figures 12.1 and 12.2 obtained shortly before his death. 80 × 80 matrix, not enhanced. The old contusions appear as hypodense areas (*arrows*).

cranial vault. On admission to our hospital, his temperature was 104.3°F., pulse 146/minute, respirations were 28/minute, and blood pressure 90/60 mm Hg. The pupils were fixed and dilated. A CT scan showed areas of lucency and hemorrhage in the right temporal lobe (Type II contusion) and a lucency in the occipital lobe (Type I contusion) with compression of the right lateral ventricle. He expired three hours later, less than 24 hours from the time of trauma.

At autopsy, there was an extensive right-sided depressed skull fracture extending from the frontal to the occipital bone. The brain showed a large contusion with surface hemorrhage on the lateral surface of the right temporal lobe. The left hemisphere weighed 718 g and the right 811 g, a 13% increase in weight on the right side. Sections of the brain, cut in the plane of the CT scanner are shown in Figures 12.4 and 12.5. In addition to the massive contusion on the right, smaller contre-coup contusions are shown in the left temporal lobe (Fig. 12.4). Petechial hemorrhages are found in the corpus callosum (Fig. 12.5) indicating a shearing injury. Figure 12.6 compares these sections with the corresponding cuts of the CT scans. The large contusion appears as an irregular hypodense area containing focal areas of hyperdensity. These correspond to areas of contusional hemorrhage and blood in the Sylvian fissure shown in black in the gross specimen. Areas of primary traumatic injury are crosshatched. The contused areas in the temporal and frontal lobes, show, in addition to petechial hemorrhages, diffuse edema of the neuropil (Fig. 12.7). These changes are not found in the uninvolved cortex (Figure 12.8). The neurons in the contused area generally have pyknotic nuclei and a cytoplasm which stains red with eosin. Although this is considered to represent an ischemic change, the "red and dead"[40] picture is, in fact, non-specific and could be the direct effect of trauma. Glial cells with necrotic nuclei are also seen but these are less prominent than the neuronal

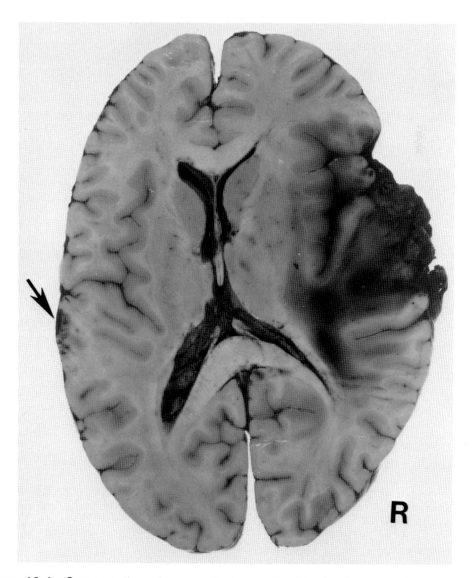

Figure 12.4 Cross-section of a recently traumatized brain showing a large temporal contusion on the right and a smaller contusion on the left (*arrow*).

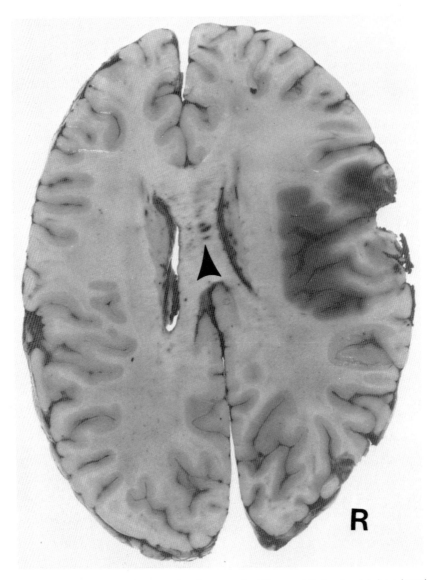

Figure 12.5 Photograph of same brain seen in Figure 12.4 at a higher level showing petechial hemorrhages in the corpus callosum (*arrowhead*) as well as the larger contusion.

changes. The contused gray matter also showed areas in which the neuropil was homogeneous (Fig. 12.9). We view these homogeneous areas as regions of total necrosis in which the astrocytes can no longer react to injury by swelling. There was a mild accompanying acute inflammation characterized by polymorphonuclear leukocytes within perivascular spaces (Fig. 12.10). In places these extended for a short distance into the tissue. In the occipital contused gray matter, these inflammatory changes were found with rare petechial hemorrhages (Figure 12.11), but no evidence of neuronal or glial cell death. Although the neuropil in this illustration appears to be mildly vacuolated, it could, in fact, not be distinguished from the gray

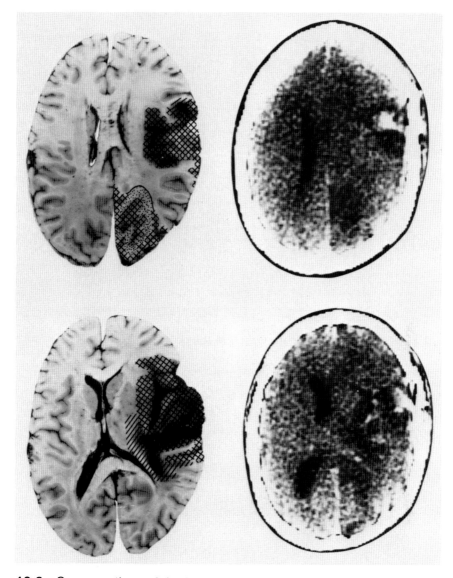

Figure 12.6 Cross-sections of the brain compared with the corresponding cuts of the CT scans. Areas of contusion identified histologically are cross hatched and areas of edema hatched and stippled. The smaller area of contusion in the left hemisphere does not appear on the CT scan and has not been included.

matter in the left occipital lobe and it was interpreted as being normal.

Contused white matter showed a more variable picture, the only constant feature being the presence of acute inflammation. In some areas, the nuclei were markedly pyknotic, and pools of PAS-positive edema fluid were present. In other areas, the nu-

clear changes were not impressive but myelin basket figures were very prominent. The most frequent change was simply pallor of the myelinated fibers with the luxol fast blue stain (Fig. 12.12).

The white matter adjacent to the massive contusion showed separation of the nerve fibers by PAS-positive edema fluid without

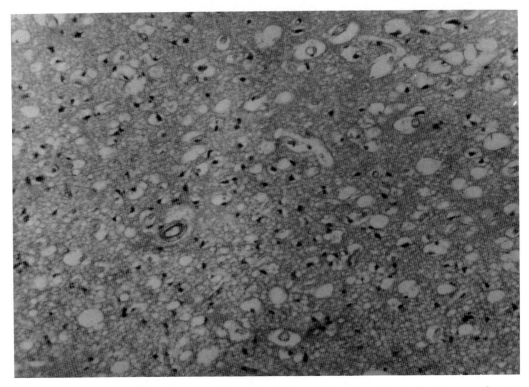

Figure 12.7 High power photomicrograph of the contused cortex in the temporal area. This and all subsequent photomicrographs are stained by the luxol fast blue-periodic acid-Schiff hematoxylin technique. The neuropil is vacuolated.

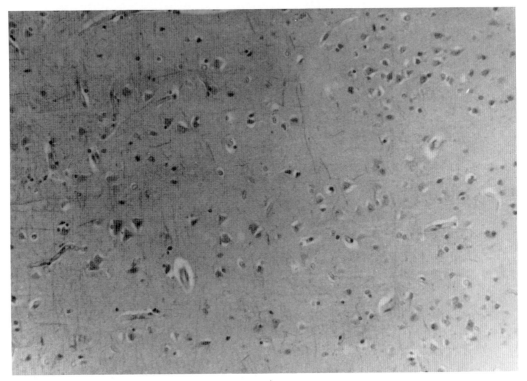

Figure 12.8 High power photomicrograph of uninvolved cortex. The neuropil is homogeneous and there is no evidence of cellular damage.

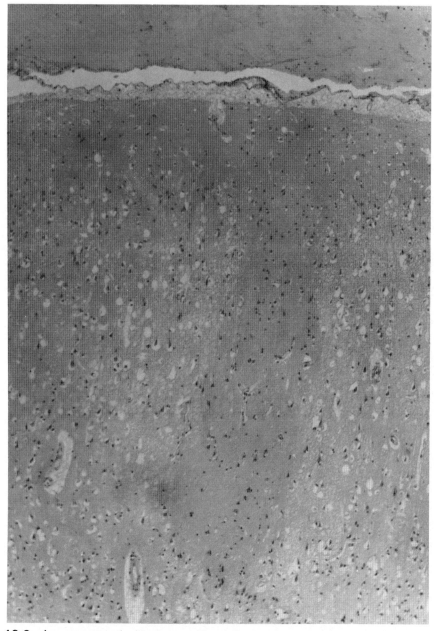

Figure 12.9 Low power photomicrograph of the temporal contusion. An area in which the neuropil is homogeneous is seen between the vacuolated areas. Both areas show marked evidence of cellular damage.

evidence of cellular damage (Figure 12.13). The nerve fibers stained well with luxol fast blue and few myelin basket figures were seen. This is the classical picture of vaso-genic edema. It is shown as a hatched area on the gross sections (Fig. 12.6). The white matter in the occipital area showed similar changes but there was no evidence of PAS-

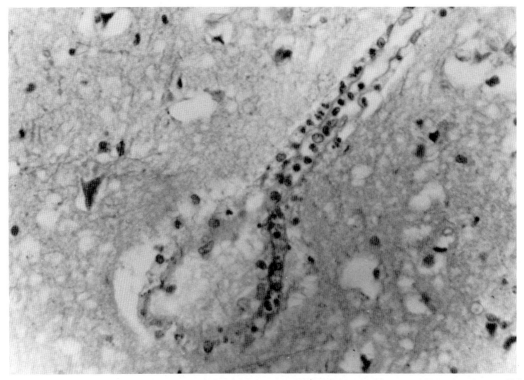

Figure 12.10 High power photomicrograph of the temporal contusion showing mild acute inflammation.

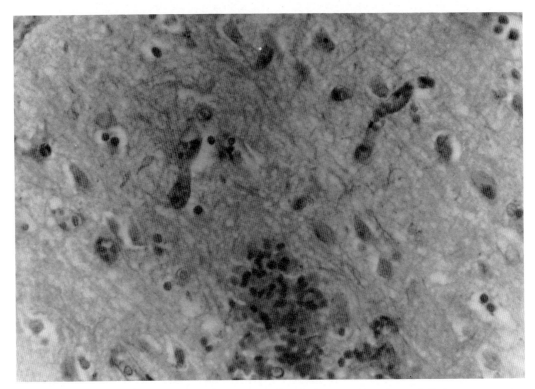

Figure 12.11 High power photomicrograph of the contused occipital gray matter showing a petechial hemorrhage without evidence of marked vacuolation of the neuropil.

positive fluid between the fibers (Fig. 12.14 and stippled area in Fig. 12.7). The individual nerve fibers did not show diminished staining. This change could only be appreciated by careful comparison with the white matter of the opposite hemisphere (Fig. 12.15). There were no inflammatory changes in this white matter.

The lateral contusion seen pathologically corresponds to a Type II contusion on CT scan.[56] The hypodensity is due to edematous changes in the contused white matter and accompanying vasogenic edema. The principal change, however, seems to be cellular swelling within the injured gray matter. If these cellular changes are attributed to anoxia, then the term *ischemic edema* could be used. However, without proof of this, the term *traumatic cellular swelling* is a better description of this condition.

Care must be taken in interpreting histological changes in gray matter, since too rapid dehydration will produce in normal tissue the same findings as in Figure 12.7.[25] For that reason, slow dehydration was used in our preparations. The fact that hypodensity was seen on CT scan in the precise region that these histological abnormalities

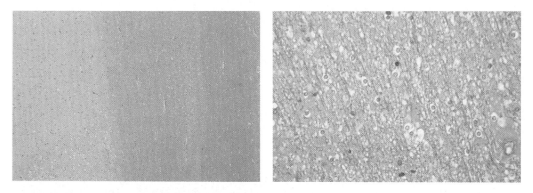

Figure 12.12 (*Left*) Low power photomicrograph of the border of the temporal contusion. The contused white matter stains less intensely than the adjacent normal white matter.

Figure 12.13 (*Right*) High power photomicrograph of the hatched edematous area in Figure 12.6. The enlarged extracellular space contains PAS-positive edema fluid.

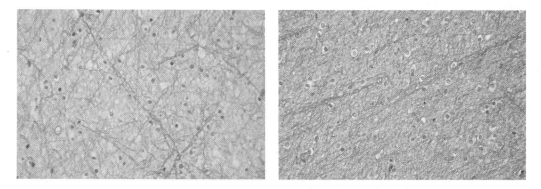

Figure 12.14 (*Left*) High power photomicrograph of the stippled edematous area in Figure 12.6. There is no stainable material in the enlarged extracellular space.

Figure 12.15 (*Right*) High power photomicrograph taken from the normal white matter of the left occipital lobe in an area comparable to Figure 12.14.

are found also argues for real, not artifactual change.

Focal edema is illustrated by the hypodensity on CT scan in the right occipital region. Judging only by the scan, the occipital lucency in Figure 12.6 might be interpreted as an occipital infarct secondary to focal swelling (Cone-Reid phenomenon). Histological examination (Figure 12.11) shows that this is not the case. The cortex had petechial hemorrhages and signs of acute inflammation, but no traumatic cellular swelling. The lucency is due to the white matter edema. The lack of inflammation in the white matter indicates that it is not part of the contusion *per se*. Rather, the edema appears to be secondary and corresponds to a Type I contusion. Since it only involves the white matter, one interpretation is that it is vasogenic edema. However, the edema lacks demonstrable protein by PAS staining, so it does not have one important characteristic of the vasogenic form. For that reason, it is best labeled as traumatic focal white matter edema until its origin is better understood.

The histologic correlations of CT Type I and Type II contusions are only for this single case. Obviously, many more cases will have to be examined before general conclusions can be drawn. This example does emphasize the importance of precise topological correlation of histology with CT changes. Simple gross comparisons[86] would have missed the occipital lobe changes, and with random histologic sections the occipital lobe edema would probably have been missed. Careful mapping is mandatory if the CT scan is going to help sort out the different types of traumatic edema.

EXPERIMENTAL CEREBRAL TRAUMA

Extradural Balloon Placement

Extradural balloon compression has been used to simulate acute epidural hematomas.[45] The original method used in cats consisted of inflating a balloon, maintaining the compression for 24 hours, and then deflating it. Gross swelling of the damaged hemisphere was found to be greatest 24 hours after decompression, and subsided by 48 hours. Examined by light microscopy, the white matter showed a spongy appearance with the Kluver technique. Unfortunately, the microscopic description was not complete. Electron microscopic study of these brains[79, 92] demonstrated passage of intravenous ferritin by pinocytosis into an enlarged extracellular space of white matter, as well as myelin and cellular breakdown. In the original paper, increased uptake of diiodofluorescein by the damaged hemisphere was reported. This was more marked in gray matter than white matter. Similar results were seen with intravenous Evans blue.[18] The latter experiments included chemical measurements. The gray matter of the compressed hemisphere showed, on a dry weight basis, an increase in water and sodium, but no decrease in potassium.

A modification of this technique has been reported in rats. A rubber bar is inserted through a 2-mm burr hole and left in place for 24 hours. Then, 24 hours after removal, the rat is sacrificed. Vital staining with Evans blue occurred at the site of implantation, and the compressed hemisphere had an increase in tissue water[108] compared to the opposite side. The whole brain had an increase in water and sodium and a decrease in potassium on a dry weight basis.[107]

One wonders if the epidural balloon model is basically an ischemic lesion[104] with restoration of blood flow after decompression.[55] The time course of the uptake of iodinated dye closely parallels the swelling accompanying human ischemic infarction[87] and the morphologic findings are consistent with ischemic damage. The compression models may have relevance for the cerebral swelling which often follows surgical evacuation of blood clots.[56]

Physical Trauma

The symptoms of concussion may be produced in animals by striking a column of water in contact with the exposed dura.[85] In rabbits, the trauma is associated with a transient exudation of serum proteins into the brain stem and cervical cord. Dogs subjected to a similar injury showed no chemical evidence of cerebral edema in the cerebral hemispheres.[22]

The only experimental models utilizing blows to the head in which hemispheric cerebral swelling has been demonstrated occurred when the head of the animal was unrestrained rather than held stationary. Diffuse cerebral swelling has been produced in the cat by delivering a blow over the occiput with a swinging pendulum at striking speeds of 34–46 feet per second.[105] The swelling appeared within 15 minutes of trauma, reached its maximum in 5–24 hours and subsided within three days. Although there were several instances of small extracerebral intracranial hemorrhages and skull fracture, none of the hemispheres showed gross or microscopic evidence of contusions. In the normal cat, the brain occupies 89% of the intracranial cavity. Following trauma, the brains occupied between 91 and 95% of the intracranial space. No evidence of ventricular dilatation or a measurable change in blood volume was found. The histologic basis for the cerebral swelling demonstrated in this model was not evident on light microscopy.

This cat model is as close as we can come on an experimental basis to the diffuse traumatic swelling observed in human CT scans. Since tissue chemical data were not included in this study, we cannot predict whether X-ray density would be changed. The lack of a clear histopathologic basis for this swelling, however, suggests that it may be isodense. Tissue chemistry, electron microscopy and CT scanning are needed to resolve these issues.

The edema associated with cerebral contusion has been studied by vital staining and specific gravity measurements of brain tissue, but has not been well characterized by histologic methods. In the impact sled model, distention of perivascular and pericellular spaces and glial swelling is mentioned but not illustrated.[51] The vital staining of the white matter found in the sled model implies the presence of PAS-positive extracellular edema fluid and would correspond to the component of vasogenic edema described in our case report (Fig. 12.13). Intravenous fluorescein in the Rhesus monkey shows the dye in the contusion and associated edematous region.[71] Large contusions produced in the cat result in a decrease in the specific gravity of the white matter 10 to 14 mm beyond the gross margin of the injury.[93] The decrease is consistent with edema fluid. The pericontusional tissue may well be the counterpart of the vitally stained white matter in the Rhesus monkey.[51] Unfortunately, the histology and vital staining of this tissue were not reported.

Focal traumatic edema has been produced in rats. After an occipital blow to the movable head, mild edema in the frontal white matter was seen.[4] Animals with gross contusion were eliminated from the study. The frontal cortex showed slight swelling of the perivascular astrocytic processes and some enlargement of the extracellular space. Interestingly, intravenous ferritin particles were found in the gray matter extracellular space, but not in the white matter. This is as close as we can come to an experimental counterpart of the Type I non-hemorrhagic contusion.

Cryogenic Cerebral Injury

The experimental prototype of vasogenic edema is that associated with focal freezing of the brain. The model has been the subject of numerous chemical and physiological investigations and is the only model of traumatic cerebral swelling that has been studied by CT scanning.[9, 84] The edema has been well characterized by light[2, 50] and electron microscopy.[3, 59] It is primarily confined to the white matter which has enlarged extracellular spaces containing PAS-positive, slightly electron opaque fluid. Intracellular swelling of glial elements in the edematous white matter and in the gray matter adjacent to the lesion has also been described. Both intravenous ferritin[57] and horseradish peroxidase[5] are demonstrable in the expanded extracellular space of the white matter.

The edema associated with the cryogenic lesion spreads from the lesion into the adjacent white matter by bulk flow.[82] When this fluid reaches the ependyma, it passes into the CSF. The clearance is dependent upon the pressure gradient between the edematous tissue and the cerebrospinal fluid. When the gradient is increased by lowering CSF pressure, clearance is enhanced and edema decreases.[83]

THERAPEUTIC STUDIES

Experimental Therapy

Assessment of the effects of therapy in experimental cerebral edema is difficult because many models exist and data obtained from one of these may not be relevant to the others. Furthermore, the CT data in man demonstrates the co-existence of several types of traumatic cerebral swelling (as was emphasized in our case report in which vasogenic edema, cellular swelling in the contusion, and non-hemorrhagic focal edema were all present). Experimental models isolate individual components of traumatic swelling. This is convenient for an understanding of pathophysiology, but therapeutic data derived from these models may have limited applicability to the clinical situation.

Balloon Compression Edema. The edema associated with compression is reduced by steroids[107, 108] and a mixture of drugs designated as "aescorin"[18] which are anti-inflammatory non-steroidal compounds. Diminished mortality has been demonstrated in monkeys treated with dimethylsulfoxide or hypertonic urea,[96] although neurological defects in surviving animals were more common in the group treated with urea. Animals treated by surgical decompression showed a decreased mortality but the quality of survival was poor.[64]

Cryogenic Edema. In the original description of cryogenic brain injury from our institution, the experimental animal was the rabbit.[41] The volume of the lesions was measured and shown to be related to survival. The mortality rate was decreased by surgical decompression, but not by intravenous hypertonic glucose. The rabbit brain, in common with rodent brains, has little white matter in relation to gray.

Edematous changes in the white matter in this experimental model were not described. Subsequent studies using the PAS technique showed that they do indeed occur, but are much less impressive than that seen in cats and dogs, which have much more white matter. Surgical decompression in the dog with a cryogenic lesion results in a marked enhancement of white matter edema.[14] There would seem to be a trade-off between reduction of intracranial pressure and the possible deleterious effects of the enhanced edema.

Numerous therapeutic studies utilizing the cryogenic lesion were described in detail in a recent publication in relation to the treatment of hemorrhagic stroke.[47] Edema was reduced by hypotension and hypothermia and increased by fever. Furosemide, pentobarbital, reserpine, and pentoxyfilline all reduced edema. Edema was not diminished by intravenous hypertonic solutions which exert their effect by dehydrating normal brain. The response to steroids was variable and seemed to depend upon the method by which the lesion is produced.

More recent work demonstrates that even massive doses of corticosteroids do not reduce the edema associated with cryogenic lesions produced by liquid nitrogen.[11] Another report showed edema reduction to low dose corticosteroids but no increase in effectiveness when the dose was increased.[89]

Suppression of cryogenic edema was reported with the proteinase inhibitor trasylol[18] and by increasing oxygen diffusion with the drug crocetin.[30] A study in the rat reported no effect on brain water with furosemide treatment.[29] In the rabbit treated 24 hours after injury, the water increment in the damaged hemisphere was reduced 38 minutes after therapy, but the decrease was not statistically significant.[39] This failure may be the result of the short time period between treatment and sacrifice.

Physical Trauma. Furosemide reduces the edema associated with experimental contusion in the cat.[95] The same group, using the same methods, reported suppression by corticosteroids only in the case of small contusions confined to the gray matter.[94] On the other hand, studies with the sled impact model in the Rhesus monkey have shown suppression of contusion related edema by corticosteroids even with large contusions.[51] All of the controls died within 18 hours with markedly increased intracranial pressure, while all of the treated animals lived to be sacrificed at 72 hours, and none of the treated animals showed as great an increase in intracranial pressure. Although this was a qualitative rather than a quantitative study, the data would imply that cerebral edema is an important factor in experimental head injury and that it can be effectively treated by steroids.

Human Therapy

Assessing the effect of anti-edema therapy in traumatized humans is difficult because cerebral edema is only one of many factors which contribute to the pathophysiology of these patients. Although difficult, clinical studies are necessary since no definite conclusions about how a given therapeutic modality will work in man can be drawn from any experimental model no matter how impressive the results. Experimental models are valuable guides which should neither be ignored nor totally relied upon.

Many of the anti-edema therapies have other effects which may be of importance. For example, steroids have a multitude of actions unrelated to reducing vasogenic edema. In the treatment of edema due to tumors, clinical improvement may occur before a significant reduction of edema is seen on the CT scan.[62] This implies that the steroids may alleviate symptoms by a direct action on the tumor or by other metabolic effects.

Another problem is the precise relationship between the edema and clinical symptoms. Recent studies in man have demonstrated normal clinical and electrical function of cerebral tissue in spite of clearly recognizable edema on the CT scan[73] and parallel findings have been demonstrated in animal models.[61, 90] This is not to say that edema is without effect, especially in situations of altered intracranial dynamics. But one must not assume that the existence of edema is necessarily injurious to a given patient or that it must always be treated if seen.

Extensive unilateral decompressive craniectomy has been advocated in the treatment of acute subdural hematomas. Initially, favorable results were reported.[81] When a larger group of patients over a longer period were studied,[17] the results were unfavorable. The overall mortality was 90% and only 4% of the patients were able to return to their previous activities. As the authors point out, the poor outcome was probably due to the immediate and extensive nature of the brain injury. It should not be taken as evidence for or against treatment of edema *per se* by decompression. Bifrontal craniotomy has been used in the treatment of traumatic cerebral swelling in man.[48, 98] This procedure has generally been abandoned because of the poor quality of survival.

Ventricular Drainage. While one does not usually think of continuous ventricular drainage as a therapy for edema in head trauma, evidence in animals indicates that edema can be lessened by this technique. Presumably, the lower pressure facilitates bulk flow of edema fluid out of the tissue into the ventricles. The phenomenon has not been studied in man, although intermittent drainage is frequently employed to reduce intracranial pressure.[72]

Hypothermia. The beneficial effects of hypothermia in head injury is an observation which dates back to antiquity. Hippocrates observed that "in fatal cases, a man will survive longer in winter than in summer, whatever be the part of the head in which the wound is situated." Controlled systemic hypothermia is not widely used today in the treatment of head injury, but it has not been wholly abandoned and it appears, at least in some patients, to be beneficial.[35] The reduction of vasogenic edema by this means has a firm experimental basis. The corollary of the proposition is certainly applicable. Since vasogenic edema is increased in hyperthermia, fever should be vigorously treated in the head injured patient.

Hypertonic Solutions. Intravenous hypertonic solutions (urea and mannitol) reduce the increased intracranial pressure in head injury patients. The effect is generally attributed to dehydration of normal brain, since vasogenic edema has been demonstrated not to be diminished by these agents. The other possibility is that the intracellular edema of gray matter contusions and the white matter edema of Type I contusions might well be dehydrated by these agents.

Corticosteroids. The most controversy has been over the question of whether or not corticosteroids are effective in the treatment of head trauma. This is not the same question as, "Do corticosteroids reduce traumatic edema?" It has been presumed that if corticosteroids were found to be effective, it would be because of a reduction in edema, but this is not necessarily the case. No controlled study on changes in traumatic edema as measured by CT techniques has yet been performed.

The more general question of the effectiveness on outcome has been addressed by many investigators. A tabulation of five clinical studies published between 1965 and 1972[27, 38, 43, 80, 88] was included in a recent experimental paper.[94] The authors concluded that overall, the investigations failed to demonstrate a positive effect of corticosteroids on morbidity and mortality in head injury.

Five additional studies more recently published are listed in Table 12.2. The first of these is an analysis of 1,000 severe head injuries from three different countries.[46] Corticosteroids in conventional doses did not affect outcome. Indeed, the authors came to the melancholy conclusion that none of the conventionally used methods for treating head trauma (osmotics, surgical decompression, tracheostomy and mechanical ventilation) had any influence on the final outcome. High dose corticosteroid therapy was not evaluated in the study.

In a second study, placebo, low dose, and high dose corticosteroids were compared. The mortality rates were 45, 41, and 23% respectively.[32] Using the chi-square analysis, these results are not statistically significant. A decrease in intracranial pressure

was reported with the high dose but not the low dose corticosteroids. These differences, based on the highest pressures recorded, are statistically significant. The same investigator later reported a statistically significant decrease in mortality in children with head trauma treated by high dose corticosteroids.[33] In both studies, the treatment groups were not randomized and the control group consisted of patients treated at an earlier time period. The studies cannot be considered definitive.

Two randomized prospective studies addressing the question of high dose corticosteroid therapy have been published. The authors of each came to opposite conclusions. A significantly higher survival rate was found in the first study,[24] but not in the second.[16] Interestingly, in the first, the better survival with corticosteroids was accompanied by a seven-fold increase in patients left in a chronic vegetative state (3.6–25.4%). On the other hand, the group with total recovery went from 3.6% with placebo to 13.4% with steroids (p < 0.01). Nevertheless, nine of 28 patients receiving placebo achieved a good outcome (good recovery, moderate disability) and 26 of 67 patients who received corticosteroids reached this level of neurological functioning. The difference in overall outcome between placebo and corticosteroid-treated groups is not statistically significant.

Furosemide. The effects of furosemide have not been extensively investigated. Experimentally, this drug has been shown to be superior to corticosteroids in the treatment of cerebral edema. In human brain tumors, a distinctly better resolution of edema occurred when furosemide is combined with corticosteroids. This was demonstrated by CT analyses and by chemical analysis of biopsies.[62] No comparable study has been done in trauma.

Considering the complexities of cerebral edema and swelling in head trauma, it would be surprising if clinical research on treatment of presumed edema had led to definitive answers. Too many different conditions have been lumped together and little attention has been paid to the actual measurement of the amount of edema or swelling on CT scan, and correlating it with

Table 12.2

Author	Type of Study	No. Cases	Selection	Drug and Dosage	Test	Results
Jennett, et al.[46]	Retrospective	1,000	Severe head injury	Dexamethasone 4 mg q6h	Mortality	Stratifying for age, coma sum, pupils, hematoma, country. No difference with steroids
Gobiet[32]	Retrospective	93	Acute head-injured children and adults	Dexamethasone high—48 mg, then 8 mg q2h low—16 mg, then 4 mg q6h	Mortality, morbidity, and ICP	Decreased mortality No steroids 45.5% Low steroid 41.5% High steroids 23% No statistically significant
Gobiet[33]	Retrospective	205	Children with acute head injury (ages 2–14)	Dexamethasone "high"—not given	Morbidity and mortality	Decreased mortality No steroids 41.7% Steroids 15.8%
Faupel[24]	Prospective, random, double-blind	95	Acute head injury	Dexamethasone high—100 mg, then 100 mg at 6 hr and then 4 mg q6h × 8 days low—12 mg IV, then 4 mg q6h × 8 days	Morbidity and mortality	Significant decrease in mortality p < .1% No steroids— 57% Low—30% High—18%
Cooper[16]	Prospective, random, double-blind	76	Severe head injury	Dexamethasone high—60 mg IV, then 24 mg q6h low—10 mg IV, then 4 mg q6h	Morbidity and mortality	No difference in mortality No steroids— 48% Low—40% High—66%

pathological changes. If different states, such as the swelling which occurs in children, can be distinguished, then treatment can be specifically tailored to the pathophysiological problem. CT scanning offers a new wealth of information which will have to be assimilated over the next decade.

References

1. Arimitsu, T., DiChiro, G., Brooks, R.A., Smith, P.M.: White-gray matter differentiation in computed tomography. J. Comput. Assist. Tomogr., 1:437–442, 1977.
2. Bakay, L., Haque, I.U.: Morphological and chemical studies in cerebral edema. I. Cold induced edema. J. Neuropath. Exp. Neurol., 23:393–418, 1964.
3. Bakay, L., Lee, J.C.: Cerebral Edema, Charles C Thomas, Springfield, Ill, 1965, pp. 12–28.
4. Bakay, L., Lee, J.C., Lee, G.C., Jiun-Rong, P.: Experimental cerebral concussion. I. An electron microscopic study. J Neurosurg, 47:525–531, 1977.
5. Baker, R.N., Cancilla, P.A., Pollock, P.S., Frommes, S.P.: The movement of exogenous protein in experimental cerebral edema. J Neuropath. Exp. Neurol., 30:668–679, 1971.
6. Bergstrom, M., Ericson, K., Levander, B., Svendsen, P., Larsson, S.: Variation with time of the attenuation values of intracranial hematomas. J. Comput. Assist. Tomogr., 1:57–63, 1977.
7. Bergvall, U., Kjellin, K.G., Levander, B., Svendsen, P., Söderström, CE: Computer tomography of the brain and spectrophotometry of the CSF in cerebral concussion and contusion. Acta Radiol., 19:705–714, 1978.
8. Christensen, E.E., Curry, T.S. III, Dowdey, J.E.: An Introduction to the Physics of Diagnostic Radiology, 2nd Ed., Lea & Febiger, Philadelphia, 1978, pp. 59–76, 329–360.
9. Clasen, R.A., Huchman, M.S., Pandolfi, S., Laing, I., Jacobs, J.: Computed tomography of vasogenic cerebral edema. In: Dynamics of Brain Edema, Pappius HM, Feindel W, Eds. Springer-Verlag, New York 1976, pp. 278–282.
10. Clasen, R.A., Huchman, M.S., Von Roenn, K.A., Pandolfi, S., Laing, I., Clasen, J.R.: Time course of cerebral swelling in stroke: a correlative autopsy and CT study. Adv. Neurol., 28:395–412, 1980.
11. Clasen, R.A., Pandolfi, S., Clasen, J.R.: Massive doses of steroids in cryogenic cerebral injury and edema. Stroke 10:670–673, 1979.
12. Clasen, R.A., Sky-Peck, H.H., Pandolfi, S., Laing, I., Hass, G.M.: The chemistry of isolated edema fluid in experimental cerebral injury. In: Brain Edema, Klatzo I., Seitelberger F., Eds. Springer-Verlag, New York, 1967, pp. 536–553.
13. Clifton, G.L., Grossman, R.G., Makela, M.E., Miner, M.E., Handel, S., Sadhu, V.: Neurologic course and correlated computerized tomography findings after severe closed head injury. J. Neurosurg., 52:611–624, 1980.
14. Cooper, P.R., Hagler, H., Clark, W.K., Barnett, P.: Enhancement of experimental cerebral edema after decompressive craniectomy: implications for the management of severe head injuries. Neurosurgery, 4:296–300, 1979.
15. Cooper, P.R., Moody, S.: Neurodiagnostic studies and the management of head injury. Comput. Tomogr., 2:197–206, 1978.
16. Cooper, P.R., Moody, S., Clark, W.K., Kirkpatrick, J., Maravilla, K., Gould, A.L., Drane, W.: Dexamethasone and severe head injury. A prospective double-blind study. J. Neurosurg., 51:307–316, 1979.
17. Cooper, P.R., Rovit, R.L., Ransohoff, J.: Hemicraniectomy in the treatment of acute subdural hematoma. re-appraisal. Surg. Neurol., 5:25–28, 1976.
18. Czernicki, Z.: Treatment of experimental brain oedema following sudden decompression, surgical wound, and cold lesion with vasoprotective drugs and the proteinase inhibitor "Trasylol." Acta Neurochir., 50:311–326, 1979.
19. Davis, K.R., Taveras, J.M., Roberson, G.H., Ackerman, R.H., Dreisbach, J.N.: Computed tomography in head trauma. Sem. Roentgenol., 12:53–62, 1977.
20. Denny-Brown, D., Russell, W.R.: Experimental cerebral concussion. Brain, 64:93–164, 1941.
21. Dublin, A.B., French, B.N., Rennick, J.M.: Computed tomography in head trauma. Radiology, 122:365–370, 1977.
22. Eichelberger, L., Kollros, J.J., Walker, A.E., Roma, M.: Water, nitrogen and electrolyte content of brain following cerebral concussion. Am. J. Physiol., 156:129–136, 1949.
23. Evans, J.P., Scheinker, I.M.: Histologic studies of the brain following head trauma. I. Post-traumatic cerebral swelling and edema. J. Neurosurg., 2:306–314, 1945.
24. Faupel, G., Reulen, H.J., Müller, D., Schürmann, K.: Double-blind study on the effects of steroids on severe closed head injury. In: Dynamics of Brain Edema. Pappius, H.M., Feindel, W., Eds. Springer-Verlag, New York, 1976, pp. 337–343.
25. Feigin, I.: Sequence of pathological changes in brain edema. In: Brain Edema, Klatzo, I., Seitelberger, F., Eds. Springer-Verlag, New York, 1967, pp. 128–151.
26. Fishman, R. A.: Cerebrospinal Fluid in Diseases of the Nervous System, W.B. Saunders Co., Philadelphia, 1980, pp. 107–128.
27. French, L.A.: The use of steroids in the treatment of cerebral edema. Bull. N.Y. Acad. Med., 42:301–311, 1966.
28. French, B.N., Dublin, A.B.: The value of computerized tomography in the management of 1000 consecutive head injuries. Surg. Neurol., 7:171–183, 1977.
29. Gaab, M., Knoblich, O.E., Schupp, J., Herrmann, F., Fuhrmeister, U., Pflughaupt, K.W.: Effect of furosemide on acute severe experimental cerebral edema. J. Neurol., 220: 185–197, 1979.
30. Gainer, J.V., Nugent, G.R.: Effect of increasing the plasma oxygen diffusivity on experimental

cryogenic edema. J. Neurosurg., 45:535–538, 1976.

31. Garcia, J.H., Conger, K.A., Morawetz, R., Halsey, Jr., J.H.: Postischemic brain edema: quantitation and evolution. Adv. Neurol., 28:147–169, 1980.

32. Gobiet, W.: The influence of various doses of dexamethasone on intracranial pressure in patients with severe head injury. In: Dynamics of Brain Edema, Pappius, H.M., Feindel, W., Eds. Springer-Verlag, New York, 1976, pp. 351–355.

33. Gobiet, W.: Advances in management of severe head injuries in childhood. Acta Neurochir., 39:201–210, 1977.

34. Gorons, S.R., Lewey, F.H., Grant, F.C.: Neurophysiological and neurohistological results following experimental head trauma produced by blasting caps. Assn. Res. Nerv. Ment. Dis., 24:201–215, 1943.

35. Gruszkiewicz, J., Doron, Y., Peyser, E.: Recovery from severe craniocerebral injury with brain stem lesions in childhood. Surg. Neurol., 1:197–201, 1973.

36. Gudeman, S.K., Miller, J.D., Becker, D.P.: Failure of high-dose steroid therapy to influence intracranial pressure in patients with severe head injury. J. Neurosurg., 51:301–306, 1979.

37. Gurdjian, E.S.: Impact Head Injury, Mechanistic, Clinical and Preventive Correlations, Charles C Thomas, Springfield, Ill., 1975, pp. 223–253.

38. Gutterman, P., Shenkin, H.A.: Prognostic features in recovery from traumatic decerebration. J. Neurosurg., 32:330–335, 1970.

39. Harbaugh, R.D., James, H.E., Marshall, L.F., Shapiro, H.M., Laurin, R.: Acute therapeutic modalities for experimental vasogenic edema. Neurosurgery, 5:656–665, 1979.

40. Hardman, J.M.: The pathology of traumatic brain injuries. Adv. Neurol., 22:15–50, 1979.

41. Hass, G.M., Taylor, C.B.; Quantitative studies of experimental production and treatment of acute closed cerebral injury. Arch. Neurol. Psychiat., 69:145–170, 1953.

42. Hounsfield, G.N.: Computerized transverse axial scanning (tomography). I. Description of system. Br. J. Radiol., 46:1016–1022, 1973.

43. Hoyt, H.J., Goldstein, F.P., Reigel, D.H., Holst, R.: Clinical evaluation of highly water-soluble steroids in the treatment of cerebral edema of traumatic origin (a double-blind study). Clin. Pharmacol. Therapeut., 13:141, 1972.

44. Huk, W., Schiefer, W.: Computerized axial tomography in cranio-cerebral trauma. In: Cranial Computerized Tomography, Lanksch, W., Kazner, E., Eds. Springer-Verlag, New York, 1976, pp. 310–317.

45. Ishii, S., Hayner, R., Kelly, W.A., Evans, J.P.: Studies of cerebral swelling. II. Experimental cerebral swelling produced by supratentorial extradural compression. J. Neurosurg., 16: 152–166, 1959.

46. Jennett, B., Teasdale, G., Fry, J., Braakman, R., Minderhoud, J., Heiden, J., Kurze, T.: Treatment for severe head injury. J. Neurol. Neurosurg. Psychiat., 43:289–285, 1980.

47. Katzman, R., Clasen, R., Klatzo, I., Meyer, J.S., Pappius, H.M., Waltz, A.G.: Brain edema in stroke. Stroke, 8:510–540, 1977.

48. Kjellberg, R.N., Prieto, Jr., A.: Bifrontal decompressive craniotomy for massive cerebral edema. J. Neurosurg., 34:488–493, 1971.

49. Klatzo, I.: Neuropathologic aspects of brain edema. J. Neuropath. Exp. Neurol., 26:1–14, 1967.

50. Klatzo, I., Piraux, A., Laskowski, E.J.: The relationship between edema, blood-brain barrier and tissue elements in a local brain injury. Neuropath. Exp. Neurol., 17:548–564, 1958.

51. Kobrine, A.I., Kempe, L.G.: Studies in head injury. I. An experimental model of closed head injury. II. Effect of dexamethasone on traumatic brain swelling. Surg. Neurol., 1:34–42, 1973.

52. Kobrine, A.I., Timmins, E., Rajjoub, R.K., Rizzoli, H.V., Davis, D.O.: Demonstration of massive traumatic brain swelling within 20 minutes after injury. J. Neurosurg., 46:256–258, 1977.

53. Koo, A.H., LaRoque, R.L.: Evaluation of head trauma by computed tomography. Radiology, 123:345–350, 1977.

54. Kuhl, D.E., Alavi, A., Hoffman, E.J., Phelps, M.E., Zimmerman, R.A., Obrist, W.D., Bruce, D.A., Greenberg, J.H., Uzzell, B.: Local cerebral blood volume in head-injured patients. Determination by emission computed tomography of 99mTc-labeled red cells. J. Neurosurg., 52:309–320, 1980.

55. Langfitt, T.W., Kassell, N.F.: Acute brain swelling in neurosurgical patients. J. Neurosurg., 24:975–983, 1966.

56. Lanksch, W., Grumme, T., Kazner, E. (translated by Dougherty, F.C.): Computed Tomography in Head Injuries, Springer-Verlag, New York, 1979.

57. Lee, J.C., Bakay, L.: Ultrastructural changes in the edematous central nervous system. II. Cold-induced edema. Arch. Neurol., 14:36–49, 1966.

58. Lindenberg, R.: Trauma of the meninges and brain. In: Pathology of the Nervous System, Vol. II. Minckler, J, Ed. McGraw-Hill, New York, 1971, pp. 1705–1765.

59. Long, D.M., Maxwell, R.E., French, L.A.: The effects of glucosteroids upon cold induced brain edema. II. Ultrastructural evaluation. J. Neuropath. Exp. Neurol., 30:680–697, 1971.

60. Manz, H.J.: The pathology of cerebral edema. Hum. Pathol., 5:291–313, 1974.

61. Marshall, L.F., Bruce, D.A., Graham, D.I., Langfitt, T.W.: Alterations in behavior, brain electrical activity, cerebral blood flow, and intracranial pressure produced by triethyl tin sulfate induced cerebral edema. Stroke, 7:21–25, 1976.

62. Meinig, G., Reulen, H.J., Simon, R.S., Schürmann, K.: Clinical, chemical, and CT evaluation of short-term and long-term antiedema therapy with dexamethasone and diuretics. Adv. Neurol., 28:471–489, 1980.

63. Miller, J.D., Gudeman, S.K., Kishore, P.S., Becker, D.P.: Computed tomography in brain edema due to trauma. In: Brain Edema—Pathology Diagnosis and Therapy, Cervós-Navarro, J., and Ferszt, R., Eds. Raven Press, New York, Advances in Neurology, 28:413–422, 1980.

64. Moody, R.A., Ruamsuke, S., Mullan, S.F.: An evaluation of decompression in experimental head injury. J. Neurosurg., 29:586–590, 1968.

65. New, P.F.J., Aronow, S.: Attenuation measurements of whole blood and blood fractions in computed tomography. Radiology, 121:635–640, 1976.

66. New, P.F.J., Scott, W.R.: Computed Tomograpy of the Brain and Orbit, Williams & Wilkins Co., Baltimore, 1975, p. 427.

67. Norman, D., Price, D., Boyd, D., Fishman, R., Newton, T.H.: Quantitative aspects of computed tomography of the blood and cerebrospinal fluid. Radiology, 123:335–338, 1977.

68. Obrist, W.D., Dolinskas, C.A., Gennarelli, T.A., Zimmerman, R.A.: Relation of cerebral blood flow to CT scan in acute head injury. In: Neural Trauma, Popp, A.J., Bourke, R.S., Nelson, L.R., Kimelberg, H.K., Eds. Raven Press, 1979, pp. 41–50.

69. Ommaya, A.K., Gennarelli, T.A.: Cerebral concussion and traumatic unconsciousness. Brain, 97:633–654, 1974.

70. Ommaya, A.K., Grubb, R.L. Jr., Naumann, R.A.: Coup and contre-coup injury: observations on the mechanics of visible brain injuries in the rhesus monkey. J. Neurosurg., 35:503–516, 1971.

71. Ommaya, A.K., Rockoff, S.D., Baldwin, M., Friauf, W.S.: Experimental concussion: A first report. J. Neurosurg., 21:249–265, 1964.

72. Papo, I., Caruselli, G., Luongo, A., Scarpelli, M., Pasquini, U.: Traumatic cerebral mass lesions: Correlations between clinical, intracranial pressure, and computed tomographic data. Neurosurgery, 7:337–346, 1980.

73. Penn, R.D.: Cerebral edema and neurological function in human beings. Neurosurgery, 6:249–254, 1980.

74. Penn, R.D.: Cerebral edema and neurological function: CT, evoked responses, and clinical examination. Adv. Neurol., 28:383–394, 1980.

75. Penn, R.D., Kurtz, D.: Cerebral edema, mass effects, and regional blood volume in man. J. Neurosurg., 46:282–289, 1977.

76. Penn, R.D., Walser, R., Ackerman, L.: Cerebral blood volume in man. Computer analysis of a computerized brain scan. J.A.M.A., 234:1154–1155, 1975.

77. Pevsner, P.H.: Computed tomography of head injury: Practice and pitfalls. In: Neural Trauma, Popp, A.J., Bourke, R.S., Nelson, L.R., Kimelberg, H.K., Eds. Raven Press, 1979, pp. 263–271.

78. Raichle, M.E.: Brain edema: Evaluation in vivo with positron emission tomography. Adv. Neurol., 28:423–427, 1980.

79. Raimondi, A.J., Evans, J.P., Mullan, S.: Studies of cerebral edema. III. Alterations in the white matter: An electron microscopic study using Ferritin as a labeling compound. Acta Neuropath., 2:177–197, 1962.

80. Ransohoff, J.: The effects of steroids on brain edema in man. In: Steroids and Brain Edema, Reulen, H.J., Schürmann, K., Eds. Springer-Verlag, New York, 1972, pp. 211–218.

81. Ransohoff, J., Benjamin, M.V., Gage, Jr., E.L., Epstein, F.: Hemicraniectomy in the management of acute subdural hematoma. J. Neurosurg., 34:70–76, 1971.

82. Reulen, H.J., Tsuyumu, M., Prioleau, G.: Further results concerning the resolution of vasogenic brain edema. Adv. Neurol., 28:375–381, 1980.

83. Reulen, H.J., Tsuyumu, M., Tack, A., Fenske, A.R., Prioleau, G.R.: Clearance of edema fluid into cerebrospinal fluid. A mechanism for resolution of vasogenic brain edema. J. Neurosurg., 48:754–764, 1978.

84. Rieth, K.G., Fujiwara, K., DiChiro, G., Klatzo, I., Brooks, R.A., Johnston, G.S., O'Connor, C.M., Mitchell, L.G.: Serial measurements of CT and specific gravity in experimental cerebral edema. Radiology, 135:343–348, 1980.

85. Rinder, L., Olsson, Y.: Studies on vascular permeability changes in experimental brain concussion. I. Distribution of circulating fluorescent indicators in brain and cervical cord after sudden mechanical loading of the brain. II. Duration of altered permeability. Acta Neuropath., 11:183–209, 1968.

86. Schellmann, B., Huk, W., Thierauf, P.: Correlations of CT-findings and neuropathological investigations in cranio-cerebral trauma. Zeit. Rechtsmedizin., 82:199–204, 1978.

87. Shaw, M., Alvord, E.C., Berry, R.G.: Swelling of the brain following ischemic infarction with arterial occlusion. Arch. Neurol., 1:161–177, 1959.

88. Sparacio, R.R., Lin T-H., Cook, A.W.: Methylprednisolone sodium succinate in acute craniocerebral trauma. Surg. Gynecol. Obstet., 121:513–516, 1965.

89. Sugiura, K., Kanazawa, C., Muraoka, K., Yoshino, Y.: Effect of steroid therapy on cerebral cold injury edema in the rat: the optimal dosage. Surg. Neurol., 13:301–305, 1980.

90. Sutton, L.N., Bruce, D.A., Welsh, F.: The effects of cold-induced brain edema and white-matter ischemia on the somatosensory evoked response. J. Neurosurg., 53:180–184, 1980.

91. Sweet, R.C., Miller, J.K., Lipper, M., Kishore, P.R.S., Becker, D.P.: Significance of bilateral abnormalities on the CT scan in patients with severe head injury. Neurosurgery, 3:16–21, 1978.

92. Tani, E., Evans, J.P.: Electron microscopic studies of cerebral swelling. I. Studies on the permeability of brain capillaries, using ferritin molecules as tracers. II. Alterations of Myelinated nerve fibers. III. Alterations in the neuroglia and the blood vessels of the white matter. Acta Neuropath., 4:507–526, 604–639, 1965.

93. Tornheim, P.A., McLaurin, R.L., Thorpe, J.F.: The edema of cerebral contusion. Surg. Neurol., 5:171–175, 1976.

94. Tornheim, P.A., McLaurin, R.L.: Effect of dexamethasone on cerebral edema from cranial impact in the cat. J. Neurosurg., 48:220–227, 1978.

95. Tornheim, P.A., McLaurin, R.L., Sawaya, R.: Effect of furosemide on experimental traumatic cerebral edema. Neurosurgery, 4:48–52, 1979.

96. de la Torre, J.C., Rowed, D.W., Kawanaga, H.M., Mullan, S.: Dimethyl sulfoxide in the treatment of experimental brain compression. J. Neurosurg., 38:345–354, 1973.

97. Unterharnscheidt, F., Higgins, L.S.: Traumatic lesions of brain and spinal cord due to nondeforming angular acceleration of the head. Texas Rept. Biol. Med., 27:127–166, 1969.

98. Venes, J.L., Collins, W.F.: Bifrontal decompressive craniectomy in the management of head trauma. J. Neurosurg., 42:429–433, 1975.

99. de Villasante, J.M., Taveras, J.M.: Computerized tomography (CT) in acute head trauma. Am. J. Roentgenol., 126:765–778, 1976.

100. Waga, S., Tochio, H., Sakakura, M.: Traumatic cerebral swelling developing within 30 minutes after injury. Surg. Neurol., 11:191–193, 1979.

101. Wasterlain, C.G., Posner, J.B.: Cerebral edema in water intoxication: I. Clinical and chemical observations. Arch. Neurol., 19:71–78, 1968.

102. Wasterlain, C.G., Torack, R.M.: Cerebral edema in water intoxication. II. An ultrastructural study. Arch. Neurol., 19:79–87, 1968.

103. Weinberg, L.A.: CT and acute head trauma. Comput. Tomogr., 3:15–28, 1979.

104. Weinstein, J.D., Langfitt, T.W., Bruno, L., Zaren, H.A., Jackson, J.L.F.: Experimental study of patterns of brain distortion and ischemia by an intracranial mass. J. Neurosurg., 28:513–521, 1968.

105. White, J.C., Brooks, J.R., Goldthwait, J.C., Adams, R.D.: Changes in brain volume and blood content after experimental concussion. Ann. Surg., 118:619–634, 1943.

106. White, J.C., Verlot, M., Selverstone, B., Beecher, H.K.: Changes in brain volume during anesthesia: The effects of anoxia and hypercapnia. Arch. Surg., 44:1–21, 1942.

107. Yamaguchi, M., Shirakata, S., Taomoto, K., Matsumoto, S.: Steroid treatment of brain edema. Surg. Neurol., 4:5–8, 1975.

108. Yamaguchi, M., Shirakata, S., Yamasaki S., Matsumoto, S.: Ischemic brain edema and compression brain edema. Water content, blood-brain barrier and circulation. Stroke, 7:77–83, 1976.

109. Zimmerman, R.A., Bilaniuk, L.T.: Computer tomography of traumatic intracerebral hemorrhagic lesions: The change in density and mass effect with time. Neuroradiology, 16:320–321, 1978.

110. Zimmerman, R.A., Bilaniuk, L.T., Bruce, D., Dolinskas, C., Obrist, W., Kuhl, D.: Computed tomography of pediatric head trauma: Acute general cerebral swelling. Radiology, 126:403–408, 1978.

111. Zimmerman, R.A., Bilaniuk, L.T., Gennarelli, T.: Computed tomography of shearing injuries of the cerebral white matter. Radiology, 127:393–396, 1978.

112. Zimmerman, R.A., Bilaniuk, L.T., Gennarelli, T., Bruce D., Dolinskas, C., Uzzell, B.: Cranial computed tomography in diagnosis and management of acute head trauma. Am. J. Roentgenol., 131:27–34, 1978.

13

Gunshot Wounds of the Brain

PAUL R. COOPER

Although the literature on missile wounds of the head sustained in war is more extensive than those incurred in peacetime conditions, shrapnel and military rifle wounds are most unusual in civilian practice and not often encountered by practicing neurosurgeons. For this reason this chapter is primarily concerned with gunshot wounds of the head seen in *civilian* practice.

The differences between civilian and military injuries are considerable. Military rifles achieve high muzzle velocities (generally 2,400–3,200 feet/second)[23]; the destruction produced by a direct hit of the head by these missiles is generally incompatible with survival and relatively few of these patients come to neurosurgical attention. The majority of patients with head wounds sustained in combat receive them from shrapnel fragments.[15, 25] The head wounds tend to be massive and often involve extensive areas of the scalp and skull. In addition, multiple systems injuries tend to be common. Civilian wounds are usually produced by handguns with muzzle velocities of less than 1,000 feet/second. The wounds are cleaner than those seen in the military and less emphasis has been placed on total debridement of intracranial bone and missile fragments to prevent future abscess formation.

It is ironic that deaths from civilian gunshot wounds of the brain in the United States since the end of World War II exceed those from the Korean and Viet Nam conflicts combined. However, the number of injuries seen in any individual neurosurgical center are few when compared to the large numbers of patients accumulated in military series. Heterogeneous management policies and small retrospective series in the literature make it difficult to draw firm conclusions about the treatment of civilian gunshot wounds. In this chapter, recommendations for the care of gunshot wounds of the brain are based on the author's experience in several large metropolitan hospitals where gunshot wounds are a relatively common occurrence. When appropriate, the experience of others in managing this type of injury is reviewed. Where relevant the military experience will be cited.

BALLISTIC PHYSICS AND PATHOPHYSIOLOGY

Ballistic Considerations

The amount of kinetic energy contained by a missile is defined by the formula, $E = \frac{1}{2}mv^2$, where m is the mass of the missile and v is its velocity.[9] Because the energy varies directly with the mass and with the square of the velocity, velocity is relatively more important in determining the energy of the missile and thus the extent of injury

Acknowledgments: Portions of this chapter have previously appeared in Contemporary Neurosurgery, number 5, 1979.

than is mass. The amount of energy imparted to the brain is dependent on the difference between the missile velocity at impact with the brain and its residual velocity upon exiting from the brain and is defined by the formula:

$$E = \tfrac{1}{2}mv_i^2 - \tfrac{1}{2}mv_r^2$$

Where v_i = the initial velocity of the missile at impact and v_r = the velocity of the missile when it leaves the head. If the missile does not exit from the skull, the energy imparted to the skull and brain is equal to the amount of energy contained in the missile at the time of impact. Thus, the lower the residual velocity the greater the energy liberated.[18] Because the energy released by the missile determines the amount of brain damage, the destructive effect may be viewed in terms of the retardation it undergoes and is defined as:

$$x = \frac{AC_d}{2_m}$$

where A is the presenting area, C_d is the drag coefficient and m is the mass of the sphere.

The amount of injury produced by a missle is increased by anything causing it to give up more of its energy intracranially. A missile which yaws (defined as a deviation of the longitudinal axis of a projectile from the line of flight) will give up more of its energy than will a missile which is tumbling. Hollow point bullets which shatter upon impact will tend to give up more of their kinetic energy to the brain and are thus more destructive than bullets which don't shatter. Similarly shotgun injuries caused by multiple pellets each with relatively small amounts of kinetic energy are extremely destructive; each pellet acts as "an independent missile and is invested with kinetic energy in accord with its size (mass) and velocity."[30] Other factors which determine the amount of kinetic energy lost by a bullet include the histological characteristics of the tissues which the bullet encounters and the tendency of a bullet to deform and produce an increase in its presenting area with a consequent increase in energy transfer to tissues.

Mechanism of Brain Injury

Under experimental conditions, immediately after tissue penetration, there is an instantaneous rise in pressure due to shock waves lasting 15–25 microseconds. The magnitude of this rise is determined by the kinetic energy of the missile and has been reported under certain circumstances to exceed 80 kg/cm^2.[6] This rise is transmitted down the neuraxis to the brain stem and may produce herniation and immediate irreversible damage in addition to the injury to the cerebral parenchyma surrounding the missile track. Death or decerebration following wounding in the absence of significant mass effect probably results from this phenomenon.[23] In experimental animals there is a second rise of the intracranial pressure (ICP) of 60–100 mm Hg within 2–5 minutes of injury. Cerebral blood flow falls and remains reduced for 6–12 hours following impact and the cerebral metabolic rate of oxygen consumption is also reduced.[8]

As the missile penetrates the brain, cerebral parenchyma in its path is crushed and spread apart, creating a permanent cavity which is slightly larger than the diameter of the missile.[23] A temporary cavity, which collapses in less than 20 milliseconds, forms adjacent to the permanent missile track. The size of this temporary cavity (and surrounding area of tissue injury) may be as much as 30 times the diameter of the missile itself and is largely dependent on the velocity of the missile.[9] The temporary cavity (and thus the area of destruction) is smaller in low velocity sounds than in high velocity ones.

Under experimental conditions, as the missile velocity is slowed by its passage through the tissues, the area of surrounding destruction is decreased, producing a conical configuration of disruption. In clinical practice, the same phenomenon does not always occur. When a missile strikes the skull, it is often deformed, causing it to yaw. An irregular cavity results from this yaw. Bone fragments are indriven at least one-third of the time and may follow a different course than that of the missile itself, creating an irregular track or even a second one (Fig. 13.1). The kinetic energy imparted to bone fragments must be less than the kinetic energy contained by the missile. For this reason bone fragments tend to be embedded in brain closer to the wound of entrance than the missile fragment.

The amount of residual energy left in civilian type missiles after penetrating the skull and traversing the brain is frequently insufficient to allow the missile to exit from the skull. After striking the inner table on the side opposite the entrance wound, the missile may ricochet back into the brain, producing a second missile track. The pattern of ricochet may be quite variable. Thus, a line drawn from the wound of entrance to the site of radiographic localization of the missile fragment is not always a reliable indicator of the missile course through the brain.

Larger caliber civilian missiles (0.38–0.45 caliber) fired at close range are more likely to possess enough kinetic energy to exit the skull. Bursting of the skull at the site of exit from a pressure wave transmitted to the brain has been described in military wounds. This probably results from transmission of pressure by both the missile and the brain at the site of exit. Experimentally, spheres filled with water burst at the site of missile exit after being struck by a high velocity missile whereas hollow spheres struck by missiles containing the same energy do not.[8] Bursting of the skull at the exit wound is seen infrequently in civilian practice, and the exit wound (although usually larger than the entrance one) is generally small.

Other pathophysiological phenomena following missile wounding are important in determining morbidity and mortality and must be recognized by the neurosurgeon in order that he may rationally plan his therapy and understand the patient's course in the post-injury and postoperative periods.

Contusion and hemorrhage may occur in areas distant from the missile track. These injuries are similar in gross appearance and location to those resulting from blunt head trauma. They occur secondary to brain displacement by the sudden pressure wave associated with intracranial missile penetration and are most commonly located in

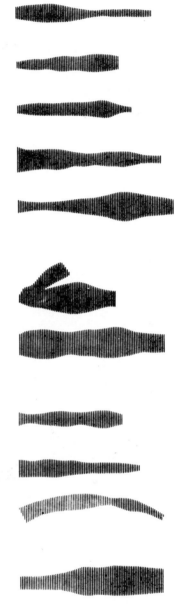

Figure 13.1. Line drawing showing irregular configuration of track caused by missile penetration in brain. Line drawings made from autopsy examination of brain specimens by Kirkpatrick and DiMaio.[23] (Reproduced with permission.)

the cortex and subcortical white matter (Fig. 13.2). Rapid increases in the ICP associated with supratentorial wounds may result in sudden downward displacement of

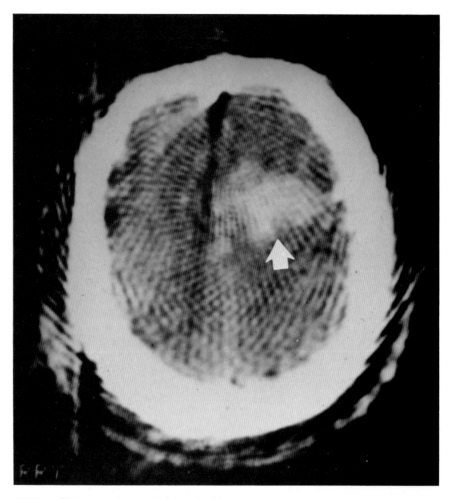

Figure 13.2. CT scan shows right-sided intracerebral hematoma (*arrow*) considerably distant from track of missile which passed through left cerebral hemisphere only.

the cerebellum through the foramen magnum, resulting in contusions of the cerebellar hemispheres and the tonsils.

White matter edema commonly occurs as soon as twelve hours after injury. Although the presence of "edema" appearing minutes after injury has been reported,[23] it is more likely that the grossly observed "swollen brain" seen in patients dying immediately after injury are hyperemic rather than edematous — a phenomenon that may be exacerbated by hypercarbia.

Hemorrhage commonly occurs along the missile track. In addition, laceration of major vessels may produce large parenchymal hematomas extending considerable distances from the site of the track. Significant hematomas may also occur in the subdural space from either tearing of bridging veins or bleeding from cortical contusions. These hematomas result from brain movement within the calvarium with tearing of bridging vessels following a shock wave or from direct missile injury to cortical or bridging vessels.

Patients who have no intracranial penetration by a missile may also have neurologic deficit as a result of cortical contusion underlying the point where the missile has struck. They may also develop extraparenchymal hematomas as a result of injury of cortical or meningeal vessels (Fig. 13.3).

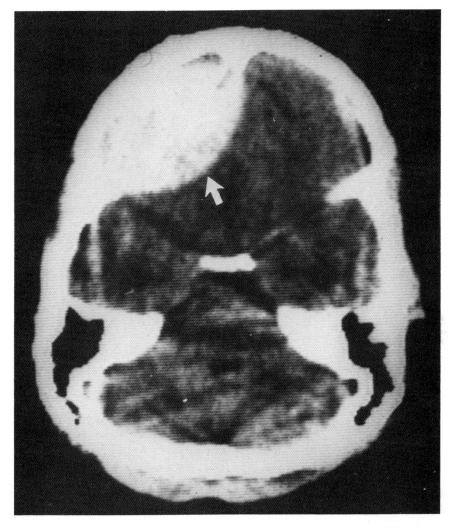

Figure 13.3.   CT scan of a patient with a large left sided acute epidural hematoma (*arrow*) who was struck in the left frontal skull by a bullet but in whom there was no intracranial penetration. Hematoma presumably originated from injury to middle meningeal artery at the time of impact.

EVALUATION, INITIAL MANAGEMENT, AND TRIAGE

Rapid neurological deterioration following gunshot wounds occurs in a high percentage of patients. Because morbidity and mortality are significantly influenced by the patient's immediate preoperative neurological status, it is imperative that the interval from injury to therapy be minimized.[29]

Ironically, triage and transport of the patient to definitive care occurs more rapidly under combat conditions than in many large cities of this country. Raimondi and Samuelson[29] noted that 60% of their patients were first seen elsewhere, resulting in an average delay in treatment of three hours. Significant neurological deterioration from expansion of intracranial hematomas occurred in 40% of these patients, with a corresponding increase in mortality. No patient improved while awaiting transfer.

Resuscitation

Upon arrival in the emergency room, neurological evaluation is performed within minutes. It should include a notation as to the patient's level of consciousness, motor responses, pupillary reactivity, and brain stem reflexes. Patients who do not have purposeful motor responses are intubated and hyperventilated to achieve an arterial pCO_2 of 25 torr. We believe that these patients are at greatest risk from elevated ICP (see Chapter 9). The finding of hypotension should arouse suspicion of systemic missile wounds with intraabdominal, intrathoracic, or long-bone injury. Hypotension may also occur from injury to scalp vessels or compound injuries involving the venous sinuses or major arterial branches.

Diagnostic Studies

Initial diagnostic studies should consist of plain anterior-posterior and lateral skull films for localization of missile and bone fragments (Fig. 13.4). Unfortunately, emergency room films are often not of sufficient quality to accurately identify many small bone fragments; the number of fragments found at operation is often greater than

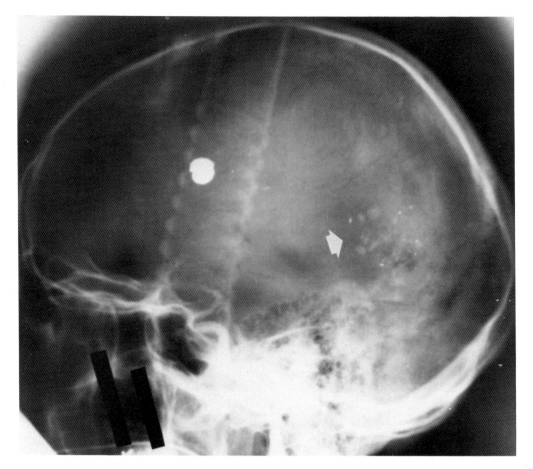

Figure 13.4. Lateral skull roentgenogram of a patient who had intracranial penetration by a low calibre missile. The wound of entrance was occipital and the bullet is located in the posterior frontal region. Bone fragments and a few very small missile fragments (*arrow*) are located more posteriorly, closer to the wound of entrance.

that suspected on plain films. However, plain films are particularly helpful in patients with gunshot wounds involving the base of the skull. Small missile particles will accurately outline the passage of the missile through basal bony structures and serve as a guide to the site of dural penetration and the location where dural repair is needed. When a large missile fragment is seen to be retained on plain films, it must be remembered that missiles with low residual energy will ricochet once they reach the inner table after traversing the brain. For this reason a line drawn from the wound of entrance to the retained missile fragment is not necessarily an accurate guide to the intracranial path of the missile.

All patients with civilian missile injuries to the brain should have definitive neurodiagnostic studies (*i.e.*, computerized tomography of the brain and/or arteriography) to define the presence and location of intra- and extraparenchymal mass lesions prior to craniotomy. There are two exceptions to this rule: (1) in patients with rapid neurological deterioration, an expanding hematoma is assumed to be present, and immediate operation without diagnostic studies is indicated (2) in patients with systemic gunshot wounds in whom arterial pressure cannot be stabilized and maintained with blood and intravenous fluids, immediate operation is indicated for control of hemorrhage. Ideally, craniotomy is performed simultaneously with either laparotomy or thoracotomy. If this is not pos-

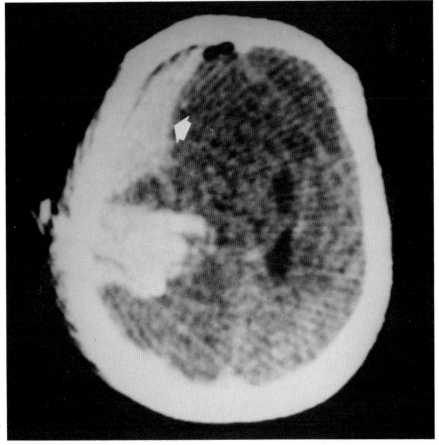

Figure 13.5. CT scan of a patient with a gunshot wound showing an anteriorly placed hematoma (*arrow*) that was located subdurally and intra-parenchymally. Posteriorly located hematoma is entirely within the parenchyma.

sible because of the nature of the systemic wounds or the operating room facilities, craniotomy is performed immediately after the systemic injury has been treated.

CT scanning is the procedure of choice for the definitive diagnostic evaluation of missile injuries and, for several reasons, has replaced cerebral angiography in this regard.[5] CT scans currently available allow scanning and computer reconstruction to be completed in less than 30 minutes. Under the most ideal circumstances, cerebral angiography may take twice as long. Additional time is consumed when bilateral angiographic studies must be performed in patients with lesions involving both hemispheres as well as posterior fossa structures. The CT scan not only identifies the presence of mass lesions, but readily distinguishes between confluent hematoma, contusion, and edema and will define the presence of hematoma along the missile track (Figs. 13.5 and 13.6). Experience with the CT scan has shown that what was previously diagnosed as swelling by angiography usually consists of hematoma. Finally, the CT scan may visualize small intracerebral bone fragments that are sometimes not seen on initial plain skull films.

If a CT scanner is not available patients should have cerebral angiography. Although the use of angiography in patients with missile injuries of the head is thought to be unnecessary by some authorities, angiography is essential to identify "distant unsuspected but surgically important mass lesions."[35] Vascular pathology, such as arterial spasm, traumatic aneurysm, and carotid-cavernous sinus fistula, can be identified only by cerebral angiography[1] (Fig. 13.7). If these lesions are suspected, angiography (must be performed in addition to CT scanning) preoperatively if the patient's condition is stable or, as is more often the case, postoperatively.

Triage

The decision to operate on a patient with a gunshot wound of the brain is often difficult. Patients who are either decerebrate or flaccid upon admission rarely survive. Of the few who do, the majority will remain vegetative. For this reason, most neurosurgeons do not consider these patients as operative candidates.[6, 19, 29] Patients who are decerebrate or flaccid from the time of impact and remain so after resuscitation with mannitol and hyperventilation have probably sustained a diffuse and irremediable injury with involvement of brain stem structures. On the other hand, patients who are initially purposeful or semi-purposeful and then deteriorate have not sustained a primary diffuse brain injury. Their clinical course is most likely accounted for by an expanding mass lesion. Operative evacuation of hematoma and contused brain is indicated in this latter group. Although overall morbidity and mortality is very high, an occasional patient will make a functional survival.

OPERATIVE MANAGEMENT

The goals of operative therapy of missile wounds of the brain are: 1) to evacuate intracranial hematoma and nonviable brain along the path of the missile, 2) to remove missile and bone fragments where feasible (without enhancing pre-existing neurological deficit) 3) to repair and close the dura and scalp in watertight fashion, and 4) to minimize elevations of ICP in the post-operative period.

Gunshot wounds of the brain are sometimes managed with debridement via small craniectomies.[15] However, large bone flaps centered over the wound of entrance have the advantage of exposing a large area of brain that may then be evaluated for viability and debrided as necessary. Moreover, large flaps allow hemorrhage to be more easily visualized and controlled. If the wound is polar (e.g., frontal or temporal tip), a large craniotomy will provide exposure for a lobectomy and internal decompression. The usefulness of this tactic is minimizing large brain shifts as a result of edema has been confirmed by CT scanning. In addition, large craniotomies permit visualization and removal of subdural hematoma. The actual incidence of intracranial hematomas varies in different series;

Hubschmann *et al.*[19] reported an incidence of 10% and emphasized that the incidence of hematoma formation is a function of the time elapsed between injury and the presentation of the patient. Thus, in series where patients are seen early after admission, the incidence is low and the highest rate of hematoma formation occurs between three and eight hours after injury.[19]

Careful attention to the missile track and bone and missile fragments is important in minimizing postoperative septic complications. The missile track should be debrided of necrotic brain, bone, and bullet fragments *when readily accessible*. In wounds that traverse multiple lobes of one hemisphere, the potential for additional iatrogenic injury in following the missile track its entire length will usually outweigh any potential benefits. When an exit wound is present, a local craniectomy and debridement is performed at this site. The dura is

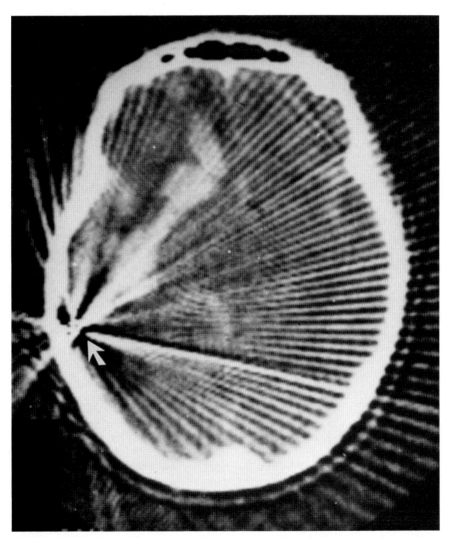

Figure 13.6. CT scan of a patient who was shot in the forehead in the midline. Scan clearly defines hematoma within the missile track. *Arrow* delineates missile at posterior end of missile track.

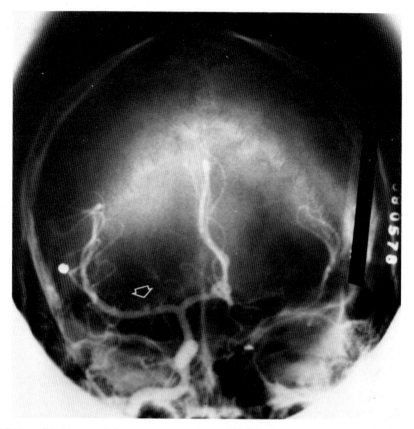

Figure 13.7. Right carotid angiogram of a patient who sustained a missile wound of the brain. The retained fragment is seen. *Arrow* points to traumatic aneurysm of proximal middle cerebral artery. Subsequent angiograms showed enlargement of the aneurysm which was treated by extra-cranial-intracranial bypass and trapping of the aneurysm.

closed (with a pericranial graft when necessary) to prevent a cerebral fungus and strangulation of the brain at the craniectomy margin.

The surgical strategy described above will sometimes result in retention of bone and missile fragments. Many neurosurgeons dealing with military wounds believe it is imperative to remove all bone fragments and any pieces of metal that are accessible. Indeed, in some military series, reoperation is advocated if retained bone fragments are radiographically evident following initial debridement.[3, 16, 27]

Abscess formation or other suppurative complications in relation to retained bone and missile fragments have been a major pre-occupation of military neurosurgeons.[16, 26] Martin and Campbell[26] recorded a parenchymal infection rate of 16% based on their World War II experience. They felt that infections were ten times more likely to occur in the presence of retained bone fragments than in their absence. Over 40% of retained bone fragments in their patients became infected and they advocated reoperation for retained bone fragments. Nevertheless, the complication rate of secondary procedures is high and consists of increased neurological deficit, enhancement of cerebral edema, infection and death. A more conservative approach has been advocated by others.[24, 29, 31]

The high incidence of suppurative complications in military wounds with retained fragments is probably explained by the greater soft tissue, bone and cerebral parenchymal injury when compared with civilian injuries.[24] The presence of necrotic brain may be as responsible for abscess formation as the presence of the bone itself (Fig. 13.8).

In short, in civilian injuries we have been more aggressive with the removal of bone than with the removal of metallic fragments and we remove bone *if it can be done without adversely affecting the patient's neurological function.* If, on the other hand, bone is embedded in the deep gray matter or in white matter underlying eloquent cortex (*i.e.*, motor, speech cortex), at a distance from the wound of entrance or in proximity to a potentially lacerated venous sinus we have not hesitated to leave it in place. We have had only one case of abscess formation as a result of this policy (Fig. 13.9). In all patients with retained fragments the CT scan may be employed for postoperative follow-up to monitor the development of cerebritis and/or abscess.

ADJUNCTS TO OPERATIVE MANAGEMENT

Anticonvulsants

There are few large series which document the incidence of epilepsy following civilian gunshot wounds of the brain. Crockard[6] reported a seizure incidence of

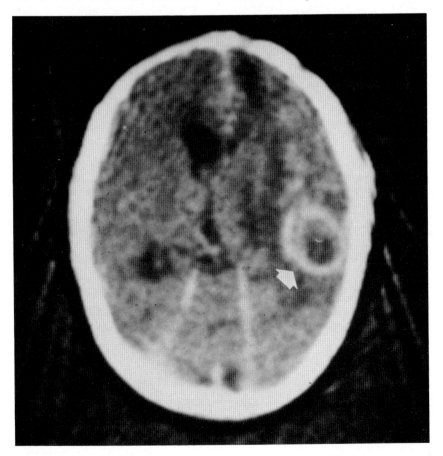

Figure 13.8. Contrast enhanced CT scan of a young boy with a gunshot wound defines a brain abscess (*arrow*) along the bullet path but not in relation to retained bone or missile fragments.

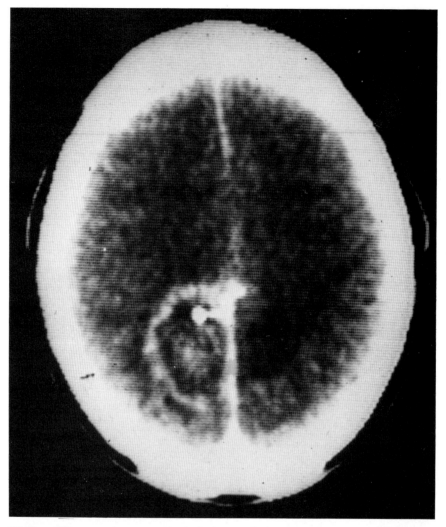

Figure 13.9. CT scan shows posteriorly located abscess near the midline. Bone fragment located within the center of the abscess was intentionally left at the time of original debridement to avoid manipulation of the posterior part of the saggital sinus which had been damaged but was being tamponaded by a depressed bone fragment. Three weeks after injury the patient presented with headache and fever. At that time the retained fragment and abscess were evacuated and the patient recovered.

35% in a civilian series and Gordon[13] cited an epilepsy rate of 40–50%. Some military reports show an incidence of late epilepsy of 35–40% or more.[2, 4, 32, 33] The actual incidence of epilepsy will vary as a function of the frequency with which patients receive prophylactic anticonvulsant therapy and the length of time between wounding and follow-up. In non-missile injuries, the presence of a dural tear is associated with a late epilepsy incidence of at least 21%.[22] Thus, it would seem logical that the true incidence of late epilepsy in civilian gunshot wounds with dural penetration and coexisting severe cerebral injury is at least 20% and perhaps as high as 35 or 40%. For this reason, anticonvulsants should be administered to all patients in the emergency room. Parenteral phenobarbital is given initially because of its immediate anticonvulsant effect. When convenient, we switch to phenytoin for long-term management.

Antibiotics

Early debridement of necrotic brain, removal of readily accessible bone and missile fragments, and meticulous dural and scalp closure are the most important factors in minimizing infectious complications in the post-operative period. The prophylactic use of antibiotics in the management of gunshot wounds is widely advocated.[13, 19, 24, 26] Nevertheless, there is no scientific evidence that antibiotic administration lowers the infection rate. It is unlikely that antibiotics will control infection if patients do not have adequate debridement of necrotic tissue, watertight dural closure and removal of all accessible missile and bone fragments. If antibiotics are given, it is important that they be agents that cross the blood-brain barrier and that they be administered in high dosages. The general principles guiding the use and choice of antibiotics are discussed in detail in Chapter 18.

Management of Elevated Intracranial Pressure

Current concepts in the management of gunshot wounds of the head emphasize the frequent occurrence of elevated ICP in the post-injury period.[6, 7] To a large extent, ICP elevations can be minimized by judicious debridement of injured cerebral tissue and evacuation of intraparenchymal and extraparenchymal hematomas. Often, however, in bihemispheric or multilobar injuries, debridement is limited by the desire to minimize neurological deficit. Edema adjacent to long missile tracks may be extensive and result in dangerous elevations of ICP. These elevations are managed according to the principles discussed in Chapter 9.

SPECIAL PROBLEMS ASSOCIATED WITH GUNSHOT WOUNDS

Craniofacial Wounds

Missile wounds that traverse the face prior to entering the intracranial compartment are relatively common. Shotgun wounds are especially likely to cause injury to both facial and intracranial structures.[30]

It can be difficult on plain X-rays to distinguish those pellets which are embedded in soft tissue from those which have penetrated intracranially. A CT scan is most useful in this regard (Fig. 13.10). When missile fragments have passed through the nose, mouth, or paranasal sinuses, brain wounds are likely to be contaminated, and the patient is at high risk of developing intracranial infectious complications.[10] Moreover, defects in the dura at the base of the frontal fossa may allow direct communication between the paranasal sinuses and the intracranial cavity, with subsequent development of cerebrospinal fluid fistulas.

The general principles of management of craniofacial wounds are similar to those described earlier. The brain wound always take precedence over the facial injuries. A frontal bone flap that is large enough to permit visualization of the frontal fossa back to the sphenoid wing is made. A bifrontal craniotomy is performed if there is any question regarding injury to the opposite frontal lobe and bony structures of the contralateral frontal fossa. Dural tears are identified via an intradural exploration. The dura is then separated from the floor of the frontal fossa and repaired primarily, if possible. A pericranial graft is utilized if the dura cannot be otherwise approximated. Bony defects of the orbital roof or cribriform plate, when large, may result in the formation of encephaloceles and should be repaired with stainless steel wire mesh. If the frontal sinus is involved by the missile wound or entered at the time of craniotomy, the mucosa is exenterated. The surgical opening in the dura is meticulously closed. Cottonoids are left in the epidural space to protect the brain during facial repair. They are removed when the repair is completed, after which the craniotomy is closed. Prophylactic antibiotics are used because of the contaminated nature of the wounds involving the paranasal sinuses.

Vascular Injuries

Injuries of the dural venous sinuses are a relatively frequent occurrence in war wounds but are less commonly seen in civilian practice.[28] Hemorrhage can be pro-

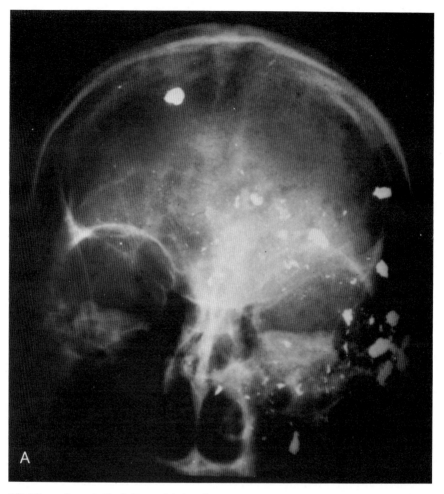

Figure 13.10.   *A* and *B*, A-P and lateral roentgenograms of a patient with a shotgun injury of the face. It is difficult to ascertain how many fragments have penetrated intracranially. CT scan (*C*) shows that only one pellet has penetrated the skull.

fuse and difficult to control. When either the dominant transverse sinus or the sagittal sinus posterior to the coronal suture is injured, obstruction to venous return can be fatal. If the bone and scalp immediately adjacent to the sinus are destroyed, the patient may exsanguinate prior to receiving medical attention. More commonly, the rent in the sinus is sealed by either hematoma or bone fragments, and hemorrhage occurs at the time of debridement. When the location of bone fragments or the path of the missile suggests the possibility of sinus injury, the surgeon must have a clear idea of his operative strategy prior to de-bridement. Wide exposure must be obtained on all sides of the suspected lesion. The bone over the sinus is removed last. If there is a small tear in the sinus, hemorrhage may be controlled by digital pressure, and hemostasis achieved with either thrombin soaked Gelfoam or muscle sewn in over the rent. With larger tears and destruction of a wall of the sinus, this technique is not adequate. If the anterior half of the sagittal sinus is involved, ligation is the procedure of choice. When the transverse sinus or posterior half of the saggital sinus is involved repair should be undertaken as described in Chapter 14.

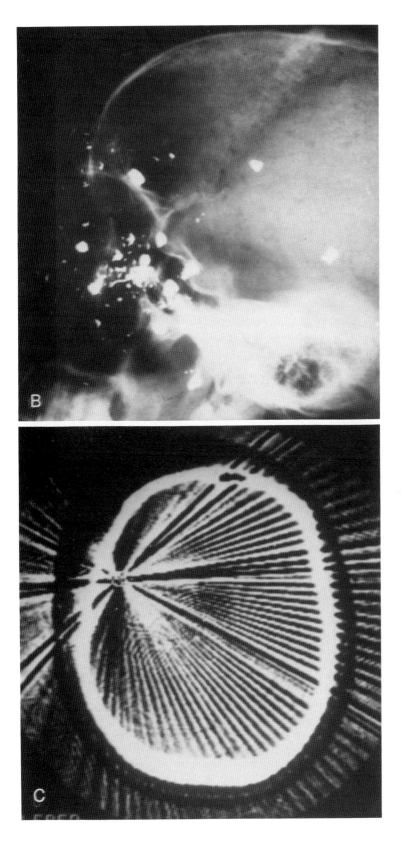

Figure 13.10 *B*

Figure 13.10 *C*

Gunshot injuries to major cerebral arteries may result in occlusion, transection with massive hemorrhage, or traumatic (false) aneurysms. Previously, these lesions were identified by arteriography in the course of the diagnostic work-up. As CT scanning in evaluating these cases becomes more widespread, it is likely that some arterial injuries will be missed in the future.

We have seen three cases of carotid-cavernous sinus fistulas following gunshot wounds involving the base of the middle fossa. This lesion should be suspected when proptosis, chemosis, and a retroorbital bruit appear in the post-traumatic period. When the patient's condition has stabilized and edema has resolved, these lesions are managed similar to carotid-cavernous sinus fistulas caused by blunt trauma.

Scalp Injuries

Destruction of large areas of the scalp is more common with wounds caused by missile fragments under military circumstances. However, civilian shotgun wounds sustained at short distances also will produce extensive scalp and bone destruction. All injured and non-viable scalp and bone must be completely debrided. The brain wound is treated as previously described. The techniques of plastic surgical closure of the scalp wound are discussed in Chapter 15. Whatever methods are used, it is essential that dural and scalp closure be watertight to prevent cerebrospinal fluid leaks and infection in the post-operative period.

Tangential Wounds

Tangential or "gutter" wounds are seen frequently in military practice.[11, 20, 21] They occur infrequently in civilian life and are seen when a missile fired at close range strikes the skull at a very oblique angle. The missile does not penetrate the skull, but causes bone to be indriven over a variable distance, depending on the angle of impact. The cortex may be extensively injured as a result, and severe neurological deficit is common. Bone may be indriven deep into the brain. Exposure is best provided by utilizing a large bone flap. The skin incision must be planned with consideration for the scalp injury caused by the tangential wound. The scalp wound, bone fragments, and devitalized brain are debrided according to principles previously outlined.

OUTCOME

The overall mortality of patients with civilian gunshot wounds of the brain is poor and has been reported to range from 30–97%.[6, 7, 12, 24, 29] In series where outcome is calculated as a percentage of *all* patients with gunshot wounds, the mortality rate will be high.[17] Relatively high in-hospital death rates will also be seen where many unsalvagable patients are rapidly transported for definitive care and die shortly after admission.[6] Low *in-hospital* death rates are seen where transport systems are inefficient and only patients who have survived several hours are admitted for care.[29]

As with other types of head injury, the single greatest determinant of outcome is the patient's level of consciousness when first seen. Patients who are alert upon admission have a very low mortality which, in most series, ranges from 0–20%.[6, 17, 19, 24, 29] Patients who are comatose rarely survive (even if they receive operation).[12, 17, 19, 29]

Another factor which influences survival is the type of the missile causing the brain injury. In general missiles which have a high kinetic energy are associated with a greater mortality than those with low velocity and/or smaller calibers. The missile course also has a bearing on mortality; missile wounds which involve only one lobe have a mortality of 35–45%,[17, 29] whereas those which injure multiple lobes or cross the midline have a mortality as high as 65–90%.[17, 29]

SUMMARY

Gunshot wounds of the brain are a relatively frequent occurrence in our society. Rapid transport to centers where definitive care may be rendered is essential. Neurological deterioration occurs rapidly, and the ultimate results are largely dependent on the patient's neurological status at the time of surgery. CT scanning has replaced angiography as the diagnostic procedure of choice and should be performed if the patient's condition is stable. Aggressive removal of missile and bone fragments must be balanced by the knowledge that it is often better to leave behind a few hard to reach fragments than to increase the patient's neurological deficit. CT scanning in the post-operative period will identify incipient abscess formation as well as new or recurrent hematomas, edema, and areas of tissue injury not evident at the time of initial scanning. Anticonvulsants are indicated in all gunshot wounds of the brain. Currently, the efficacy of antibiotic and corticosteroid administration is not clear. It does appear that control of ICP in the post-operative period has a salutary influence on mortality and morbidity. Judicious debridement of injured brain and lobectomy of noneloquent areas of the brain coupled with medical management of ICP will maximizes the quality of recovery and increase the number of patients surviving.

References

1. Adeloye, A., Odeku, E.L.: The radiology of missile head wounds. Clin. Radiol., 22:312–321, 1971.
2. Ascroft, P.B.: Traumatic epilepsy after gunshot wounds of the head. Br. Med J., 1:739–744, 1941.
3. Carey, W., Young, H.F., Rish, B.L., Mathis, J.L.: Follow-up study of 103 American soldiers who sustained a brain wound in Vietnam. J. Neurosurg., 41:542–549, 1974.
4. Caveness, W.F.: Onset and cessation of fits following craniocerebral trauma. J. Neurosurg., 20:570–583, 1963.
5. Cooper, P.R., Maravilla, K., Cone, J. Computerized tomographic scan and gunshot wounds of the head: indications and radiographic findings. Neurosurgery, 4:373–380, 1979.
6. Crockard, H.A.: Bullet injuries of the brain. Ann. Roy. Coll. Surg. Engl. 55:111–123, 1974.
7. Crockard, H.A.: Early intracranial pressure studies in gunshot wounds of the brain. J. Trauma, 15:339–347, 1975.
8. Crockard, H.A., Brown, F.D., Johns, L.M., Mullan, S.: An experimental cerebral missile injury model in primates. J. Neurosurg, 46:776–783, 1977.
9. DeMuth, W.E.: Bullet velocity as applied to military rifle wounding capacity. J. Trauma 9:27–38, 1969.
10. Dillon, J.D., Jr., Meirowsky, A.M.: Facio-orbito-cranial missile wounds. Surg. Neurol., 4:515–518, 1975.
11. Dodge, P.R., Meirowsky, A.M.: Tangential wounds of scalp and skull. J. Neurosurg., 9:472–483, 1952.
12. Goodman, J.M., Kalsbeck, J.: Outcome of self-inflicted gunshot wounds of the head. J. Trauma, 5:636–642, 1965.
13. Gordon, D.S.: Missile wounds of the head and spine. Br. Med. J., 1:614–616, 1975.
14. Hagan, R.E.: Early complications following penetrating wounds of the brain. J. Neurosurg., 34:132–141, 1971.
15. Hammon, W.M.: Analysis of 2187 consecutive penetrating wounds of the brain from Vietnam. J. Neurosurg., 34:127–131, 1971.
16. Hammon, W.M.: Retained intracranial bone fragments: analysis of 42 patients. J. Neurosurg., 34:142–144, 1971.
17. Hernesniemi, J.: Penetrating craniocerebral gunshot wounds in civilians. Acta Neurochir., 49:199–205, 1979.
18. Hopkinson, D.A.W., Marshall, T.K.: Firearm injuries. Br. J. Surg. 54:344–353, 1967.
19. Hubschmann, O., Shapiro, K., Baden, M., Shulman, K.: Craniocerebral gunshot injuries in civilian practice—prognostic criteria and surgical management: experience with 82 cases. J. Trauma, 19:6–12, 1979.
20. Jacobs, G.B., Berg, R.A.: Tangential wounds of the head. J. Neurosurg., 32:642–646, 1970.
21. Jefferson, G.: The physiological pathology of gunshot wounds of the head. Br. J. Surg., 7:262–289, 1919.
22. Jennett, B.: Epilepsy after non-missile head injuries. Year Book Medical Publishers, Chicago, 1975.
23. Kirkpatrick, J.B., DiMaio, V.: Civilian gunshot wounds of the brain. J. Neurosurg., 49:185–198, 1978.
24. Lillard, P.L.: Five years experience with penetrating craniocerebral gunshot wounds. Surg. Neurol., 9:79–83, 1978.
25. Maltby, G.L.: Penetrating craniocerebral injuries. J. Neurosurg., 3:239–249, 1946.
26. Martin, J., Campbell, E.H.: Early complications following penetrating wounds of the skull. J. Neurosurg., 3:58–73, 1946.
27. Mathews, W.E.: The early treatment of craniocerebral missile injuries: experience with 92 cases. J. Trauma, 12:939–954, 1972.
28. Meirowsky, A.M.: Wounds of dural sinuses. J. Neurosurg., 10:496–514, 1953.
29. Raimondi, A.J., Samuelson, G.H.: Craniocerebral gunshot wounds in civilian practice. J. Neurosurg., 32:647–653, 1970.
30. Sights, W.P.: Ballistic analysis of shotgun injuries to the central nervous system. J. Neurosurg., 31:25–33, 1969.
31. Sukoff, M.H., Helmer, F.A., Plaut, M.R.: Retained intracranial fragments following missile injuries. Bull L. A. Neurol. Soc., 36:64–71, 1971.

32. Wagstaffe, W.W.: The incidence of traumatic epilepsy after gunshot wounds of the head. Lancet, 2:861–862, 1928

33. Watson, C.W.: The incidence of epilepsy following cranio-cerebral injury. Proc. Assoc. Res. Nerv. Ment. Dis., 26:516–528, 1947.

34. Yashon, D., Jane, J.A., Martonffy, D., White, R.J.: Management of civilian craniocerebral bullet injuries. Am. Surg., 38:346–351, 1972.

35. Yashon, D., Jane, J.A., White, R.J. Arteriographic observations in craniocerebral bullet wounds. J. Trauma, 8:238–255, 1968.

14

Intracranial and Cervical Vascular Injuries

NEAL F. KASSELL
DAVID J. BOARINI
HAROLD P. ADAMS, JR.

INTRODUCTION

In this chapter, injuries to arterial and venous structures in the head as well as the neck are discussed. Injuries to vascular structures in the neck are included because there is often extension of the injury to involve intracranial vessels or thrombotic or embolic complications of intracranial vessels occur secondary to the neck injury.

The true incidence of vascular injury associated with head and neck trauma is difficult to accurately estimate. Various reports in the literature describe a wide range of incidence depending upon the definition of vascular trauma, the method of diagnosis, and the type of patient being seen. Perhaps the best recent estimate of vascular injuries was given by El Gindi *et al.*[30] in a review involving 2,000 cases of civilian head injuries. Excluding intracranial hematoma and GI bleeding, El Gindi *et al.* reported a 4.2% incidence of vascular injuries. This estimate may be somewhat conservative due to the difficulty in diagnosing certain vascular injuries. The clinical manifestations of vascular trauma may occur simultaneously with those from a direct injury to the brain or their appearance may be delayed. Vascular injuries can occur with both major and minor trauma to the head and neck, and the pathogenesis can involve a variety of different mechanisms. Because the symptoms and signs of the direct effect of head injury are similar to those which result from cerebral ischemia caused by vascular injury, it can be difficult to recognize associated vascular injury in trauma patients. In addition to the difficulties in reaching a clinical diagnosis, a recent problem in the roentgenographic diagnosis of these abnormalities has arisen due to the widespread use of the CT scan. Most arterial and venous injuries cannot be accurately diagnosed by the CT scan, particularly during their early course. Because angiography has been replaced as the primary diagnostic examination of patients with head injury, our recognition of vascular trauma will increasingly depend upon accurate clinical diagnosis. The relative rarity, difficulty in recognition, and high morbidity and mortality associated with these lesions demand that the involved clinician be aware of the syndromes of vascular injury and be on the lookout for them, if favorable outcomes are to be obtained.

ARTERIAL INJURIES

Arterial Occlusions

Post-traumatic arterial thrombosis occurs as a result of intimal damage, regardless of whether the inciting injury is blunt or sharp. The injury must be sufficient to form a nidus for thrombosis. Sharp injuries in the neck can do this by completely transecting the vessel, by causing a vessel laceration with disruption of the intima, or by formation of a compressive extravascular clot.

The causes of blunt traumatic injuries of the arteries of the head and neck are frequently similar or interrelated. Whether occlusions are caused by a thrombotic or embolic phenomenon is often unclear. Furthermore, the relative etiologic importance of vasospastic occlusion or dissection in these cases is difficult to estimate. The neurological manifestations of these entities may be indistinguishable and the site of occlusion may not be clinically identifiable. Even if arteriography is performed and an occlusive syndrome is diagnosed and documented, it may not be possible to define where the pathology originated due to the occurrence of both antegrade and retrograde propagation of thrombosis in posttraumatic occlusions. If a thrombotic occlusion is identified only in the neck, then the origin is clearly in that location. In occlusions where a thrombus is found in both the cervical and intracranial arteries, the primary site of injury is usually in the neck. In those instances in which a thrombus is only found in intracranial arteries, it is often difficult to determine the primary site of pathology. In an autopsy review of eight cases of middle cerebral artery occlusions following trauma, four had intracranial dissecting aneurysms, one had a recent primary thrombosis, another had a recent embolic thrombosis, and two were found to be entirely normal.[28] The rarity of this disorder makes it impossible to generalize regarding its pathogenesis.

Penetrating Neck Injuries. Penetrating neck injuries are an uncommon occurrence. Even rarer are penetrating wounds with injury to major arterial structures supplying the brain. Jones, in a review of 274 cases of penetrating injuries of the neck, found only 12 cases of carotid artery involvement and four cases of vertebral involvement.[48] In most major series of penetrating trauma involving the carotid arteries, the common carotid artery is injured more frequently than the internal carotid artery.[22] The mechanism of injury varies depending upon the population involved. In military series, injuries were caused by gunshot or fragment wounds. In civilian practice, knife wounds, small caliber gunshot wounds, and a variety of other low velocity injuries predominate.

Pathologically these lesions may be divided into those that disturb vessel patency and those that do not. The major vessels may escape injury altogether or the laceration may be partial and may not result in a significant disruption of cerebral blood flow. On the other hand, penetrating injuries may cause vessel occlusion by transection (Fig. 14.1), laceration with a compressive hematoma or partial vessel wall injury with subsequent thrombosis. This last category is particularly common with high velocity missile injuries which may cause complete occlusion of the lumen without disruption of the vessel wall. If the artery is occluded, the development of neurological signs and symptoms will then depend upon the extent of collateral circulation, the subsequent propagation of thrombus, and the occurrence of distal embolization.

The diagnosis of cervical arterial laceration is usually straightforward with clear evidence of external bleeding or hematoma formation and an open wound in the neck. If there is no associated head injury and the patient develops a focal ischemic neurological deficit, compromise of the luminal integrity of a major artery supplying the brain can be assumed. However, if the patient has sustained significant head trauma, it may be difficult to determine if the neurological impairment is a result of the primary brain injury or is ischemic in nature and related to the arterial injury. The diagnosis becomes extremely difficult in a patient with a penetrating injury that has occluded an artery without causing laceration of the vessel and subsequent hemorrhage. Accordingly, all patients with penetrating neck injuries accompanied by neurological deficits should have immediate angiography unless external or intratracheal hemorrhage or other life-threatening injury requires immediate surgery. Furthermore, it is probably judicious to perform angiography prior to surgical exploration in patients with a penetrating neck injury who

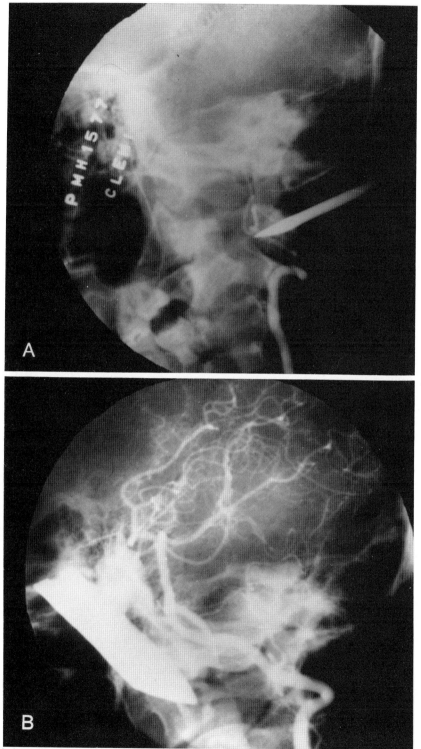

Figure 14.1. *A*, vertebral angiogram shows nearly complete occlusion of vertebral artery by knife. *B*, angiogram of opposite vertebral artery shows excellent filling of posterior circulation and reflux down nearly occluded opposite vertebral artery. At operation, the occluded vertebral artery was ligated and the knife was removed. The patient recovered without neurological deficit.

277

are neurologically asymptomatic, if circumstances allow. This is particularly true for a wound which may involve arterial structures near the base of the skull and therefore be difficult to explore or reconstruct. Likewise, a pre-operative angiogram is especially desirable for low neck wounds which may involve the arterial structures in the chest and require sternotomy for adequate proximal exposure.

Exploration of penetrating injuries that violate the platysma is a long-standing surgical principle. If the vessel lumen remains patent in spite of arterial injury, then simple repair is indicated. The critical therapeutic decision, however, is whether or not vascular reconstruction should be undertaken if an occlusive arterial injury is discovered. In recent years, technical advances in vascular surgery have made most of the wounds encountered in civilian practice accessible to reconstruction. Even extensive wounds resulting from high velocity gunshots or major associated blunt trauma can often be repaired with the use of bypass grafts.

Asymptomatic carotid occlusions as a result of trauma should be reconstructed unless mitigating circumstances prevent operation. The mortality rate following vascular reconstruction for carotid injuries from penetrating wounds in patients who did not have a neurological deficit preoperatively is less than 4%. Post-operative ischemic deficits occur in less than 2% of these cases.[15, 22, 69]

The treatment of an asymptomatic vertebral artery occlusion is less straightforward and, in addition to the neurological status of the patient, the accessibility of the occluded portion of the vertebral artery must be taken into account.

Reconstructive surgery in patients with pre-operative neurological deficits always presents the danger of converting a bland infarct into a hemorrhagic one. In two small series, nine of 18 such patients died from neurological sequelae after reconstruction and five of 18 patients went on to experience permanent neurological deficits.[15, 22] Although it is uncertain what role the reconstruction had in these outcomes, these authors did demonstrate that the revascularization of carotid occlusions in patients with penetrating injury and neurological deficit results in morbidity and mortality rates of approximately 80%. It was the conclusion of these authors that an occluded carotid or vertebral artery in a patient with neurological deficit should be treated by ligation only.

While these conclusions are appropriate for patients with profound and long-standing neurological deficits, others may be benefited by revascularization. Minor or evolving deficits as well as profound deficits seen in the very acute period may be reversible. Clear guidelines for their treatment are not yet available. When a penetrating neck wound is further complicated by impact injury to the brain, it becomes important to differentiate between a neurological deficit caused by the head injury and the vascular injury. A decision to reconstruct an artery must be based on the surgeon's judgment of the etiology of the deficit.

In summary, neck wounds that penetrate the platysma require: 1) careful neurological examination, 2) angiography in all cases if time permits and particularly if there has been bleeding that would suggest arterial injury, 3) operative exploration, 4) debridement and ligation if the artery has been occluded and there is profound and persistent neurological deficit, and 5) reconstruction of an occluded artery in patients without neurological deficit. In the presence of arterial occlusion with minor or hyperacute deficit, the best form of treatment is unclear and cases must be individualized. Further discussion of alternate revascularization is presented at the end of the section on blunt trauma occlusions.

Arterial Occlusion from Blunt Trauma. The incidence of blunt trauma causing arterial occlusion in the head and neck is difficult to estimate. Undoubtedly a large number of these cases are unsuspected and never diagnosed. El Gindi's report on 2,000 head injuries included five cases of internal carotid artery occlusion in the neck and five cases of occlusion of a major intracranial vessel, for an overall incidence of one-half of 1%.[36] In a 1978 review Aarabi and McQueen[1] were able to find 117 documented cases of traumatic occlusions. This included 94 cases of vessel occlusion in the neck and 23 intracranially. In 1980, Krueger and Okazaki[52] reported a search of the literature which revealed 37 cases of vertebral-basilar occlusion following neck manipulations.

Post-traumatic vessel occlusion is much less common than occlusion secondary to atherosclerosis. Unfortunately, the differing pathogenesis makes comparison of the experience with atherosclerotic occlusions difficult. Similarly, iatrogenic intra-operative occlusion of the carotid artery differs from post-traumatic occlusions in its presentation and treatment.

Occlusions from blunt injury to neck vessels occur in several patterns. Cervical carotid artery injury is usually caused by a direct blow or by contusion of the artery against the transverse process of a vertebra, most commonly C-2. Numerous studies, both pathological and roentgenographic, have shown that the transverse process of C-2 can be positioned so as to impinge upon the carotid artery, especially with rotation and hyperextension of the neck.[9, 14] The vertebral artery is also most commonly injured at the level of the C-2 vertebra, probably during extreme rotation and stretching of the vessels over a bony prominence of C-1 or C-2.[16, 18, 35, 38, 65, 68, 76, 101, 105] (Fig. 14.2). Vertebral artery occlusion may be associated with a cervical fracture at any level above C-6.[63] In these situations, the vertebral artery is occluded by compression from the dislodged bony element or from pressure caused by an enlarging hematoma in the foramen transversarium.

The clinical diagnosis of blunt traumatic arterial occlusion is often difficult. Trauma that results in cervical carotid artery occlusion is often minimal, and there may be no external signs of injury to the neck.[9, 79] The traumatic event is usually followed by a symptom-free interval, most frequently lasting less than 24 hours.[8, 34, 124] However, during this time there may be transient ischemic attacks, formation of a neck hematoma, or development of a Horner's syndrome.[146] Once occlusion occurs, rapid onset of focal neurologic deficits may result if there is ensuing ischemia. Although the resultant focal deficit may be severe, the patient's level of consciousness is not significantly affected immediately after an ischemic insult. The preserved level of consciousness serves to distinguish occlusive stroke from an expanding intracranial mass lesion which virtually always causes early obtundation.[39] At times the patient's condition prior to the ischemic event may not allow this distinction to be made. Moreover, large infarctions may result in obtundation several days after the injury because of secondary edema in the infarcted area.

Vertebral artery injuries in the neck often manifest themselves soon after the initial traumic event and a wide variety of brainstem syndromes has been described as a result of traumatic vertebral occlusion.[52, 103, 109] The time course of the development of ischemic symptoms is variable; in some instances gradual progression of neurologic deficits occurs while others show immediate, severe, and unremitting neurological deficits.

The delay in the appearance of neurological deficit in patients with arterial occlusions of neck vessels is due to several factors. Even when the initial injury causes intimal damage, a certain amount of time may be required before a thrombus forms at the site. The time of appearance of sympwtoms depends upon two additional factors: extension of the clot or hemodynamic insufficiency. The extension of the clot may occur as a continuous propagation of the thrombus, the expansion of an occlusive dissection, or propagation by embolization. Hemodynamic insufficiency may result immediately after proximal occlusion or may take place later during hypotension from any cause.[40, 52, 63]

The mortality rate for traumatic carotid thrombosis in the neck has been reported to be between 40 and 90%, with the vast majority of survivors having permanent neurological deficits.[46, 74] Fewer cases of traumatic vertebral occlusion have been documented, but the mortality rate in a literature review of 37 cases reached 19%. If the vertebral arteries are occluded bilaterally, the mortality increases to 46%.[52] The morbidity among survivors of traumatic vertebral occlusion appears to be less severe

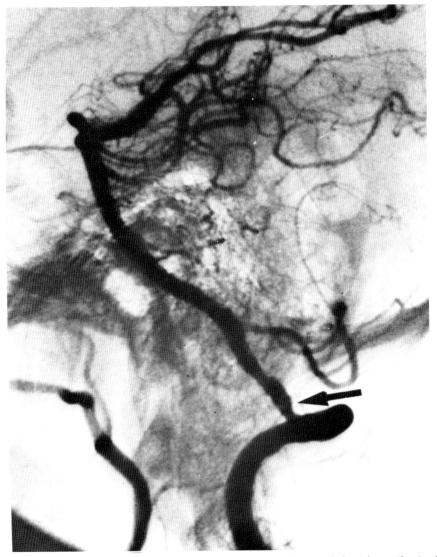

Figure 14.2. Vertebral angiogram. *Arrow* shows persistent defect in patient who presented with bilateral posterior cerebral infarction following chiropractic manipulation.

than with carotid occlusions. This may be because vertebral collateral flow, particularly with unilateral occlusion, is frequently sufficient to prevent a major infarction.

The variable time-course and protean manifestations of post-traumatic arterial occlusions require a high degree of suspicion on the part of the clinician if the diagnosis is to be made. Traumatic arterial thrombosis needs to be considered, particularly in patients who have sustained minor

head injury accompanied by a focal deficit but who maintain a normal level of consciousness. If the CT scan does not reveal a cause for delayed neurological deterioration in a patient with head injury, Doppler examination or arteriography must be carried out to identify arterial occlusion. The directional Doppler is an easily used, rapid, noninvasive instrument that is highly accurate.[2, 12] Unfortunately, a very high cervical or intracranial occlusion may not be detectable by Doppler examination. When angiography is indicated, the entire brachiocephalic system must be examined in a search for occlusions as well as any irregularity which might be the origin of intracranial emboli. Thrombi, emboli, and dissection are frequently indistinguishable by arteriography. The exception is the demonstration of a true double lumen diagnostic of dissecting aneurysm.[53, 126]

The traditional treatment for blunt injury occlusions of vessels in the neck has been anti-coagulation.[74, 101, 124] This is based upon theoretical considerations and anecdotal observations, but there has been no controlled study to evaluate the efficacy of this therapy. Despite such treatment, the majority of the symptomatic patients are left with permanent neurological sequelae. Furthermore, anti-coagulation is not without danger. Frequently the head injury is severe enough to prohibit anti-coagulation because of the risk of intracranial hemorrhage. In patients with arterial dissections, anti-coagulation may predispose to extension of the false channel and even intracranial rupture.[126] Anti-coagulation should be reserved for patients with mild head injury without having the classical radiologic signs of dissection. The best treatment of an incidentally discovered, asymptomatic, traumatic occlusion has not been determined, and the decision to anti-coagulate in such cases remains a matter of individual judgement.

The utility and timing of surgical revascularization in acute stroke with occlusion of a major artery in the neck continues to be controversial, whether vascular occlusion results from trauma or atherosclerotic disease. In patients with an acute post-traumatic stroke, it is well accepted that surgery should not be attempted if the deficit has been present beyond 24 hours and should probably not be undertaken later than six hours. This suggests that the presence of a profound, fixed neurological deficit in itself may contraindicate thrombectomy. As with penetrating trauma, blunt injuries with mild or fluctuating deficits as well as any injury which can be operated upon within the first few hours may benefit from oper-

ative reconstruction and therapy must therefore be individualized.

Intracranial Arterial Occlusion. The mechanism by which intracranial arteries become occluded after head trauma is often less clear than the mechanism in neck injuries. Undoubtedly a certain number can be explained by direct injury of a vessel against bony prominences or dural edges. Vascular trauma often occurs in association with basal skull fractures and there is frequently significant evidence of contusion of contiguous cerebral parenchyma as well. For example, an anterior cerebral artery may occlude at the edge of the falx in association with a frontal lobe contusion, or the carotid artery may thrombose at its exit from the carotid canal in association with a fracture in that vicinity. Some of these injuries may occur in association with relatively minor head trauma far from any bony prominence or dural edge. A certain number of these occlusions are due to embolic phenomena secondary to injury of vessels in the neck and several well-documented cases have shown irregularities in the lumen of vessels in the neck in patients with middle cerebral artery occlusions occurring shortly after neck trauma.[40] Some occlusions, however, probably are caused by stretch injury of intracranial vessels occurring during the shifting of intracranial contents which takes place during the acceleration-deceleration phase of head injury.

Intracranial vessel occlusion, like carotid occlusion in the neck, generally manifests itself after an asymptomatic period of less than 24 hours, although much longer intervals have been noted.[1, 29, 40, 102, 103] Like extracranial occlusions, intracranial occlusions are also associated with the onset of severe focal deficits without a concomitant decrease in the level of consciousness.[39]

With traumatic occlusion of intracranial arteries, the mortality and morbidity rates depend both upon the vessel involved and the severity of the original trauma. Mortality ranges from 33 to 80%.[1, 28, 40, 59, 102] Most survivors of intracranial occlusion are left with permanent neurological sequelae.[28, 102]

As with vascular injuries in the neck, diagnosis requires angiography. The early CT scan will be normal, although later scans will show evidence of infarction.

The treatment of intracranial and combined intracranial-cervical occlusions is both controversial and disappointing. The efficacy of anti-coagulation is unproven and contraindicated when there is severe impact injury to the brain. Various methods are being investigated to improve the brain's tolerance to ischemia and to improve collateral blood flow.[54] Attempts to protect the brain from permanent ischemic deficits for longer periods of time, by using mannitol, barbiturates, and DMSO, are still clinically unproven.

The place for extracranial/intracranial bypass early in the course of these post-traumatic occlusions has not yet been clarified.[28, 29, 102, 126] As with thrombectomy, the danger of revascularizing an ischemic area is present with bypass. The use of intracranial or extracranial ligation to prevent extension of a dissection or propagation of a thrombosis has also been suggested. This treatment has rarely been used and its usefulness is not known. The results of middle cerebral embolectomy in the early stages of acute symptomatic occlusion have been well documented in only a few cases and the mortality approximates 33%.[29] Whether surgical intervention is indicated prior to six hours after the onset of deficit is unclear. In view of the great difficulty in performing such a procedure within six hours of the occurrence of occlusion, surgical intervention is rarely indicated in blunt head injuries.

Supportive measures in the face of such ischemic events should be employed as with any ischemic stroke. The maintenance of adequate blood volume and pressure, as well as the use of steroids and dehydrating agents is indicated to control intracranial pressure elevations.

Traumatic aneurysms

Traumatic Arterial Aneurysms in the Neck. Traumatic arterial aneurysms in the neck are rare. In a report of 2,000 patients with head injury, El Gindi et al.[30] noted only one instance of traumatic aneurysm of a cervical artery. Raphael et al.,[91] in an analysis of 2,300 aneurysms throughout the body, found seven involving the carotid system in the neck, only one of which was traumatic. In two series of penetrating neck wounds sustained in military combat, traumatic carotid artery aneurysms were reported to have occurred in 0.4 and 1.7% of patients.[95, 110]

Penetrating injuries are the most common cause of traumatic arterial aneurysms in the neck, although in rare instances they can develop following blunt trauma.[23, 110] They are most commonly "false" aneurysms with hematomas forming at least part of the wall of the aneurysm. They usually become symptomatic between two and eight weeks after trauma although they may become manifest any time from immediately after the injury to as late as 30 years after the incident.[41, 95] These aneurysms rarely rupture and if they do, it is usually into the oropharyngeal space with exsanguinating hemorrhage.[117]

The most common symptom is a neck mass which may or may not be pulsatile. Less commonly present are focal neurological deficits (secondary to emboli from a mural thrombosis in the sac or delayed thrombosis of the carotid artery), local compression of the trachea, esophagus, or lower cranial nerves, bruit, and non-specific symptoms such as headache and neck pain (carotidynia).[89, 94, 110, 117] Progressive symptoms of respiratory embarrassment, lower cranial nerve palsies and embolic neurologic deficits comprise the usual course of untreated lesions.[91, 110, 117] The diagnosis may be anticipated by the presence of a pulsatile mass in the neck with a bruit and is confirmed by angiography.

In the past, treatment has included proximal carotid ligation or trapping and various wrapping and banding procedures.[115] The present treatment of choice is excision of the aneurysm and either primary or prosthetic arterial repair. When this cannot be technically accomplished, carotid ligation or trapping of the aneurysm preceded by an extracranial to intracranial arterial bypass should be considered.

Traumatic Aneurysms at the Base of the Skull. Aneurysms involving the carotid artery in its extracranial portion at the base of the skull or in its petrous and cavernous portions are rare. Only 69 well-documented cases have been identified.[62] Post-traumatic aneurysms in the neck, which are contiguous to the base of the skull are essentially the same as those in the more proximal portion of the internal carotid artery, with the exception that they are almost universally inaccessible for aneurysmorrhaphy.

Traumatic aneurysms of the cavernous and petrous portions of the internal carotid artery differ from those in the neck, both in their symptomatic presentation and in their treatment. These aneurysms are often associated with basilar skull fracture and frequently occur following a severe head injury caused by a motor vehicle accident.[45, 114] A smaller number have been reported as a result of gunshot wounds or other penetrating head injuries.[58, 62] The mechanism of injury is similar to that involved in the development of a carotid-cavernous fistula and it is possible that some of these aneurysms of the base of the skull may represent spontaneous closure of low-flow carotid-cavernous fistulas.

Because these aneurysms are extradural and encased in bone, the majority remain asymptomatic and are discovered incidentally on angiograms. Most often, symptoms appear after a silent interval from the time of injury and consist of epistaxis, cranial nerve palsy, pain, or distal embolization.[62, 116]

An identifiable syndrome of skull base aneurysms of the internal carotid artery begins with delayed epistaxis.[62] Nasal hemorrhage usually occurs at the time of the injury, and either stops spontaneously or following packing. In almost all instances an ipsilateral injury to the optic nerve occurs as well. Several weeks to months after the injury, severe epistaxis occurs. While epistaxis usually results from rupture of the lesion into the nasopharynx or paranasal air sinuses, bleeding from the nose can result by rupture of the aneurysm into the middle ear. Approximately one-half of the delayed hemorrhages occur within four hours of trauma. These post-traumatic aneurysms differ from congenital aneurysms of the internal carotid artery of the skull base in that they will stop spontaneously after their initial hemorrhage, while congenital aneurysms tend to bleed severely until operative intervention is undertaken.

Cranial nerve involvement by traumatic aneurysms of the base of the skull is relatively common. The optic nerve is most frequently involved, and visual loss or visual field defects can be documented in more than 80% of cases. In nearly 40% of cases, third nerve function may be impaired and cranial nerves IV, V and VI are involved in 10–15% of cases.

Because of their location intracranial rupture of these lesions is extremely rare. Surgical therapy is undertaken because of progressive enlargement producing pain or cranial nerve dysfunction or to prevent delayed epistaxis. Asymptomatic aneurysms which have never ruptured should be watched closely for enlargement with serial angiography or CT scan. Treatment consists of proximal ligation or an extracranial/intracranial trapping procedure. Proximal ligation is adequate for these lesions unless they have produced epistaxis in which case trapping is safer. The risks of iatrogenic carotid occlusion may be reduced with the concomitant use of an extracranial/intracranial arterial bypass. Recently, detachable balloons have been used to occlude these aneurysms. If the lesion is accessible and its configuration allows placement of a balloon, the procedure is useful. Although reported numbers are small, the results with bypass and balloons have been encouraging.[108, 111, 116]

Intracranial Traumatic Aneurysms. Post-traumatic intracranial aneurysms are unusual. El Gindi et al.[30] reported only seven cases in his study of 2,000 head injuries. There were only two post-traumatic intracranial aneurysms in more than 3,000 penetrating head wounds reported from the Korean and Vietnam wars.[20, 100] In civilian practice, 61% of post-traumatic intracranial aneurysms followed closed head injury, 24% followed penetrating injury, and 15% were iatrogenically produced during neurosurgical or otolaryngological procedures.[4, 7, 33, 55, 81, 125]

The pathology of intracranial traumatic aneurysms differs from traumatic aneurysms of other arteries. In large arteries throughout the rest of the body, the adventitia represents the strongest layer of the arterial wall. Intracranial arteries, on the other hand, have their greatest strength within the internal elastic membrane and media.[3, 119] While other arteries, especially the aorta, frequently have tears in the outer layers and subsequently develop aneurysms, intracranial traumatic aneurysms result either from rupture of the intima and the internal elastic membrane (with consequent formation of a true aneurysm), or from transection of the vessel wall with subsequent tamponade hematoma and false aneurysm formation.[67, 87, 99, 119] In one review of the pathology of intracranial traumatic aneurysms, 19 of 23 cases were found to be false aneurysms while only four were true aneurysms.

The event associated with aneurysm formation is usually severe trauma. Greater than 90% of the patients who go on to form such aneurysms lost consciousness at the time of the trauma and more than half sustained a skull fracture.[7, 33, 97] The mechanism is probably a direct contusion of the carotid artery against the base of the skull, the middle cerebral artery against the sphenoid wing, or the anterior cerebral artery against the edge of the falx. Gunshot wounds may also cause injury to the arterial wall with aneurysm formation (Fig. 14.3).

Approximately 40% of these aneurysms rupture and produce subarachnoid hemorrhage and the vast majority (85–90%) occur within three weeks of the time of the trauma.[7, 33, 99] The most common site is the middle cerebral artery, followed by the anterior cerebral and the internal carotid arteries.[7, 33, 97] As in other cases of vascular injuries from trauma, the increasing use of the CT scan to evaluate patients with head injury may result in failure to diagnose this entity unless subarachnoid hemorrhage produces an intracranial hematoma large enough to be identified on the scan. These aneurysms are easily differentiated on angiography from congenital berry aneurysms by their location. Traumatic aneurysms are frequently found near the cortical surface and not at major arterial bifurcations.[7]

The treatment of these lesions is obliteration. This is difficult because there is often no available neck. Distal cortical aneurysms can generally be resected, clipped, or excised without great risk of neurologic deficit. Proximal post-traumatic aneurysms, however, present several problems regarding surgical exposure. In addition to frequently lacking a clippable neck, the high incidence of false aneurysms makes intra-operative rupture frequent. Even minimal brain retraction may dislodge the clot which forms the wall of the aneurysm and uncontrollable bleeding may ensue.

Despite these difficulties, the recommended treatment is exploration and, if possible, clipping.[97] If a clippable neck is not found or cannot be fashioned, an encircling clip may be used. If this is not possible, the aneurysm may be coated with acrylic or gauze. For those aneurysms which can neither be clipped nor manipulated sufficiently for coating, trapping or proximal ligation supplemented with intracranial/extracranial arterial bypass must be used.

The operative mortality of traumatic aneurysms is approximately 20%, which compares favorably with 30–70% mortality rate if they are left untreated.[7, 11, 20, 30, 33, 84, 97] Mortality correlates with two factors: the severity of the primary trauma and the occurrence of delayed subarachnoid hemorrhage. In one series of patients with aneurysms found incidentally on an angiographic evaluation for intracranial hematoma, the mortality rate was 16%. In patients whose aneurysms ruptured before diagnosis, the mortality rate was 41%.[33] With the decline in the use of angiography for routine post-traumatic evaluation, the possibility of delayed recovery or secondary deterioration on the basis of an intracranial post-traumatic aneurysm must be kept in mind. If the CT scan does not reveal an obvious etiology for the deterioration, angiography is warranted to confirm the presence of an aneurysm.[84]

ARTERIOVENOUS FISTULAS

Fistulas in the Neck

Traumatic arteriovenous (AV) fistulas involving the carotid or vertebral arterial systems in the neck are rare. Among 558

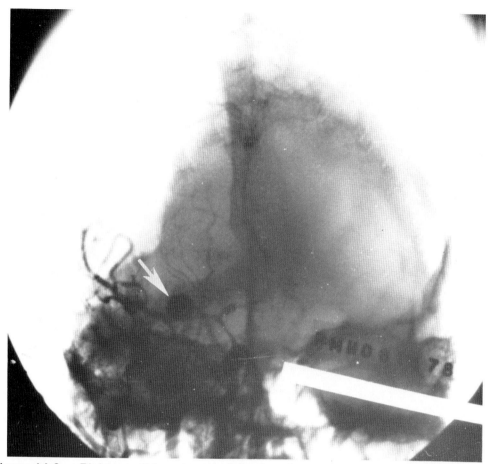

Figure 14.3. Right carotid angiogram following decompressive craniectomy and removal of subdural hematoma in a patient with gunshot wound of the right hemisphere. Large aneurysm (*arrow*) of the proximal middle cerebral artery is visualized. There is, as well, considerable vasospasm of the internal carotid, middle cerebral, and anterior cerebral arteries.

AV fistulas and false aneurysms reported from the Vietnam War, only eight involved the internal or common carotid artery and six involved the vertebral artery.[92] Nagashima *et al.*[75] reviewed the incidence of AV fistulas of the vertebral artery and was able to find only 60 cases of traumatic fistulas. Nineteen of these were iatrogenically induced. The majority of traumatic carotid fistulas involve the common carotid artery and the jugular vein. Approximately 75% of vertebral artery injuries involve the second portion of the artery which lies within the foramina transversaria of the cervical spine.

Sixteen percent of vertebral fistulas involve the third portion lying distally to the arch of C-1, and the remainder (approximately 9%) involve the first portion of the vertebral artery.[75] Vertebral injuries resulting in AV fistulas most usually involve the vertebral venous plexus as well. Occasionally multiple arteries or veins are involved.

Fragment or gunshot wounds are the most common etiology of AV fistulas in military series. In a civilian setting, stab wounds and low caliber gunshot wounds predominate (Fig. 14.4). Iatrogenic causes, including carotid endarterectomy and per-

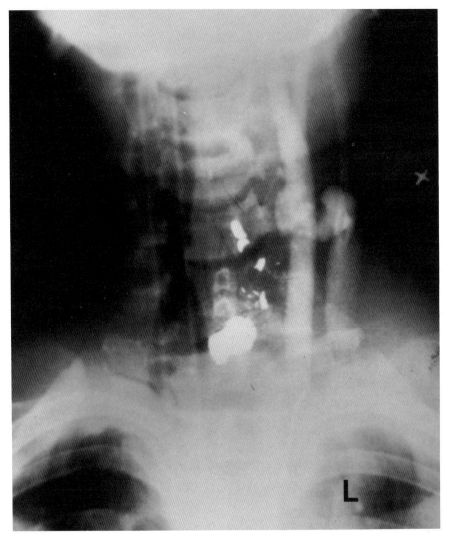

Figure 14.4.   Left carotid angiogram demonstrating fistula between common carotid artery and jugular vein in a patient with a gunshot wound of the neck. Operative closure of the fistula was uneventful.

cutaneous angiography, have also been reported.[44]

The diagnosis of AV fistulas is usually not difficult. A pulsatile mass accompanied by a bruit is noted. The bruit is often loud and may be heard by the patient. Neurological symptoms are secondary to a steal phenomenon or result from direct compression of neural structures by the enlarged vertebral vein plexus. Mass effect is common with vertebral artery injuries and may

cause cervical cord or lower brainstem compression. Cardiac failure from high flow AV fistulas has been reported.

Once these fistulas become symptomatic, they tend to enlarge progressively and spontaneous thrombosis is uncommon. Therefore, operative treatment is recommended. Prior to intervention, high quality angiography of the brachiocephalic vessels is required. Because numerous feeding and draining vessels may exist, multiple views with rapid sequence filming and subtraction techniques are necessary to identify the precise location of fistulous connections. Even then, particularly when the vertebral artery is involved, the entire fistula may not be defined roentgenographically.

As with AV fistulas anywhere in the body, a procedure for complete obliteration should be initially attempted. Incomplete obliteration leads to recurrence, and a second operation is always more difficult because of the development of additional collateral pathways. Several therapeutic modalities are available. Proximal ligation is almost always ineffective in eliminating the fistula. A trapping procedure with ligation and distal occlusion either in the neck or intracranially is somewhat more successful, particularly with carotid-jugular fistulas. However, such a procedure entails the danger of occlusion of a major artery to the brain.[80]

Optimal treatment consists of obliteration of the fistula with preservation of normal arterial blood flow. The majority of carotid fistulas are amenable to direct surgical repair with preservation of carotid blood flow. The arterial supply usually comes from the carotid artery and contributions from muscular branches are unusual. The most common location for these fistulas is between the common carotid artery and the jugular vein, and surgical exposure is usually straightforward. The fistula should be isolated and excised, followed by either primary or vein patch graft repair of the carotid artery.

Fistulas between the vertebral artery and vertebral venous plexus, often involve multiple arterial and venous components and are more difficult to approach operatively. Ligation and trapping procedures for vertebral fistulas are often unsuccessful because of the presence of multiple feeding channels. Direct surgical repair, particularly to the vertebral artery within the transverse processes, requires a difficult surgical exposure. Fistulas which originate from C-1 to C-3 may be approached posteriorly via a sub-occipital craniectomy allowing the vertebral artery to be traced proximally from its intradural portion to the location of the fistulous connection which

can then be obliterated. Fistulas from C-4 to C-6 are more easily approached anteriorly. The venous plexus is often greatly dilated, and isolation of the fistulous communication can be so complex as to preclude complete visualization. Because of the frequent failure of ligation and the difficulty of direct repair, embolization of these fistulas is increasingly popular.[21]

Balloons and particles of acrylic emboli are used alone or in combination with another procedure.[37, 96] Methods vary but generally involve distal ligation followed by embolization of the fistula and proximal ligation. Materials including muscle plugs, gelfoam, acrylic, and detachable balloons have been used successfully. This technique is very useful in the elimination of the fistula if embolization is complete. The disadvantage is that preservation of the blood flow via the feeding artery is not maintained.

The best approach is embolization with preservation of the patency of the parent artery. With this technique, detachable balloons or other material may be introduced into the fistula itself causing subsequent obliteration. When fistulas are too extensive to permit complete occlusion, embolization may reduce the shunt sufficiently to make direct surgical repair much simpler. These techniques are also applicable to those carotid fistulas which are too complex or too close to the base of the skull to allow for direct excision.[70] Both Debrun and Serbienko have reported treatment of AV fistulas with a high rate of patency of the parent vessel, almost complete success in obliteration of the fistula, and minimal complications.[25, 26, 104]

Treatment of these lesions by excision, embolization, or balloon occlusion generally results in a good outcome. However, the occurrence of major neurological impairment from steal or compression by the fistulas is fairly low and one must take this into account before advising repair. Obliteration of the fistula with preservation of the parent artery is clearly the optimal treatment, but in cases where this cannot be accomplished, trapping and embolization procedures appear to be acceptable alternatives.

Intracranial Fistulas

The incidence of traumatic intracranial AV fistulas, other than carotid-cavernous fistula, is low. The Cooperative Aneurysm Study did not report a single case of traumatic AV fistula and no single series has reported more than five such cases.[88] Most traumatic AV fistulas involve the meningeal vessels, usually from the middle meningeal artery to a meaningeal vein.[77] These generally follow penetrating trauma or a depressed fracture and are frequently associated with an intracranial hematoma. Fistulas between meningeal vessels and one of the major dural sinuses or between cortical arteries and veins have also been reported.[82]

Intracranial AV fistulas usually have a delayed presentation with subarachnoid, subdural, or epidural hemorrhage, or a bruit. They are often found incidentally at the time of angiography or during removal of an intracranial hematoma.[122] Angiographic diagnosis is usually straightforward, but on occasion scalp AV fistulas have been confused with meaningeal or cortical AV fistulas.[42] A search of the literature in 1980, by Feldman et al.,[31] for traumatic dural fistulas revealed only three cases of symptomatic intracranial fistulas. The magnitude of danger and the incidence of later intracranial hemorrhage from these lesions is unknown.

Treatment consists of obliteration of the fistula. Those involving dural arteries only are easily treated by embolization of the external carotid artery. If embolization is unsuccessful, direct excision should be carried out. Fistulas involving intracranial vessels require direct surgical treatment. Although proximal ligation has been successful, the superficial location of these lesions generally makes them accessible to complete removal, which is the preferred method of therapy. Those that drain into a major venous sinus require proximal ligation only.[32]

Carotid-cavernous Fistulas

Carotid-cavernous fistulas are the most well recognized of all post-traumatic vascular injuries. The distinctive clinical syndrome and the difficulty in treating these fistulas has led to widespread reporting of the entity. Although it is an uncommon disorder, considerable interest has centered upon its treatment.

Carotid-cavernous fistulas are of traumatic origin in 60–80%[60, 71] of cases; the remainder occur spontaneously. Although fistulas occasionally result from mild head injury, more often they follow a severe impact with an associated basilar skull fracture. Epidemiological studies suggest that there is probably little relationship between post-traumatic carotid-cavernous fistula and congenital aneurysms of the cavernous portion of the internal carotid artery. The age and sex of the patient with traumatic fistulas parallel that of the head trauma population.[71] In contrast to spontaneous carotid-cavernous fistulas which occur predominantly in older women, carotid-cavernous fistulas of traumatic origin are most often found in younger men.

As the internal carotid artery emerges from the base of the skull, it passes through the multiseptated cavernous sinus before piercing the dura and entering the subarachnoid space. Within the cavernous sinus, the meningohypophyseal trunk (the artery of the cavernous sinus), and one or two capsular arteries exit from the internal carotid artery. Occasionally a persistent trigeminal artery is present as well. A traumatic carotid-cavernous fistula arises when the intracavernous portion of the internal carotid artery or one of these branches is lacerated and ruptures into the venous channels of the cavernous sinus. If the hemorrhage is contained by the septae within the cavernous sinus and does not rupture into a venous channel, a false aneurysm may result.

The clinical diagnosis of carotid-cavernous fistula is generally straightforward. The syndrome includes, in order of frequency: proptosis, chemosis, bruit, ophthalmoplegia, deterioration of vision, and headache.[73] Patients may complain of a swishing sound in the head and a bruit may be confirmed by auscultation. The Doppler stethoscope may be helpful in confirming the presence of a carotid-cavernous fistula in an unconscious patient or in instances where the flow is too low to produce sounds detectable by a conventional stethoscope. A false aneurysm of the intracavernous internal carotid artery may be differentiated from a carotid-cavernous fistula by the absence of a bruit or chemosis, although the other findings may be present.

Carotid-cavernous fistulas may be of sufficient magnitude to divert antegrade blood flow from the proximal internal carotid artery into the venous circulation; and may also produce a steal in which blood from the intracranial internal carotid artery flows in a retrograde direction into the cavernous sinus through the fistula. However, cerebral ischemia is rare despite the steal effect.[71]

Deterioration in vision is the most common serious complication of carotid-cavernous fistula and occurs in approximately 10% of patients. The visual loss may occur at the time of trauma or be delayed and progressive.[71, 73] It may result from injury to the optic nerve or it may be of ischemic origin. The ischemia results from decreased flow from the arterial side or from venous congestion in the retina from the high venous pressure. Once visual function is lost, there is little chance of its recovery.

Proptosis is the most common sign of carotid-cavernous fistula and may be associated with visual loss. As the proptosis increases, it may become grotesquely disfiguring, cause exposure keratitis, and produce blindness. In the absence of visual loss, total ophthalmoplegia may render the eye useless.

The CT scan is not helpful in the diagnosis of carotid-cavernous fistula and arteriography is the diagnostic procedure of choice. In order to fully elucidate the nature of a fistula, multiple projections, magnification, and subtraction techniques, and rapid film sequences are important. Selective cross circulation studies from the opposite carotid artery and the vertebral artery are often helpful in defining the precise anatomical relationships of the fistula.

The natural history of carotid-cavernous fistula is discouraging. Approximately 40–50% of these patients will develop progressive, irreversible monocular blindness.[73] Al-though these fistulas have been observed to close, spontaneous remission of traumatic carotid-cavernous fistulas is uncommon and the usual history is one of progressive monocular blindness, intolerable bruit, and progressively disfiguring proptosis. These symptoms justify attempts to obliterate the fistula unless there are medical contraindications. There is no advantage of a prolonged waiting period between the detection of a fistula and attempts at surgical occlusion. If there is no indication of resolution of the fistula at the time the acute effects of the head injury have resolved, treatment should be undertaken.

The objective of treatment of carotid-cavernous fistulas is the elimination of the communication between the arterial and venous circulation while preserving the lumen of the internal carotid artery. The latter consideration is often secondary since, as previously noted, fistulas may be shunting blood away from the brain and obliteration of the fistula, even if it is accompanied by occlusion of the internal carotid artery, might increase ipsilateral hemispheric blood flow.

There are numerous descriptions of surgical treatments of carotid-cavernous fistulas.[13] These range from simple carotid ligation in the neck to exotic, direct visualization and obliteration of the fistula intracranially while the patient is under deep hypothermia and cardiopulmonary arrest.[71, 83, 85, 86] In the past several years, treatment of carotid-cavernous fistula has improved considerably. The current methods can be divided into approaches from the arterial and venous sides of the fistula. The simplest arterial approach is balloon occlusion of the internal carotid artery at the level of the fistula. This can be done by direct exposure of the carotid artery in the neck and the use of a Fogarty catheter (as described by Prolo and Hanbery[90]) or percutaneously, using detachable balloon catheters. While this is an effective form of treatment, it has the disadvantage of carotid occlusion with possible distal propagation or embolization of thrombus.

Another approach which has been described is the placement of a detachable balloon directly into the AV fistula with preservation of carotid blood flow. There has been progressive improvement in the technology of balloon catheterization and advances in instrumentation have made the majority of these fistulas accessible to experienced technicians.[26, 27, 72] Detachable balloon systems with or without acrylic embolization have been shown to be effective and result in few complications.[78] Debrun has had a cure rate of carotid-cavernous fistulas of nearly 100% with carotid patency of 85% in patients using balloon occlusion[26, 27] (Figs. 14.5 and 14.6). The major disadvantage of this technique is that it is only appropriate for large fistulas which will allow for the placement of balloons. A small neck or a severely kinked proximal carotid artery will make placement of a balloon impossible. Further experience and continued technical improvements will almost certainly lead to even better results.

Approaches to the venous side involve both balloon techniques and direct occlusion. Direct surgical approaches were originally described by Parkinson[83] and involved hypothermia and cardiopulmonary bypass (Fig. 14.7). The current techniques as evolved by Campbell (as described by Debrun[24]) and Mullan.[73] Campbell's approach uses direct opening of the posterior cavernous sinus and packing with thrombogenic material. Mullan has described the obliteration of the sinus by anterior packing via the ophthalmic vein (Figs. 14.8 and 14.9)

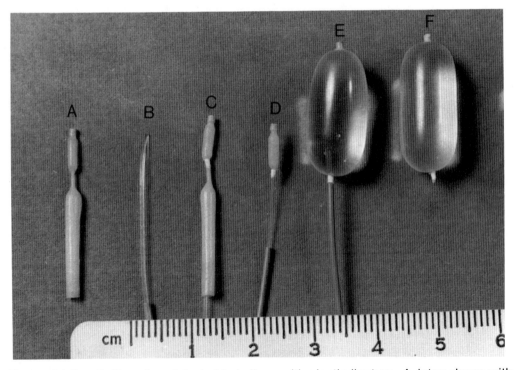

Figure 14.5.   Self-sealing detachable balloon with elastic ligature. *A*, latex sleeve with narrowed portion 0.3 mm in diameter. Silver index in place in the teat like distal portion; *B*, Teflon catheter "A" 0.4 mm internal diameter, 0.6 mm external diameter; *C*, the sleeve is ligated over catheter "A" with latex thread and its proximal portion is then cut away; *D*, the proximal portion of the sleeve has been cut away. Polyethylene coaxial catheter "B" is visible; *E*, to detach the balloon, catheter B is slid up over catheter A into contact with the base of the balloon. Catheter B thus holds the balloon in place while catheter A is pulled back out of the balloon to detach it; *F*, the latex ligature immediately closes the aperture of the balloon which is detached. (Courtesy Gerard DeBrun, M.D.)

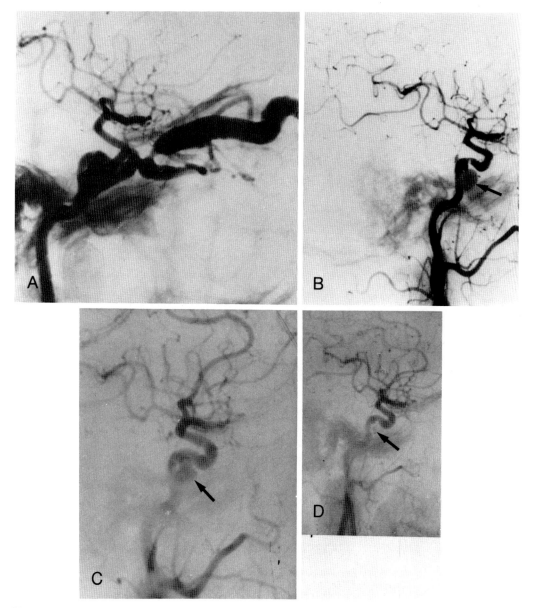

Figure 14.6.   A post-traumatic carotid-cavernous sinus fistula. Pre-treatment (*A*) and post-treatment (*B*) using an iodine-inflated balloon (*arrow*). *C*, the fistula was occluded, but a false aneurysmal pouch formed in place (*arrow*). *D*, this was later occluded with a silicone-inflated balloon. (Reprinted with permission from Gerard DeBrun, M.D., *et al.*: J. Neurosurg., 49:635–649, 1978.)

or the introduction of thrombogenic wire into the posterior sinus. Mullan's method used in 33 cases resulted in no mortality or progression of visual loss. The use of balloons *via* the internal jugular vein has only recently been introduced. In cases where the arterial opening of the fistula is inadequate to allow placement of a detachable balloon, this method may offer an alternate approach.

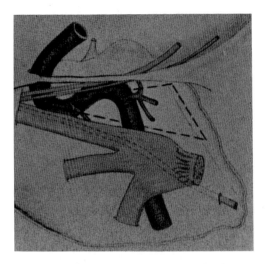

Figure 14.7. Diagram of the left triangular space of the cavernous sinus with the third and fourth nerves above and the first division of the fifth nerve and sixth nerve below showing how an incision placed within this triangular space affords access to the parasellar portion of the carotid artery and its branches while avoiding incision of the cranial nerves. (Reproduced by permission from Dwight Parkinson, M.D.: Carotid-cavernous fistula: direct repair with preservation of the carotid artery. Technical note. J. Neurosurg., 38:99–106, 1973.)

It would appear from these more recent reports that either the Campbell or Mullan operations for direct approach or a balloon obliteration should make virtually all carotid-cavernous fistulas amenable to surgical treatment. Wide-necked lesions would seem to be more easily treated with a balloon technique while lesions with a narrow neck or tortuous proximal vessels may require open surgical obliteration.

VENOUS SINUS INJURIES

Depending upon the nature of the traumatic event, injuries to the cerebral venous sinuses result in hemorrhage and/or thrombosis. El Gindi reported 18 cases of dural tear and 15 cases of dural thrombosis among the 2,000 patients that he reviewed.[36]

Dural Venous Sinus Laceration

Laceration of the dural sinuses is virtually always related to a skull fracture. In civilian practice, road accidents and bullet wounds account for the majority of lacerations, whereas in war, sinus injury occurs as a result of missile wounds.

The clinical presentation of the patient with a lacerated dural venous sinus depends upon the mechanism of injury. If it is related to an open, comminuted fracture, the most obvious sign is external hemorrhage. This is frequently a dramatic injury, with many victims exsanguinating before definitive therapy can be established. However, if it is related to a closed fracture, the patient may present with signs and symptoms of an epidural hematoma, either shortly after the injury or, more often, after a delay of several days.

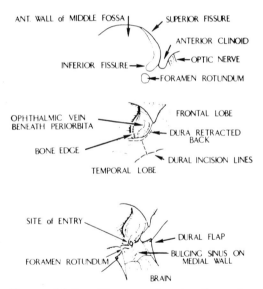

Figure 14.8. Diagram showing the anterior extradural technique. *Upper,* the foramen rotundum is located. *Center,* the bone between fissures is drilled out. *Lower,* an incision is made at the point of entry into the sinus. (Reproduced by permission from Sean Mullan, M.D.: Treatment of carotid-cavernous fistulas by cavernous sinus occlusion. J. Neurosurg., 50:131–144, 1979.)

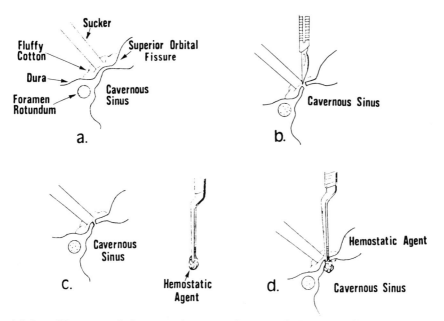

Figure 14.9. Diagram of the anterior extradural technique. *a,* Schematic transverse section at point of entry of the vein into the sinus. *b,* A very small incision is made. *c,* Bleeding is prevented by pressure of cotton-occluded sucker. *d,* Piecemeal insertion of small thrombogenic plugs into the sinus. (Reproduced by permission from author, Sean Mullan, M.D.: Treatment of carotid-cavernous fistulas by cavernous sinus occlusion. J. Neurosurg., 50:131–144, 1979.)

The diagnosis of laceration of the dural sinus causing hemorrhage is usually self-evident. Typically, a patient with a scalp laceration in the region of the sagittal or transverse sinus presents with profuse venous hemorrhage. Inspection, palpation, or skull X rays will demonstrate a comminuted fracture, either depressed or elevated. The situation is somewhat more complicated if the bleeding is less dramatic. In a case with a laceration in the vicinity of a cerebral venous sinus, the surgeon must avoid being lulled into a false sense of security by the absence of severe bleeding. A mere change in head position or the movement of a bony fragment may result in a torrential venous hemorrhage. In any instance where such an injury is a possibility, steps to reduce the dangers from sinus laceration must be taken until the diagnosis is clarified.

When such an injury is suspected, intracranial venous pressure should be lowered by placing the head in a neutral position and elevating it to the point where the bleeding just stops or is reduced to a minimum. Care should be taken to avoid elevating the head too high because of the risk of air embolization.[66] Packing the wound with sponges soaked in antibiotic solution decreases the chances for air embolus and helps to tamponade the hemorrhage. Large bore IV catheters should be placed to make rapid fluid resuscitation possible. Colloid and crystalloid solutions should be used and a large quantity of whole blood should be cross matched. Whole blood must be obtained in excess of that required for simple resuscitation since sudden losses during surgery must be anticipated. Arterial and central venous lines (or preferably Swan-Ganz catheter) should be placed and the patient must be taken to the operating room as soon as possible. Adequate skull films are essential and, if conditions permit, a CT scan should also be performed. Arteriography is of little help in the acute setting. In situations where the bleeding is minor and can be completely stopped with elevation of the head, it may be reasonable to debride and cleanse the wound and perform a primary closure of the scalp without attempting to elevate the fracture. This might be particularly appropriate if the injury involves a small depression over the posterior two-thirds of the sagittal sinus or the torcula. In these instances, patients must be observed carefully for signs of developing epidural hematoma or a sinus thrombosis.

At the beginning of any operative repair a precordial Doppler and/or an end-tidal CO_2 analyzer should be used for detection of air emboli. Special care should be taken to maintain a head position that will not compromise venous outflow. The operative approach must be planned to insure sufficient exposure of the proximal and distal sinus in order to control bleeding. The pa-

tient must also be positioned so that a vein graft may be taken, should it be required to repair the injury. Once wide exposure is obtained, the injury can be evaluated.

With sagittal sinus injuries, the variability of the rolandic inflow and collateral venous circulation dictates the exact point at which the sinus becomes essential.[43] In most instances, the anterior one-third to one-half of the saggital sinus can be occluded without significant ill effects (Fig. 14.10).[50] In dealing with injuries of the transverse sinus, there is more difficulty in deciding whether or not the sinus is expendable. A clearly dominant sinus should not be sacrificed, but pre-operative angiograms are generally not available. Therefore, transverse sinus damage should be treated as an injury to an essential venous structure with every effort made to preserve patency.

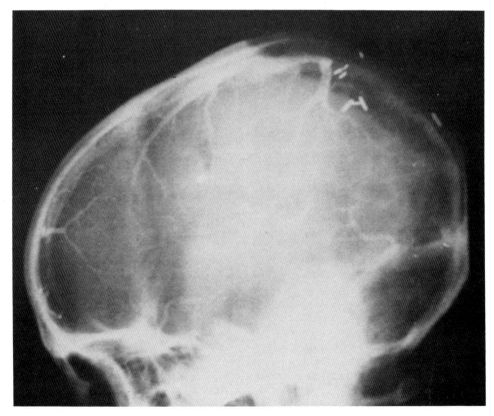

Figure 14.10. Sinogram demonstrating traumatic occlusion of posterior sagittal sinus. (Courtesy of John Kapp, M.D., Ph.D.)

Once the sinus is fully exposed, hemorrhage must be controlled to allow careful inspection and debridement in a bloodless field. Minor injuries may be controlled by direct pressure. Larger injuries and transections require more extensive measures. Although it is possible to obtain proximal and distal control with parasagittal dural incisions and sinus clamping, the preferred method is an internal shunt device (Fig. 14.11). These shunts utilize heparinized tubing with an inflatable balloon at each end.[49] The balloons are inserted into the sinus and inflated and serve the dual purpose of controlling hemorrhage and allowing continued venous blood flow. Once control is obtained in this manner, repair may be carried out without undo haste and in a bloodless operating field.

Primary repair should be carried out any time 50% or more of the sinus lumen can be preserved.[50] If the laceration is too extensive for primary repair, reconstruction with a patch graft should be attempted. In the past, muscle stamp grafts and fascia have been used with reasonably good success. More recently, vein patch grafts have been found to give superior results. If the sinus is completely transected and tissue loss is too great to permit primary repair then a reverse saphenous vein graft is the treatment of choice.[50, 93, 107] If a thrombosis is found in the lumen of the sinus, thrombectomy should be performed and thorough irrigation with heparin carried out.

The mortality in injuries of the venous sinuses is related to the primary brain injury and the location of the sinus involved. When the injury involves the anterior one-half of the sagittal sinus, a mortality rate of less than 5% can be expected. The mortality rate for lacerations of the posterior one-half of the sagittal sinus approaches 35%, but can probably be significantly reduced with the use of contemporary techniques, particularly vein grafts. There is also a high mortality (25%) from lacerations of the transverse sinus. Injuries to other sinuses including the straight sinus, the inferior sagittal sinus, and the petrosal sinus are more dif-

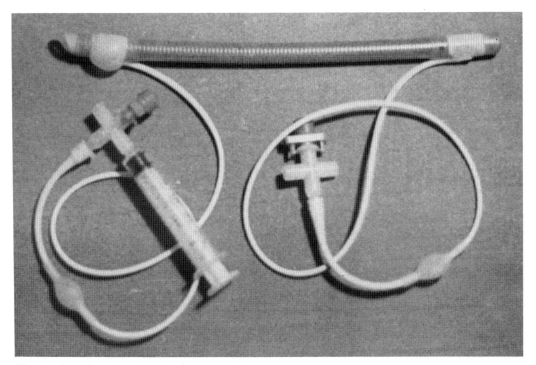

Figure 14.11.   Internal shunt for use in sinus repairs (see description in text). (Courtesy of John Kapp, M.D., Ph.D.)

ficult to evaluate because these injuries are seldom reported. In any case, the primary brain injury is the most important factor governing outcome for patients with such injuries.[50, 66, 93]

The management of acute epidural hematomas, caused by lacerations of the dural venous sinus, is discussed in Chapter 11. Sinus lacerations causing subacute or chronic epidural hematomas are easier to deal with because, in most instances, the rent in the sinus will have become clotted by the time the patient develops symptoms of a mass lesion. In these instances, an attempt should be made to remove the bulk of the hematoma without disturbing the clot directly over the sinus. However, one must be prepared for the possibility of sudden hemorrhage requiring surgical repair of the laceration.

Dural Venous Sinus Thrombosis

Dural venous sinus thrombosis most often results from a depressed skull fracture, although it occasionally occurs after blunt head injury without skull fracture or with only a linear or diastatic fracture.[19, 51] The clinical manifestations of this disorder depend upon the sinus which is involved. Traumatic thromboses of the anterior sagittal sinus or the non-dominant transverse sinus are usually asymptomatic and go unrecognized in the majority of cases. Thrombosis of the posterior sagittal sinus or dominant transverse sinus may result in venous infarction with severe brain swelling and intracranial hypertension. Propagation of the thrombus into cortical veins is not uncommon.

Seizures are particularly frequent and postictal paralysis often fails to resolve. Signs of bilateral cerebral hemisphere dysfunction, particularly paraplegia or quadriplegia, are common.[19] Mortality and morbidity are high and patients who survive may develop chronically increased intracranial pressure.

In patients with severe head injury with brain contusion and depressed levels of consciousness, the early diagnosis of sinus thrombosis is difficult because its clinical presentation is not distinctive. A CT scan may demonstrate sinus thrombosis or hemorrhagic infarction and edema.[17, 118] However, hemorrhage, infarction, and edema may also occur as a direct effect of the primary injury. Angiography is helpful, but occasionally it is difficult to visualize the area of thrombosis with certainty. The situation is further complicated by the congenital variability of the dural sinuses including hypoplasia or even absence of a sinus.

The diagnosis of sinus thrombosis should be strongly suspected in a patient who has an injury in the region of a major dural sinus (particularly a depressed fracture) and who then develops seizures followed by profound focal neurological deficits. This is particularly true if a hemorrhagic infarction is demonstrated by CT scan. Therapy in the acute period is directed at controlling seizures, reducing brain swelling with hyperventilation, mannitol and ventricular drainage of CSF, and improving the rheological characteristics of the blood. Anticoagulation has been used in some patients with non-traumatic cortical thrombophlebitis and sinus thrombosis, but the efficacy of this therapy is unclear. When sinus thrombosis occurs following head injury, anti-coagulation is almost always contraindicated, both because of the initial brain injury and because of the propensity for anti-coagulation to cause hemorrhagic infarction.[19] The value of thrombectomy for sinus thrombosis is unresolved. The difficulty in making the diagnosis of sinus thrombosis rarely allows thrombectomy to be carried out soon after its occurrence unless there is a concomitant open injury. Because the sinuses are multi-septated and contain a delicate endothelium, the surgeon is often unable to completely remove the thrombus and recurrent thrombosis is frequent.[19]

Less than 5% of patients who survive initial injury and sinus thrombosis develop chronic, increased, intracranial pressure.[10, 30, 51] In most instances, this is a benign syndrome and can be adequately treated with steroids and acetazolamide. Occasionally, patients do not respond to this treatment and have continued papilledema and visual loss. Surgical therapy, most commonly decompressive anterior temporal lobectomy, has been used for these cases. In 1980, Sindou et al.[106] reported a case of progressive, medically refractory loss of vision secondary to bilateral transverse sinus occlusion. He performed a bypass graft of the transverse sinus to the external jugular vein with excellent results. This technique holds promise in the treatment of such refractory cases.

TRAUMATIC VASOSPASM

Cerebral vasospasm is the angiographically demonstrable narrowing of the lumen of the major cerebral arteries which occurs following subarachnoid hemorrhage. It may be associated with a syndrome of progressive ischemic neurological deficit which usually develops insidiously 5–10 days following subarachnoid hemorrhage. Cerebral vasospasm is most often noted after spontaneous subarachnoid hemorrhage caused by the rupture of an intracranial aneurysm. The spasm can be demonstrated angiographically in as many as 80% of patients with aneurysmal subarachnoid hemorrhage, and signs of cerebral ischemia occur in 40% of these patients.

Traumatic subarachnoid hemorrhage occurs far more often than spontaneous subarachnoid hemorrhage; a reflection of the much higher incidence of head trauma than ruptured aneurysms. More than 75% of all head injury patients show clinical signs of meningeal irritation or lumbar puncture evidence of hemorrhage.[36, 56, 112, 120, 121]

Mechanical injury alone does not appear to cause long-term vasospasm.[6, 113] Rather, the arterial luminal narrowing is probably related to the volume of clotted blood adhering to the arteries in the subarachnoid space. Rupture of an aneurysm of the circle of Willis allows a large volume of blood to be injected directly into the basal cisterns. In contrast, however, subarachnoid hemorrhage following trauma is deposited diffusely in the cerebrospinal fluid throughout the subarachnoid space.

In certain circumstances, more severe subarachnoid hemorrhage like that following aneurysmal rupture, does occur, usually from arterial laceration, but in these instances the injury is usually severe and patients do not survive long enough to develop vasospasm. Furthermore, the survivors of such a head injury are frequently so severely injured that the diagnosis of further neurological deficits due to vasospasm is difficult.[61] It is also likely that in many patients who develop vasospasm, the arterial narrowing is not recognized, as the initial angiogram is performed within 48 hours of head injury and luminal narrowing does not reach its peak until 5–9 days. In addition, with the increasing use of the CT scanner, angiography is being performed less frequently in patients with head injury.

Cerebral vasospasm should be suspected in patients who deteriorate neurologically 5–9 days following a head injury. The most common symptoms are drowsiness, the insidious onset of a focal neurologic deficit, or increasing headache. These symptoms may occur with normal intracranial pressure and in the absence of a mass lesion.[64]

The CT scan will assist in differentiating vasospasm from subdural hematoma, contusion, or delayed intracerebral hematoma. Furthermore, if the initial CT scan performed near the time of injury showed no thick layering of blood within the subarachnoid space, vasospasm is less likely to occur. Nevertheless, the definitive diagnostic procedure is still angiography.

The treatment of post-traumatic vasospasm follows the same principles as the treatment of vasospasm following aneurysmal rupture. There are no effective means for dilating the narrowed arteries. Accordingly, efforts must be made to improve cerebral circulation in an attempt to reverse the ischemic consequences of the arterial narrowing. Arterial pO_2 should be maintained above 60 torr and pCO_2 between 30 and 40 torr. Circulating blood volume is kept in the high normal range with use of blood, colloid, and crystalloid solutions as needed. Cardiac output and systemic arterial pressure are kept elevated with fluid volume control and dopamine. Mannitol is often helpful, not only for lowering the intracranial pressure and improving the cerebral perfusion pressure, but also to improve the rheological characteristics of blood.

Using this regimen, approximately two-thirds of patients with ischemic neurological deficits from vasospasm following aneurysmal subarachnoid hemorrhage will have a permanent reversal of their neurological impairments. There is insufficient experience in treating patients with post-traumatic vasospasm to comment on the effectiveness of this protocol in the traumatic setting. Because of the complications of brain injury and the limitations upon hypervolemia-hypertensive therapy in the traumatized and swollen brain, it would be expected that overall results in patients with traumatic vasospasm might be inferior to those seen with ruptured aneurysm.

References:

1. Aarabi, B., McQueen, J.D.: Traumatic internal carotid occlusion at the base of the skull. Surg. Neurol., 10:233–236, 1978.
2. Ackerman, R.H.: Noninvasive carotid evaluation. Current concepts of cerebrovascular disease. Stroke, 15:7–10, 1980.
3. Acosta, C., Williams, P.E. Jr., Clark, K.: Traumatic aneurysms of the cerebral vessels. J. Neurosurg., 36:531–536, 1972.
4. Alexander, E. Jr., Adams, J.E., Davis, C.H. Jr.: Complications in the use of temporary intracranial arterial clip. J. Neurosurg., 20:810–811, 1963.
5. Arseni, C., Maretsis, M., Horvath, L.: Posttraumatic intracranial arterial spasm: report of three cases. Acta Neurochir., 24:25–35, 1971.
6. Arutiunov, A.I., Baron, M.A., Majorova, N.A.: The role of mechanical factors in the pathogenesis of short-term and prolonged spasm of the cerebral arteries. J. Neurosurg., 40:459–472, 1974.
7. Asari, S., Nakamura, S., Yamada, O., Beck, H., Sugatani, H., Nigashi, T.: Traumatic aneurysm of peripheral cerebral arteries. J. Neurosurg., 46:795–803, 1977.
8. Batzdorf, U., Bentson, J.R., Machleder, H.I.: Blunt trauma to the cervical carotid artery. Neurosurgery, 5:195–201, 1979.
9. Bauer, R., Sheehan, S., Meyer, J.S.: Arteriographic study of cerebrovascular disease. Arch. Neurol., 4:119–131, 1961.
10. Beller, A.J.: Benign post-traumatic intracranial hypertension. J. Neurol. Neurosurg. Psychiat., 27:149–152, 1964.
11. Benoit, B.G., Wortzman, G.: Traumatic cerebral aneurysms. Clinical features and natural history. J. Neurol. Neurosurg. Psychiat., 36:127–138, 1973.
12. Berguer, R., Higgins, R., Nelson, R.: Noninvasive diagnosis of reversal of vertebral artery blood flow. N. Engl. J. Med., 302:1349–1351, 1980.
13. Black, P., Uematsu, S., Perovic, M., Walker, A.E.: Carotid-cavernous fistula: a controlled embolus technique for occlusion of fistula with preservation of carotid blood flow. J. Neurosurg., 38:113–118, 1973.
14. Boldrey, E., Maass, L., Miller, E.: The role of atlantoid compression in the etiology of internal carotid thrombosis. J. Neurosurg., 13:127–139, 1956.
15. Bradley, E.L., III: Management of penetrating carotid injuries: an alternative approach. J. Trauma, 13:248–255, 1973.
16. Brown, B. St. J., Tatlow, W.E.T.: Radiographic studies of the vertebral arteries in cadavers. Radiology, 81:80–88, 1963.
17. Buonanno, F.S., Moody, D.M., Ball, M.R., Laster, D.W.: Computed cranial tomographic findings in cerebral sinovenous occlusion. J. Comp. Asst. Tomogr., 2:281–290, 1978.
18. Carpenter, S.: Injury of neck as cause of vertebral artery thrombosis. J. Neurosurg., 18:849–853, 1961.
19. Carric, A.W., Jaffé, F.A.: Thrombosis of superior sagittal sinus. J. Neurosurg., 11:173–182, 1954.
20. Chadduck, W.M.: Traumatic cerebral aneurysm due to speargun injury. Case report. J. Neurosurg., 31:77–79, 1969.
21. Chou, S.N., French, L.A.: Arteriovenous fistula of vertebral vessels in the neck. J. Neurosurg., 22:77–80, 1965.
22. Cohen, A., Brief, D., Mathewson, C.: Carotid artery injuries. J. Surgery, 120:210–214, 1970.
23. Davidson, K.C., Weiford, E.C., Dixon, G.D.: Traumatic vertebral artery pseudoaneurysm following chiropractic manipulation. Radiology, 115:651–652, 1975.
24. Debrun, G., Fox, A., Drake, C.: Comments to intravascular use of isobutyl 2-cyanoacrylate. 2. Neurosurgery, 8:55, 1981.
25. Debrun, G., Legre, J., Kasbarian, M., Tapias, P.L., Caron, J.P.: Endovascular occlusion of vertebral fistulae by detachable balloons with conservation of the vertebral blood flow. Radiology, 130:141–147, 1979.
26. Debrun, G., Lacour, P., Caron, J.P., Hurth, M., Comoy, J., Keravel, Y.: Detachable balloon and calibrated-leak balloon techniques in the treatment of cerebral vascular lesions. J. Neurosurg., 49:635–649, 1978.
27. Debrun, G., Lacour, P., Caron, J.P., Hurth, M., Comoy, J., Deravel, Y., Laborit, G.: Experimental approach to the treatment of carotid cavernous fistulas with an inflatable and isolated balloon. Neuroradiology, 9:9–12, 1975.
28. Dujovny, M., Laha, R.K., Decastro, S., Briani, S.: Post-traumatic middle cerebral artery thrombosis. J. Trauma, 19:774–779, 1979.
29. Duman, S., Stephens, J.W.: Post-traumatic middle cerebral artery occlusion. Neurology, 13:613–616, 1963.
30. El Gindi, S., Salama, M., Tawfik, E., Nasr, H.A., El Nadi, F.: A review of 2,000 patients with craniocerebral injuries with regard to intracranial haematomas and other vascular complications.

Acta Neurochir., 48:237–244, 1979.

31. Fein, J.M., Flamm, E.: Planned intracranial revascularization before ligation for traumatic aneurysm. Neurosurgery, 5:254–258, 1979.

32. Feldman, R.A., Hieshima, G., Giannotta, S.L., Gade, G.F.: Traumatic dural arteriovenous fistula supplied by scalp, meningeal, and cortical arteries: case report. Neurosurgery, 6:670–674, 1980.

33. Fleischer, A.S., Patton, J.M., Tindall, G.T.: Cerebral aneurysms of traumatic origin. Surg. Neurol., 4:233–239, 1975.

34. Frantzen, E., Jacobsen, H.H., Therkelsen, J.: Cerebral artery occlusions in childhood due to trauma to the head and neck. Neurology, 11:695–700, 1961.

35. Fraser, R.A.R., Zimbler, S.M.: Hindbrain stroke in children caused by extracranial vertebral artery trauma. Stroke, 6:153–159, 1975.

36. Freidenfelt, H., Sundström, R.: Local and general spasm in the internal carotid system following trauma. Acta Radiol. I, New Ser. Diag., 278–283, 1963.

37. Goodman, S.J., Hasso, A., Kirkpatrick, D.: Treatment of vertebrojugular fistula by balloon occlusion. Case report. J. Neurosurg., 43:362–367, 1975.

38. Hardin, G.A., Poser, C.M.: Rotational obstruction of the vertebral artery due to redundancy and extraluminal cervical fascial bands. Ann. Surg., 158:133–137, 1963.

39. Higazi, I.: Post-traumatic carotid thrombosis. J. Neurosurg., 20:354–359, 1963.

40. Hollin, S.A., Sukoff, M.H., Silverstein, A., Gross, S.W.: Post-traumatic middle cerebral artery occlusion. J. Neurosurg., 25:526–535, 1966.

41. Hunt, J.L., Snyder, W.H.: Late false aneurysm of the carotid artery: repair with extra-intracranial arterial bypass. J. Trauma, 19:198–200, 1979.

42. Hyshaw, C., DiTullio, M., Renaudin, J.: Superficial temporal arteriovenous fistula. Surg. Neurol., 12:46–48, 1979.

43. Jaeger, R.: Observations on resection of the superior longitudinal sinus at and posterior to the rolandic venous inflow. J. Neurosurg., 8:103–109, 1951.

44. Jamieson, K.G.: Case reports and technical note. Vertebral arteriovenous fistula caused by angiography needle. J. Neurosurg., 23:620–621, 1965.

45. Janon, E.A.: Traumatic changes in the internal carotid artery associated with basal skull fractures. Radiology, 96:55–59, 1970.

46. Jernigan, W.R., Gardner, W.C.: Carotid artery injuries due to closed cervical trauma. J. Trauma, 11:429–435, 1971.

47. Johnson, A.C., Graves, V.B., Pfaff, J.P.: Dissecting aneurysm of intracranial arteries. Surg. Neurol., 7:49–52, 1977.

48. Jones, R.F., Terrell, J.C., Salyer, K.E.: Penetrating wounds of the neck: An analysis of 274 cases. J. Trauma, 7:228–237, 1967.

49. Kapp, J.P., Gielchinsky, I., Petty, C., McClure, C.: An internal shunt for use in the reconstruction of dural venous sinuses. J. Neurosurg., 35:351–354, 1971.

50. Kapp, J.P., Gielchinsky, I., Deardourff, S.L.: Operative techniques for management of lesions involving the dural venous sinuses. Surg. Neurol., 7:339–342, 1977.

51. Kinal, M.E.: Traumatic thrombosis of dural venous sinuses in closed head injuries. J. Neurosurg., 27:142–145, 1967.

52. Krueger, B.R., Okazaki, H.: Vertebral-basilar distribution infarction following chiropractic cervical manipulation. Mayo Clin. Proc., 55:322–332, 1980.

53. Kunze, S., Schiefer, W.: Angiographic demonstration of a dissecting aneurysm of the middle cerebral artery. Neuroradiology, 2:201–206, 1971.

54. Laha, R.K., Dujovny, M., Barrionuevo, P.J., DeCastro, S.C., Hellstrom, H.R., Maroon, J.C.: Protective effect of methyl prednisolone and dimethyl sulfoxide in experimental middle cerebral artery embolectomy. J. Neurosurg., 49:508–516, 1978.

55. Lassman, L.P., Ramani, P.S., Sengupta, R.P.: Aneurysms of peripheral cerebral arteries due to surgical trauma. Vasc. Surg., 8:1–5, 1974.

56. Leeds, N.E., Reid, N.D., Rosen, L.M.: Angiographic changes in cerebral contusions and intracerebral hematomas. Acta Rad. Diag., 5:320–327, 1966.

57. Linell, E.A., Tom, M.I.: Traumatic arterial lesions and cerebral thrombosis. Can. M.A.J., 81:808–813, 1959.

58. Lister, J.R., Sypert, G.W.: Traumatic false aneurysm and carotid-cavernous fistula: a complication of sphenoidotomy. Neurosurgery, 5:473–475, 1979.

59. Loar, C.R., Chadduck, W.M., Nugent, G.R.: Traumatic occlusion of the middle cerebral artery. Case report. J. Neurosurg., 39:753–756, 1973.

60. Love, L., Marsan, R.E.: Carotid cavernous fistula. Angiology, 25:231–236, 1974.

61. MacPherson, P., Graham, D.I.: Arterial spasm and slowing of the cerebral circulation in the ischaemia of head injury. J. Neurol. Neurosurg. Psychiat., 36:1069–1072, 1973.

62. Mahmoud, N.A.: Traumatic aneurysm of the internal carotid artery and epistaxis. J. Laryngol. Otol., 93:629–656, 1979.

63. Marks, R.L., Freed, M.M.: Nonpenetrating injuries of the neck and cerebrovascular accident. Arch. Neurol., 28:412–414, 1973.

64. Marshall, L.F., Bruce, D.A., Bruno, L., Langfitt, T.W.: Vertebrobasilar spasm: a significant cause of neurological deficit in head injury. J. Neurosurg., 48:560–564, 1978.

65. Mehalic, T., Farhat, S.M.: Vertebral artery injury from chiropractic manipulation of the neck. Surg. Neurol., 2:125–129, 1974.

66. Meirowsky, A.M.: Wounds of dural sinuses. J. Neurosurg., 10:496–514, 1953.

67. Menezes, A.H., Graf, C.J.: True traumatic aneurysm of anterior cerebral artery. Case report. J. Neurosurg., 40:544–548, 1974.

68. Miller, R.G., Burton, R.: Stroke following chiropractic manipulation of the spine. J.A.M.A., 229:189–190, 1974.

69. Monson, D.O., Saletta, J.D., Freeark, R.J.: Ca-

rotid vertebral trauma. J. Trauma, 9:987–997, 1969.

70. Morawetz, R.B., McDowell, H.A., Richardson, J.V.: Obliteration of an internal carotid-internal jugular fistula using a Prolo catheter. Surg. Neurol., 10:276–278, 1978.

71. Morley, T.P.: Appraisal of various forms of management in 41 cases of carotid-cavernous fistula. Current Controversies in Neurosurgery, W.B. Saunders Co., Philadelphia, 1976, pp. 217–236.

72. Mullan, S., Duda, E.E., Patronas, N.J.: Some examples of balloon technology in neurosurgery. J. Neurosurg., 52:321–329, 1980.

73. Mullan, S.: Treatment of carotid-cavernous fistulas by cavernous sinus occlusion. J. Neurosurg., 50:131–144, 1979.

74. Murray, D.S.: Post-traumatic thrombosis of the internal carotid and vertebral arteries after nonpenetrating injuries of the neck. Br. J. Surg., 44:556–561, 1957.

75. Nagashima, C., Iwasaki, T., Kawanuma, S., Sakaguchi, A., Kamisasa, A., Suzuki, K.: Traumatic arteriovenous fistula of the vertebral artery with spinal cord symptoms. Case report. J. Neurosurg., 46:681–687, 1977.

76. Nagler, W.: Vertebral artery obstruction by hyperextension of the neck: report of three cases. Arch. Phys. Med. Rehab., 54:237–240, 1973.

77. Nakamura, K., Tsugane, R., Ito, H., Obata, H., Narita, H.: Traumatic arterio-venous fistula of the middle meningeal vessels. J. Neurosurg., 25:424–429, 1966.

78. Ohta, T., Nishimura, S., Kikughi, H., Toyama, M.: Closure of carotid-cavernous fistula with polyurethane foam embolus. J. Neurosurg., 38:107–112, 1973.

79. Olafson, R.A., Christoferson, L.A.: The syndrome of carotid occlusion following minor craniocerebral trauma. J. Neurosurg., 33:636–639, 1970.

80. Olson, R.W., Baker, H.L., Svien, H.J.: Arteriovenous fistula: a complication of vertebral angiography. J. Neurosurg., 20:73–75, 1963.

81. Overton, M.C., Calvin, T.H.: Iatrogenic cerebral cortical aneurysm. Case report. J. Neurosurg., 24:672–675, 1966.

82. Pakarinen, S.: Arteriovenous fistula between the middle meningeal artery and the sphenoparietal sinus. A case report. J. Neurosurg., 23:438–439, 1965.

83. Parkinson, D.: Carotid-cavernous fistula: direct approach with repair of fistula and preservation of the artery. Current Controversies in Neurosurgery, W.B. Saunders Co., Philadelphia, 1976, pp. 237–249.

84. Parkinson, D., West, M.: Traumatic intracranial aneurysms. J. Neurosurg., 52:11–20, 1980.

85. Parkinson, D.: A surgical approach to the cavernous portion of the carotid artery. J. Neurosurg., 23:474–483, 1965.

86. Parkinson, D.: Carotid cavernous fistula: direct repair with preservation of the carotid artery. J. Neurosurg., 38:99–106, 1973.

87. Paul, G.A., Shaw, C.M., Wray, L.M.: True traumatic aneurysm of the vertebral artery. J. Neurosurg., 53:101–105, 1980.

88. Perret, G., Nishioka, H.: Report on the cooperative study of intracranial aneurysms and subarachnoid hemorrhage: Sec. VI, Arteriovenous malformations. J. Neurosurg., 25:467–490, 1966.

89. Pinkerton, J.A., MacGee, E.E., Romine, K.G.: Traumatic aneurysm of the intrathoracic left carotid artery with cerebral embolization. J. Trauma, 17:975–977, 1977.

90. Prolo, D.J., Hanbery, J.W.: Treatment of carotid-cavernous fistula with catheter and balloon. Current Controversies in Neurosurgery, W.B. Saunders Co., Philadelphia, 1976, pp. 250–254.

91. Raphael, H.A., Bernatz, P.E., Spittell, J.A., Ellis, F.H.: Cervical carotid aneurysms: treatment by excision and restoration of arterial continuity. Am. J. Surg., 105:771–778, 1963.

92. Rich, N.M., Hobson, R.W., Collins, G.J.: Traumatic arteriovenous fistulas and false aneurysms: a review of 558 lesions. Surgery, 78:817–828, 1975.

93. Rish, B.L.: The repair of dural venous sinus wounds by autogenous venorrhaphy. J. Neurosurg., 35:392–395, 1971.

94. Rittenhouse, E.A., Radke, H.M., Sumner, D.S.: Carotid artery aneurysm. Arch. Surg., 105:786–789, 1972.

95. Robinson, N.A., Flotte, C.T.: Traumatic aneurysms of the carotid arteries. Am. Surg., 40:121–124, 1974.

96. Rothman, S.L.G., Pratt, A.G., Kier, E.L., Allen, W.E.: Traumatic vertebral-carotid-jugular arteriovenous aneurysm. J. Neurosurg., 41:92–96, 1974.

97. Rumbaugh, C.L., Bergeron, R.T., Talalla, A., Kurze, T.: Traumatic aneurysms of the cortical cerebral arteries. Radiology, 96:49–54, 1970.

98. Sato, O., Bascom, J.F., Logothetis, J.: Intracranial dissecting aneurysm. J. Neurosurg., 35:483–487, 1971.

99. Sadar, E.S., Jane, J.A., Lewis, L.W., Adelman, L.S.: Traumatic aneurysms of the intracranial circulation. Surg. Gynecol. Obstet., 137:59–67, 1973.

100. Salar, G., Mingrino, S.: Traumatic intracranial internal carotid aneurysm due to gunshot wound. Case report. J. Neurosurg., 49:100–102, 1978.

101. Schneider, R.C., Lemmen, L.J.: Traumatic internal carotid artery thrombosis secondary to nonpenetrating injuries to the neck. J. Neurosurg., 9:495–507, 1952.

102. Schoter, I.: Cerebral artery occlusion due to trauma. Advances in Neurosurgery, Vol. 3. Springer-Verlag, Berlin, 1975, pp. 401–404.

103. Sedzimir, C.B.: Head injury as a cause of internal carotid artery thrombosis. J. Neurol. Neurosurg. Psychiat., 18:293–296, 1955.

104. Serbinenko, F.A.: Balloon catheterization and occlusion of major cerebral vessels. J. Neurosurg., 41:125–145, 1974.

105. Simeone, F.A., Goldberg, H.I.: Thrombosis of the vertebral artery from hyperextension injury to the neck. Case report. J. Neurosurg., 29:540–544, 1968.

106. Sindou, M., Mercier, P., Bokor, J., Brunon, J.:

Bilateral thrombosis of the transverse sinuses: Microsurgical revascularization with venous bypass. Surg. Neurol., 13:215–220, 1980.

107. Sindou, M., Mazoyer, J.F., Fischer, G., Piolat, J., Fourcade, C.: Experimental bypass for sagittal sinus repair. J. Neurosurg., 44:325–330, 1976.

108. Sindou, M., Grunewald, P., Guegan, Y., Redondo, A., Rey, A.: Cerebral revascularization with extra-intracranial anastomoses for vascular lesions of traumatic, malformative and tumorous origin. Acta Neurochir. Suppl., 28:282–286, 1979.

109. Smith, R.A., Estridge, M.N.: Neurologic complications of head and neck manipulations. J.A.M.A., 182:130–133, 1962.

110. Solheim, K.: Common carotid artery aneurysm after blunt trauma. J. Trauma, 19:707–709, 1979.

111. Spetzler, R.F., Owen, M.P.: Extracranial-intracranial arterial bypass to a single branch of the middle cerebral artery in the management of a traumatic aneurysm. Neurosurgery, 4:334–337, 1979.

112. Suwanwela, C., Suwanwela, N.: Intracranial arterial narrowing and spasm in acute head injury. J. Neurosurg., 36:314–323, 1972.

113. Symon, L.: An experimental study of traumatic cerebral vascular spasm. J. Neurol. Neurosurg. Psychiat., 30:497–505, 1967.

114. Teal, J.S., Bergeron, R.T., Rumbaugh, C.L., Segall, H.D.: Aneurysms of the petrous or cavernous portions of the internal carotid artery associated with nonpenetrating head trauma. J. Neurosurg., 38:568–574, 1973.

115. Thompson, J.E., Austin, D.J.: Surgical treatment of cervical carotid aneurysms. A.M.A. Arch. Surg., 74:81–88, 1957.

116. VanDellen, J.R.: Intracavernous traumatic aneurysms Surg. Neurol., 13:203–207, 1980.

117. Wemple, J.B., Smith, G.W.: Extracranial carotid aneurysm. J. Neurosurg., 24:667–671, 1966.

118. Wendling, L.R.: Intracranial venous sinus thrombosis. Diagnosis suggested by computed tomography. Am. J. Roentgenol., 130:978–980, 1978.

119. White, J.C., Sayre, G.P., Whisnant, J.P.: Experimental destruction of the media for the production of intracranial arterial aneurysms. J. Neurosurg., 18:741–745, 1961.

120. Wilkins, R.H., Alexander, J.A., Odom, G.L.: Intracranial arterial spasm: a clinical analysis. J. Neurosurg., 29:121–134, 1968.

121. Wilkins, R.H., Odom, G.L.: Intracranial arterial spasm associated with craniocerebral trauma. J. Neurosurg., 32:626–633, 1970.

122. Wilson, C.B., Cronic, F.: Traumatic arteriovenous fistulas involving middle meningeal vessels. J.A.M.A., 188:953–957, 1964.

123. Wolman, L.: Cerebral dissecting aneurysms. Brain, 82:276–291, 1959.

124. Woodhurst, W.B., Robertson, W.D., Thompson, G.B.: Carotid injury due to intraoral trauma: case report and review of the literature. Neurosurgery, 6:559–563, 1980.

125. Yamaura, A., Makino, H., Hachisu, H., Takemiya, S.: Secondary aneurysm due to arterial injury during surgical procedures. Surg. Neurol., 10:327–333, 1978.

126. Yonas, H., Agamanolis, D., Takaoka, Y., White, R.J.: Dissecting intracranial aneurysms. Surg. Neurol., 8:407–415, 1977.

15

Scalp Injuries; Reconstruction of Skull Defects

DANIEL C. BAKER
HAROLD GEWIRTZ

SCALP INJURIES

Anatomical Considerations

The scalp is composed of five layers: a superficial covering of skin, a subcutaneous layer, a tough fascial layer of galea, a layer of loose connective tissue and the pericranium. The skin of the scalp is thick in the occipital area and thinner in the frontal, temporal, and mastoid regions. The scalp adheres to the superficial fascia and is firmly attached to the underlying occipitofrontalis muscle. The galea is continuous with the fascia overlying the frontal and occipital muscles and serves as their origin. The subgaleal layer of loose connective tissue permits free movement of the scalp over the cranium and is the plane where avulsion occurs in scalping injuries.

The peculiar anatomical organization of the layers of the scalp is of particular significance in lacerations; when the galea is cut transversely, the wound tends to enlarge because the frontalis and occipitalis muscles draw the galea aponeurotica apart. In contradistinction to the gaping of transverse wounds of the galea, little separation of the wound edges occurs after sagittal cuts.

The pericranium or external periosteum is a thin fibrous membrane containing blood vessels and is loosely attached to the cortex of the outer table of the skull except at the suture lines where it is fairly adherent. A very rich network of arteries, veins, and lymphatics courses through the subcutaneous layer (Fig. 15.1) which is divided into multiple fat lobules by the interlacing fibrous sheets. These septa limit vessel retraction following injury and are partly responsible for the profuse hemorrhage often associated with scalp lacerations. A knowledge of the vascular supply of the scalp is essential in selecting the flaps to be used in the repair of defects and in deciding the direction of scalp incisions. The vessels which supply the scalp are peripheral, so it is usually possible to design a flap with a vascular pedicle. Because of the abundant blood supply of the scalp, large flaps can be shifted on relatively small pedicles.

Contusions

Contusions of the scalp generally heal readily. Occasionally localized hematomas will form in the subgaleal space. When these collections are large they can be aspirated with a large bore needle using sterile technique. This will minimize the chance of formation of an encapsulated seroma which could eventually erode the outer table of the skull.

Lacerations

In contradistinction to the extensive shaving of hair which is a necessary preparation for intracranial operations, most plastic surgeons believe that simple scalp lacerations do not require the shaving of hair. Trimming a few hairs from the wound

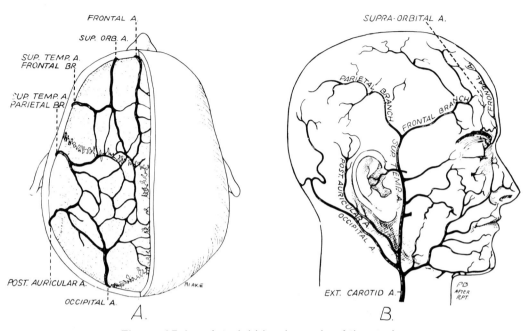

Figure 15.1. Arterial blood supply of the scalp.

edges is usually sufficient preparation and avoids an embarrassing bald patch. When infection occurs in a scalp laceration, it is usually caused by inadequate debridement of foreign material or necrotic tissue rather than hair in the wound.

Scalp lacerations should always be probed or palpated with a finger to assess for an underlying skull fracture. Irrigation with sterile saline solution beneath the flaps will help cleanse dirt and foreign material. Bleeding is usually easily controlled with pressure, and most bleeding stops with proper suturing. The galea is not closed as a separate layer. In view of the potentially contaminated nature of these wounds, closure in a single layer (including the galea) with a synthetic, monofilament suture is recommended. Scar revisions, such as Z-plasties, are deferred and the wound is closed in the simplest manner possible.

Traumatic Avulsion of the Scalp

Small, Partial Losses with an Intact Pericranium. Treatment of partial scalp loss depends upon the extent of the loss and the presence or absence of pericranium. If the pericranium is intact and viable, the simplest and most reliable technique is the use of a split-thickness graft taken from the avulsed scalp itself, the thigh or buttock. If the graft is taken from a portion of the avulsed scalp, it should not be expected to grow hair.

Small, Partial Losses with a Destroyed Pericranium. Skin grafts cannot be expected to supply a permanent coverage over denuded skull when the periosteum has been lost. Although a split-thickness skin graft can be applied to the denuded bone for temporary coverage, it is rarely lasting. In the absence of pericranium, the use of a local scalp flap is necessary. This is fashioned by establishing a plane of cleavage between the cranial periosteum (pericranium) and the galea aponeurotica. After the flap is transposed into the defect, a split-thickness graft is used to cover the donor defect if closure by direct approximation or by an additional adjacent flap is not possible (Figs. 15.2–15.6).

In a classic note, Gillies[16] described the use of bipedicle, rotation, and transposition flaps for reconstruction of small scalp wounds. This technique has been extended recently by Orticochea who described three-flap[46] and four-flap[45] techniques for closure of defects up to 11 × 11 cm (Fig.

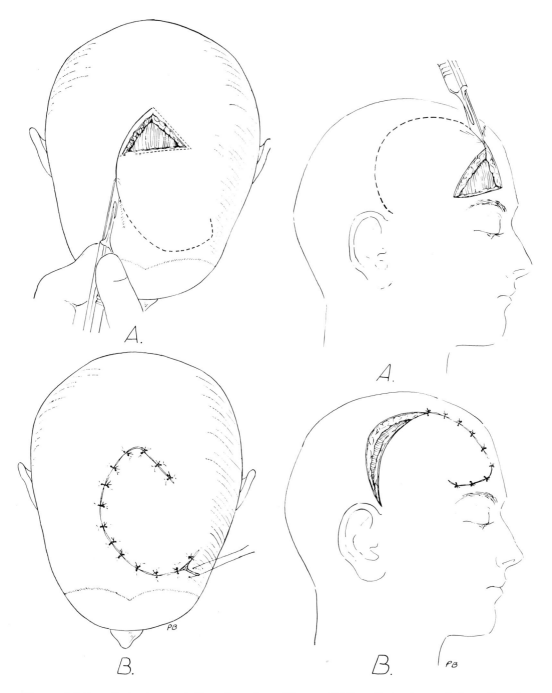

Figure 15.2. Swinging rotation flap for closure of scalp defect. *A*, design of rotation flap. *B*, rotation flap placed over defect: closure of secondary defect by V-Y method.

Figure 15.3. Swinging rotation flap including superficial temporal vessels in pedicle.

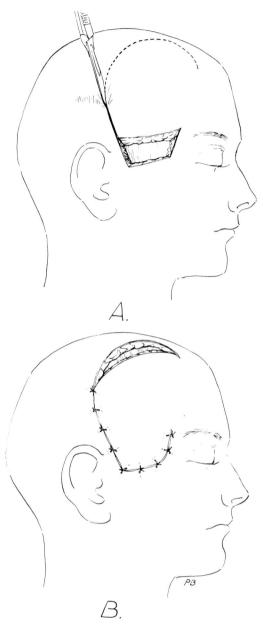

A.

B.

Figure 15.4. Retrograde rotation flap designed with broad pedicle, which is necessary to insure vascularization of flap because branches of superficial temporal vessels are severed.

15.7). A variant of this technique employs the Crane principle of Millard, which uses a pedicle flap for transfer of subcutaneous tissue and subsequent over-grafting with split skin.[39] The use of this technique to repair certain defects in the frontal region was described by Hamilton and Royster.[18] Other techniques for closure of frontal scalp defects are seen in Figures 15.8 and 15.9. With the introduction of microsurgical techniques, the use of distant pedicle flaps is currently uncommon, although good results have been achieved using this technique in the past.[10]

Another technique for the treatment of partial scalp loss including the pericranium is the decortication of the outer cortex and either immediate or late application of a split-thickness skin graft. The decision often depends upon the amount of bleeding from the bone. This technique has been described by Jensen and Petersen[24] and Koss *et al.*,[29] but except for very small defects, it produces wounds that tend to break down and often require later flap coverage.

Total Scalp Avulsion

Total scalp avulsions usually occur at the level of the subgaleal aponeurotic tissue, but may also include part of the pericranium. The history of these injuries has been reviewed by Davis[13] and Koss *et al.*,[29] who stressed that the injury became common with the industrial revolution.

The initial controversy involved whether or not to replace the avulsed tissue as a graft. Davis[13] described 21 attempts, without success; Kazanjian and Webster[26] had several patients in whom healing occurred by secondary intention, and noted that these were all cosmetically unacceptable, unstable, and caused upper lid ectropion. Osborne[47] used the avulsed scalp as the donor site for the split-thickness grafts. Because of universally unsuccessful attempts at replantation, the standard technique for the treatment of scalping injuries became the use of split-thickness skin grafts over pericranium.[6, 53, 65]

A solitary exception to the above is the description by Lu[34] of replacement of four-fifths of a hair-bearing scalp as a composite graft. The scalp later grew adequate hair, evidence of at least full thickness take.

Microsurgical Scalp Replantation. The advent of microvascular surgery has revolutionized total scalp replantation. Miller *et al.*[41] reported the first successful

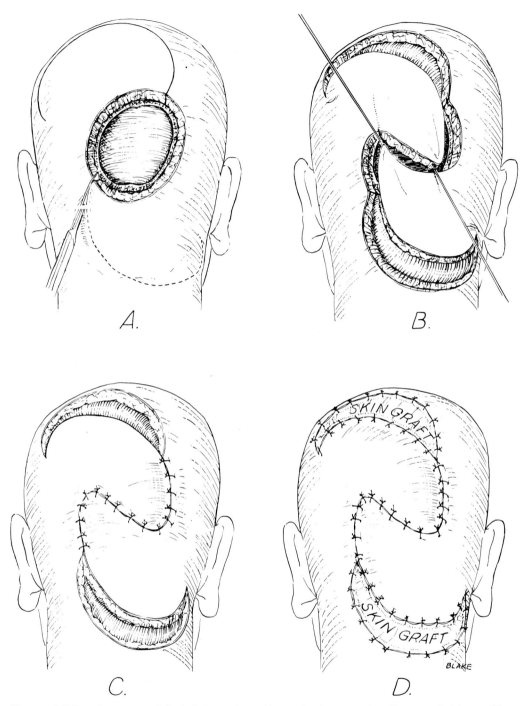

A.

B.

C.

D.

BLAKE

Figure 15.5. Large occipital defect closed by swinging rotation flaps and skin grafting.

scalp replantation, performing 13 anastomoses using vein grafts. Buncke et al.[4] later reported two successful cases and documented luxurious growth of hair in six months, and Van Beek and Zook[62] performed a partial scalp replantation in a four-year-old boy, completing four anastomoses, and noted that the vessels were so

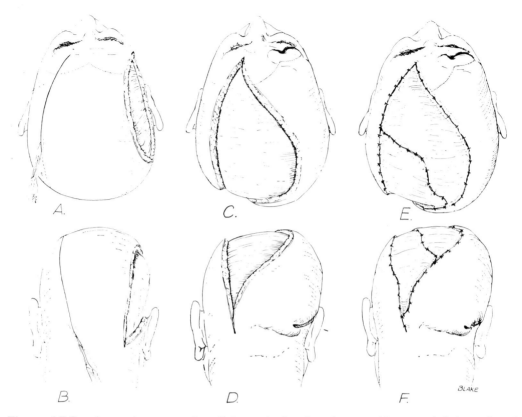

Figure 15.6. Large transposed pedicle scalp flap for closure of temporal defect. *A* and *B*, design of large pedicle scalp flap. *C* and *D*, flap transposed over defect. *E* and *F*, secondary defect covered by skin grafts applied over pericranium. (Figs. 15.5 and 15.6 from J. M. Converse: Surgical closure of scalp defects. In: Correlative Neurosurgery, E. A. Kahn, R. C. Schneider, E. C. Crosby, J. A. Taren, Eds. Charles C Thomas, Springfield, Ill., 1969.)

small that arteries could not be distinguished from each other or veins. Spira[61] also described a successful replant in a male, and Nahai et al.[43] demonstrated that an entire scalp could be replanted with only a single artery and vein.

This demonstration of successful replantations of acute scalping injuries has led to the reconstruction of scalp defects due to trauma, osteoradionecrosis, tumor, and burns by microvascular free flap transfer. Buncke et al.[4] and Chater et al.[7] successfully used a groin flap based upon the superficial circumflex iliac artery, and Maxwell et al.[38] used a free latissimus dorsi myocutaneous flap anastomosed to the superficial temporal artery. Harii et al.[21] used a free dorsalis pedis flap for reconstruction of a unilateral frontal defect. Another variation is the free transfer of omentum covered with split thickness skin. McLean and Buncke,[36] employing microsurgical revascularization techniques, covered a bare cranial defect with a free omental transplant anastomosed to the superficial temporal artery and vein; the omentum, in turn, was covered with a skin graft. This technique was repeated by Ikuta[22] and Harii.[20] Ohmori[44] treated post-burn alopecia with free temporo-parieto-occipital flaps based on the contralateral posterior branch of the superficial temporal artery in three patients.

RECONSTRUCTION OF SKULL DEFECTS

Following head injury, portions of the calvarium may be removed to achieve an external decompression[51] or because contaminated fragments of a depressed fracture are unsuitable for replacement. The goal of repair of these bony defects is to restore the integrity of the calvarium, to protect the brain and, when necessary, to render skull deformities cosmetically acceptable. Thus, the need for cranioplasty is determined both by the location and the

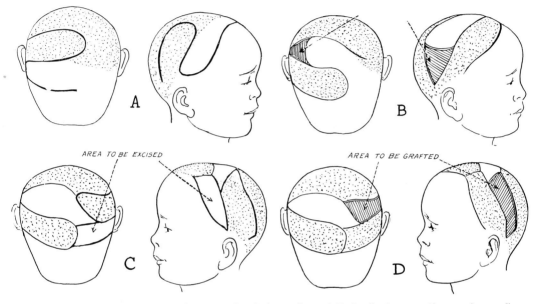

Figure 15.7. Repair of hairless scalp defect. *A* and *B*, in first operation, a large flap from right occipital region was transposed to temporal region and donor area was closed by shifting skin of bald area and applying skin graft. *C* and *D*, in next operation, another rectangular flap of hair-bearing skin was transposed from left occipitoparietal region.

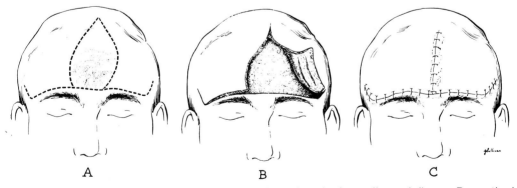

Figure 15.8. Rotation flaps for closure of forehead. *A*, outline of flaps. *B*, vertical incisions are made through frontalis muscle to permit stretching flap. *C*, approximation of flaps.

size of the defect. Skull defects less than 4–5 cm in diameter behind the hairline generally do not need repair, whereas the deformity created by even a small loss of

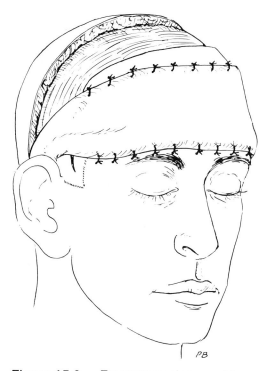

Figure 15.9. Emergency closure of frontal defect with bipedicle temporal scalp flap. Flap is nourished by superficial temporal vessels on each side, thus permitting narrow pedicles. Scalp defect is temporarily skin grafted. A preauricular pedicle may also be employed.

bone over the forehead may require cranioplasty.

Reconstruction of bony defects of the calvarium can be achieved with autogenous bone or prosthetic materials. Both have their advantages and disadvantages (Table 15.1) and in this century each has been popular at various times. Initially, reconstruction with autogenous bone was favored, followed by the use of prosthetic materials after World War I, and a subsequent revival of the use of autogenous bone in the 1950's.

Alloplastic Materials

After World War I, a number of alloplastic materials became popular. Weiford and Gardner,[63] Lane and Wester,[30] and Lewis et al.[31] all reported series where tantalum was used. In each there was a high incidence of infection necessitating removal in as many as 22% of patients.[30] Moreover, the radiodensity of tantalum limited subsequent diagnostic evaluations.

Simpson[59] reported the use of titanium and Black et al.[1] used aluminum in 61 patients but this latter prosthesis suffered from being insufficiently rigid. Scott et al.[55] used stainless steel and reported long-term results[56] in 70 patients—9% of whom required removal of the plate for infection or seizures. It is unlikely, however, that the occurrence of seizures was a consequence of the prosthetic material. Rather, the patient's initial injury most likely determined the frequency of subsequent epilepsy. Scott et al.,[56] attributed most of their infections to inadequate soft tissue coverage. Al-

Table 15.1
A Comparison of Autogenous Bone and Synthetic Material for Cranioplasty

Synthetic Materials	
Advantages	*Disadvantages*
1. Simpler to use; smooth contour	1. Greater infection rate
2. No donor site morbidity	2. Can be fractured
	3. ? induce seizures
	4. Radioopaque

Autogenous Bone	
Advantages	*Disadvantages*
1. Diminished infection rate	1. Can be difficult to contour
2. Grows with the patient	2. Resorption
	3. Donor site morbidity

though 16% of patients had unpleasant sensations at the site of the cranioplasty and 9% had chronic headaches, it is unlikely that the nature of the material was responsible for these sequelae.

White[64] described late complications in 151 cranioplasties. There was a 10.6% incidence of complications with lucite and 12.3% with tantalum. Like Scott et al.,[56] he stressed the importance of soft tissue coverage in assuring success. He made no mention of the use of perioperative antibiotics which has lowered the infection rate when used with the insertion of other prosthetic materials.

More recently, plastic materials have been used. Courtemanche and Thompson,[12] and Brown et al.[3] both reported the use of silastic blocks. Although these may be shaped to produce a satisfactory cosmetic result, this material is soft and provides insufficient protection of the brain.

Methyl-methacrylate implants have been used extensively by neurosurgeons over the past 35 years.[2, 5, 60] The material is mixed at the operating table and polymerizes *in situ*, permitting the surgeon to shape the prosthesis to the three-dimensional contours of the skull. The infection rate has been lower than that for other materials.[19, 52] A disadvantage of the acrylic is that, although it is firm, it is somewhat brittle and may fracture with trauma.[23] To obviate this problem, a prosthesis of stainless steel mesh and acrylic has been employed.[15] The use of these two materials in combination gets around the problem of the brittleness of the acrylic and the lack of rigidity of the stainless steel mesh. A preformed wire mesh-acrylic plate has also been used.[11] This saves operating time and allows the prosthesis to be fashioned to fit the exact three-dimensional contours of the skull.

In short, neurosurgeons, for the most part, favor synthetic cranioplastic materials. Although these substances have the disadvantage of being a foreign body and are never incorporated into living tissue, they are easily shaped to fit the contours of the skull. Unless the cranioplasty material incites an intense foreign body reaction, the infection rate is low and is dependent on operative technique and the presence of adequate soft tissue coverage.

Autogenous Bone Grafts

With the advent of the Second World War there was a renewed interest in the use of autogenous grafting. Kazanjian and Converse[25] used tibial-osteo-periosteal grafts for reconstruction of osteomyelitic frontal bone but the use of iliac bone and split-rib grafts became more popular than this technique.

Longacre and deStefano[32, 33] have been the principal proponents of split rib grafting. If the periosteum is left intact, the entire rib may be removed and split and the bone will regenerate. These authors[32] described 118 rib grafts using this technique without infection or graft loss. Unfortunately, a major problem with the use of rib grafts is attaining a smooth surface and cosmetically acceptable result (Figure 15.10).

To a certain extent, iliac bone grafts circumvent these disadvantages as a single long piece of bone without interstices can be used. The infection rate is low, and successful series have been reported by several authors.[9, 17, 27, 28, 35, 37, 49] Macomber[37] and Pickerill[49] have both stressed the importance of adequate soft tissue coverage for successful grafting.

Other autogenous cranioplasty techniques include the use of bone dust[28] and adjoining intact calvarium. The former technique has the disadvantage of having a high rate of resorption. Use of the outer table as a graft was first described by Muller in 1890.[42] Santoni-Rugiu[54] used outer table osteoperiosteal grafts leaving the inner table *in situ*. Psillakis et al.[50] used a similar technique for frontal reconstruction. They removed the entire thickness of bone and then replaced the inner table at the donor site and used the outer table for a graft.

Frontal Bone Reconstruction

The proximity of the frontal sinus creates special problems in the reconstruction of the frontal bone. If the frontal sinus is in contact with the defect, the wound is potentially contaminated due to communica-

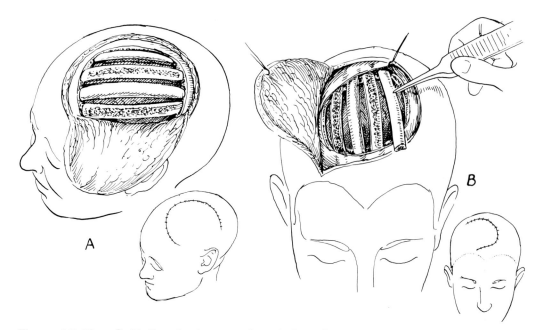

Figure 15.10. Split-rib onlay bone graft technique (Longacre and DeStafano, 1957). *A* and *B*, split ribs placed across two different types of cranial defects.

tion with the nose via the nasofrontal duct. The incidence of infection rises when using prosthetic materials in the frontal region. For this reason, autogenous materials are strongly recommended for reconstructive procedures in this area. To prevent muco-pyocele, the frontal sinus must be totally obliterated and the nasofrontal duct occluded.[8] Iliac bone graft is well suited to this area as it produces a smooth contour and the iliac crest can be left attached to recreate the supraorbital ridge.

In summary, there are advantages and disadvantages to both autogenous bone and prosthetic material. In both, satisfactory soft tissue coverage is essential for successful cranioplasty.

References

1. Black, S.P.W., Kam, C.C.M., Sights, W.P. Jr.: Aluminum cranioplasty. Technical note. J. Neurosurg., 29:562–564, 1968.
2. Blatt, I.M., Failla, A.: Acrylic implants for frontal bone defects. Milit. Med., 137:22–25, 1972.
3. Brown, J.B., Fryer, M.P., Randall, P., Lu, M.: Silicones in plastic surgery: laboratory and clinical investigations, a preliminary report. Plast. Reconstr. Surg., 12:374–376, 1953.
4. Buncke, H.J., Rose, E.H., Brownstein, M.J., Chater, N.L.: Successful replantation of two avulsed scalps by microvascular anastomoses. Plast. Reconstr. Surg., 61:666–672, 1978.
5. Cabanela, M.E., Coventry, M.B., MacCarty, C.S., Miller, W.E.: The fate of patients with methyl methacrylate cranioplasty. J. Bone Joint Surg., 54A:278–281, 1972.
6. Caldwell, E.H.: Complete scalp avulsion. Arch. Surg., 111:159–161, 1976.
7. Chater, N.L., Buncke, H.J., Alpert, B.: Reconstruction of extensive tissue defects of the scalp by microsurgical composite tissue transplantation. Surg. Neurol., 7:343–345, 1977.
8. Converse, J.M.: Technique of bone grafting for contour restoration of the face. Plast. Reconstr. Surg., 14:332–346, 1954.
9. Converse, J.M., Campbell, R.M.: Bone grafts in surgery of the face. Surg. Clin. North Am., 34:375–401, 1954.
10. Converse, J.M., Campbell, R.M., Watson, W.L.: Repair of large radiation ulcers situated over the heart and the brain. Ann. Surg., 133:95–103, 1951.
11. Cooper, P.R., Schechter, B., Jacobs, G.B., Rubin, R.C., Wille, R.L.: A pre-formed methyl methacrylate cranioplasty. Surg. Neurol., 8:219–221, 1977.
12. Courtemanche, A.D., Thompson, G.B.: Silastic cranioplasty following craniofacial injuries. Plast. Reconstr. Surg., 41:165–170, 1968.
13. Davis, J.S.: Scalping accidents. Johns Hopkins Hosp. Rep., 16:257–362, 1911.
14. Delangenière, H., Lewin, P.: A general method of

repairing loss of bony substance and reconstructing bones by osteoperiostal grafts taken from the tibia. Surg. Gynecol. Obstet., 30:441–447, 1920.

15. Galicich, J.A., Hovind, K.A.: Stainless steel mesh-acrylic cranioplasty. J. Neurosurg., 27:376–378, 1967.

16. Gillies, H.: Note on scalp closure. Lancet, 2:310–313, 1944.

17. Grocott, J.: Experiences in cranial bone grafting. Br. J. Plastic Surg., 5:51–59, 1952–53.

18. Hamilton, R., Royster, H.P.: Reconstruction of extensive forehead defects. Plast. Reconstr. Surg., 47:421–424, 1971.

19. Hammon, W.N., Kempe, L.G.: Methyl methacrylate cranioplasty. Acta Neurochirurg., 25:69–77, 1971.

20. Harii, K.: Clinical application of free omental flap transfer. Clin. Plast. Surg., 5:273–281, 1978.

21. Harii, K., Ohmori, K., Ohmori, S.: Successful clinical transfer of ten free flaps by microvascular anastomoses. Plast. Reconstruct. Surg., 53:259–270, 1974.

22. Ikuta, Y.: Autotransplant of omentum to cover large denudation of the scalp. Case report. Plast. Reconstr. Surg., 55:490–493, 1975.

23. Jackson, I.J., Hoffmann, G.T.: Depressed comminuted fracture of a plastic cranioplasty. J. Neurosurg., 13:116–117, 1956.

24. Jensen, F., Petersen, N.C.: Repair of denuded cranial bone by bone-splitting and free-skin grafting. J. Neurosurg., 44:728–731, 1976.

25. Kazanjian, V.H., Converse, J.M.: Reconstruction after radical operation for osteomyelitis of the frontal bone. Experience in eighteen cases. Arch. Otol., 31:94–112, 1940.

26. Kazanjian, V.H., Webster, R.C.: The treatment of extensive losses of the scalp. Plast. Reconstr. Surg., 1:360–385, 1946.

27. Kiehn, C.L., Grino, A.: Iliac bone grafts replacing tantalum plates for gunshot wounds of the skull. Am. J. Surg., 85:395–400, 1953.

28. Korlof, B., Nylen, B., Rietz, K.-A.: Bone grafting of skull defects. A report on 55 cases. Plast. Reconstr. Surg., 52:378–383, 1973.

29. Koss, N., Robson, M.C., Krizek, T.J.: Scalping injury. Plast. Reconstr. Surg., 55:439, 1975.

30. Lane, S., Webster, J.: A report on the early results in tantalum cranioplasty. J. Neurosurg., 4:526–529, 1947.

31. Lewin, W., Graham, M.P., Northcroft, G.B.: Tantalum in the repair of traumatic skull defects. Br. J. Surg., 36:26–41, 1948–49.

32. Longacre, J.J., de Stefano, G.A.: Further observations on the behavior of autogenous split-rib grafts in reconstruction of extensive defects of the cranium and face. Plast. Reconstr. Surg., 20:281–296, 1957.

33. Longacre, J.J., de Stefano, G.A.: Reconstruction of extensive defects of the skull with split rib grafts. Plast. Reconstr. Surg., 19:186–200, 1957.

34. Lu, M.M.: Successful replacement of avulsed scalp. Plast. Reconstr. Surg., 43:231–234, 1969.

35. McClintock, H.G., Dingman, R.O.: The repair of cranial defects with iliac bone. Surgery,

30:955–963, 1951.

36. McLean, D.H., Buncke, H.J. Jr.: Autotransplant of omentum to a large scalp defect, with microvascular revascularization. Plast. Reconstr. Surg., 49:268–274, 1972.

37. Macomber, D.W.: Cancellous iliac bone in depressions of forehead, nose, and chin. Plast. Reconstr. Surg., 4:157–162, 1949.

38. Maxwell, G.P., Stueber, K., Hoopes, J.E.: A free latissimus dorsi myocutaneous flap. Case report. Plast. Reconstr. Surg., 62:462–466, 1978.

39. Millard, D.R.: The Crane principle for the transport of subcutaneous tissue. Plast. Reconstr. Surg., 43:451–462, 1969.

40. Millard, D.R., Yates, B.M.: Practical variations of cranioplasty. Am. J. Surg., 107:802–809, 1964.

41. Miller, G.G., Anstee, E.J., Snell, J.A.: Successful replantation of an avulsed scalp by microvascular anastomoses. Plast. Reconstr. Surg., 58:133–136, 1976.

42. Müller, W.: Zure Frage der temporären Schädel-resektion an Steele der Trepanation. Zentrabl Chir., 17:65–66, 1890.

43. Nahai, F., Hurteau, J., Vasconez, L.O.: Replantation of an entire scalp and ear by microvascular anastomoses of only 1 artery and 1 vein. Br. J. Plastic Surg., 31:339–342, 1978.

44. Ohmori, K.: Free scalp flap. Plast. Reconstr. Surg., 65:42–49, 1980.

45. Orticochea, M.: Four flap scalp reconstruction technique. Br. J. Plastic Surg., 20:159–171, 1967.

46. Orticochea, M.: New three-flap scalp reconstruction technique. Br. J. Plast. Surg., 24:184–188, 1971.

47. Osborne, M.P.: Complete scalp avulsion: rational treatment. Report of case; experimental basis for production of free, hair bearing grafts from avulsed scalp itself. Ann. Surg., 132:198–213, 1950.

48. Phemister, D.B.: The fate of transplanted bone and regenerative power of its various constituents. Surg. Gynecol. Obstet., 19:303–333, 1914.

49. Pickerill, H.P.: Note on cranial autoplasty. Br. J. Surg., 35:204–207, 1947–48.

50. Psillakis, J.M., Nocchi, V.L.B., Zanini, S.A.: Repair of large defect of frontal bone with free graft of outer table of parietal bones. Plast. Reconstr. Surg., 64:827–830, 1979.

51. Ransohoff, J., Benjamin, M.V., Gage, E.L. Jr., Epstein, F.: Hemicraniectomy in the management of acute subdural hematoma. J. Neurosurg., 34:70–76, 1971.

52. Rietz, K.-A.: The one-stage method of cranioplasty with acrylic plastic with a follow-up study. J. Neurosurg., 15:176–182, 1958.

53. Robinson, F.: Complete avulsion of the scalp. Br. J. Plastic Surg., 5:37–50, 1952–53.

54. Santoni-Rugiu, P.: Repair of skull defects by outer table osteoperiosteal free grafts. Plast. Reconstr. Surgery, 43:157–161, 1969.

55. Scott, M., Wycis, H.T.: Experimental observations on the use of stainless steel for craniopasty. A comparison with tantalum. J. Neurosurg., 3:310–317, 1946.

56. Scott, M., Wycis, H., Murtagh, F.: Long term

evaluation of stainless steel cranioplasty. Surg. Gynecol. Obstet., 115:453–462, 1962.

57. Seydel, H.: Eine neue methode, grosse Knochendefekte des Schädels zu deckon. Zentrabl. Chir., 16:209–211, 1889.

58. Shehadi, S.I.: Skull reconstruction with bone dust. Br. J. Plast. Surg., 23:227–234, 1970.

59. Simpson, D.: Titanium in cranioplasty. J. Neurosurg., 22:292–293, 1965.

60. Small, J.M., Graham, M.P.: Acrylic resin for the closure of skull defects. Preliminary report. Br. J. Surg., 33:106–113, 1945–46.

61. Spira, M., Daniel, R.K., Agris, J.: Successful replantation of totally avulsed scalp, with profuse regrowth of hair. Case report. Plast. Reconstr. Surg., 62:447–451, 1978.

62. VanBeek, A.L., Zook, E.G.: Scalp replantation by microsurgical revascularization. Case report. Plast. Reconstr. Surg., 61:774–777, 1978.

63. Weiford, E.C., Gardner, W.J.: Tantalum cranioplasty. Review of 106 cases in civilian practice. J. Neurosurg., 6:13–32, 1949.

64. White, J.C.: Late complications following cranioplasty with alloplastic plates. Ann. Surg., 128:743–755, 1948.

65. Wynn, S.K.: Free pattern skin graft in total scalp avulsion. Plast. Reconstr. Surg., 7:225–236, 1951.

16

Special Considerations of the Pediatric Age Group

DEREK A. BRUCE

Through infancy and childhood, the brain develops from a friable, unmyelinated, unprogrammed mass with enormous plasticity to the rather rigid heavily myelinated adult brain with little or no plasticity. It is hardly surprising that the effects of head injury vary tremendously, not only between adult and child, but also among infants, children, and adolescents. The type and degree of injury varies greatly in children of different ages and is dissimilar from that occurring in late adolescence and adulthood. Thus, the type of pathology that is seen, the clinical course and recovery are all likely to be different at these different ages. Finally, the measurement of recovery will be more difficult in children since the patient's preinjury potential is unknown and, while good recovery may occur, this may be accompanied by a significant loss of potential.

BIRTH INJURY

It is impossible to obtain accurate information on the incidence of birth injuries. Many of these are minor and involve only the cranium. The ping-pong fracture, a small or large area of focal depression, where the skull is inbent in a fashion similar to a ping-pong ball, is a fairly frequent finding in the neonate who has undergone prolonged labor. The overlying skin is usually quite normal and there is no subgaleal hematoma. These fractures are probably the result of pressure on the scalp from the mother's bony pelvis and are not due to the obstetrical application of forceps. While a few of these fractures may resolve by themselves over the first few days, the larger ones will not, and are best treated surgically. The operation is minor and consists of a small skin incision at the margin of the fracture site. A burr hole is placed, a long periosteal elevator is passed under and past the central portion of the depression and the dent is gently elevated. These injuries are not associated with any late sequelae and the brain is not injured.

The most severe head injuries in the neonatal age group are the result of ineptly or inappropriately applied forceps. In our experience, these injuries occur as the result of mid- or high-forceps application. In order of frequency, the pathology involves the bone, the dura, and the brain. Linear skull fractures are common and unless extensive, require no therapy. Depressed fractures occur and occasionally bone fragments may be driven directly into the brain. In contradistinction to the ping-pong fracture, these lesions are associated with contusions or lacerations of the overlying skin and subgaleal hematomas. The full effects of these lesions on the brain may not become clear for six months or more after delivery. Even when the motor cortex is involved, hemiparesis may not become obvious until four to six months of age. A guarded prognosis is therefore appropriate. The most severe injuries involve a combination of linear skull fracture, often extensive and involving the base of the brain, with laceration of dural sinuses and subarachnoid hemorrhage. These children are born with low Apgar scores, scalp contusions or laceration, and frequently bleeding from the ears. Following delivery, they may rapidly go into shock and die. At autopsy, there are no surgically treatable lesions, only severe basilar fractures with subarachnoid bleeding and sinus laceration. Treatment is directed at preventing shock by giving blood and controlling the ICP with ventilatory support.

Subarachnoid Hemorrhage

There is a spectrum of birth injuries that occurs, not as a result of obstetrical mismanagement, but as a result of distortion of the cranium and its dural attachments during the molding of the head that accompanies delivery. These occur in full-term babies and the commonest of these is subarachnoid hemorrhage. There are frequently no clinical manifestations, and while the incidence of sequelae is low, a small percentage of these children will develop delayed hydrocephalus from six weeks to three months of age. More serious lesions are associated with lacerations of the tentorium and subdural, infratentorial or subarachnoid hemorrhage (Fig. 16.1). These rarely need operative treatment and,

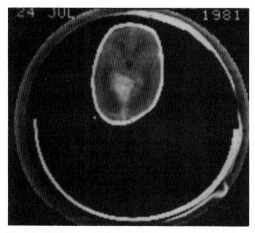

Figure 16.1. Infratentorial hemorrhage in newborn.

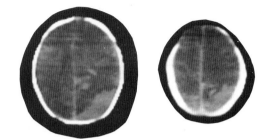

Figure 16.2. Neonate with large right posterior and small left posterior subdural hematoma with intraventricular and intraparenchymal hemorrhage.

unless very severe, are usually associated with a good outcome.

Subdural and Epidural Hematoma

Acute subdural or epidural hemorrhage[1, 19, 31, 33, 35] can occur at birth. Subdural hemorrhage is usually interhemispheric and does not require surgical evacuation unless there is neurological deterioration. It can occur in isolation or in association with multiple intracerebral hematomas (Fig. 16.2). In the latter case, a bleeding disorder should be suspected and must be carefully sought. Subdural hematomas do occur in the posterior fossa in neonates[2, 31] and are difficult to diagnose except by the use of the CT scan. Posterior fossa craniotomy and evacuation of the lesion is required if there is progressive deterioration. In general, acute subdural hematomas in the newborn period, if large enough to require operative intervention, should be evacuated using a craniotomy and not by burr hole drainage. Because the neonatal brain is unmyelinated, it is very liquid and herniation of brain through a burr hole can occur if operation is attempted through small dural openings. Subdural taps will usually miss the posterior and laterally-located hematomas and play little role in the acute management of these children.

Epidural hematomas, while uncommon, also occur in the neonatal age group, usually as a result of forceps injury, but one-fifth will show no evidence of skull fracture.[14, 33] The diagnosis of intracranial hematoma is suspected when there is a deteriorating level of consciousness and a full fontanelle, and is best confirmed by the CT scan. Evacuation of the hematoma, when required, is best performed *via* a craniotomy opening with careful replacement and wiring of the bone flap.

Intracerebral Hemorrhage

Intracerebral hemorrhage can occur in the full-term child and usually presents with seizures within the first 24 hours of birth and a deteriorating level of neurological function. When large intracerebral hematomas are identified, they should be removed; the subsequent appearance of neurological deficit is dependent on the site of the hematoma (Fig. 16.3).

Treatment

The technique of intracranial surgery in children of this age is a little different than that used in older children. The brain is extremely soft and friable and the pia-arachnoid easily peels from the underlying

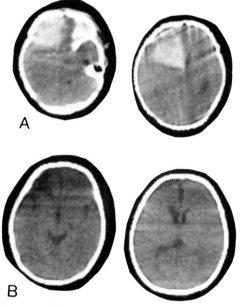

Figure 16.3. Neonate with large left frontal intracerebral hematoma. *A*, acute scan; *B*, CT scan taken several months post-evacuation showing normal size ventricles and left frontal encephalomalacia.

cortex. Because of this, small suctions with a low vacuum should be used when resecting contused areas to avoid aspirating normal brain tissue. The small vessels of the white matter tend to burst and shrink and then retract producing continued bleeding. Therefore, low settings on the bipolar cautery with continuous irrigation are necessary. Craniectomy should be avoided and a well beveled bone flap used to prevent later cosmetic deformities. The skin incision should never enter the forehead and should be well behind the hairline. Dural closure should be watertight. Skin closure is done with a single layer of running nylon sutures. In the posterior fossa, the lateral or prone position must be used and no effort made to position the child in a sitting position. The majority of hemorrhages are lateral and lateral craniectomy, which leaves the dura mater over the cisterna magna intact, is preferred. The incidence of postoperative hydrocephalus is then significantly diminished. Late complications of these lesions are focal neurological deficits, seizures (although with prophylactic antiseizure medication for a year, this has not been a major problem), and the delayed development of porencephaly and/or hydrocephalus.

FIRST YEAR OF LIFE

Subgaleal Hematoma

In the first year of life, head injuries are common. However, most are minor and the mechanism is usually that of a fall. Subgaleal hematomas occur frequently in this group of children. The lump is often not noticed for several days. The child then presents with a soft boggy swelling, occasionally in association with a linear skull fracture. The extent of the swelling may increase, spreading under much of the scalp. Frequently because of the liquid feel, these are diagnosed as cerebrospinal fluid collections with leakage through the fracture. They are, of course, liquefied subgaleal blood which can spread circumferentially around the entire skull. Although some physicians believe these lesions should be aspirated in adults, it is my belief that in children they should be left alone. They should not be aspirated since this predisposes to infection and removes iron which can lead to later anemia. Compressive dressings do not work because the bleeding has usually stopped by the time the patient is seen. The only risk is of sufficient blood loss into the subgaleal space to produce anemia and occasionally a transfusion will be necessary. These lesions usually resolve and in children aspiration is rarely necessary or indicated. Skull fractures are common in this age group but cerebral injury is quite uncommon. Seizures occurring within the first hour after injury are quite common group but the later onset of a seizure is uncommon and long term anticonvulsant medication is usually not necessary.

Infant Concussion Syndrome

Following mild head injury, there is a characteristic syndrome that is seen: some minutes to hours after the fall, consciousness rarely having been lost, the baby becomes very sleepy, pale and begins vomiting. Examination usually reveals a pale child with tachycardia, clammy skin, normal blood pressure, no evidence of focal neurological deficit, and a soft fontanelle. The level of consciousness varies from spontaneous movements of all extremities to deep stupor with only pain responses. Fractures are often seen on skull X-ray but are most valuable as an indicator of increased intracranial pressure (ICP); if there is evidence of splitting of the sutures a CT scan should be obtained. In the great majority of children with the infant concussion syndrome (90% or more), no evidence of suture splitting is seen and no intracranial mass lesion is present. The vomiting usually subsides rapidly, but occasionally hospitalization and administration of intravenous fluids is necessary for at least 24 hours.

Epidural Hematoma

The most likely lesion to be encountered in the presence of elevated ICP is an epidural hematoma. This usually results from a fall from a height onto a hard surface or, in two cases we have seen, children falling down steps while in a walker.

Acute epidural hematoma in infancy is associated with anemia and shock; a large amount of blood can accumulate in the head because of the compressibility of the brain and can be much greater than the 10% of the intracranial space that can be acutely occupied in adults. Moreover, in a small child, 150 cc may represent 40% of the blood volume. If an associated skull fracture is present, the hematoma can decompress into the subperiosteal or subgaleal space permitting even greater blood loss. Plain X-rays will show splitting of the sutures and the CT scan will provide a definitive diagnosis. The CT scan, we believe, can also demonstrate continued bleeding (Fig. 16.4). The location of epidural hematomas in this age group is more likely to be parietal than temporal and a diagnostic study is advised wherever possible. Operation should be performed using a craniotomy flap and not by craniectomy.

Growing Skull Fracture

The only late effect we have seen after the infant concussion syndrome has been

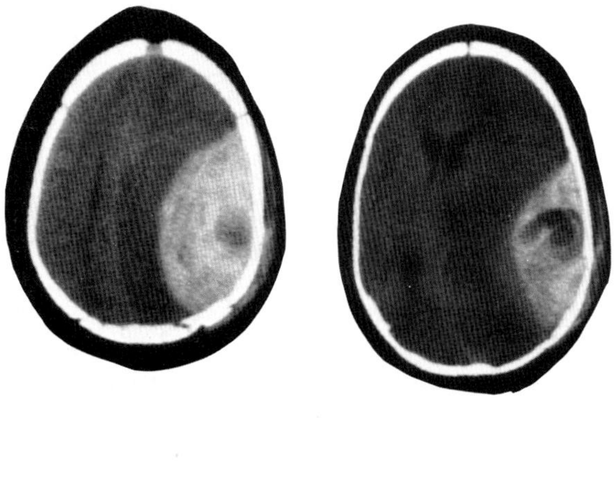

Figure 16.4 Large acute epidural in 4-month-old child. Area of decreased density in center of hematoma suggests continuous active hemorrhage. Large midline shift and decreased density of surrounding brain suggests infarction.

an occasional growing fracture.[16, 17] In these cases, the initial trauma has fractured the skull and torn the underlying dura with a small contusion of the brain. There is rarely focal neurological deficit but over weeks or months there is gradual herniation of the brain out through the fracture site with an increase in size of the fracture on X-ray and usually bulging of the overlying scalp. Because of this, all children with large linear skull fractures should have the area clinically examined 2–3 months later to check for evidence of a growing fracture. If there is any skin bulging, repeat X-rays should be taken. If the X-ray shows an increase in the separation of the fracture edges, then an operation should be performed. A scalp flap over the site of the growing fracture is fashioned. The bone is rongeured to expose the dural tear. Herniated brain is excised and the dura mater repaired with a graft, if needed.

Diffuse Brain Injury

Severe head injuries in this age group are usually the result of child abuse.[22] A shaking injury is the most frequent one we encounter.[11, 12] Pathologically, the pattern is that of tearing of the anterior bridging veins, petechial hemorrhage throughout the white matter, and deep grey structures with shearing of myelin and axons, frequently contusions of the corpus callosum, subarachnoid hemorrhage, and acute intracranial hypertension. These children are often brought to the hospital after hours of coma because the parent is afraid of the consequences. The children may have received several previous but less major injuries and, thus, the damage may be cumulative. Clinically, there is rarely a good history of a single traumatic episode. The story is usually of a minor injury, then sleepiness followed by a sudden deterioration. Often, the child has been reported to have been shaken in an effort to "bring him around." Occasionally, episodes of stiffening or crying out are described.

On examination, there is often no evidence of external trauma other than bruising of the upper arms. Patients with severe injuries present either: 1) in deep coma with decerebrate posturing or flaccidity, fixed dilated pupils and apnea or bradypnea with an extremely tense fontanelle or 2) arousable to painful stimulation, move all extremities, breathe well and spontaneously, and have a full fontanelle. Both groups of children have retinal hemorrhages on funduscopic examination.

In the former group with Glasgow Coma Scores of 3 or 4, the management is immediate hyperventilation with 100% oxygen using an ambu bag and mask followed by tapping of the lateral margins of the fontanelle with a 19- or 21-gauge short spinal needle. Usually, 10–15 cc of bloody, nonclotting fluid can be obtained from either side. This often produces a dramatic improvement in the neurological state: the pupils become responsive, spontaneous ventilation begins, and there is often a decrease in the degree of decerebrate rigidity. At present, we believe that this fluid is a combination of subdural and localized subarachnoid hemorrhage and cerebrospinal fluid. The children are then intubated with precautions to avoid intracranial hypertension (hyperventilation, hyperoxygenation, muscle relaxant, and pentothal) and are then transported for CT scan. The CT scan rarely shows a large subdural collection and we have not had to perform craniotomy on any of these children over the last 5 years. The most frequent finding is a posterior inter-hemispheric collection of blood[36] often with a slight decreased density suggesting early infarction in the distribution of the posterior cerebral arteries. The pathology consists of subarachnoid and subdural hemorrhage plus severe brain swelling. This combination results in a massive increase in ICP with tentorial herniation and posterior cerebral compression.

In children with coma scores of 5 or more, an immediate CT scan should be obtained. This rarely shows an operable lesion and the pattern is usually similar to that described above for the sicker children. In both groups, careful monitoring of ICP is necessary since secondary swelling is common and delayed death due to intracranial hypertension can occur. If the children survive, there is a high incidence of focal atrophy; intellectual development is frequently impaired, and focal neurological deficit may be present. In the group with Glasgow Coma Scores better than 4 on admission, recovery is the rule although, once again, focal deficits, particularly homonymous hemianopsia are common.

The incidence of ischemia in the distribution of major vessels is unusually high in the severely head injured child less than one year of age. Infarctions may be associated with child abuse or follow other forms of trauma. The commonest site is in the posterior cerebral distribution and this is assumed to occur as a result of severe transient intracranial hypertension occurring around the time of trauma with a compression of one or both posterior cerebral arteries as they cross the tentorium. The next most frequent areas are the proximal anterior cerebral artery distribution and the middle cerebral artery territories. These occur early in the course of the injury and are probably secondary to intracranial hypertension. It is not clear whether vascular torsion or spasm plays any role in the genesis of these ischemic lesions. Blood flow studies, several days after trauma, show patent major cerebral vessels suggesting that traumatic dissection or occlusion are not the causes of the infarction. Whatever the cause, the destructive effects in the hemisphere are major with massive areas of loss of cerebral substance (Fig. 16.5). Interestingly, despite this CT scan finding, the degree of neurological deficit may be quite minor.

A final pathological lesion that occurs exclusively in the infant is that of clefts within the white matter. These occur as a result of blunt trauma and have been described pathologically.[21] They are not grossly hemorrhagic pathologically or on the CT scan and are presumed to result from separation of the poorly myelinated white matter. The CT scan pattern has been well described.[25] These lesions frequently resolve spontaneously and do not require operative therapy. The influence of these lesions in later development are unknown, but it is likely that outcome is determined less by the presence of these small focal injuries than by the amount of diffuse brain injury sustained.

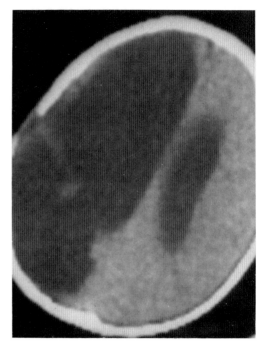

Figure 16.5. Massive left-sided porencephaly in 9-month-old child following severe head trauma with infarction in the anterior and middle cerebral distribution.

Chronic Subdural Hematoma

Chronic subdural hematomas are rare in our hospital setting. No craniotomy for this lesion has been done in the last five years. The usual presentation in infancy is that of a child with an enlarging head. There is rarely a history of trauma. Indications for surgery are signs of increased intracranial pressure, vomiting, and a bulging fontanelle. If these are not present, no therapy is generally required. In children with signs of increased ICP, we usually perform bilateral subdural peritoneal shunts.[23]

CHILDREN OVER ONE YEAR OF AGE

Before describing the specific ways in which children's responses to head injury differ from those of adults, it is important once again to consider the effects of different mechanisms of injury. Children who sustain a road traffic accident are usually pedestrians or bicycle riders. The accidents usually occur in an urban or suburban area and frequently the involved automobile is trying to stop. Thus, the input force would be considerably less than that delivered when a vehicular accident occurs at high speed. In children, the neurological state has to be viewed in the context of the mechanism of injury (e.g., a child who is decerebrate on admission following an automobile accident has a good chance of recovery, whereas a child with a similar neurological picture on admission after a fall of three stories or more is less likely to recover and will probably die). It is not surprising that the mechanism of injury affects outcome and it is important to realize that early prognosis cannot be based on the Glasgow Coma Score alone and that the addition of information concerning the mechanism of injury, the presence of shock,[20] the initial ICP and the initial CT scan can help the physician make a more accurate estimate of outcome early during the course of hospitalization. In our own experience, if the ICP is over 40 torr following intubation and treatment with pentothal and hyperventilation, the mortality in the absence of a surgical lesion is 100%.

Epidural Hematomas

In children less than five years of age, epidural hematomas rarely present with the classic pattern of a lucid period followed by rapid neurological deterioration occurring within hours of injury.[15] Most children at this age never become deeply unconscious but present with the onset of papilledema within 24 hours of injury, bradycardia, continued moderate lethargy and sometimes with prolonged vomiting over several days. Skull X-rays may be helpful; splitting of the sutures consistent with increased ICP or a linear fracture is seen in about 50% of patients. Bradycardia in this age group, even if unaccompanied by other findings, is an indication for a CT scan. Early diagnosis using the CT scan and evacuation of the lesion will result in full recovery in almost every instance and the mortality rate should be close to zero.

In our experience, 10% of epidural hematomas in children are subacute or chronic. The clinical presentation is that of prolonged mild lethargy following injury and the onset of vomiting within 3–5 days of trauma. Careful funduscopic examination will usually reveal papilledema. These chronic hematomas present from 5–20 days after trauma and they appear on the CT scan as an area of mildly increased density with an enhancing inner membrane, which represents the dura and granulation tissue. After proper evacuation and removal of the granulation tissue, these lesions do not recur and the brain rapidly expands to fill in the epidural space.

Acute Diffuse Brain Swelling

The acute onset of severe brain swelling or "malignant" edema is well recognized in children and has been equated with the pediatric concussion syndrome. (see also Chapters 6 and 12) The clinical picture is that of a child who sustains a relatively minor injury. Minutes to hours later, there develops a progressively decreasing level of consciousness,[17, 29] pallor, often sweating and vomiting, and occasionally focal neurological deficit. At this point, further clinical deterioration may cease with resolution of all signs or there may be progression to deep obtundation and coma with dilated pupils, apnea, and death. A similar picture has been described but with focal signs (e.g., unilateral pupillary enlargement and hemiplegia). In adults, this would most likely be due to an expanding mass lesion, such as an epidural hematoma. In children, this is rarely the case and most frequently diffuse swelling of one or both cerebral hemispheres is found. This is important since operation is contraindicated for this condition.

If the outcome is fatal, autopsy will usually reveal a severely swollen brain without any underlying primary lesion.[20] Since this picture is not associated with immediate loss of consciousness, it is not surprising that diffuse white matter lesions are not seen. Of the first 147 children we examined following head trauma, 30% had a CT scan appearance of diffuse bilateral hemispheric swelling with loss of CSF spaces (particularly the perimesencephalic cistern) and ventricular compression. Fifty percent of children with severe head injuries (*i.e.*, Glasgow Coma Scores of 8 or less) had a CT scan which showed diffuse swelling. Forty percent of all children with diffuse swelling had a Glasgow Coma Score of 5 or less; 40%, 6 to 8; and 20% 9 to 15.[4] Sixty percent of patients had no lucid interval and were immediately unconscious, 34% had a period of recovery of consciousness or did not initially lose consciousness. With adequate resuscitation and good intensive care, no patient with a lucid period died. In those who were comatose with no lucid period, five died and autopsy on three of these children revealed the presence of diffuse immediate impact injury.[4]

Acute brain swelling can occur with or without an underlying primary brain injury and, therefore, the unconscious child with this pattern on scan is likely to benefit from ICP monitoring in order to identify and treat any elevation in ICP. In those patients who have a lucid period, control of the acute brain swelling will result in an excellent outcome but, if left untreated, an occasional child who could have been salvaged will develop a massive elevation of ICP and die. In these patients who are never unconscious, monitoring of ICP or controlled ventilation is unnecessary.

The etiology of acute brain swelling is unknown. CT studies in these patients show an increased white matter density during the acute phase suggesting that the swelling is not due to cerebral edema but perhaps to an increase in cerebral blood volume.[4] Studies of local cerebral blood volume have not included adequate numbers of children to be certain whether or not local cerebral blood volume is elevated during the acute stages,[18] but cerebral blood flow studies, both regional and global, show that there is a significant brain hyperemia with the cerebral blood flow being much higher than that required to sustain oxygen metabolism of the brain manifest by a high jugular bulb PaO_2.[7] We believe that these findings support the hypothesis that the acute brain swelling is due to acute vascular congestion of the brain and not an increase in brain water content. With time (2–5 days after injury), however, especially in patients with diffuse impact injury, there is an increase in multifocal edema and secondary increases in ICP. When these occur, the pathology is usually that of true brain edema and appropriate therapy can be given.

With an understanding of acute brain swelling and the knowledge of the frequency with which it occurs in children, the emergency care of the acutely head injured child is focused on hyperventilation. This will rapidly decrease cerebral blood flow and cerebral blood volume and lower the ICP. In children with no significant underlying brain lesions, rapid and complete recovery will occur if intracranial hypertension is controlled. In children with diffuse impact injury, initial control of the hyperemia will maintain a normal ICP, but in this group of children, delayed elevation of ICP due to true cerebral edema can occur and long term rehabilitation may be necessary. Nonetheless, the likelihood of a good outcome is high.

INTRACRANIAL HYPERTENSION

Intracranial hypertension is common in children with severe head injury whether or not a mass lesion is present. The ICP may be elevated early or after several days. Of those patients with an ICP over 40 torr, the outlook is extremely poor. At the present time, ICP monitoring is performed in children with admission Glasgow Coma Scores of 5 or less. In children with a Glasgow Coma Score of 6–8, ICP monitoring is not usually required unless the CT scan shows a mass lesion with herniation or displacement of brain. Because of the early onset of intracranial hypertension in some patients, we believe that the ICP should be monitored from the time of admission and now tend to do this during resuscitation in the emergency room. In children in coma and shock or those with Glasgow Coma Scores of 5 or less, we insert the ICP monitor in the energency room along with an arterial line and endotracheal intubation. Transport for CT scanning is then done with portable monitoring of the ICP, systemic arterial pressure, and end-tidal PCO_2.

The medications available to treat elevated ICP are the same in children as in adults (see also Chapter 9) but different emphasis is placed on the selection of therapy and the time it is most likely to be beneficial. Hyperventilation is the mainstay of early resuscitation in childhood. Because of cerebral congestion, this is the most effective therapy and can be readily instituted by a bag and mask and by paramedical technicians at the scene of the accident. If rapid deterioration of neurological status occurs in a child, immediate intubation with all precautions to prevent elevations of ICP, including hyperventilation with 100% oxygen, intravenous sodium pentothal, pancuronium, and cricoid pressure during intubation followed by hyperventilation to a PCO_2 in the range of 20–22 torr should be first performed. If pupillary dilatation does not reverse, or if signs of herniation continue, further pentothal or mannitol in a dose of 0.5 g/kg should be given and a CT scan obtained. The *routine* use of mannitol is not advised since an increase in cerebral blood flow will occur[6] that may, at least transiently, aggravate the intracranial hypertension. This can be avoided by prior hyperventilation. When severe hyperventilation is used, a jugular bulb catheter is recommended to monitor jugular bulb PaO_2. If this remains above 20–25 torr, we believe it is safe to continue the hyperventilation.

After the first 24 hours, there is a phase when the congestion resolves and true cerebral edema appears.[5, 28] During this time, methods of brain dehydration may prove useful in controlling intracranial hypertension. This period of elevated ICP may require increased blood osmolality up to 320 milliosmols/100 cc, prolonged hyperventilation with a $PaCO_2$ in the 18–20 torr range, intermittent diuretic administration (*e.g.*, furosemide), head-up position, two-thirds fluid maintenance, and possibly hypothermia and barbiturates. This may last from 10–14 days in more severely injured children and withdrawal of therapy must be done in a slow stepwise fashion. Barbiturates, when used in large doses, are danger-

ous in childhood and careful monitoring of ICP, arterial pressure, central venous pressure, end-tidal CO_2, blood gases, central venous pressure, temperature, and urine output are necessary. It is occasionally necessary to determine cardiac output and the capability to perform this test must be available.[9, 28] In children with severe head injury, where ICP cannot be controlled by other means, barbiturates (usually pentobarbital) are used in doses adequate to maintain the ICP below 15 torr and not necessarily to levels high enough to flatten the EEG. The usual blood levels required vary from 2.5–3.5 mg%. It is our belief that barbiturate therapy is helpful as an ancillary measure in controlling the ICP in those children with the highest and most refractory elevations, particularly those who have evidence of diffuse swelling on CT scan (see also Chapter 9).

If the ICP again rises after withdrawal of one mode of therapy, then reinstitution of that modality may be necessary for several more days. During the period from the fifth to the fourteenth day of injury, repeat CT scan may show moderate enlargement of the ventricles, the subarachnoid spaces, or both (Fig. 16.6). At this time, ventricular or lumbar CSF withdrawal will serve to maintain a normal ICP and allow cessation of other therapies.[5, 26]

We have found an elevated ICP over 20 torr in 75% of children with Glasgow Coma Scores of 5 or less, irrespective of the presence of a mass lesion. In our experience, the 15 primary deaths out of 145 patients with Glasgow Coma Scores of 8 or less were all due to elevated ICP in the first few hours. The ICP was over 40 torr in all patients at the time the monitor was inserted. Nine of these 15 patients had a recorded neurological exam that would have predicted survival early in the course of their injury but rapidly deteriorated, developed fixed dilated pupils, and often apnea. If this mortality is to be reversed, more active immediate management and rapid transfer to a center capable of handling major pediatric trauma will be necessary.

All of the injuries that occur following adult head trauma also occur in children.

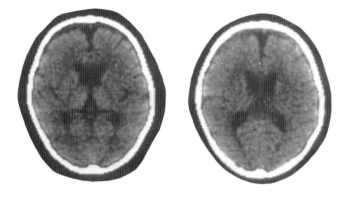

Figure 16.6 Four-year-old 3 weeks post-head trauma showing mild ventricular dilatation, bilateral frontal CSF collections and mild cortical atrophy.

However, in children the incidence of the various lesions is different and, therefore, the early resuscitative efforts will be slightly different with an emphasis on airway control and hyperventilation as opposed to agents like mannitol. Because of the importance of intracranial hypertension in children following head injury, ICP monitoring for several days is necessary in those children with Glasgow Coma Scores of 5 or less (*i.e.*, abnormal flexion posturing or worse). The intensive efforts to control the ICP must be prolonged over many days and at each different pathological stage (swelling, edema, expanded CSF spaces), the correct therapeutic combinations must be selected. If this is done well, the majority of children will recover. Children with lesser degrees of injury (*i.e.*, those with Glasgow Coma Scores of 6 or more) should not die of their head injury, but may succumb as a result of systemic trauma.[24]

OUTCOME FROM SEVERE HEAD INJURY

The recovery rate from severe head trauma in childhood remains considerably better than that of adults.[3, 10, 13] In our own experience in children admitted with decerebrate posturing (Glasgow Coma Score of 4) the mortality rate is 13%, and 80% make a good recovery or are left moderately disabled. For those patients who are in coma and flaccid, the mortality rate is 50%, and 44% are moderately disabled. In this group, if the patient has been continuously apneic from injury or for more than a few minutes prior to arrival in our emergency room, all have died, are vegetative, or are severely disabled. However, those with spontaneous

ventilation will often make a useful recovery and few are left severely disabled. Children who are admitted with a Glasgow Coma Score of 6 or more should not die and should make a good recovery.[8]

The period of recovery from coma and subsequent rehabilitation are difficult ones for the family and they require the continuous support and encouragement of medical and paramedical personnel. Even once formal rehabilitation is over, neuropsychological testing suggests that significant defects in the performance I.Q. are to be expected, often with auditory and visual perceptive difficulties (see also Chapter 20). All of these very severely injured children need good neuropsychological and psychosocial evaluation prior to their return to school and will require a special education program designed for their individual needs. All patients and their families require long-term support from a cadre of neurosurgeons, pediatricians, psychologists and physical medicine personnel. Nonetheless, with a comprehensive approach to the emergency care, critical acute care, and rehabilitation follow-up, the mortality and morbidity from severe head trauma in children can be decreased to less than 20% and mortality can be virtually eliminated in those with Glasgow Coma Scores of 5 or better.

References

1. Alvarez-Garijo, J.A., Gomila, D.T., Aytes, A.P., Mengual, M.V., Martin, A.A.: Subdural hematomas in neonates. Surgical Treatment. Child's Brain, 8:31–38, 1981.
2. Blank, N.K., Strand, R., Gilles, F.H., Palakshappa, A.: Posterior fossa subdural hematomas in neonates. Arch. Neurol., 35:108–111, 1978.
3. Brink, J.D., Imbus, C., Woo-Sam, J.: Physical re-

covery after severe closed head trauma in children and adolescents. J. Pediatr., 97:721–727, 1980.

4. Bruce, D.A., Alavi, A., Bilaniuk, L.T., Dolinskas, C., Obrist, W., Uzzell, B.: Diffuse cerebral swelling following head injuries in children: the syndrome of "malignant brain edema." J. Neurosurg., 54:170–178, 1981.

5. Bruce, D.A., Berman, W.A., Schut, L.: Cerebrospinal fluid pressure monitoring in children: Physiology, pathology and clinical usefulness. In: Advances in Pediatrics, Vol. 24, Barnes, L.A., Ed. Year Book Medical Publishers, Inc., Chicago, 1977, pp. 233–290.

6. Bruce, D.A., Langfitt, T.W., Miller, J.D., Schutz, H., Vapalahti, M.P., Stanek, A., Goldberg, H.I.: Regional cerebral blood flow, intracranial pressure, and brain metabolism in comatose patients. J. Neurosurg., 38:131–144, 1973.

7. Bruce, D.A., Obrist, W., Zimmerman, R., Bilaniuk, L., Dolinskas, C., Kuhl, D., Schut, L.: The pathophysiology of acute severe brain swelling following pediatric head trauma. Acta Neurol. Scand. (Suppl. 74): 62:VI-4, 89, 1980.

8. Bruce, D.A., Raphaely, R.C., Goldberg, A.I., Zimmerman, R.A., Bilaniuk, L.T., Schut, L., Kuhl, D.E.: Pathophysiology, treatment and outcome following severe head injury in children. Child's Brain, 5:174–191, 1979.

9. Bruce, D.A., Raphaely, R.A., Swedlow, D., Schut, L.: The effectiveness of iatrogenic barbiturate coma in controlling increased ICP in 61 children. In: Intracranial Pressure IV, Shulman, K., Marmarou, A., Miller, J.D., Becker, D.P., Hochwald, G.M., Brock, M. Eds. Springer-Verlag, Berlin, 1980, pp. 630–632.

10. Bruce, D.A., Schut, L., Bruno, L.A., Wood, J.H., Sutton, L.N.: Outcome following severe head injuries in children. J. Neurosurg., 48:679–688, 1978.

11. Caffey, J.: On the theory and practice of shaking infants. Its potential residual effects of permanent brain damage and mental retardation. Am. J. Dis. Child., 124:161–169, 1972.

12. Caffey, J.: The whiplash shaken infant syndrome: manual shaking by the extremities with whiplash-induced intracranial and intraocular bleeding linked with residual permanent brain damage and mental retardation. Pediatrics, 54:396, 1974.

13. Carlsson, C.-A., von Essen, C., Lofgren, J.: Factors affecting the clinical course of patients with severe head injuries. Part 1, Influence of biological factors. Part 2, Significance of post-traumatic coma. J. Neurosurg., 29:242–251, 1968.

14. Carter, A.E.: Extradural haemorrhage in a child, without skull fracture, following minor trauma. J. Neurosurg., 17:155–156, 1960.

15. Hendrick, E.B., Harwood-Hash, D.C.F., Hudson, A.R.: Head injuries in children. A survey of 4465 consecutive cases at the Hospital for Sick Children, Toronto, Canada. Clin. Neurosurg., 11:46–65, 1964.

16. Ito, H., Miwa, T., Onodra, Y.: Growing skull fractures of childhood. With reference to the importance of the brain injury and its pathogenetic consideration. Child's brain, 3:116–126, 1977.

17. Kingsley, D., Till, K., Hoare, R.: Growing fractures of the skull. J. Neurol. Neurosurg. Psych., 41:312–318, 1978.

18. Kuhl, D.E., Alavi, A., Hoffman, E.J., Phelps, M.E., Zimmerman, R.A., Obrist, W.D., Bruce, D.A., Greenberg, J.H., Uzzell, B.: Local cerebral blood volume in head-injured patients: determination by emission computed tomography of ^{99m}Tc-labeled red cells. J. Neurosurg., 52:309–320, 1980.

19. Lefkowtiz, L.L.: Extradural hemorrhage as a result of birth trauma. Arch. Pediatr., 53:404–407, 1936.

20. Lindenberg, R., Fisher, R.S., Durlacher, S., Lovitt, W.J. Jr., Freytag, E.: The pathology of the brain in blunt head injuries of infants and children. Proceedings of the Second International Congress of Neuropathology. Excerpta Medica, Amsterdam, 1:477–479, 1955.

21. Lindenberg, R., Freytag, E.: Morphology of brain lesions from blunt trauma in early infancy. Arch. Pathol., 87:298–305, 1969.

22. McClelland, C.Q., Rekate, H., Kaufman, B., Persse, L.: Cerebral injury in child abuse: a changing profile. Child's Brain, 7:225–235, 1980.

23. McLaurin, R.L.: Management of chronic subdural hematomas in infancy. In: Pediatric Neurological Surgery, M.S. O'Brien, Ed. Raven Press, New York, 1978, pp. 135–146.

24. Mayer, T., Walker, M.L., Shasha, I., Matlak, M., Johnson, D.G.: Effect of multiple trauma on outcome of pediatric patients with neurologic injuries. Child's Brain, 8:189–197, 1981.

25. Ordia, I.J., Strand, R., Gilles, F., Welch, K.: Computerized tomography of contusional clefts in the white matter in infants. Report of 2 cases. J. Neurosurg., 54:696–698, 1981.

26. Papo, I., Caruselli, G., Luongo, A.: CSF withdrawal for the treatment of intracranial hypertension in acute head injuries. Acta. Neurochir., 56:191–199, 1981.

27. Pickles, W.: Acute general edema of the brain in children with head injuries. N. Engl. J. Med., 242:607–611, 1950.

28. Raphaely, R., Swedlow, D., Downes, J., Bruce, D.A.: Management of severe pediatric head trauma. Ped. Clin. North Am., 27:715–727, 1980.

29. Schnitker, M.T.: A syndrome of cerebral concussion in children. J. Pediatr., 35:557–560, 1949.

30. Schut, L., Bruce, D.A.: Recent advancements in the treatment of head injuries. Ped. Ann., 5:80–104, 1976.

31. Serfontein, G.L., Stein, S.: Posterior fossa subdural hemorrhage in the newborn. Pediatrics, 65:40–43, 1980.

32. Sulamaa, M., Vara, P.: An investigation into the occurrence of perinatal subdural haematoma: its diagnosis and treatment. Acta. Obstet. Gynecol. Scand., 31:400–412, 1952.

33. Takagi, T., Nagai, R., Wakabayashi, S., Mizawa, I., Hayashi, K.: Extradural hemorrhage in the newborn as a result of birth trauma. Child's Brain, 4:306–318, 1978.

34. Volpe, J.J.: Neonatal intracranial hemorrhage. Clin. Perinatol., 4:77–102, 1977.

35. Zimmerman, R.A., Bilaniuk, L.T., Bruce, D., Schut, L., Uzzell, B., Goldberg, H.I.: Interhemispheric acute subdural hematoma: a computed tomographic manifestation of child abuse by shaking. Neuroradiology, 16:39–40, 1978.

17

Medical Complications of Head Injury

LAWRENCE H. PITTS

Abnormalities of extraneural organ systems are common after cerebral trauma and are a function of several factors: the severity of head injury, the age, and general health of the victim. Undoubtedly, some extra-central nervous system involvement secondary to head injury is not recognized clinically, but is very common in head-injured patients and is a frequent cause of mortality. In this chapter some of the extraneural effects of non-traumatic central nervous system (CNS) injury generally and of craniocerebral trauma specifically will be examined.

PULMONARY COMPLICATIONS

The adverse effect of respiratory insufficiency on outcome has been recognized for many years. Table 17.1 lists some of the pulmonary abnormalities seen in patients with CNS injury. Manual or mechanical ventilation, used to improve outcome in bulbar poliomyelitis in the 1950's,[70] was also first used for the management of severe head injury during that period.[76] Although we now consider the viewpoint to be overly simplistic, some authors[45, 76] felt that maintenance of adequate blood oxygenation would produce a good outcome in many patients with severe head injury who did not die immediately following trauma. Their emphasis was placed appropriately

The author thanks Beverly J.H. McGehee for preparation of the manuscript, and Neil Buckley for editorial assistance.

because maintenance of normal blood gas values is essential for optimal outcome from severe head injury.

Abnormal Respiratory Patterns

Patients with acute brain damage frequently have abnormal breathing patterns.[93] Plum and Posner[98] suggested that certain definite breathing patterns could be of localizing value. While it is true that medullary and pontine lesions often produce irregular breathing, there is no statistically significant relationship between a particular lesion site and a specific breathing pattern, and the same patient may have more than one pattern at different times.[93] Poor outcome is associated significantly with abnormal breathing only when tachypnea (greater than 25 breaths a minute) is associated with spontaneous hyperventilation ($pACO_2$ pressure below 30 torr),[93, 118] a combination which frequently accompanies pneumonia or systemic metabolic acidosis. Hyperventilation independent of pneumonia or acidosis also may arise from loss of cortical inhibition of respiration.[71]

Hypoxemia

Hypoxemia frequently occurs secondary to severe head injury; at admission, pAO_2 is below 80 torr in nearly 50% of patients,[12, 110] and below 65 torr in 20–30% of patients.[64, 83, 87, 110] Causes of this early hypoxemia are unclear, although aspiration, obstruction of the airway by the tongue or foreign body, or chest wall inju-

Table 17.1
Pulmonary Abnormalities in Head Injury

Apnea
Hypoventilation
Hyperventilation
Ventilation-perfusion imbalance
Aspiration
Fat embolism (in multiple injuries)
Brain embolism
Decreased pulmonary compliance
Atelectasis
Pneumonia
Neurogenic pulmonary edema

ries can be implicated in some patients. Concussion alone routinely causes hypoventilation which generally resolves rapidly[48] but can be prolonged. Overwhelming neurogenic pulmonary edema can occur almost instantaneously after devastating brain injuries,[109] but there is as yet no evidence that increased lung water causes the hypoxia sometimes present at the time of initial medical care in head injured patients.

Hypoxia that occurs hours to days after injury may arise from any of the causes described above. Focal atelectasis and pneumonia contribute significantly to diminished blood oxygenation. However, hypoxia may exist in many patients with normal chest X-rays, possibly due to unexplained imbalances between pulmonary perfusion and ventilation.[37, 81, 105, 122] Atelectasis is not solely responsible for the imbalance; lung functional residual capacity may be normal in head injured patients[105] and mechanical lung hyperinflation may not restore pulmonary venous pO_2 to normal levels.[86] Schumacker et al.[105] have suggested that an active bronchiolar constriction causes an increased resistance of small airways with decreased alveolar ventilation; a failure of compensatory vascular constriction then produces insufficient ventilation of perfused alveoli with lowered pulmonary venous pO_2. Increased inspired oxygen or mechanical ventilation usually improves pO_2, but the two therapies may not have an additive beneficial effect.[105] Moreover, mechanical hyperventilation may not lessen the development of ventilation-perfusion abnormalities.[38, 39]

Neurogenic Pulmonary Edema. The existence of "neurogenic pulmonary edema" (NPE) is disputed only by those who have not seen the sudden appearance of copious amounts of frothy pink sputum in patients suffering from acute CNS disorders. NPE has been reported in a variety of experimental and clinical disorders including head injury,[24, 29, 85, 109] seizures,[113] subarachnoid hemorrhage (SAH),[15] and acute hydrocephalus.[36] Although survival after the onset of NPE is not uncommon, some patients die of progressive respiratory failure in the face of a stable or improving neurologic status.

Hypothalamic lesions caused fatal pulmonary edema and congestion in cats,[19] and pre-optic area lesions caused NPE in rats.[40] These findings would appear to implicate the hypothalamus in the formation of NPE. Increasing intracranial pressure (ICP) caused NPE in dogs, cats, and primates,[30, 54, 97] although NPE did not appear uniformly in all animals. Chen and colleagues[17] studied the effects of direct cerebral compression in rats coupled with combinations of decerebration, vagotomy, spinal cord transection, and adrenalectomy and concluded that NPE was produced by overactive sympathetic vasomotor mechanisms in the medulla and, perhaps, in the spinal cord. Their data did not explain the possibility of activation by medullary mechanisms. Most hypotheses that attempt to explain the formation of NPE include the following sequential factors: a massive sympathetic discharge with venoconstriction, increased circulating blood volume, and left heart failure with increasing pulmonary artery pressure and capillary injury with extravasation of fluid into the pulmonary alveoli,[34, 75, 104, 114] along with some extravasation of red blood cells. While increased sympathetic tone commonly plays a role in NPE formation, it has been shown in cats[55] and in humans[96] that lung water content can increase in the absence of elevated systemic or pulmonary artery pressures. These data suggest that pulmonary capillary "leakiness" can cause NPE.

We have determined lung water volumes over several days in 14 patients with severe head injury. We employ thermal dilution and cardio-green dye are techniques with injection into the superior vena cava or pulmonary artery[74]; differences between the mean transit times of the two indicators gives a reliable measure of lung water content *in vivo*.[73] Because of the invasive nature of this technique, control values from normal humans are not available. But a number of studies in humans with multisystem trauma or burns who had no apparent pulmonary dysfunction suggests that normal human lung water volumes are essentially of the same magnitude proportionally as for normal experimental animals. Figure 17.1 shows mean lung water volumes for head-injured patients in our study, normal values for dogs, and data for a group of patients with serious burns. Virtually all head-injured patients had elevated lung water volumes that averaged about 50% above "normal" values. Burn patients generally

EXTRAVASCULAR LUNG WATER

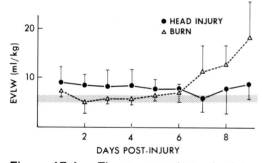

Figure 17.1. The mean and standard deviation for values of extravascular lung water (EVLW) measured *in vivo* in two groups of patients after either head injury (○) or severe burns (△) and (because data are not available for normal humans) in dogs without lung disease (*shaded area*). EVLW was significantly higher in head-injured patients than in burn patients (p < 0.02) for the first five days after injury. At that time, lung water values for head-injured patients became normal or were moderately elevated, while some burn patients developed markedly elevated lung water concurrent with the onset of sepsis.

had normal lung water volumes until 5 to 7 days after injury, after which sepsis often complicated their clinical status and apparently contributed to increased lung water.

In our study, head-injured patients had different degrees of pulmonary shunting of blood, but only modest hypoxemia, which was readily corrected by increasing the amount of inspired oxygen. No patient had pulmonary artery or systemic hypertension and none had clinically evident NPE. However, the uniform increase in lung water in these patients suggests that clinically apparent NPE is only an extreme example of the effects of increased extravascular lung water, which appears to be a common and often clinically unrecognized complication in head-injured patients.

Treatment of Pulmonary Complications

Treatment of pulmonary dysfunction in patients with severe craniocerebral trauma is similar to the treatment of pulmonary problems that may result from any trauma although a few special precautions must be taken.[38] Early hypoxia and hypercarbia usually respond promptly to intubation and mechanical ventilation after pulmonary toilet is achieved. Aspiration is treated with intubation and suctioning only; steroids do not prevent the subsequent development of pneumonia or decrease its severity. Appropriate antibiotics are begun when pneumonia is diagnosed by chest X-ray and sputum analysis. Broad spectrum antibiotic coverage is selected initially (*e.g.*, penicillin and tobramycin), and a specific regimen is selected as rapidly as possible based on identification of a specific organism. Mild-to-moderate hypoxia, whether due to atelectasis, pulmonary venous shunting, ventilation/perfusion imbalances, increased lung water, or other unknown abnormalities, usually responds to increases in inspired oxygen.

Positive end-expiratory pressure (PEEP) may further improve oxygenation, and should be used if NPE develops.[60] However, caution must be exercised in the use of PEEP because its use may increase ICP[2, 3, 68, 85] and decrease systemic arterial pressure and cardiac output.[61] Because such adverse effects of PEEP are difficult to predict in an individual patient, ICP and cardiac output should be monitored carefully when PEEP is employed.

Dehydration with hyperosmotic agents or diuretics is routinely employed in the management of head injured patients and may minimize an increase in lung water and the formation of NPE although increased lung water commonly occurs despite dehydration.[96]

CARDIAC ABNORMALITIES

A number of CNS lesions can produce virtually any EKG abnormality that may reflect either minor or severe cardiac pathology[1] (Table 17.2). SAH in humans[26, 28, 46, 108, 119] and in animals,[31] stroke,[43] meningitis, intracranial tumors, abscesses[25, 52] and head injury in animals[32, 35, 50, 58] and in humans[51, 116] may be accompanied by atrial, atrio-ventricular (AV), nodal, or ventricular arrhythmias, AV dissociation, and unifocal or multifocal extrasystoles. There may be no intrinsic cardiac lesion even when significant EKG changes are found after rupture of a cerebral aneurysm.[7] However, SAH can produce myocardial changes ranging from necrosis of individual muscle fibers and small foci of inflammatory cells to extensive myocardial hemorrhage and necrosis.[28, 46] Although no detailed study has been done that evaluated myocardial pathology

Table 17.2
Electrocardiographic Abnormalities in CNS Disease

Common
   Prolonged Q-T interval
   Large upright or deeply inverted T wave
   Bradycardia
   Prominent U wave
   Elevated S-T segment
   Peaked P wave

Less Common
   Shortened Q-T interval
   Prolonged or shortened P-R interval
   Increased QRS voltage
   Presence of Q wave
   Notched T wave
   Atrial or ventricular arrhythmias

after head injury, EKG changes seen in head-injured patients are the same as those seen in patients with other catastrophic CNS dysfunction. Myocardial damage probably occurs in some cases of severe head injury, although it usually does not cause any clinically obvious cardiac disease.

The mechanisms that cause changes in heart function and possibly cause myocardial damage are probably related to the same sympathetic hyperactivity that cause the pulmonary problems described in the previous section. Brief electrical stimulation of the hypothalamus in cats produced striking arterial hypertension and EKG changes consisting of S-T segment depression, ectopic beats, and T-wave inversion that reverted quickly to normal after cessation of stimulation; there was no myocardial damage. However, prolonged bilateral hypothalamic stimulation produced myocardial infarction in one-half of the cats tested.[82] Stimulation of the midbrain reticular formation in cats produced typical arterial hypertension and EKG alterations. Microscopic examination showed myocardial inflammation and damage including diffuse myofibrillar degeneration and subendocardial and transmural infarction.[46] Adrenalectomy did not prevent the lesions, which suggests that a direct neural effect on the heart causes hemorrhage and necrosis. Transection of the cervical spinal cord abolished the EKG changes seen with hypothalamic stimulation, but bilateral vagotomy had no effect.[100] However, vagal stimulation in dogs produced EKG changes and myocardial damage that were blocked by atropine.[79] Atropine also diminished EKG abnormalities after experimental head injury in mice.[58]

Despite the occasional report of the influence of the vagus nerve on CNS-induced cardiac changes, the sympathetic nervous system plays a more influential role. Patients with SAH secondary to the rupture of an aneurysm had significantly elevated plasma levels of epinephrine and norepinephrine[33]; patients whose levels decreased did well, but patients whose levels remained elevated had poor outcomes.[9] Oral administration of propranolol, a competitive inhibitor of catecholamine beta-receptors, diminished EKG abnormalities after SAH in patients, although pathologic Q waves were not abolished in one patient.[26] In a prospective double-blind study in 80 patients who suffered SAH, 12 patients died; six had received a placebo and six had received a combination of propranolol and phentolamine. All six patients who died and who received a placebo had abnormal EKG's and necrotic myocardial lesions, while none who received propranolol-phentolamine had abnormal EKG's and/or myocardial necrosis.[88] These findings strongly imply that the sympathetic nervous system mediates the influence of CNS damage on the heart.

Head injury can produce cardiovascular alterations including EKG and blood pressure changes (Fig. 17.2). Blows to the skull vertex of mice caused nodal rhythms, variable RR intervals, T-wave changes, incomplete AV blocks, dropped P-waves, bradycardia or tachycardia, and premature ventricular systoles. Pretreatment with atropine generally prevented the arrhythmias

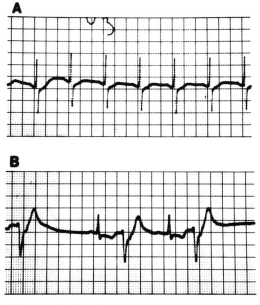

Figure 17.2. Abnormal electrocardiograms after head injury vary from minor, non-specific S-T segment and T-wave changes (A) to major arrythmias (B) and, in rare circumstances, may reflect myocardial infarction.

and T-wave changes, but hearts were not examined for pathological evidence of myocardial damage.[58] Intracerebral or subarachnoid blood injected into mice produced myocardial hemorrhage and/or necrosis that was entirely blocked by pretreatment with reserpine and markedly attenuated by pre-treatment or by adrenalectomy before blood was injected.[50] Severe impact injuries in monkeys consistently caused immediate bradycardia and hypotension that were unaffected by adrenergic blockade but were prevented by pretreatment with atropine. However, a return to preimpact heart rate and blood pressure occurred more rapidly in monkeys with intact sympathetic nervous systems, indicating that early changes are vagally mediated and later responses involve sympathetic innervation.[32]

EKG changes in head-injured humans were described nearly 50 years ago in a report of a young patient with no cardiovascular disease who had persistent atrial fibrillation after minor head trauma.[13] A later and more extensive study reported an increased incidence of peaked P waves and prolonged Q-T intervals in head-injured patients compared to patients with limb injuries or to normal controls.[51] The EKG abnormalities were more pronounced in those head-injured patients who were also comatose. Less specific changes (including most of those listed in Table 17.2) were noted in head-injured and limb-injured patients and were felt to be a nonspecific EKG manifestation to trauma. Patients with acute subdural hematomas frequently develop new arrhythmias in the postoperative period, most of which are ventricular in origin. On occasion, ventricular tachycardia or fibrillation has been noted. Patients with more severe EKG abnormalities had poorer outcomes; both EKG changes and outcome may be the result of more severe brain trauma.[116]

Although no extensive evaluation of myocardial damage has been made in humans who die from head injury, EKG changes are essentially the same as those seen with other CNS catastrophies in which severe myocardial damage is evident. Thus, while overt cardiac problems are rare in head-injured patients, overactivity of the autonomic nervous system may well cause malfunctioning of the heart and may affect blood pressure regulation which can jeopardize the homeostasis needed for neural recovery after craniocerebral trauma.

Treatment of Cardiac Complications

Usually, cardiac changes are not as severe in head-injured patients as in those with other CNS disorders such as SAH. Minor EKG changes can be followed with serial cardiograms and determination of cardiac enzyme levels to ensure that there has not been substantial myocardial damage after head injury. Occasional hazardous cardiac dysrrhythmias may require intravenous lidocaine or other antiarrhythmic drugs. If myocardial failure develops, the patient may require digitalization, and fluid balance and cardiac output must be monitored carefully.

SHOCK

Brain damage generally does not produce sustained hypotension, although transient hypotension may develop.[32] An obvious exception to this general clinical finding is observed in patients with an overwhelming cerebral injury that causes terminal hypotension from rapid failure of medullary vasopressor centers. Therefore, shock (arterial pressure below 90 torr) seen early after head injury must be assumed to be hypovolemic in origin and sources of blood loss in the chest, abdomen, or, occasionally, in the legs must be carefully sought and treated appropriately. Plain films of the chest, pelvis, and femurs will usually disclose unsuspected hemothorax or other possible sources of bleeding into the pelvis or thighs, any of which can account for blood loss to 2 to 3 liters or more.[21] Peritoneal lavage is effective in diagnosing intraperitoneal hemorrhage from injuries to abdominal viscera. Computerized tomographic (CT) scans of the abdomen can reveal intra- or retroperitoneal bleeding and intravenous pyelography may show renal injuries directly or retroperitoneal hemorrhage indirectly by ureteral obstruction or deviation. The evaluation and treatment of systemic hemorrhage is discussed more fully in Chapter 3.

In a review of 400 head-injury victims with a range of severity of injury, shock was present in only 2% of patients and an evident cause was recognized in all but one patient. In 70 cases of fatal head injury, shock was present in 7% of patients.[57] Higher incidences of shock, ranging from 10–18%, have been reported in patients with more severe head injuries.[83, 91, 101, 123] Among those who survive head injury, hypotensive patients take longer to become oriented and have lengthier hospitalizations than matched normotensive control patients. When hypoxia and hypotension were both present, patients were less likely to resume normal work after injury than matched controls.[101]

At our institution, one-third of patients with coma-producing head injury are in shock during the first 24 hours after injury (Table 17.3). Most patients in shock have one or more major injuries of the face, chest, abdomen, or limbs. However, 20% of patients with head injury only had shock within the first 24 hours after injury. In these latter patients, shock occurred as a preterminal event or as a result of catastrophic brain damage and early medullary failure.

We have found that shock significantly increases mortality in patients in traumatic coma, from 50% in those head-injured patients without early shock to 82% if shock is present. Only 6% of patients with head injury without shock die within 6 hours of injury, while 34% of patients with head injury and hypotension die within 6 hours. Table 17.4 lists the influence of shock and mortality on injuries to one or more extracranial organ systems.

Clearly, shock represents a major hazard for the patient with severe head injury. Patients with early hypotension must be resuscitated vigorously with electrolyte solutions or whole blood (if available) when hemorrhage has been documented. Details of the resuscitation of the multiply-injured patient are discussed in Chapters 2 and 3. An algorithm we have found useful for evaluation and treatment of the multiply injured patient is seen in Figure 17.3.

Although it is not established that shock

Table 17.3
Head Injury and Shock[a]

	Shock Present	Shock Absent	Total
Head injury only	40	167	207
Any other major injury	74	60	134
One other major injury	26	33	59
Two other major injuries	24	21	45
Three other major injuries	16	6	22
Four other major injuries	8	0	8
Total (one or more major injury)	114	227	341

[a] Patients with severe head injuries are defined as surviving six or more hours of traumatic coma or who die within 6 hours of injury. Shock is defined as an arterial pressure below 90 mm Hg in the first 24 hours after injury. Major multi-system injuries are defined as injuries to the face, chest, trunk, or limbs that would require hospitalization independent of the head injury.

Table 17.4
Multisystem Injuries: Shock and Death

	Shock	Death
	%	
Head injury plus one other injury	44	48
Head injury plus two other injuries	47	66
Head injury plus three other injuries	73	66
Head injury plus four other injuries	100	78

MULTIPLE INJURIES AND SHOCK

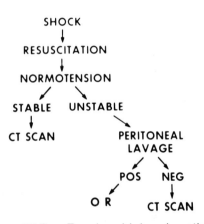

Figure 17.3. For head-injured patients with multiple injuries and shock, immediate resuscitation is initiated and a chest X-ray obtained. If a normal blood pressure can be restored rapidly and then maintained, intracranial studies then can be performed. If the blood pressure remains unstable, we perform peritoneal lavage to investigate possible intra-abdominal sources of bleeding; if the "peridial" is positive, a laporatomy is done. However, if peritoneal dialysis is negative, attempts to sustain the blood pressure are continued while we either obtain intracranial studies to determine the extent of cerebral injury or proceed directly to the operating room for intracranial exploration. Craniotomy and abdominal or thoracic surgery are often performed simultaneously at our institution.

causes or worsens outcome after head injury, it profoundly influences cerebral perfusion. Hypotension can lead directly to cerebral ischemia, which may destroy or injure brain that has not been damaged by direct injury.

COAGULATION

Clotting disorders have been described after a variety of cerebral insults including stroke,[6] surgery for excision of a brain tumor,[80] placement of ventricular catheters,[107] and head injury of many types.[20, 44, 65, 117] Between 40 and 70% of head-injured patients have depressed levels of clotting factors.[65, 117] Abnormal clotting may be due to a consumption coagulopathy and cause either increased hemorrhage[66] or vascular occlusion.[14]

Brain has the highest level of thromboplastin of any body tissue,[4] and destruction of cerebral tissue and disruption of the blood-brain barrier can release large quantities of thromboplastin into the circulation and activate "extrinsic" pathways for blood clotting (Fig. 17.4). Released thromboplastin is converted to thrombin which in turn converts plasma fibrinogen to fibrin, causing the disseminated intravascular coagulation (DIC) seen with these cerebral insults. Thrombin also promotes conversion of plasminogen to plasmin, the factor that facilitates the breakdown of formed fibrin to "fibrin split products," which are hematologic markers for DIC. When most of the circulating fibrinogen is activated and becomes fibrin, the body loses a major hemostatic protective mechanism and generalized hypocoagulation ensues.

If a bleeding diathesis should occur, the diagnosis of DIC should be established quickly so that appropriate therapy can be initiated. Clotting time can be determined in the operating room or on the ward by placing several milliliters of blood in a glass tube that does not contain anticoagulants; the tube is tilted every 30–60 seconds until a clot forms. The normal clotting time is less than 8–10 minutes, and a clotting time longer than 12 minutes is very suggestive of DIC and would warrant treatment. A more definitive diagnosis can be made by measuring the levels of circulating fibrin split products, which always will be elevated in patients with DIC. Prothrombin times may be more readily available on an emergency basis in some hospitals and provide a presumptive diagnosis of DIC if the prothrombin time exceeds 25 seconds.

Treatment of Coagulopathies

Symptomatic coagulopathies present their greatest problems soon after head injury, particularly when surgery is necessary to treat intracranial hemorrhage. Low fibrinogen levels, caused by DIC or chronic liver disease, can be corrected by administration of 2–4 units of fresh frozen plasma or whole blood. Severe continued bleeding might warrant the use of platelets or fresh (less than 24 hours old) whole blood. The effectiveness of treatment can be determined by repeated measurements of the clotting time, which will return to normal if adequate fibrinogen has been replaced. Such treatment can be lifesaving during surgical and medical management of head injury, and may prevent the delayed intracranial bleeding sometimes seen after trauma.[65]

FLUID AND ELECTROLYTE DISTURBANCES

Corticosteroids

Many factors influence salt and water regulation in patients with head injury. Levels of endogenous glucocorticoids increase in response to stress, infection, and surgery including craniotomy[11]; exogenous corticosteroids may be given therapeutically. Corticosteroids act in several ways to regulate the body's salt and water content. In patients undergoing craniotomy for excision of tumor, dexamethasone increases urine output, but even greater amounts of sodium, potassium, and chloride are excreted, which produce a decrease in serum sodium levels and, consequently, of osmolarity.[106] Corticosteroid administration may also unmask latent diabetes mellitus with increased urine volume and glucose loss.

Antidiuretic Hormone

Antidiuretic hormone (ADH) markedly increases the permeability of the distal renal tubule to water and urea,[72] which promotes the retention of free water and leads to systemic hyponatremia. Head injury and its treatment may affect ADH secretion in a number of ways and may lead to fatal brain edema if not treated appropriately. Early resuscitation often involves infusion of 2–4 liters of electrolyte solutions, particularly if multiple injuries and hypovolemic shock are present. Surgery and anesthesia[27] or SAH[63, 121] can produce hyponatremia and hypoosmolarity consistent with inappropriate ADH secretion. Norepinephrine levels increase with trauma[22] and can markedly suppress the release of ADH from the posterior pituitary; conversely, experimental increases in ICP markedly increased ADH secretion in monkeys.[41] Dehydration caused by osmotic agents or other diuretics will produce an appropriate secretion of ADH in an attempt to maintain a normal blood volume. SAH in humans[89] or in animals[90] produces an undefined

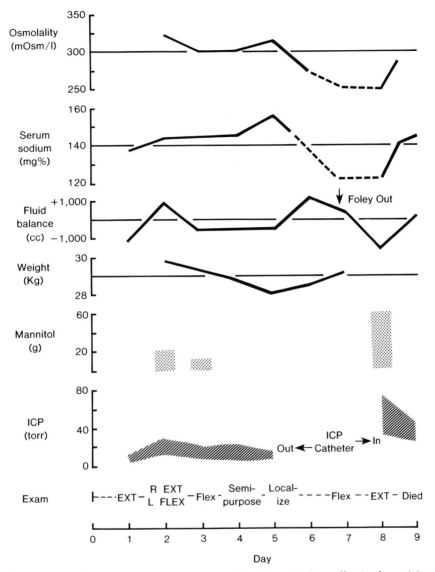

Figure 17.4. This figure depicts the potentially devastating effect of post-traumatic hyponatremia, probably due to inappropriate antidiuretic hormone secretion. This 8-year-old child suffered a severe head injury that required early removal of a subdural hematoma. Postoperative ICP control below 20 torr was achieved with relatively low doses of mannitol on days 2 and 3; there were associated weight loss and negative fluid balance and modest elevations in serum sodium and osmolality. The child showed steady neurologic improvement, the ICP catheter was removed on day 5, and nasogastric feedings begun. Weight gain and a positive fluid balance were noted on day 6 but serum sodium and osmolality values were "lost in the lab." Significant hyponatremia and hypoosmolality were not appreciated until day 8, by which time the patient had deteriorated significantly. Despite reinstitution of ICP monitoring and aggressive attempts at ICP control, high ICP's persisted and the child died on day 9, presumably because of brain swelling that resulted from retention of free water.

"cerebral salt wasting syndrome" that can cause a natriuresis with an appropriate secondary ADH secretion. Thus, many factors associated with head injury may lead to altered secretion of ADH.

In addition to an osmotic diuresis from steroid-induced glycosuria, inappropriately high urine output may be caused by a reduction in ADH secretion resulting in diabetes insipidus (DI) secondary to damage to the pituitary and is seen in some cases of severe head injury,[47, 69, 92] although injuries to the pituitary, pituitary stalk, or hypothalamus do not always produce DI.[42, 59, 84] Excretion of large volumes of urine are not necessarily due to DI; normal diuresis of fluids retained after resuscitation or as a response to stress usually gives rise to a large urine output, at times in excess of 1,000 cc/hour. The serum sodium level is the critical distinguishing factor; diuresis of retained fluids will cease as serum sodium and osmolarity approach normal, while the diuresis of DI will continue despite abnormally high serum sodium levels. Because of the multiplicity of factors affecting electrolyte and fluid balance, careful monitoring of serum sodium and potassium levels and osmolarity is mandatory and will provide the basis for rational management of these problems.

Treatment of Fluid and Electrolyte Disturbance

Treatment of fluid imbalance requires frequent assessment of fluid and electrolyte status. Daily body weight should be recorded, and intake and output balance noted every 8–12 hours in the first week or so after a severe head injury. Urine sodium levels should be measured daily, and serum sodium levels should be determined daily or more frequently if the patient has an altered mental status. Hyponatremia is treated best and most safely by fluid restriction to 10–20 cc/kg body weight of normal saline per day. Occasionally diuretics (*e.g.*, furosemide 10–40 mg for adults) or 3% normal saline may be used when fluid restriction alone fails to correct hyponatremia.

A marked increase in urinary output may be due to DI and is treated effectively by 3–5 units of aqueous vasopressin given subcutaneously. However, vasopressin should be used only when serum sodium levels are above 148 mEq/liter, because a large urine output can represent a normal diuresis. Prolonged DI arising from hypothalamic or pituitary injury can be treated by desmopressin acetate nasal spray after initial management with aqueous vasopressin. In most head-injured patients, fluid and electrolyte imbalances return to normal within 1–2 weeks after injury.

METABOLIC ALTERATIONS IN HEAD INJURY

In general, trauma increases metabolism[62] and produces a catabolic state with a negative nitrogen balance that is caused by muscle breakdown.[120] Changes in metabolism are roughly proportional to the severity of injury.[67, 112] Negative nitrogen balance was thought to be a result of tissue mobilization to provide energy for injury repair, but studies have shown that protein contributes less than 20% of the caloric expenditure after injury, and that the majority of energy is provided by fatty acid metabolism.[67] Trauma induces elevation of catecholamines[18, 22, 99] and initiates muscle glycogenolysis, both of which cause blood glucose levels to increase.[111] Hemorrhage elevates glucagon levels[49] which stimulates liver gluconeogenesis and glycogenolysis which in turn convert carbohydrate stores to circulating glucose. Insulin levels are elevated, but not to the extent that would be expected from the amount of hyperglycemia, perhaps because insulin production is inhibited by circulating catecholamines.

Higgins *et al.*[53] described a variety of metabolic disorders in patients with traumatic coma that included proteinuria, hypoproteinemia, glucosuria, and hyperglycemia. McLaurin *et al.*,[77, 78] described the appearance of multiple metabolic changes after head injury or elective intracranial surgery and confirmed the existence of a post-traumatic catabolic condition with a negative nitrogen balance that resulted in a loss of as much as 300 g of muscle per day despite nasogastric feedings. He reported that this catabolism lasted 10 days or more and was unaffected by the presence or absence of multiple injuries, although the severity of cerebral injury seemed to correlate with the degree of catabolism. Dietary nitrogen supplements did not eliminate the catabolism, but the negative nitrogen balance was reduced when 1,000 calories or more per day were administered.

Although sodium retention is prolonged in patients with severe head injury, sodium retention is more variable than nitrogen loss. There was a sodium retention but an even greater free-water retention that caused progressive hyponatremia consistent with either an inappropriate ADH secretion or with a "cerebral salt-wasting syndrome"[94] with subsequent appropriate secretion of ADH to counteract hypovolemia.

Treatment of Metabolic Alterations

The catabolism seen with traumatic coma cannot always be reversed. A brief, initial hypermetabolic state is well tolerated by most patients, but establishment of good nutrition is important to reduce the frequency and severity of sepsis. Most comatose head-injured patients tolerate nasogastric feedings well, and after early fluid retention has stopped, 3,000–4,000 calories a day may be delivered by a nasogastric tube. In patients in whom gastrointestinal absorption is not adequate, hyperalimentation by central intravenous lines offers another route, although this generally requires large volumes of fluid that may exacerbate hyponatremia if the patient is still retaining free-water in excess of sodium.

SEPTICEMIA

Patients who survive more than two days after major trauma are at risk of sepsis and multiple organ failure, both of which can lead to death.[10, 23] In one series, over one-half of the deaths from general trauma that occurred later than two days after injury and 78% of deaths after one week, were due to sepsis.[5]

Patients in traumatic coma have a significant risk of developing severe infec-

tions.[56] It is necessary to monitor these patients intensively by invasive techniques that, unfortunately, provide routes for bacterial contamination. Endotracheal intubation or tracheostomy, with frequent tracheal suctioning, provide the ideal route for pulmonary bacterial contamination. The increased water content of the lungs routinely seen in these patients[96] may be accompanied by other lung dysfunction that may lead to an increased risk of pneumonia.

Indwelling urethral catheters required to monitor fluid balance increase the risk of urinary tract infections. Systemic and pulmonary arterial catheters or venous catheters are necessary for the administration of fluids and medications and for monitoring hydrodynamic status, but can be sources of bacterial contamination of the blood stream. Scalp lacerations, compound skull fractures, and craniotomies for treatment of intracranial mass lesions increase the incidence of wound infections, meningitis,[102, 103] and brain abscesses, which is further increased by the use of various ICP monitors (see also Chapter 18).

All these infections occur in severely head-injured patients with alarming frequency (Table 17.5), and often increase both morbidity and mortality. It has been stated that increases in mortality that are seen with advancing age are due almost exclusively to systemic sepsis rather than to the cerebral injury.[8, 16] While sepsis certainly is more common in older patients,

Table 17.5
Infectious Complications of Severe Head Injury[a]

	%
Pneumonia	64
Urinary tract infection	23
Wound infection	
ICP catheter site	0
Scalp	3
Infected intravenous site	9
Any wound	26
Septicemia	13
CNS infection	3

[a] Data collected from 207 consecutive patients admitted with traumatic coma who survived longer than three days after injury.

outcome in younger patients also has been affected adversely by infection.

Treatment of Sepsis

Prevention of sepsis is more important than its treatment. Meticulous care must be taken with all monitoring catheters. Any systems known to have been contaminated must be replaced immediately. CSF or urine must be drained into closed systems (see also Chapter 10) and dressed appropriately. Any leakage of blood or CSF from wound edges must be stopped promptly, and the wound(s) reclosed if necessary.

Despite these precautions, infection occurs in a substantial number of patients. When the patient becomes febrile, blood, urine, and sputum are cultured. We generally do not culture ventricular or lumbar CSF from patients whose fevers begin early after injury unless there is strong likelihood of CNS contamination from compound cranial wounds or basilar skull fractures and we almost never culture lumbar or cervical CSF in the face of intracranial hypertension or a significant midline shift of the intracranial contents (see also Chapter 18). After samples for culture are obtained, we begin broad spectrum antibiotic coverage (*e.g.*, penicillin 16 million units a day, nafcillin, 8 g/day and tobramycin or gentamycin 240 mg/day). In hospitals with a high incidence of penicillinase-producing *Staphylococcus aureus*, vancomycin 2 g/day is administered until the organism is identified and its sensitivity determined at which time a specific, effective antibiotic is chosen. If no organism or source of sepsis is identified, but the patient's temperature returns to normal, a 7–10 day course of the broad spectrum coverage is given. If no organism is found and fever continues, antibiotics are stopped after 2–3 days and repeat samples for culture are obtained. Other sources of fever, such as drug reactions and atelectasis must be considered and, if possible, eliminated. A very aggressive approach to treatment of sepsis is required to reduce morbidity and mortality.

CONCLUSIONS

The frequency of extra-CNS complications after head injury makes it almost certain that disordered brain function contributes significantly to their genesis. Until we better understand how the brain influences other organ systems and, specifically, discover ways to prevent these multisystem insults, we must rely on the meticulous application of currently available and accepted methods of therapy for the treatment of head-injured patients. Haphazard attempts to prevent these problems or unwarranted delay in their treatment will contribute to the continued high morbidity and mortality seen in this group of patients. Fortunately, brain-body interactions are being investigated actively, and we can anticipate a clearer delineation of the underlying pathologic mechanisms. In the near future it is likely that there will be substantial improvement in the treatments for medical complications of severe head injury.

References

1. Abildskov, J.A., Miller, K., Burgess, M.J., Vincent, W.: The electrocardiogram and the central nervous system. Prog. Cardiovasc. Dis., 13:210–216, 1970.
2. Aidinis, S.J., Lafferty, J., Shapiro, H.M.: Intracranial responses to PEEP. Anesthesiology, 45:275–286, 1976.
3. Apuzzo, M.L.J., Weiss, M.H., Petersons, V., Small, R. B., Kurze, T., Heiden, J.S.: Effect of positive end expiratory pressure ventilation on intracranial pressure in man. J. Neurosurg., 46:227–232, 1977.
4. Astrup, T.: Assay and content of tissue thromboplastin in different organs. Thromb. Diath. Haemorrh., 14:401–416, 1965.
5. Baker, C.C., Oppenheimer, L., Stephens, B., Lewis, F.R., Trunkey, D.D.: Epidemiology of trauma deaths. Am. J. Surg., 140:144–150, 1980.
6. Bang, N.U., McDowell, F.: Cerebral infarctions and blood clotting. Trans. Am. Neural Assoc., 91:84–86, 1966.
7. Beard, E.F., Robertson, J.W., Robertson, R.C.L.: Spontaneous subarachnoid hemorrhage simulating acute myocardial infarction. Am. Heart J., 58:755–759, 1959.
8. Becker, D.P., Miller, J.D., Ward, J.D., Greenberg, R.P., Young, H.F., Sakalas, R.: The outcome from severe head injury with early diagnosis and intensive management. J. Neurosurg., 47:491–502, 1977.
9. Benedict, C.R., Loach, A.B.: Sympathetic nervous system activity in patients with subarachnoid hemorrhage. Stroke, 9:237–244, 1978.
10. Blaisdell, F.W., Lewis, F.R.: Respiratory distress syndrome of shock and trauma: post-traumatic respiratory failure. In: Major Problems in Clinical

Surgery, Vol. 21. 1977, pp. 69–72. W.B. Saunders Co., Philadelphia.

11. Bouzarth, W.F., Shenkin, H.A., Gutterman, P.: Adrenal cortical response to neurosurgical problems, noting the effects of exogenous steroids. In: Steroids and Brain Edema, Reulen, H.J., Schürmann, K., Eds. Springer-Verlag, Berlin, 1972, pp. 183–194.

12. Brackett, C.E.: Respiratory complications of head injury. In: International Symposium on Head Injuries, Gillingham, R., Obrador, L., Eds. Williams and Wilkins, Baltimore, 1971, pp. 255–265.

13. Bramwell, C.: Can head injury cause auricular fibrillation? Lancet, 1:8–10, 1934.

14. Buonanno, F.S., Cooper, M.R., Moody, D.M., Laster, D.W., Ball, M.R., Toole, J.F.: Neuroradiologic aspects of cerebral disseminated intravascular coagulation. Am. J. Neuroradiol., 1:245–250, 1980.

15. Carlson, R.W., Schaeffer, R.C., Michaels, S.G., Weil, M.H.: Pulmonary edema following intracranial hemorrhage. Chest, 75:731–734, 1979.

16. Carlsson, C.A., von Essen, C., Löfgren, J.: Factors affecting the clinical course of patients with severe head injuries. J. Neurosurg., 29:242–251, 1968.

17. Chen, H.I., Sun, S.C., Chai, C.Y.: Pulmonary edema and hemorrhage resulting from cerebral compression. Am. J. Physiol., 224:223–229, 1973.

18. Chien, S.: Role of the sympathetic nervous system in hemorrhage. Physiol. Rev., 47:214–288, 1967.

19. Clark, G., Magoun, H.W., Ranson, S.W.: Hypothalamic regulation of body temperature. J. Neurophysiol., 2:61–90, 1939.

20. Clark, J.A., Finelli, R.E., Netsky, M.G.: Disseminated intravascular coagulation following cranial trauma. J. Neurosurg., 52:266–269, 1980.

21. Clarke, R., Fisher, M.R., Topley, E., Davies, J.W.L.: Extent and time of blood-loss after civilian injury. Lancet, 2:381–386, 1961.

22. Clifton, G.L., Ziegler, M.G., Grossman, R.G.: Circulating catecholamines and sympathetic activity after head injury. Neurosurgery, 8:10–14, 1981.

23. Clowes, G.H.A. Jr.: Pulmonary abnormalities in sepsis. Surg. Clin. North Am., 54:993–1013, 1974.

24. Cohen, H.B., Gambill, A.F., Eggers, G.W.N.: Acute pulmonary edema following head injury. Two case reports. Anesth. Analg., 56:136–139, 1977.

25. Connor, R.C.R.: Heart damage associated with intracranial lesions. Br. Med. J., 3:29–31, 1968.

26. Cruickshank, J.M., Neil-Dwyer, G., Lane, J.: The effect of oral propranolol upon the ECG changes occurring in subarachnoid haemorrhage. Cardiovasc. Res., 9:236–245, 1975.

27. Deutsch, S., Goldberg, M., Dripps, R.D.: Postoperative hyponatremia with the inappropriate release of antidiuretic hormone. Anesthesiology, 27:250–256, 1966.

28. Doshi, R., Neil-Dwyer, G.: A clinicopathological study of patients following subarachnoid hemorrhage. J. Neurosurg., 52:295–301, 1980.

29. Ducker, T.B.: Increased intracranial pressure and pulmonary edema. I. Clinical study of 11 patients. J. Neurosurg., 28:112–117, 1968.

30. Ducker, T.B., Simmons, R.L.: Increased intracranial pressure and pulmonary edema. II. The hemodynamic response of dogs and monkeys to increased intracranial pressure. J. Neurosurg., 28:118–123, 1968.

31. Estanol, B.V., Loyo, M.V., Mateos, J.H., Foyo, E., Cornejo, A., Guevara, J.: Cardiac arrhythmias in experimental subarachnoid hemorrhage. Stroke, 8:440–447, 1977.

32. Evans, D.E., Alter, W.A. III, Shatsky, S.A., Gunby, E.N.: Cardiac arrhythmias resulting from experimental head injury. J. Neurosurg., 45:609–616, 1976.

33. Feibel, J.H., Campbell, R.G., Joynt, R.J.: Myocardial damage and cardiac arrhythmias in cerebral infarction and subarachnoid hemorrhage: Correlation with increased systemic catecholamine output. Trans. Am. Neurol. Assoc., 101:242–244, 1976.

34. Fein, A., Grossman, R.F., Jones, J.G., Overland, E., Pitts, L.H., Murray, J.F., Staub, N.C.: The value of edema fluid protein measurement in patients with pulmonary edema. Am. J. Med., 67:32–38, 1979.

35. Fernando, O.U., Mariano, G.T., Jr., Gurdjian, E.S., Hodgson, V.R.: Electrocardiographic patterns in experimental cerebral concussion. J. Neurosurg., 31:34–40, 1969.

36. Findler, G., Cotev, S.: Neurogenic pulmonary edema associated with a colloid cyst in the third ventricle. J. Neurosurg., 52:395–398, 1980.

37. Froman, C.: Alterations of respiratory function in patients with severe head injuries. Br. J. Anaesth., 40:354–360, 1968.

38. Frost, E.A.M.: The physiopathology of respiration in neurosurgical patients. J. Neurosurg., 50:699–714, 1979.

39. Frost, E.A.M., Arancibia, C.U., Shulman, K.: Pulmonary shunt as a prognostic indicator in head injury. J. Neurosurg., 50:768–772, 1979.

40. Gamble, J.E., Patton, H.D.: Pulmonary edema and hemorrhage from preoptic lesions in rats. Am. J. Physiol., 172:623–631, 1953.

41. Gaufin, L., Skowsky, W.R., Goodman, S.J.: Release of antidiuretic hormone during mass-induced elevation of intracranial pressure. J. Neurosurg., 46:627–637, 1977.

42. Gnehm, H.E., Bernasconi, S., Zackmann, M.: Posttraumatic anterior pituitary insufficiency in childhood. Helv. Paediat. Acta, 34:529–535, 1979.

43. Goldstein, D.S.: The electrocardiogram in stroke: relationship to pathophysical type and comparison with prior tracings. Stroke, 10:253–259, 1979.

44. Goodnight, S.H., Kenoyer, G., Rapaport, S.I.: Defibrination after brain-tissue destruction. A serious complication of head injury. N. Engl. J. Med., 290:1043–1047, 1974.

45. Gordon, E.: Controlled respiration in the management of patients with traumatic brain injuries. Acta Anaesth. Scand., 15:193–208, 1971.

46. Greenhoot, J.H., Reichenbach, D.D.: Cardiac injury and subarachnoid hemorrhage. A clinical, pathological, and physiological correlation. J.

Neurosurg., 30:521–531, 1969.

47. Griffin, J.M., Hartley, J.H. Jr., Crow, R.W., Schatten, W.E.: Diabetes insipidus caused by craniofacial trauma. J. Trauma, 16:979–984, 1976.

48. Grubb, R.L., Naumann, R.A., Ommaya, A.K.: Respiration and cerebrospinal fluid in experimental cerebral concussion. J. Neurosurg., 32:320–329, 1970.

49. Halmagyi, D.F.J., Neering, I.R., Lazarus, L., Young, J.D., Pullin, J.: Plasma glucagon in experimental posthemorrhagic shock. J. Trauma, 9:320–326, 1969.

50. Hawkins, W.E., Clower, B.R.: Myocardial damage after head trauma and simulated intracranial hemorrhage in mice. The role of the autonomic nervous system. Cardiovasc. Res., 5:524–529, 1971.

51. Hersch, C.: Electrocardiographic changes in head injuries. Circulation, 23:853–860, 1961.

52. Hersch, C.: Electrocardiographic changes in subarachnoid hemorrhage, meningitis and intracranial space-occupying lesions. Br. Heart J., 26:785–793, 1964.

53. Higgins, G., O'Brien, J.R.P., Lewin, W., Taylor, W.H.: Metabolic disorders in head injury. Lancet, 1:61–67, 1954.

54. Hoff, J.T., Nishimura, M.: Experimental neurogenic pulmonary edema in cats. J. Neurosurg., 48:383–389, 1978.

55. Hoff, J.T., Nishimura, M., Garcia-Uria, J., Miranda, S.: Experimental neurogenic pulmonary edema. Part 1: The role of systemic hypertension. J. Neurosurg., 54:627–631, 1981.

56. Hoffman, E.: Mortality and morbidity following road accidents. Ann. Roy. Coll. Surg. Engl., 58:233–240, 1976.

57. Illingworth, G., Jennett, W.B.: The shocked head injury. Lancet, 2:511–514, 1965.

58. Jacobson, S.A., Danufsky, P.: Marked electrocardiographic changes produced by experimental head injury. J. Neuropathol. Exp. Neurol., 13:462–475, 1954.

59. Jambart, S., Turpin, G., de Gennes, J.L.: Panhypopituitarism secondary to head trauma: evidence for a hypothalamic origin of the deficit. Acta Endocrinol., 93:264–270, 1980.

60. James, H.E., Tsueda, K., Wright, B., Young, A.B., McCloskey, J.: The effect of positive end-expiratory pressure (PEEP) ventilation in neurogenic pulmonary oedema. Acta Neurochir., 43:275–280, 1978.

61. Jardin, F., Farcot, J.C., Boisante, L., Curien, N., Margairaz, A., Bourdarias, J.P.: Influence of positive end-expiratory pressure on left ventricular performance. N. Engl. J. Med., 304:387–392, 1981.

62. Johnston, I.D.A.: The metabolic and endocrine response to injury: a review. Br. J. Anaesth., 45:252–255, 1973.

63. Joynt, R.J., Afifi, A., Harbison, J.: Hyponatremia in subarachnoid hemorrhage. Arch. Neurol., 13:633–638, 1965.

64. Katsurada, K., Yamada, R., Sugimoto, T.: Respiratory insufficiency in patients with severe head injury. Surgery, 73:191–199, 1973.

65. Kaufman, H.H., Moake, J.L., Olson, J.D., Miner, M.E., du Cret, R.P., Pruessner, J.L., Gildenberg, P.L.: Delayed and recurrent intracranial hematomas related to disseminated intravascular clotting and fibrinolysis in head injury. Neurosurgery, 7:445–449, 1980.

66. Kaufman, H.H., Olson, J.D., Makela, M.E., Pruessner, J.L., Moake, J.L., Miner, M.E., Haar, F.L., Gildenberg, P.L.: Disseminated intravascular coagulation and fibrinolysis in head injury. Presented at the American Association of Neurological Surgeons meeting, Boston, April, 1981.

67. Kinney, J.M., Long, C.L., Duke, J.H.: Carbohydrate and nitrogen metabolism after injury. In: Energy Metabolism in Trauma, Porter, R., Knight, J., Eds. Ciba Foundation Symposium, London, 1970, pp. 103–126.

68. Kosnik, E.J., Paul, S.E., Rossel, C.W., Sayers, M.P.: Central neurogenic pulmonary edema: with a review of its pathogenesis and treatment. Child's Brain, 3:37–47, 1977.

69. Landau, H., Adin, I., Spitz, I.M.: Pituitary insufficiency following head injury. Israel J. Med. Sci., 14:785–789, 1978.

70. Lassen, H.C.A.: A preliminary report on the 1952 epidemic of poliomyelitis in Copenhagen with special reference to the treatment of acute respiratory insufficiency. Lancet, 1:37–41, 1953.

71. Leitch, A.G., McLennan, J.E., Balkenhol, S., Loudon, R.G., McLaurin, R.L.: Mechanisms of hyperventilation in head injury: case report and review. Neurosurgery, 5:701–707, 1979.

72. Lester, M.C., Nelson, P.B.: Neurological aspects of vasopressin release and the syndrome of inappropriate secretion of antidiuretic hormone. Neurosurgery, 8:735–740, 1981.

73. Lewis, F., Elings, V.: Microprocessor determination of lung water using thermal-green dye double indicator dilution. Surg. Forum, 29:182–184, 1978.

74. Lewis, F., Elings, V., Sturm, J.: Bedside measurement of lung water. J. Surg. Res., 27:250–261, 1979.

75. Luisada, A.A.: Mechanism of neurogenic pulmonary edema. Am. J. Cardiol., 20:66–68, 1967.

76. Maciver, I.N., Frew, I.J.C., Matheson, J.G.: The role of respiratory insufficiency in the mortality of severe head injury. Lancet, 1:390–393, 1958.

77. McLaurin, R.L.: Metabolic changes accompanying head injury. Clin. Neurosurg., 12:143–160, 1966.

78. McLaurin, R.L., King, L.R., Flam, E.B., Budde, R.B.: Metabolic response to craniocerebral trauma. Surg. Gynecol. Obstet., 110:282–288, 1960.

79. Manning, G.W., Hall, G.E., Banting, F.G.: Vagal stimulation and the production of myocardial damage. Can. Med. Assoc. J., 37:314–318, 1937.

80. Matjasko, M.J., Ducker, T.B.: Disseminated intravascular coagulation associated with removal of a primary brain tumor. J. Neurosurg., 47:476–480, 1977.

81. Maxwell, J.A., Goodwin, J.W.: Neurogenic pulmonary shunting. J. Trauma, 13:368–373, 1973.

82. Melville, K.I., Blum, B., Shister, H.E., Silver,

M.D.: Cardiac ischemic changes and arrhythmias induced by hypothalamic stimulation. Am. J. Cardiol., 12:781–791, 1963.

83. Miller, J.D., Sweet, R.C., Narayan, R., Becker, D.P.: Early insults to the injured brain. J.A.M.A., 240:439–442, 1978.

84. Miller, W.L., Kaplan, S.L., Grumbach, M.M.: Child abuse as a cause of post-traumatic hypopituitarism. N. Engl. J. Med., 302:724–728, 1980.

85. Milley, J.R., Nugent, S.K., Rogers, M.C.: Neurogenic pulmonary edema in childhood. J. Pediatr., 94:706–709, 1979.

86. Moss, I.R., Wald, A., Ransohoff, J.: Respiratory functions and chemical regulation of ventilation in head injury. Am. Rev. Resp. Dis., 109:205–215, 1974.

87. Naeraa, N.: Blood-gas analysis in unconscious neurosurgical patients on admission to hospital. Acta Anaesth. Scand., 7:191–199, 1963.

88. Neil-Dwyer, G., Walter, P., Cruickshank, J.M., Doshi, B., O'Gorman, P.: Effect of propranolol and phentolamine on myocardial necrosis after subarachnoid haemorrhage. Br. Med. J., 2:990–992, 1978.

89. Nelson, P.B., Seif, S.M., Maroon, J.C., Robinson, A.G.: Hyponatremia in patients with subarachnoid hemorrhage—a study of vasopressin and blood volume. Presented at the American Association of Neurological Surgeons Annual Meeting, New York, April, 1980.

90. Nelson, P.B., Seif, S., Sekhar, L., Robinson, A.: Hyponatremia with natriuresis in subarachnoid hemorrhage. Presented at the American Association of Neurological Surgeons, Annual Meeting, Boston, April, 1981.

91. Newfield, P., Pitts, L.H., Kaktis, J., Hoff, J.: The influence of shock on mortality after head trauma. Crit. Care Med., 8:254, 1980.

92. Notman, D.D., Mortek, M.A. Moses, A.M.: Permanent diabetes insipidus following head trauma: observations on ten patients and an approach to diagnosis. J. Trauma, 20:599–602, 1980.

93. North, J.B., Jennett, S.: Abnormal breathing patterns associated with acute brain damage. Arch. Neurol., 31:338–344, 1974.

94. Peters, J.P., Welt, L.G., Sims, E.A.H., Orloff, J., Needham, J.: A salt-wasting syndrome associated with cerebral disease. Trans. Assoc. Am. Phys., 63:57–64, 1950.

95. Pitts, L.H.: Unpublished data.

96. Pitts, L.H., Lewis, F., Christianson, J., Kaktis, J.V.: Neurogenic pulmonary edema. Presented at the American Association of Neurological Surgeons Annual Meeting, New York, 1980.

97. Pitts, L.H., Severinghaus, J.W., Mitchell, R.A., Hoff, J.T.: The role of increased intracranial pressure in the production of neurogenic pulmonary edema. In: Intracranial Pressure II, Lundberg, N., Pontén, U., Brock, M., Eds. Springer-Verlag, Berlin, 1975, pp. 319–323.

98. Plum, F., Posner, J.B.: Diagnosis of Stupor and Coma, 3rd Ed. F.A. Davis Co., Philadelphia, 1980, pp. 32–41.

99. Porte, D., Graber, A.L., Takeshi, K., Williams,

R.H.: The effect of epinephrine on immunoreactive insulin levels in man. J. Clin. Invest., 45:228–236, 1966.

100. Porter, R.W., Kamikawa, K., Greenhoot, J.: Persistent electrocardiographic abnormalities experimentally induced by stimulation of the brain. Am. Heart J., 64:815–819, 1962.

101. Price, D.J.E., Murray, A.: The influence of hypoxia and hypotension on recovery from head injury. Injury, 3:218–224, 1972.

102. Reilly, P.L., Adams, J.H., Graham, D.I., Jennett, B.: Patients with head injury who talk and die. Lancet, 2:375–377, 1975.

103. Rose, J., Valtonen, S., Jennett, B.: Avoidable factors contributing to death after head injury. Br. Med. J., 2:615–618, 1977.

104. Sarnoff, S.J., Sarnoff, L.C.: Neurohemodynamics of pulmonary edema. II. The role of sympathetic pathways in the elevation of pulmonary and systemic vascular pressures following the intracisternal injection of fibrin. Circulation, 6:51–62, 1952.

105. Schumacker, P.T., Rhodes, G.R., Newell, J.C., Dutton, R.E., Shah, D.M., Scovill, W.A., Powers, S.R.: Ventilation-perfusion imbalance after head trauma. Am. Rev. Resp. Dis., 119:33–43, 1979.

106. Shenkin, H.A., Gutterman, P.: The analysis of body water compartments in postoperative craniotomy patients. Part. 3: The effects of dexamethasone. J. Neurosurg., 31:400–407, 1969.

107. Shurin, S., Rekate, H.: Disseminated intravascular coagulation as a complication of ventricular catheter placement. J. Neurosurg., 54:264–267, 1981.

108. Shuster, S.: The electrocardiogram in subarachnoid hemorrhage. Br. Heart J., 22:316–320, 1960.

109. Simmons, R.L., Martin, A.M. Jr., Heisterkamp, C.A. III, Ducker, T.B.: Respiratory insufficiency in combat casualties: II. Pulmonary edema following head injury. Ann. Surg., 170:39–44, 1969.

110. Sinha, R.P., Ducker, T.B., Perot, P.L.: Arterial oxygenation—findings and its significance in central nervous system trauma patients. J.A.M.A., 224:1258–1260, 1970.

111. Stoner, H.B., Barton, R.N., Little, R.A., Yates, D.W.: Measuring the severity of injury. Br. Med. J., 2:1247–1249, 1977.

112. Stoner, H.B., Heath, D.F.: The effects of trauma on carbohydrate metabolism. Br. J. Anaesth., 45:244–251, 1973.

113. Terrence, C.F., Rao, G.R., Perper, J.A.: Neurogenic pulmonary edema in unexpected, unexplained death of epileptic patients. Ann. Neurol., 9:458–464, 1981.

114. Theodore, J., Robin, E.D.: Pathogenesis of pulmonary edema. Lancet, 2:749–751, 1975.

115. Tranbaugh, R., Lewis, F.: Pulmonary edema: mechanisms and etiologies. In: Physiologic Problems in Surgery: Cardiopulmonary resuscitation, Proctor, H.J., Ed. Lippincott, Philadelphia (in press).

116. Vander Ark, G.D.: Cardiovascular changes with acute subdural hematoma. Surg. Neurol., 3:305–308, 1975.

117. van der Sande, J.J., Veltkamp, J.J., Boekhout-Mussert, R.J., Bouwhuis-Hoogerwerf, M.L.: Head injury and coagulation disorders. J. Neurosurg., 49:357–365, 1978.

118. Vapalahti, M., Troupp, H.: Prognosis for patients with severe brain injuries. Br. Med. J., 3:404–407, 1971.

119. Weintraub, B.M., McHenry, L.C.: Cardiac abnormalities in subarachnoid hemorrhage: a resume. Stroke, 5:384–392, 1974.

120. Williamson, D.H., Farrell, R., Kerr, A., Smith, R.: Muscle-protein catabolism after injury in man, as measured by urinary excretion of 3-methyl-histi-

dine. Clin. Sci. Mol. Med., 52:527–533, 1977.

121. Wise, B.L.: Syndrome of inappropriate antidiuretic hormone secretion after spontaneous subarachnoid hemorrhage—a reversible cause of clinical deterioration. Neurosurgery, 3:412–414, 1978.

122. Yen, J.K., Rhodes, G.R., Bourke, R.S., Powers, S.R., Newell, J.C., Popp, A.J.: Delayed impairment of arterial blood oxygenation in patients with severe head injury. Preliminary report. Surg. Neurol., 9:323–327, 1978.

123. Youmans, J.R.: Causes of shock with head injury. J. Trauma, 4:204–209, 1964.

18

Infectious Complications of Head Injury

SHELDON LANDESMAN
PAUL R. COOPER

In this chapter important concepts relating to antimicrobial therapy of central nervous system (CNS) infection will be presented, selected material on the activity, toxicity, and utility of antibiotics used to treat central nervous system infections will be detailed, and the specific management of brain abscess, meningitis, subdural empyema and cranial osteomyelitis will be discussed. A full discussion of the *sytemic* infectious complications associated with head trauma (pneumonia, urinary tract infection, septicemia, etc.) is presented in Chapter 17.

BASIC PRINCIPLES OF ANTIMICROBIAL THERAPY OF CENTRAL NERVOUS SYSTEM INFECTIONS

Blood-brain and Blood-cerebrospinal Fluid Barrier

The structure of the vascular components of the CNS inhibits the passage of many antibiotics into the cerebrospinal fluid (CSF) and the extracellular fluid (ECF) of the brain parenchyma.[54]

Passage of many compounds from the choroid plexus into the CSF is blocked by the basement membrane and tight junctions of the capillary endothelial cells and the absence of trans-endothelial channels (blood-brain barrier). Close approximation of astrocytic foot processes to the capillary endothelium further impairs passage of antibiotics from the capillary lumen into the ECF of the brain.[41, 42, 54] Although the anatomy of the blood-brain and blood-CSF barriers are not identical, their physiologic effects are similar: antibiotics that enter the CSF sparingly are also limited in their ability to enter the brain parenchyma; conversely, antibiotics with poor parenchymal penetration enter the CSF with difficulty. For the remainder of this discussion, the blood-brain and blood-CSF barriers will be used interchangeably unless otherwise noted.

The characteristics of an antibiotic that influence its passage into the CSF include its lipid solubility, degree of ionization, protein binding, and serum levels. Compounds that are lipid soluble, poorly ionized at physiological pH, poorly protein bound and can be given so as to achieve high *sustained* serum levels will pass readily into the CSF. Antibiotics that lack these properties will penetrate into the CSF poorly. Inflammatory processes (meningitis, encephalitis) will, in general, enhance the passage of antibiotics into the CSF. Unfortunately, the actual increase in concentration achieved as a result of inflammation may not always be of therapeutic significance.[54]

Antibacterial Activity of Antibiotics

The *in vitro* activity of antimicrobial agents is determined by the minimal concentration of the agent that is required to inhibit growth of a specific bacteria. This is referred to as the minimal inhibitory concentration (MIC) of the antibiotic and will vary according to the type of bacteria. It may also vary for bacteria of the same species. For example, the MIC of cephalothin for *Escherichia coli* may be 2–16 μg/ml for 70% of the isolates tested; the remaining 30% may require 32 μg/ml or more before they are inhibited. Since cephalothin levels of 32 μg/ml are not easily achieved for any length of time in the blood, all *E. coli* with an MIC of 32 μg/ml would be considered resistant to the antibiotic. Another example would be *enterobacteria* sp., almost all of which are resistant to cephalothin (MIC equal or greater than 64 μg/ml). A routine susceptibility report for *E. coli* isolated from a patient will usually, but not always, report the organism as susceptible, whereas a similar report on an enterobacter isolate will list the organism as resistant.

An antibiotic that is capable of killing an organism at a concentration similar to that required to inhibit its growth is considered bactericidal. The lowest concentration of the antibiotic at which bacterial destruction occurs is termed the minimum bactericidal concentration (MBC) for that organism. For example, the MIC of penicillin G for most strains of *Streptococcus pneumoniae* (pneumococcus) is 0.03 μg/ml; the minimal bactericidal concentration for these organisms is 0.03–0.06 μg/ml. This is equal to, or one dilution higher than, the MIC. Therefore, penicillin is considered a bactericidal drug against the pneumococcus. As a rule, all β-lactam antibiotics (penicillins and cephalosporins) are bactericidal drugs.

Antibiotics that inhibit the growth of an organism at one concentration (the MIC) but require a considerably higher concentration to kill the organism are considered bacteriostatic agents. An important example is the activity of chloramphenicol against *E. coli*. Most strains of *E. coli* are inhibited by 4–8 μg/ml of chloramphenicol. However, 120 μg/ml of chloramphenicol or more may be required to kill the same organisms.[46] The divergence of the MIC and MBC is characteristic of bacteriostatic agents. Chloramphenicol is particularly important because it is used to treat meningitis. It is a peculiar characteristic of chloramphenicol that it is bactericidal against

the common meningeal pathogens such as the pneumococcus, the meningococcus and *Haemophilus influenzae*, but is bacteriostatic against some of the common pathogens of Gram-negative meningitis such as *Klebsiella pneumoniae* and *E. coli*. This property of chloramphenicol has important implications for the therapy of Gram-negative meningitis and will be discussed subsequently.

Host Defenses in the CSF

The efficacy of any antibiotic in treating an infection is, in part, dependent upon a number of host factors such as complement, antibody, polymorphonuclear leukocytes, etc. Of particular importance is the fact that complement and antibody levels in the CSF are lower than they are in the serum.[55, 57] This localized impairment of CSF defense mechanisms mandates the use of bactericidal rather than bacteriostatic agents for the successful therapy of meningitis.[46, 55, 57] Chloramphenicol is an important example of this principle. This drug is bactericidal against the pneumococcus and is effective (although not the agent of choice) in the treatment of pneumococcal meningitis. On the other hand, the drug is bacteriostatic against Gram-negative organisms (*E. coli* and klebsiella) and is less effective in the treatment of Gram-negative bacillary meningitis.[11]

SPECIFIC ANTIMICROBIAL AGENTS: SPECTRUM OF ACTIVITY, CNS PENETRATION, AND CLINICAL USAGE

In this section, only those antibiotics that are clinically useful in treating CNS infections will be discussed. Each antibiotic will be examined in terms of its spectrum of activity, CNS penetration, clinical application, and toxicity. Additional material on the use of these agents will be found in the discussion of specific CNS infections.

Penicillins

Penicillins are β-lactam compounds that contain a 6-aminopenicillanic nucleus to which a variety of radical groups (R-groups) have been attached. Different R-group substitutions result in changes in the spectrum of activity, resistance to penicillinase, and protein binding. All penicillins are bactericidal drugs; the MBC, therefore, is equal to or only one dilution higher than the MIC. Penicillin probably acts by inhibiting the synthesis of the bacterial cell wall which results in the death of the organism.[61]

Penicillin G. The minimal toxicity of penicillin G and its high activity against susceptible organisms make it the antibiotic of choice for organisms that are susceptible to it. Its spectrum, however, is limited to certain organisms. Susceptible organisms (MIC equal to or less than 0.025 μg/ml) commonly encountered in CNS infections include the pneumococcus, *Neisseria meningitidis*, all streptococci except the enterococcus, non-penicillinase producing staphylococci, and oropharyngeal anaerobes (peptococcus, peptostreptococcus, fusobacteria and bacteriodes sp. other than *Bacillus fragilis*).[17, 61]

The penetration of penicillin G into the CSF is poor even when meningeal inflammation is present. A peak CSF level of only 1.5–2.0 μg/ml can be expected when conventional doses of penicillin G (24 million units/day given as two million units every two hours in adults or 300,000–400,000 units/kg/day in divided doses in children) are used to treat bacterial meningitis.[25] Fortunately, even this low level is greater than the MBC of the common organisms for which penicillin is the drug of choice (*e.g.*, the MBC of pneumococcus and aerobic streptococci are 0.02 μg/ml or less). When meningeal inflammation decreases, the concentration of penicillin that is found in the CSF will also decrease, although for sensitive organisms the concentration will remain at bactericidal levels. It is important, therefore, to maintain a full dosage schedule of the drug as the patient's meningitis improves. If the dose of penicillin is decreased as the patient recovers, the combined effect of decreased dose and decreased CSF penetration may result in inadequate therapy and clinical relapse.

The penetration of penicillin G into the brain parenchyma and intracranial abscess has not been well studied. Information from reports in the literature is of limited utility because of variations in the administered dose of penicillin G, timing and the processing of CSF samples, and the degree of CNS inflammation. However, from the data that is available it would appear that therapeutic concentrations of penicillin G can be achieved in brain parenchyma and in brain abscess pus when 20–40 million units of penicillin are administered and the organism causing the infection (oral anaerobes, aerobic streptococci) are susceptible to the drug.[15, 17]

The toxicity of penicillin G is generally limited to allergic phenomena (rash, hives, bronchospasm, urticaria and anaphylaxis). Rarely, in patients given massive doses of the drug, seizures and myoclonic jerks may appear. Penicillin is excreted by the kidney. Total daily dose must therefore be decreased in patients with impaired renal function.

Nafcillin and Oxacillin. When penicillin G first became available, most strains of *Staphylococcus aureus* were susceptible to the drug. Within ten years, however, *S. aureus* resistant to penicillin G were common within the hospital environment.

Today, 85–95% of all *S. aureus* isolates (either community or hospital acquired) are penicillinase-producers and therefore are not susceptible to penicillin G. Modification of the R-groups attached to the basic 6-aminopenicillanic molecule has resulted in several semi-synthetic penicillins (nafcillin, oxacillin, methicillin) that are resistant to the enzymic degradation induced by staphylococcal penicillinase. These agents are now considered the initial treatment of choice for all *S. aureus* infections. The semi-synthetic penicillins are also active against such Gram-positive cocci as the pneumococcus and Group A streptococcus. They are less effective than penicillin, however, and should not be used when culture-documented infections with these organisms are present. Documented or suspected *S. aureus* infection, therefore, is the principal reason for the use of the semi-synthetic penicillins.

Nafcillin and oxacillin can be used interchangeably. The MBC of S. aureus to these drugs is generally 1 µg/ml or less. Nafcillin, when given in doses of 12–16 g/day (150–200 mg/kg/day) will result in levels in the CSF that exceed the MBC of most S. aureus isolates.[20, 28, 49] Sparse and inconclusive data are available on the penetration of nafcillin into brain abscess pus. Although methicillin does penetrate into the CNS, it is rarely used because high dose intravenous administration of the drug results in a significant incidence of nephritis.

Nafcillin, in a dose of at least 12g/day, is the drug of choice for the treatment of meningitis and brain abscess caused by S. aureus or S. epidermidis. Situations where S. aureus or S. epidermidis are suspected pathogens include: brain abscess secondary to trauma, meningitis in a patient who has had a recent neurosurgical procedure, and/or patients with a CNS shunt or catheter in place, or hospital-acquired meningitis in a patient who has been hospitalized for greater than 72 hours and meets any of the first two conditions.

Excretion of these drugs occurs mainly via the biliary tract and only minimal reduction in dosage is required in patients with severe renal insufficiency. Toxicities of both drugs are similar to penicillin G. In addition, reversible neutropenia has been noted in a small but significant number of persons who receive high dose nafcillin (12 g/day) for prolonged periods of time. Hepatitis is a rare, but well-documented, side effect of prolonged high-dose oxacillin therapy.

Ampicillin. Ampicillin is active against H. influenzae, selected Gram-negative organisms (E. coli and Proteus mirabilis) and Gram-positive organisms such as pneumococci and aerobic and anaerobic streptococci.[3] Within the hospital environment, approximately 50–75% of E. coli and P. mirabilis isolates are susceptible to ampicillin. Ampicillin is the drug of choice in the management of meningitis secondary to H. influenzae. However, this organism is infrequently encountered in adults with head injury-associated infections. Gram-negative bacilliary meningitis caused by certain strains of E. coli can, on occasion, be treated successfully with ampicillin. For the most part, other agents (moxalactam and cefotaxime) are preferred in the treatment of Gram-negative bacilliary meningitis (see subsequent sections). Therefore, neurosurgeons will have little use for ampicillin in the treatment of CNS infections.

Ampicillin does penetrate into the CNS in therapeutic concentrations. Overturf reported CSF levels of 4.5 µg/ml in patients with meningitis.[43] The penetration of ampicillin into brain tissue and brain abscess pus has also been studied. Levels of 0–2 µg/ml in brain tissue and 3.5–4 µg/ml in brain abscess pus have been reported by Kramer et al.[13] and DeLouvois et al.,[15] respectively. Ampicillin may therefore be used as a substitute for penicillin in the treatment of brain abscesses.

For therapy of brain abscess, ampicillin should be administered in doses of 12 g/day in adults and 200–400 mg/kg/day in children. The drug is excreted by the kidneys and dose modification is necessary for patients with renal insufficiency.

Ticarcillin and Carbenicillin. These drugs have a spectrum of activity that is broader than that of ampicillin. They are active against E. coli, Proteus sp. and H. influenzae. They are effective in the treatment of certain pseudomonas infections and they are used principally for this purpose.

These drugs penetrate into the CNS if large doses are administered and meningeal inflammation is present. CSF levels of carbenicillin of 3–50 µg/ml or more have been documented in a few patients with severe meningeal inflammation. Gram-negative bacillary meningitis caused by Pseudomonas aeruginosa can be treated with high-dose intravenous administration of carbenicillin or ticarcillin plus an intraventricular or intrathecally-administered aminoglycoside, (e.g., tobramycin, gentamicin, amikacin).

Because these agents are less active on a weight basis than other penicillin-type drugs, large doses must be administered in order to achieve effective tissue levels. The adult dose is 18–36 g/day of ticarcillin and 30–40 g/day of carbenicillin when normal renal function is present. Each gram of ticarcillin or carbenicillin contains 5 mEq of sodium. Thirty grams of these drugs will result in a sodium load of 150 mEq. Caution is therefore advised in administration of these agents to patients with congestive heart failure.

Piperacillin. Piperacillin is a new penicillin that is two to four times more active than ticarcillin against *P. aeruginosa*. The drug has recently been released and will probably replace ticarcillin and carbenicillin as the standard anti-pseudomonal penicillin.

CSF levels of 15–20 μg/ml of piperacillin have been reported in the few patients given the drug for *P. aeruginosa* meningitis. Adult dose is 12–24g/day.

Aminoglycosides

The aminoglycoside antibiotics (kanamycin, gentamicin, tobramycin and amikacin) possess broad-spectrum bactericidal activity against Gram-negative organisms (klebsiella, *E. coli*, *Proteus* sp., *Enterobacter* sp., *P. aeruginosa*, etc.) isolated within a hospital environment. Amikacin is effective against 95–98% of these organisms. Kanamycin is less active; *P. aeruginosa* and many other Gram-negative enteric organisms (klebsiella, proteus) isolated within hospitals are resistant to this drug.[17]

Peak therapeutic serum levels of gentamicin and tobramycin are 6–8 μg/ml. Amikacin, which has slightly different pharmacokinetic properties has a peak therapeutic serum level in the range of 20–25 μg/ml. Susceptible organisms are inhibited (MIC) or killed (MBC) by 0.025–2.0 μg/ml of gentamicin or tobramycin and 1–8 μg/ml of amikacin. The dosage of gentamicin and tobramycin is 1.3 μg/kg of lean body weight every 8 hours if the creatinine is 1 mg% or less. When the creatinine is greater than 1 mg%, downward adjustments are made in daily dosage.

The broad Gram-negative spectrum of the aminoglycosides ought to make them useful drugs in the treatment of Gram-negative bacillary meningitis. Because they do not penetrate the blood-brain or blood-CSF barrier, their usefulness as therapeutic agents for Gram-negative bacillary meningitis is severely limited. At standard doses, the CSF concentration of gentamicin rarely exceeds 1 μg/ml even in the presence of severe meningeal inflammation. When these agents are administered via the lumbar intrathecal route (4–8 mg of gentamicin or tobramycin or 10–15 mg of amikacin daily) high concentrations are found in the lumbar CSF but very little drug is found in the ventricles where the active site of inflammation (ventriculitis) is often located. Satisfactory ventricular concentration is obtained only by direct intraventricular administration.[27, 45] For these reasons, aminoglycosides, once the mainstay of therapy for Gram-negative bacilliary meningitis, are now considered adjunctive or secondary agents for this disease.

Aminoglycosides are characterized by a narrow therapeutic-toxic ratio and a low therapeutic index. Toxicity occurs even when the drugs are used properly and serum levels remain within the therapeutic range. Reversible acute tubular necrosis occurs in 10–20% of patients, although on rare occasions the renal insufficiency is irreversible. Eighth nerve toxicity (labrynthitis and/or high frequency hearing loss) are also well-known side effects and are enhanced when aminoglycosides are administered with other ototoxic drugs such as furosemide.

Cephalosporins

Cephalosporins are β-lactam antibiotics whose structure, mode of action, and side effects are similar to penicillin. As a rule, *all* cephalosporins are resistant to *S. aureus* β-lactamase and therefore possess a fair degree of activity against *S. aureus*, although this activity varies from agent to agent. Cephalosporins are not first line anti-staphylococcal agents and are used to treat staphylococcal infection only in those situations where a semi-synthetic penicillin (oxacillin or nafcillin) cannot be used because of penicillin allergy.

The proliferation of new cephalosporins may be confusing to clinicians trying to make an intelligent choice among the competing products. Perspective on these agents is possible if they are viewed as first, second, and third generation modifications of the same product.

The first generation cephalosporins (cephalothin and cefazolin) have a limited degree of activity against Gram-negative enteric organisms. klebsiella, *E. coli* and some *Proteus* sp., are usually susceptible (MIC's of susceptible organisms range from 4–16 µg/ml).[17, 18, 59] Within the hospital environment, however, many klebsiella and *E. coli* are resistant and enterobacter, serratia, *P. Aeruginosa* are uniformly resistant to these agents. The first generation cephalosporins do not penetrate into the CSF in significant quantities and cannot be used for the therapy of meningitis.

The second generation cephalosporins (cefamandole and cefoxitin) have increased activity against many Gram-negative isolates when compared to the first generation agents. Many cephalothin-resistant klebsiella, *E. coli*, enterobacter and proteus are susceptible to these newer drugs although serratia and *P. aeruginosa* remain resistant.[31] Cefoxitin and cefamandole penetrate into the CSF in significant quantities when the meninges are inflamed. CSF cefoxitin levels of 15–30 µg/ml have been documented in patients with Gram-negative meningitis. Nevertheless, because the MIC and MBC of these drugs against Gram-negative organisms such as *E. coli* and *Klebsiella* range from 4–32 µg/ml, these agents rarely exceed therapeutic concentrations in the CSF.[33, 39]

The third generation cephalosporin-type antibiotics (cefotaxime and moxalactam) represent a significant advance in the treatment of Gram-negative infections in general and Gram-negative bacilliary meningitis in particular. These agents differ from other cephalosporins by virtue of their very broad spectrum of activity *and* potency.[18, 40]

Moxalactam possesses marked activity against nearly all important Gram-negative pathogens. *Klebsiella, E. coli, P. mirabilis, P. vulgaris, H. influenzae, N. meningitidis, Enterobacter*, and *Serratia* are usually susceptible to 0.5 µg/ml or less. *P. aeruginosa* is less susceptible to this drug; 16–64 µg/ml of moxalactam are required to inhibit this organism. Gram-positive organisms are also sensitive to moxalactam but at higher concentrations than for Gram-negative bacilli. The pneumococcus (MIC's of 0.25–1.0 µg/ml), group-A *streptococci* (MIC's of 0.12–1.0 µg/ml) and *S. aureus* (MIC's of 2–8 µg/ml) are susceptible at readily achievable levels.[18]

Moxalactam has unusual pharmacokinetic properties in that it has a long half-life (two hours), a low degree of protein binding, and is capable of achieving high sustained serum levels with intravenous administration of only 4–6 g/day. Normal dosage is between 4–12 g/day depending on the severity of the infection. The major route of excretion is the kidney and as little as 1 g/day may result in sufficient blood levels in the presence of renal failure.

Recent studies by Landesman *et al*.[32, 33] document high CSF levels of moxalactam when the drug is administered by the intravenous route. In the presence of meningeal inflammation, moxalactam CSF levels of 7–35 µg/ml are achievable. Because of its marked potency against Gram-negative bacilli and its ability to penetrate into the CSF, moxalactam is an extraordinarily useful drug in the treatment of Gram-negative meningitis caused by susceptible organisms.

Chloramphenicol

Chloramphenicol was the first broad-spectrum antibiotic to be introduced into clinical use. The drug is active against a wide variety of organisms: *S. aureus*, aerobic streptococci, and Gram-negative enteric bacilli. Salmonella and shigella are usually susceptible to therapeutic concentrations of the drug. Chloramphenicol is also highly active against all the common pathogenic anaerobes including anaerobic streptococci, fusobacteria, clostridia and all *bacteroides* species.

It is readily absorbed from the gastrointestinal tract and serum levels with oral administration (10–15 µg/ml) of a 1 g dose closely approximate those achieved with intravenous administration. The normal dose is 50 mg/kg/day but can be increased to 100 mg/kg/day in patients with life-threatening disease. The drug is metabolized in the liver and its inactive metabolites are excreted by the kidney. Dose reductions do not have to be made for patients with renal insufficiency. In patients with severe hepatic disease, however, the dose should be drastically reduced or the drug avoided.

The drug is lipid soluble and passes readily into the CSF. CSF levels are 30–70% of those achieved in the serum and may reach a peak of 25–30 μg/ml when high doses of the drug are administered (even in the absence of meningeal inflammation).

Neurosurgeons use chloramphenicol as therapy for three different intracranial suppurative diseases: 1) Gram-negative bacillary meningitis, 2) brain abscess, and 3) subdural empyema. As noted in the section on basic principles and as will be further discussed in the section on meningitis, chloramphenicol is not a useful drug in the therapy of Gram-negative bacillary meningitis because the levels achieved in the CSF are not bactericidal against enteric pathogens. However, chloramphenicol is useful as adjunctive therapy of brain abscess and subdural empyema because concentrations of the drug are sufficient to effect clinical cure after surgical drainage of purulent material.

MENINGITIS

Meningitis secondary to head injury has a variable pathogenesis and a complex bacteriology. Factors such as the site and source of the injuries to the neuraxis, the time from injury to the development of meningitis, the presence of a foreign body, brain abscess, CSF fistula or recent neurosurgical procedure, all influence the incidence, bacteriology, therapy and prognosis of meningitis.

Meningitis Following Basal Skull Fracture (Post-traumatic Meningitis)

Following head injury, a basal skull fracture and adjacent dural tear may result in contamination of the intracranial contents by the bacterial flora of the nasopharynx or external environment. This abnormal communication may be manifest by CSF rhinorrhea or otorrhea. Occasionally, however, there is no CSF fistula and the only evidence for the communication is the development of meningitis in a person with a history of head trauma. Meningitis arising in this fashion (whether or not a CSF leak

is present) has been termed post-traumatic meningitis (PTM) and is almost always caused by *Streptococcus pneumoniae* (pneumococcus).[2, 22, 44] A further discussion of the anatomy and pathogenesis of basal skull fractures and cerebrospinal fluid fistulas is found in Chapter 5.

The nature of the cranial trauma and the interval between the trauma and the onset of the meningitis are important in predicting the bacteriology of the meningitis. In patients with a CSF leak and skull fracture who develop meningitis within three days of injury, the organism is almost always the pneumococcus. Penicillin G in a daily dose of 24 million units (two million units every two hours) is standard therapy.[2, 22, 44, 51] The penicillin-allergic patient may be treated with chloramphenicol (6 g/day). In children (aged six months–six years), PTM may be caused by *H. influenzae* and therapy, therefore, would be ampicillin and chloramphenicol if the Gram's stain is not diagnostic.

Patients with open and/or contaminated head wounds who develop meningitis after the third day of hospitalization are more likely to be infected with Gram-negative organisms and/or *S. aureus*. Moxalactam for Gram-negative organisms or nafcillin for *S. aureus* would therefore be optimal therapy.

Gram-negative Bacilliary Meningitis

Operation for head injury (particularly in the presence of open, contaminated wounds) and the presence of ventricular drains or catheters predispose the patient to development of gram-negative bacilliary meningitis (GNBM). The most common pathogens are *E. coli* and klebsiella. Less frequently, serratia, proteus and *P. aeruginosa* are the causative agents.[11]

Armengand[3] and Landesman[33] have recently formulated a major principle to guide the therapy of GNBM: because of impaired immune defenses within the CNS, inhibition of a Gram-negative organism by an antibiotic may not result in a cure; therefore, the selection of an antimicrobial agent to treat meningitis should optimally be based on the ability of the antibiotic to attain a concentration in the CSF higher than the minimal levels needed to *kill* the responsible organism. For example, this objective of bacterial destruction is readily achieved when penicillin is used to treat pneumococcal meningitis. Although penicillin G does not penetrate into the CSF exceptionally well, it is very active against the pneumococcus; the MBC of penicillin G to the organism is 0.04 μg/ml or less. Accordingly, at standard dosages, penicillin levels in the CSF (1–1.5 μg/ml) exceed the MBC of the pneumococcus by 40–50 times. Therefore, bactericidal levels of penicillin are present in the CSF during the entire course of the meningitis and penicillin is an effective form of therapy for this disease.

The situation is different for the pathogens causing GNBM (principally *E. coli* and *Klebsiella*). The mortality of this disease is high (40–90%) and optimal therapy requires an antibiotic that is very active against the infecting pathogen (*i.e.*, low MIC's/MBC) and diffuses readily into the CSF. Although the antibiotics currently recommended for the treatment of GNBM (aminoglycosides and/or chloramphenicol) have been successful on occasion, the high mortality and morbidity of the disease attests to the need for a better therapeutic agent.

In particular, although chloramphenicol is frequently used to treat GNBM, achievable CSF levels of this drug (20–30 μg/ml) are well below the MBC of most Klebsiella and *E. coli* isolates.[55] Concentrations of chloramphenicol needed to kill the growth of most Klebsiella and *E. coli* are 8–128 μg/ml or greater.[45] In view of these facts, the extremely poor results that are seen when chloramphenicol is used to treat GNBM is not surprising.[11]

Because of the general disappointment with chloramphenicol therapy, alternative treatments have been devised. Aminoglycosides (gentamicin, tobramycin, amikacin) are highly active against enteric pathogens including *P. aeruginosa*. The MBC of these agents to Klebsiella, *E. coli*, *Proteus* sp. and *P. aeruginosa* is generally between 0.5 and 2 μg/ml. Unfortunately, intravenous administration of these drugs results in CSF levels no greater than 1 μg/ml. Parenteral therapy with these agents, therefore, is often inadequate because CSF levels of the drug generally do not exceed the MBC of the infecting organism.[27, 45]

Lumbar intrathecal administration of aminoglycosides will produce adequate concentrations of drug within the spinal subarachnoid space but will not usually result in bactericidal concentrations within the ventricle. Because ventriculitis is a common accompaniment of meningitis, *intrathecal* therapy with aminoglycosides may not result in cure.[27, 45] It is for this reason that the intraventricular administration of aminoglycosides is the only reliable method of delivering adequate amounts of antibiotics to the site of infection in patients with GNBM.

Another factor that decreases the effectiveness of aminoglycosides is their use in combination with chloramphenicol. Straughbaugh, working with an experimental rabbit model of *Proteus mirabilis* meningitis, demonstrated that chloramphenicol inhibits the bactericidal activity of gentamicin within the CSF, and that the two drugs should not be used together in the treatment of meningitis.[56] Clinical data derived from a recent New York City study of GNBM point toward the same conclusion. In a review of all cases of GNBM reported to the New York City Health Department, the mortality was 90% for those cases treated with chloramphenicol and gentamicin, but only 60% for those cases treated with gentamicin alone.[11]

Ampicillin may also be used to treat a limited number of cases of GNBM. Approximately 60–70% of *E. coli* are susceptible to this agent and CSF levels will usually (but not always) exceed the MBC of the drug to the organism. Other pathogens that cause GNBM such as klebsiella, proteus, and serratia are resistant to the drug.

Moxalactam and cefotaxime are two agents that have recently been introduced for the therapy of GNBM. They are bactericidal (MBC's = 0.2 μg/ml or less for most *Klebsiella*, *E. coli*, Serratia, *Proteus* sp., and Enterobacter) and penetrate well into the CSF when administered parenterally.[18, 33, 40] CSF levels of 5–35 μg/ml of moxalactam can be achieved when the drug is given in a dose of 6 g/day.[32] Higher levels are obtained when the dose is raised to 12 g/day.

The initial experience with these agents is encouraging. Landesman et al.[33] recently reviewed a series of 35 patients treated with either moxalactam or cefotaxime alone or in combination with other drugs; the cure rate was 88% in patients treated with the new agents alone, and 87% in patients treated with these new agents plus standard therapy. Based upon these data and subsequent additional experience it appears that moxalactam and perhaps cefotaxime are the best therapeutic agents currently available to treat GNBM.[33]

In a patient with documented or suspected GNBM, 6–12 g of moxalactam should be administered intravenously daily. The higher dose is recommended when partially resistant organisms (MIC = 0.5–1 μg/ml) are suspected or documented. If P. aeruginosa is the pathogen, then 18 g of piperacillin intravenously plus intraventricular amikacin (10 mg daily) are recommended as optimal therapy. If intraventricular therapy is not feasible, then intrathecal amikacin (10–15 mg daily) is recommended. P. aeruginosa is less susceptible than other Gram-negative organisms to moxalactam. In all cases, culture and susceptibility testing should be done to guide antimicrobial therapy.

Meningitis Associated with External Shunts and Catheters

The insertion of a foreign body such as a shunt, ventriculostomy catheter, or intracranial pressure monitoring device into the intracranial space predisposes to meningitis. S. aureus and S. epidermidis are the common organisms causing shunt and catheter-associated meningitis.[53] Both organisms are usually susceptible to nafcillin. The addition of rifampin to nafcillin may help to cure infections that are recalcitrant to therapy with nafcillin alone. When S. epidermidis is resistant to nafcillin, the antibiotic combination of vancomycin and rifampin is recommended. GNBM may also occur as a complication of intracranial foreign bodies. Treatment with appropriate antibiotics according to the previously outlined principles and removal of the shunt or catheter are usually required for successful treatment of the meningitis.

Empiric Approach to the Neurosurgical Patient with Meningitis

A knowledge of the epidemiology and bacteriology of meningitis combined with evaluation of appropriate laboratory data will greatly aid the neurosurgeon in his initial management of the patient with meningitis before the results of culture and susceptibility determinations are reported. In deciding upon specific therapy, the following procedures may be useful:

1) Decide if the meningeal symptoms could be related to an underlying suppurative process (brain abscess or subdural empyema) which would contraindicate a lumbar puncture. If such is the case, an emergency CT scan should be performed. Empiric antibiotic therapy without the aid of a lumbar puncture may be started along the guidelines suggested in the subsequent section on brain abscess and subdural empyema. If a mass lesion is not a consideration, then a lumbar puncture should be done immediately.

2) CSF, once obtained, should be immediately cultured. Culture data is the single most important piece of information in the management of the patient.

3) A Gram's stain, cell count, and protein determination of the CSF should be performed.

4) The type of injury and the interval between the injury and the onset of meningitis, in part, determine the bacteriology and therefore, the therapy of the disease. The Gram's stain, however, will dictate initial therapy. If Gram-positive lancet-shaped diplococci are visualized in a patient with CSF rhinorrhea who has had a closed head injury within 72 hours, then penicillin G is the appropriate therapy. If the CSF Gram's stain from a patient who recently had a craniotomy and is at least four days following cranial trauma shows Gram-negative bacilli, then appropriate therapy for GNBM (i.e., moxalactam) would be required. If large Gram-positive cocci are seen, than nafcillin would be appropriate therapy.

When the Gram's stain is negative, antimicrobial therapy is determined by the epidemiological circumstances of the particular case. Patients with CSF leaks and cranial fractures may be treated with penicillin G if the meningitis develops within 72 hours of injury. After 72 hours, or after surgery, initial empiric therapy should cover both *S. aureus* and Gram-negative bacilli. High-dose nafcillin and moxalactam would, therefore, be appropriate initial therapy. If *P. aeruginosa* is suspected, then amikacin may be added. After culture and susceptibility data become available therapy is modified as needed.

BRAIN ABSCESS

Etiology

The etiology of brain abscess is diverse. Most commonly, this lesion arises as a result of a contiguous infection from the ear or paranasal sinuses. Less commonly, brain abscess is secondary to an infection at a site distant from the brain.[5, 8, 10, 21, 34, 50] In patients with head injury, brain abscess may occur in the following circumstances: 1) When bone fragments from a compound depressed skull fracture penetrate the brain and are not removed; 2) when bone or missile fragments are not removed from the cerebral parenchyma in patients with intracranial gunshot wounds; and 3) following operation for removal of contused brain or intracranial hematoma.

Bacteriology

The bacteriology of brain abscess is, to a large extent, determined by the original focus of infection. Abscesses that are secondary to middle ear, mastoid, or other sinus infection are usually caused by a variety of aerobic and anaerobic streptococci and other pharyngeal anaerobes (*Bacteroides* sp., veillonella). Gram-negative organisms (*E. coli*, klebsiella, proteus, pseudomonas) and staphylococci are uncommon isolates in patients with middle ear and sinus infections as the underlying cause of the abscess. The situation is reversed in those cases of brain abscess which develop following head trauma and/or neurosurgical procedures. In these cases, *S. aureus* and Gram-negative organisms are the usual isolates; streptococci and anaerobic organisms are less common.[8, 16, 24]

The relationship between the bacteriology and precipitating cause is not absolute; streptococci and bacteroides have been isolated from brain abscesses occurring after head injury, and head trauma that involves the paranasal sinuses or the ear can result in a brain abscess that contains *S. aureus*, Gram-negative organisms (both aerobes and anaerobes).

Operative cultures of brain abscesses are often sterile. This is due, in large part, to poor bacteriological technique in the culture, isolation and identification of anaerobic organisms. When meticulous aerobic and anaerobic bacteriologic techniques are employed, nearly all abscesses will yield organisms.[16, 24] Specimens should be cultured immediately and placed in the proper carrier medium (both aerobic and anaerobic) for delivery to the bacteriology laboratory.

Clinical Signs and Symptoms

In patients with penetrating injuries of the brain or following craniotomy for evacuation of mass lesions, brain abscess should be one of the diagnoses considered when a patient who has been stable or improving develops signs of infection, increased intracranial pressure, focal neurological deficit, or depression of the level of consciousness. Clinical diagnosis of brain abscess may be difficult, especially in the early stages of the disease, and a high index of suspicion is needed to avoid missing the diagnosis. Signs and symptoms of an acute infectious process (fever, elevated erythrocyte sedimentation rate, leukocytosis) may be minimal or entirely absent. Fever is present in no more than 50% of cases, even when the disease is fully developed.[10, 16, 37] Headache is present in 70–90% of patients, and is often (but not always) associated with an altered state of consciousness. Nausea and vomiting are also commonly seen. Focal neurological findings are a valuable aid when present, but are documented less than 50% of the time.[50] Nucchal rigidity, seizures, and hemiparesis are present in one-quarter to one-half of all cases. Papilledema is not consistently present and the frequency with which it is seen varies with the chronicity of the lesion.

Diagnosis

Lumbar Puncture. Lumbar puncture should not be performed if brain abscess is suspected; it is rarely diagnostic and may result in cerebral herniation and death if an abscess is present.[10, 21, 50] If a lumbar puncture is performed in the presence of a brain abscess, the pressure will almost always be elevated, the protein may be normal or only slightly elevated, and the glucose will be normal or nearly so. The cell count will be normal or show a mild pleocytosis with mononuclear and polymorphonuclear cells. Garfield reviewed 200 cases of brain abscess, 140 of whom had a lumbar puncture before definitive treatment of the abscess was initiated.[21] Forty-one of the patients had significant deterioration in their level of consciousness during the subsequent 48 hours. Twenty-five of these patients died. Of the 41 patients, 11 were either fully alert or only mildly drowsy prior to the lumbar puncture and only two of the eleven had papilledema. Carey et al.,[10] reported that a lumbar puncture was the proximate cause of death in 5 of 62 patients with brain abscess. All five had a single abscess, were neurologically stable prior to the lumbar puncture, and deteriorated rapidly following the procedure. In those situations where meningitis cannot be distinguished from brain abscess on clinical grounds, a CT scan should be done. If the scan does not show an abscess, then lumbar puncture may safely be performed.

Radiologic Techniques. In the post-traumatic period, plain skull roentgenograms may be useful in suggesting the presence of an abscess. Retained bone or metallic fragments in patients with gunshot or missile wounds should suggest the possibility of an abscess when the patient has the appropriate clinical signs, even though the injury might have taken place in the distant past. A depressed, unelevated fracture should also suggest the presence of brain abscess as should "air" density located within the cerebral parenchyma.

Technetium brain scanning is an accurate and relatively easy means of diagnosing and localizing a brain abscess. The scan becomes positive when there is a disruption of the blood-brain barrier and radioactive technetium accumulates in brain tissue. This disruption is known to occur in patients with intracranial suppurative disease. Accumulation of technetium also occurs in the presence of cerebral inflammation (cerebritis) and does not require the presence of a localized collection of pus for the scan to be abnormal. Crocker et al.[14] reported 100% accuracy in localizing cerebral abscess using technetium scanning. Typically, the brain scan will exhibit a focal spherical accumulation of radioactivity with a lesser uptake within the center of the lesion which cannot be distinguished with certainty from a tumor. When the scan is interpreted within the context of clinical data, the differentiation of brain abscess from cerebral tumor may be easier.

Until recently, angiography was considered the definitive procedure for the localization of a brain abscess. When an abscess is present, angiography will usually show an avascular mass. There are no angiographic findings that are pathognomonic and the clinician will have to infer that the mass is an abscess based upon clinical circumstances. Bhatia et al.[5] were able to localize 25 of 27 cases using angiography. However, in a study reported by Crocker et al.,[14] although 8 of 11 abscesses were lateralized by angiography, only 5 were correctly localized.

The CT scan is now the procedure of choice for the diagnosis of brain abscess. Several studies have demonstrated that CT scanning can correctly lateralize and localize greater than 95% of cerebral abscesses. The CT scan can also aid in the decision of when to intervene surgically by differentiating focal cerebritis without capsule formation from a fully formed well-encapsulated abscess. In addition, the CT scan is an excellent tool for diagnosing small secondary abscesses which cannot be identified by other techniques.[4, 12, 29, 60]

The intravenous injection of contrast material is essential in making the diagnosis of cerebral abscess and the few failures to accurately diagnose brain abscess that have been reported were due, in part, to the failure to utilize enhancement techniques. After injection of contrast, most abscesses will show a ring pattern of enhancement of the abscess capsule with a low-density center (Fig. 18.1). Serial CT scans may then be used to determine the optimal time for surgical intervention. Recent data would indicate that the increased diagnostic accuracy of the CT scan has resulted in a significant decrease in mortality when outcome from brain abscess using the scanner is compared to that reported during the angiography era.[48]

Treatment of Brain Abscess

The treatment of brain abscess is controversial; the timing of operation, the optimal operative therapy, the nature and duration of the antibiotic therapy, and the role of antibiotics without operation are hotly debated. The various treatments are not necessarily mutually exclusive and each may be appropriate in specific situations.

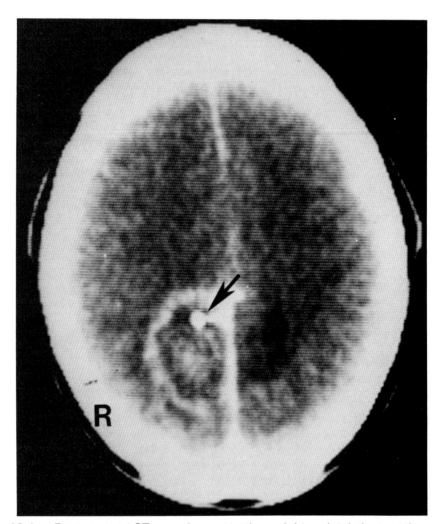

Figure 18.1.   Post-contrast CT scan demonstrating a right parietal abscess three weeks following gunshot wound. Note the ring-like enhancement of the abscess capsule. *Arrow*, retained bone fragment.

Nonoperative Therapy. Rosenblum *et al.*[48] have listed the indications for primary antibiotic treatment of brain abscess: 1) patients who are poor operative risks; 2) patients with multiple abscesses; 3) patients with abscesses in inaccessible areas of the dominant hemisphere; 4) patients with co-existing meningitis or ependymitis; and 5) patients with hydrocephalus who might need a shunt that could become infected during operative treatment of the abscess. The choice of antibiotic therapy should be based on culture of blood, CSF, or fluid aspirated from the abscess.

A brain abscess that develops after head trauma or operation for a traumatically induced intracranial mass lesion may contain a variety of organisms. *S. aureus*, aerobic and anaerobic streptococci, and Gram-negative enteric organisms are common isolates from purulent material. In the absence of positive cultures, antimicrobial therapy must cover a broad spectrum. Penicillin G (24 million units daily) and chloramphenicol (4–6 g/daily) are the mainstays of therapy. These agents are effective and reasonably safe. Penicillin G is active against aerobic and anaerobic streptococci as well as a variety of Gram-negative anerobes. Chloramphenicol penetrates the brain well and has excellent activity against oral anaerobes as well as some activity against enteric Gram-negative organisms. Neither penicillin nor chloramphenicol are primary anti-staphylococcal agents. While awaiting culture reports it may be necessary to add an anti-staphylococcal agent such as nafcillin (12–16 g/daily) to the initial therapeutic regimen. After culture and sensitivity data have become available, antibiotic therapy may be changed depending on the antibiotic susceptibility of the organisms.

Corticosteroids may be useful in the treatment of brain abscess by causing the resolution of brain edema and they may be appropriately used to decrease dangerously elevated intracranial pressure. When utilized, they should be discontinued as soon as possible as they may decrease the chances of encapsulation of the abscess and hinder antibiotic penetration.[48]

Operation has been considered the definitive form of therapy for brain abscess. Antibiotics have traditionally been considered as an adjunctive form of therapy for brain abscess. It is only recently, however, with the advent of the CT scan, that antibiotic therapy as the *definitive treatment* of brain abscess has become feasible. All patients who have antibiotic therapy for brain abscess should have weekly contrast-enhanced scans early in their course (and then progressively less frequently) to document the resolution of the abscess. Antibiotic treatment should last for two to four weeks *after* the CT scan has returned to normal. If the abscess seems to enlarge, or fails to show a decrease in size within the first month, operation is indicated. Similarly, patients who evidence neurological deterioration or who otherwise do not tolerate this regimen, should be treated by operation.

Operative Therapy. In spite of the usefulness of antibiotic therapy as the treatment of certain carefully selected patients with brain abscess, *operative therapy remains the treatment of choice in the vast majority of patients with brain abscess.* Patients who are receiving appropriate antibiotics can deteriorate without warning. Such patients have a poor prognosis even if surgery is immediately performed as outcome is related to neurological status at the time of operation. Since there is little evidence that surgery, *per se*, contributes to mortality, the abandonment of surgery as the definitive treatment of brain abscess is not recommended.

Operation is *always* the treatment of choice for the patient who has a brain abscess contiguous to a metallic or bony foreign body. Resolution of the abscess is unlikely to occur unless the abscess is drained and the foreign body removed. Similarly, operation is the preferred treatment for patients who show rapid deterioration or those who are relatively stable with an encapsulated abscess in an accessible location. In patients who are stable with an area of cerebritis or in those whose CT scan does not show an enhancing capsule with a low-density center, a trial of antibiotics may be appropriate to encourage encapsulation. Antibiotic choice is determined by the principles outlined in the previous section. Once the capsule has formed, operative therapy is indicated.

The type of operative treatment of brain abscess is controversial.[5, 21, 50] Needle aspiration has been proposed as a safe, relatively atraumatic treatment of brain abscess.[21, 38] Its proponents claim that it is a particularly appropriate treatment for deep lesions, for abscesses located near the motor region, or in the dominant temporal lobe. A burr hole is made at a site close to the abscess. The dura is opened and the pia-arachnoid is cauterized. A small caliber brain needle connected to a syringe is directed toward the location of the abscess and the contents of the abscess are aspirated. The aspirated pus is cultured for both aerobic and anaerobic organisms. Antibiotics are started before the procedure according to previously outlined principles, and are changed as necessary when culture and Gram's stain reports become available. The patient is followed with weekly CT scans to ensure that the abscess is resolving. Antibiotics are continued for two weeks after the CT scan demonstrates abscess resolution. Occasionally, a second or third aspiration is necessary.

The major advantage of this technique is that it avoids resection and operation on edematous (but viable) brain. Occasionally, the exact location of the abscess is difficult to ascertain, but in these cases the same problem will be encountered should direct surgical extirpation be attempted. Although serial aspirations may be necessary, the vast majority of abscesses will resolve when the procedure is combined with antibiotic treatment. Care must be taken not to pass the needle through the abscess cavity into the ventricle lest the ventricle and subarachnoid space be contaminated by the purulent contents of the abscess. When abscess formation occurs in relation to bone or missile fragments embedded in cerebral parenchyma, ultimate resolution of the abscess will occur only with removal of the foreign bodies and needle aspiration is not appropriate.

A major criticism of needle aspiration is that the patient must be followed very closely and that rapid deterioration can theoretically occur at any time until the abscess is clearly shown to be getting smaller.

Operative removal of the abscess *via* craniotomy is probably the treatment preferred by a majority of neurosurgeons. It is particularly well suited to an encapsulated abscess in silent areas of the brain. The goal of craniotomy is total excision of the abscess and its capsule—intact, if possible. This is often not feasible, because the capsule may be incomplete and ruptures while it is being removed. Moreover, when the abscess is large, or in areas that are anatomically important, it is probably wisest to drain the abscess by excising only a portion of the circumference of the capsule. Antibiotics are begun at least several hours before the operative procedure and are continued for 10–14 days in the post-operative period.

SUBDURAL EMPYEMA

Pathogenesis

Penetrating wounds of the skull, chronic sinusitis, ICP monitoring devices, craniofacial injuries, cranial osteomyelitis, or infection of a subdural hematoma may result in subdural empyema. It may also be seen following operation for traumatically induced mass lesions.[1, 6, 13, 26]

The extent of infection in the subdural space is influenced by gravity and anatomical boundaries. Subdural empyema is usually found over the convexity of the cerebral hemispheres or the parafalceal region. It is rarely seen in the basal areas of the skull where the subdural space is compressed by the weight of the brain. Established infection usually spreads posteriorly and medially. On rare occasions, pus may spread over the tentorium cerebelli.

Microbiology

The microbiology of subdural empyema has not been well-studied.[1, 26, 63] The best available data comes from Yoshikawa *et al.*,[63] who reviewed 327 cases of subdural empyema reported in the English literature. Aerobic streptococci (35%) and staphylococci (17%) were the most common organisms isolated. Anaerobic bacteria (12%), pneumococci (2%), and miscellaneous organisms (12%) were also encountered. Cultures were reported as sterile in 27% of cases.

Yoshikawa emphasized that anaerobes are the major pathogens in subdural empyema and that their incidence is probably underestimated in the literature because their identification requires sophisticated and meticulous techniques for isolation and recovery. When trauma is the antecedent event resulting in subdural empyema, other organisms (*S. aureus* and enteric Gram-negative bacilli) may be the responsible agent. Trauma that involves the sinuses may result in a subdural empyema that contains anaerobes, aerobic streptococci, staphylococci, and/or Gram-negative bacilli.[26] Because multiple pathogens may be present in the purulent material, careful culture and evaluation of the Gram stain are essential in determining optimal antimicrobial therapy.

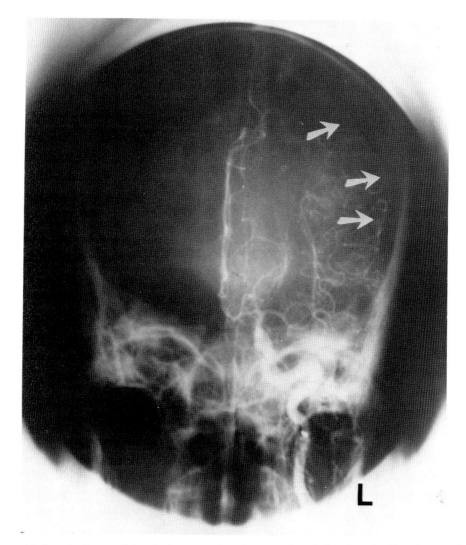

Figure 18.2.   Left carotid arteriogram showing small subdural collection (*arrows*) and spasm of intracranial vessels with a left to right shift of the anterior cerebral artery. Patient had severe focal neurological deficit and obtundation out of proportion to the size of the subdural collection. At craniotomy a subdural empyema was found.

At operation, a few milliliters of purulent material should be placed in a stoppered syringe (to prevent oxygen from destroying anerobic bacteria) and brought directly to the laboratory. The bacteriologist should be told that both *aerobic* and *anaerobic* cultures are needed.

Clinical Findings; Diagnosis

The clinical course of subdural empyema is rapid and evolves over 3–7 days. Fever, headache, vomiting, and meningeal signs are common in the early stages of the disease and the clinical picture may suggest bacterial meningitis. During this early stage, the CSF is usually sterile and may show a mild pleocytosis, elevated protein, and a normal glucose. There is a gradual deterioration in the level of consciousness with rapid progression to stupor and coma if the patient remains untreated. A focal motor deficit or dysphasia is seen in nearly every case. Seizures, both focal and generalized, and papilledema are present in 40–50% of the cases. In advanced stages, the clinical picture is that of a patient with a depressed level of consciousness, fever and focal neurological signs. Late in the course of the disease, overt meningitis may develop.[1, 13, 26, 36]

Diagnosis may be made by cerebral angiography (Fig. 18.2) or CT scan (Fig. 18.3). Angiography will show an avascular area between the cortical vessels and the inner table of the skull. Spasm of vessels at the base of the brain is sometimes seen and is presumably due to irritation of the vessels by pus. CT scan will show a hypodense collection often with severe edema of the underlying brain.

Treatment

Operation. The time between the onset of neurological findings and definitive surgical therapy is the single most important determinant of outcome in patients with subdural empyema.[9] Renaudin and Frazee[47] recently reported 23 cases of subdural em-

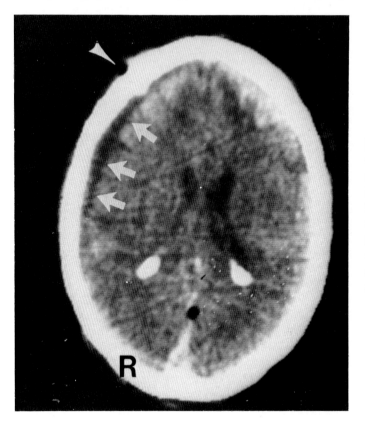

Figure 18.3 CT scan reveals a right sided hypodense subdural collection (*arrows*) in a patient who had a subarachnoid bolt (*arrowhead*) placed for ICP monitoring following a closed head injury. *Single arrow head*, bone defect at site of bolt placement.

pyema seen over the past 20 years. Of patients who had operation within 72 hours after the onset of neurologic dysfunction, nine did well and one was disabled. Of 13 patients operated on between 3 and 30 days after the onset of neurologic findings, four did well, four were disabled, and five died. Surgical therapy, therefore, should not be withheld if, in the appropriate clinical setting, CT scan or angiogram are not diagnostic.[1, 3, 36, 47] Delay until the CT scan shows a well-defined, clear-cut collection in the subdural space may seriously compromise the patient's outcome.

Operative treatment consists of multiple burr holes or craniotomy and drainage of the pus.[1, 6, 26, 34, 47] The subdural space should be irrigated with antibiotic solution. For small liquid collections of pus, drainage via burr holes may be satisfactory. However, when parafalceal collections are present, or the subdural collection is thick and tenacious, evacuation of pus is best achieved via craniotomy.[6]

Antibiotics. As soon as the diagnosis of subdural empyema is made, treatment with antibiotics should be started. Therapy should be designed to cover the potential pathogens causing the empyema (oropharyngeal anaerobes, aerobic streptococci, S. aureus and enteric Gram-negative bacilli). Standard therapy consists of nafcillin (12–16 g/day) for S. aureus and chloramphenicol (4–6 g/day) for oral anaerobes, aerobic streptococci and enteric Gram-negative organisms. Penicillin G (24 million units/day) may be added to chloramphenicol and nafcillin for additional coverage of anaerobic streptococci. In the patient with mild penicillin allergy, cefotaxime (12 g/day) and chloramphenicol may be used. In the patient with severe penicillin allergy (hives, giant urticaria, bronchospasm, anaphylaxis), all β-lactam antibiotics, including cephalosporins, should be avoided. In this circumstance, vancomycin (2 g/day) and chloramphenicol may be used although the activity of chloramphenicol against Gram-negative organisms is suboptimal. Therapy should be continued for two to four weeks after surgical drainage.

Several points regarding the therapy of subdural empyema deserve special empha-

sis. First, antimicrobial therapy is only adjunctive to the primary operative treatment of the disease and will not by itself result in cure of the empyema. Second, Gram's stain, culture (aerobic and anaerobic), and susceptibility data are essential in determining appropriate antibiotic treatment. The recommendations listed in the above paragraph are only for initial empiric therapy and antibiotic treatment may have to be changed when Gram's stain, culture, and susceptibility data are available. Third, although cefotaxime may be used because it penetrates the CSF well and has excellent activity against S. aureus and Gram-negative organisms, clinical experience with this new drug is sparse and for now its use should be reserved for patients allergic to penicillin.

CRANIAL OSTEOMYELITIS

Osteomyelitis of the skull is usually a complication of craniotomy.[9] Less often, contamination or inadequate debridment of open skull wounds will lead to osteomyelitis. In a retrospective review of 18 cases of cranial osteomyelitis reported by Bullitt and Lehman,[9] craniotomy preceded the development of osteomyelitis in 12 cases, three cases followed head injury, two occurred after irradiation, and one was associated with chronic sinusitis.

Signs and symptoms are usually local and consist of pain, tenderness and swelling over the infected bone. Fever, leukocytosis and an elevated sedimentation rate are less common. The presence of systemic signs of infection often signify an underlying collection of pus (subdural empyema).

Skull films will show evidence of osteomyelitis in over 50% of patients (Fig. 18.4). If the skull films are negative, then a technetium bone scan should be done. It may give evidence of osteomyelitis when skull films are normal. However, previous operation or trauma to the cranium may result in uptake in the absence of infection and the usefulness of this diagnostic test is therefore limited. When osteomyelitis occurs after a craniotomy, the primary treatment is removal of the entire bone flap. Scalp drainage, if present, should be cul-

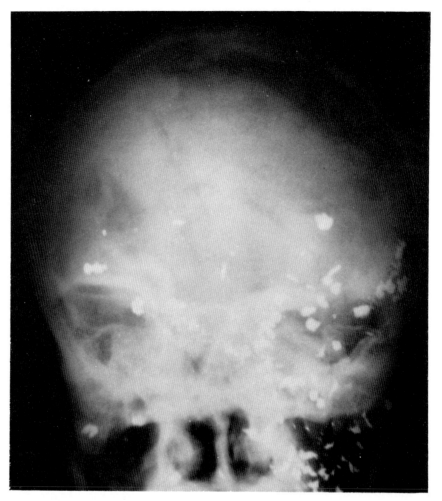

Figure 18.4. A-P skull roentgenogram showing osteomyelitis in a patient who had a shotgun wound of the skull and face nine years before. Angiography showed an epidural mass which at operation was pus.

tured and antibiotics started prior to operation on the basis of a Gram's stain of wound drainage. After bone removal, the wound is irrigated with an antibiotic solution and the scalp is closed in a single layer with wire or monofilament nylon sutures.

In patients who develop osteomyelitis of the skull following trauma (but unrelated to previous craniotomy), craniectomy of infected bone should be performed based on skull film evidence of osteomyelitis. At least 5–10 mm of bone should be debrided beyond the area of osteomyelitis observed at operation.

Optimal antimicrobial therapy of osteomyelitis is facilitated by determination of the MIC of different antibiotics to the organism causing infection. Antibiotics which have a low MIC to the causative pathogen and achieve a high level in serum and bone are desirable.

High-dose nafcillin (12 g/day) is adequate therapy for *S. aureus* infection. Antibiotic therapy for Gram-negative organisms is determined by susceptibility data. Moxalactam (6–12 g/day) may be a reasonable first choice for the therapy of Gram-negative osteomyelitis because of its broad

Gram-negative spectrum and potency. There is, however, insufficient clinical data available at this time on its efficacy in the treatment of osteomyelitis. Optimal duration of therapy has not been determined. It is likely that infection will clear shortly after removal of the infected bone even without antibiotic treatment. However, it has been our policy to continue intravenous antibiotics in these patients for 7–10 days following operative debridement.

References

1. Anagnostopoulos, D.I., Gortvai, P.: Intracranial subdural abscess. Br. J. Surg., 60:50–52, 1973.
2. Applebaum, E.: Meningitis following trauma to the head and face. J.A.M.A., 173:1818–1822, 1960.
3. Armengaud, M., Auvergnat, J.-Ch., LeNet, R., Massip, P., Tho, T.C.: Des concentrations des antibiotiques dans le LCR au cours des traitements des méningites bactériennes aiguës. Med. Hyg., 30:398–401, 1979.
4. Berg, B., Franklin, G., Cuneo, R., Boldrey, E., Strimling, B.: Neurosurgical cure of brain abscess: early diagnosis and follow-up with computerized tomography. Ann. Neurol., 3:474–478, 1978.
5. Bhatia, A., Tendon, P.N., Banerji, A.K.: Brain abscess—an analysis of 55 cases. Int. Surg., 58:565–568, 1973.
6. Bhondari, Y.S., Sarkuri, N.B.: Subdural empyema—a review of 37 cases. Neurosurgery, 32:35–39, 1970.
7. Black, P., Graybill, J.R., Charache, P.: Penetration of brain abscess by systemically administered antibiotics. J. Neurosurg., 38:705–709, 1973.
8. Brewer, N.S., MacCar, C.S.: Brain abscess: A review of recent experience. Ann. Int. Med., 82:571–576, 1975.
9. Bullitt, E., Lehman, R.A.W.: Osteomyelitis of the skull. Surg. Neurol., 11:163–166, 1979.
10. Carey, M.E., Chou, S.N., French, L.A.: Experience with brain abscess. J. Neurosurg., 36:1–9, 1972.
11. Cherubin, C.E., Marr, J.S., Sierra, M.F., Becker, S.: Listeria and Gram-negative bacillary meningitis in New York City 1972–1979. Frequent causes of meningitis in adults. Am. J. Med. 71:199–210, 1981.
12. Claveria, L.E., duBoulay, G.H., Mosely, I.F.: Intracranial infections: investigation by computerized axial tomography. Neuroradiology, 12:59–71, 1976.
13. Coonrod, J.D., Dans, P.E.: Subdural empyema. Am J. Med., 53:85–91, 1972.
14. Crocker, E.F., McLaughlin, A.F., Morris, J.G., Benn, R., McLeod, J.G., Allsop, J.L.: Technetium brain scanning in the diagnosis and management of cerebral abscess. Am. J. Med., 56:192–200, 1974.
15. deLouvois, J., Hurley, R.: Antibiotic concentration in intracranial pus: a study from a collaborative project. In: Chemotherapy, Vol. 4, "Pharmacology of Antibiotics," Williams, J.D., Geddes, A.M., Eds.

Plenum Press, New York, 1975, pp. 61–71.
16. deLouvois, J.: The bacteriology and chemotherapy of brain abscess. J. Antimicrob. Chemother., 4:395–413, 1978.
17. Everett, E.D., Strausbaugh, L.J.: Antimicrobial agents and the central nervous system. Neurosurgery, 6:691–714, 1980.
18. Fass, R.J.: In vitro activity of LY127935. Antimicrob. Agents Chemother., 16:503–509, 1979.
19. Fenstermacher, J.D., and Rall, D.P.: Physiology and Pharmacology of Cerebrospinal Fluid. In: International Encyclopedia of Pharmacology and Therapeutics. Peteis, G., Ed. Pergamon Press, Oxford, 1972, p. 35–81.
20. Fossieck, B.E., Jr., Kane, J.G., Diaz, C.R., Parker, R.H.: Nafcillin entry into human cerebrospinal fluid. Antimicrob. Agents Chemother., 11:965–967, 1977.
21. Garfield, J.: Management of supratentorial abscess: A review of 200 cases. Br. Med. J., 2:7–11, 1969.
22. Hand, W.L., Sanford, J.P.: Post-traumatic bacterial meningitis. Ann. Intern. Med., 72:869–874, 1970.
23. Hawley, B., Gump, D.W.: Vancomycin therapy of bacterial meningitis. J. Dis. Child, 126:261–264, 1973.
24. Heinman, H.S., Brande, A.I.: Anaerobic infection of the brain. Am. J. Med., 35:682–697, 1963.
25. Hieber, J.P., Nelson, J.D.: A pharmacologic evolution of penicillin in children with purulent meningitis. New Engl. J. Med., 297:410–413, 1977.
26. Hitchcock, E., Andreadis, A.: Subdural empyema: A review of 29 cases. J. Neurol. Neurosurg. Psychiat., 27:422–434, 1964.
27. Kaiser, A.B., McGee, Z.A.: Aminoglycoside therapy of gram-negative bacillary meningitis. New Engl. J. Med., 293:1215–1220, 1975.
28. Kane, J.G., Parker, R.H., Jordan, G.W., Hoeprich, P.D.: Nafcillin concentration in cerebrospinal fluid during treatment of staphylococcal infections. Ann. Intern. Med., 87:307–311, 1977.
29. Kanzer, E.: Effects of computerized axial tomography on the treatment of cerebral abscess. Neuroradiology, 12:57–58, 1976.
30. Kramer, P.W., Griffith, R.S., Campbell, R.L.: Antibiotic penetration of the brain. J. Neurosurg., 31:295–302, 1969.
31. Kucers, A., McK Bennett, N.: The Use of Antibiotics. 3rd Ed. J.P. Lippincott, Co., Philadelphia, 1979.
32. Landesman, S.H., Corrado, J.L., Cleri, D., Cherubin, C.E.: Diffusion of a new beta-lactam (LY127938) into the cerebrospinal fluid. Am. J. Med., 17:675–678, 1980.
33. Landesman, S.H., Corrado, J.L., Shah, P., Armengaud, M., Barza, M., Cherubin, C.E.: The current and historical roles of the cephalosporin antibiotics in the treatment of meningitis with special emphasis on their use in Gram-negative bacilliary meningitis. Am. J. Med. 71:693–703, 1981.
34. LeBeau, J., Creissard, P., Haripse, L., Redono, A.: Surgical treatment of brain abscess and subdural empyema. J. Neurosurg., 38:198–203, 1973.

35. List, C.F.: Interhemispheral subdural suppuration. J. Neurosurg., 7:313–324, 1950.
36. Luken, M.G., and Whelan, M.A.: Recent diagnostic experience with subdural empyema. J. Neurosurg., 52:764–771, 1980.
37. Morgan, H., Wood, M.W., Murphey, F.: Experience with 88 consecutive cases of brain abscess. J. Neurosurg., 38:698–704, 1973.
38. Mount, L.A.: Conservative surgical therapy of brain abscess. J. Neurosurg., 7:385–389, 1950.
39. Nair, S.R., Cherubin, C.E., Weinstein, M.: Penetration of cefoxitin into cerebrospinal fluid and treatment of meningitis caused by gram-negative bacteria. Rev. Infect. Dis., 1:134–141, 1979.
40. New, H.C., Aswapokee, N., Aswapokee, P., Kwung, P.F.: HR-756, A new cephalosporin active against gram-positive and gram-negative aerobic and anaerobic bacteria. Antimicrob. Agents Chemother., 15:273–281, 1979.
41. Oldendorf, W.H.: Blood-brain barrier permeability to drugs. Ann. Rev. Pharmacol., 4:239–248, 1974.
42. Oldendorf, W.H.: The Nervous System, Vol. 1, Tower, D.B., Ed. Raven Press, New York, 1975, p. 279–289.
43. Overturf, G.D., Steinberg, E.A., Underman, A.E., Wilkins, J., Leedom, J.M., Mathies, A.W., Wehrle, P.F.: Comparative trial of carbenicillin and ampicillin therapy for purulent meningitis. Antimicrob. Agents Chemother., 11:420–426, 1977.
44. Raaf, J.: Post-traumatic cerebrospinal fluid leaks. Arch. Surg., 95:648–651, 1967.
45. Rahal, J.J., Hyams, P.J., Simberkoff, M.S., Rubinstein, E.: Combined intrathecal and intramuscular gentamicin for gram-negative meningitis. New Engl. J. Med., 290:1394–1398, 1974.
46. Rahal, J.J., Simberkoff, M.S.: Bactericidal and bacterostatic action of chloramphenicol against meningeal pathogens. Antimicrob. Agents Chemother. 16:13–18, 1979.
47. Renaudin, J.W., Frazee, J.: Subdural empyema—importance of early diagnosis. Neurosurgery, 7:477–479, 1980.
48. Rosenblum, M., Hoff, J.T., Norman, D., Edwards, M.S., and Berg, B.O.: Nonoperative treatment of brain abscesses in selected high-risk patients. J. Neurosurg., 52:217–225, 1980.
49. Ruiz, D.E., Warner, J.F.: Nafcillin treatment of staphylococcus aureus meningitis. Antimicrob. Agents Chemother., 9:554–555, 1976.
50. Samson, D., and Clark, K.: A current review of brain abscess. Am. J. Med., 54:201–210, 1974.
51. Sanford, J.P., Luby, J.P., Jones, S.R.: Bacterial meningitis complicating cranio-spinal trauma. J. Trauma, 13:895–900, 1973.
52. Sathe, S.: Personal communication.
53. Schoenbaum, S.C., Gardner, P., Shillito, J.: Infections of cerebrospinal fluid shunts; epidemiology, clinical manifestations and therapy. J. Infect. Dis., 131:543–552, 1975.
54. Selkow, J.B., Barling, R.W.A.: The cerebrospinal fluid penetration of antibiotics. J. Antimicrob. Ther., 4:204–227, 1978.
55. Simberkoff, M.S., Moldover, N.H., and Rahal, J.J.: Absence of detectable bactericidal and opsonic activities in normal and infected human cerebrospinal fluid. J. Clin. Lab. Med., 95:362–372, 1980.
56. Strausbaugh, L., Sande, M.: Factors influencing the therapy of experimental *Proteus mirabilis* meningitis in rabbits. J. Infect. Dis., 137:251–260, 1978.
57. Tofte, R.W., Peterson, P.K., Kim, Y., and Quie, P.C.: Opsonic activity in normal human cerebrospinal fluid for selected bacterial species. Infect. Immun., 26:1093–1098, 1979.
58. Torres, H., Yorzagary and Ch. West, L.: Subdural empyema: Angiographic and clinical considerations. Neurochirugia., 13:201–211, 1980.
59. Turck, M., Belcher, D., Ronald, A., Smith, R., Wallace, J.: New cephalosporin antibiotic-cephaloridine-clinical and laboratory evaluation. Arch. Intern. Med., 119:50–59, 1967.
60. Weisberg, L.A.: Computed tomography in the diagnosis of intracranial disease. Ann. Intern. Med., 91:87–105, 1979.
61. Wilkowske, C.J.: The Penicillins. Mayo Clin. Proc., 52:616–624, 1977.
62. Wood, P.H.: Diffuse subdural suppuration. J. Laryng., 66:496–515, 1952.
63. Yoshikawa, T.T., Chow, A.W., Guze, L.B.: Role of anaerobic bacteria in subdural empyema. Am. J. Med., 58:99–104, 1975.

19

Behavioral Sequelae of Head Injury

THOMAS J. BOLL

Until very recently the *severely* head injured have been the almost exclusive focus of surgeons, neurologists, psychologists, sociologists, economists, epidemiologists, and physiatrists interested in neural trauma. Despite the greater amount of interest in severe as opposed to mild injury, current data suggest that the incidence of mild and moderate head injury is inadequately appreciated.

In 1980, Annegers *et al.*[2] stated "although head trauma is a major cause of morbidity and mortality, epidemiologic study has lagged because of difficulties in identifying and classifying cases and lack of standardized definition of the injuries." The United States Bureau of the Census reported that 9,759,000 head injuries occurred in 1975.[9] The majority of these were minor and were frequently dismissed as not germane to a proper discussion of head injury. Data and arguments to be presented later in this chapter suggest that such dismissal may, at least for some segment of this group, be mistaken. Despite the disparities in criteria of severity, patients with "mild" trauma account for the majority of reported head injuries.[20] Even among hospital admissions Jagger[26] reports that 80% of patients have Glasgow Coma Scale scores of 12 or above.

If for no other reason than sheer numbers, patients with head injuries rated as mild must be taken into account in any chapter on sequelae of head injury. In the past, the most usual approach has been to dismiss this group and concentrate on patients who are likely to experience obvious head injury-related difficulties in some aspect of their behavior. An example of this is the definition of concussion in Merritt's Textbook of Neurology[41] which includes a presumption of no structural damage to the brain and which results in recovery "with no residuals." Concussion is viewed as a transient loss of consciousness which is totally reversible. Therefore, if symptoms fail to fit this pattern they are due to undiagnosed and more serious structural damage or the patient is considered to be neurotic. Having thus disposed of this group, attention can then be directed to those head-injured patients whose severity of injury has provided clear evidence of focal and/or diffuse brain damage and resultant behavioral effects. These effects are usually separated into "cognitive-intellectual-ability" on one hand and personality-emotional on the other.

The subsequent discussion in this chapter will deal first with the behavioral sequelae of moderate and severe head injury. Relatively more space than is customary will be devoted to the sequelae of apparently mild injury both because this subject has received so little attention in the past and because mild injury is so much more common than is severe injury.

BEHAVIORAL SEQUELAE OF MODERATE AND SEVERE HEAD INJURY

Failure to Recognize Behavioral Sequelae

The medical advances reviewed in preceding chapters of this book have produced an increasing number of survivors of serious head injury. The quality of their survival has been over-estimated, however. This is so because those caring for the seriously injured start with a patient who is functioning at a very low level. Almost anything, including survival itself, is seen as progress or improvement. Patients who progress from danger of death to medical stability and independence have, in one very real sense, enjoyed significant recovery and have vastly improved.

For the patient and his family, however, success and recovery mean a return to the previous manner of life functioning. Thus, without intending to do so and without giving inaccurate information, the acute care physician or surgeon conveys an impression of the patient in terms that suggest a far more optimistic situation than is likely to pertain immediately and even for some time to come, if at all.

Overestimation of the quality of survival is due to the nature of the pattern of recovery following head injury. Recovery from head injury may be characterized by amazingly good physical return, physical/neurological and electroencephalographic normality, and medical stability. Add to this the youth of the typical head-injured patient and a picture emerges of a superficially intact individual who may or may not complain but whose deficits will require expertise to even identify let alone adequately appreciate. It is hardly surprising that when such a patient does complain of difficulties in relating to his environment, factors other than those of a purely neurological nature are quickly considered by his family and physicians. Assumptions about inadequate motivation as the explaining factor are routinely incompatible, not only with the patient's past life, but also with the great preponderance of data now available to document the presence of very real mental deficits in seemingly healthy patients.[17, 48] The patient's mental status may seem quite intact and yet more specific examination will reveal deficits that make a return to past intellectual tasks quite impossible.

Table 19.1 is a list of personal-social-emotional reactions frequently seen follow-

Table 19.1
Personal-Social-Emotional Sequelae of Moderate-Severe Head Injury

Hoarding	Restlessness
Boredom	Grandiosity
Denial of problems	Sleep problems
Euphoria	Social crudeness
Irritability	Silliness
Social withdrawal	Decreased libido
Suspiciousness	Lability of affect
Hostility	Disinhibition
Lack of foresight	Reduced initiative
Anxiety	Blunting of emotion

ing head injury. This list includes reactions reported by family members even when the patient denies all difficulties and changes. In fact, denial of deficits and especially denial of personality problems is itself a reasonably frequent occurrence. This stubborn insistence that all is well has the effect of leading the patient into ill-advised activities, leading the physician astray in his attempt to assess outcome if other data are not sought, and leaving the family alone and without help to cope with deficits about which all others seem unaware or indifferent.

In describing patients after severe head injury, Maciver et al.[40] stated that "the majority of patients who survive make a good physical recovery and will also make a rapid return to nearly normal mental state." Jennett,[28, 29] in commenting on such over-optimism, pointed out that many survivors show serious disability. It is necessary, however, to be able to recognize serious deficits when present before they can be properly managed. The tendency of some to underestimate difficulties is epitomized by the comments of Jacobson.[25] "The patient may stop his improvement at any level from coma to a stage of complete alertness with normal intellectual function except for *minor deficits* such as *memory, judgement and creative thinking*" (italics mine).

Time Course of Recovery of Cognitive Deficits

Table 19.2 lists some of the cognitive deficits associated with head injury which may be present long after physical recovery is complete and the patient's medical status is normal. The deficits are listed in order of their ability to disrupt function and in the length of time needed for recovery. The period of recovery may, in fact, extend for many years in individual instances, but the rate is most rapid during the early phase and these estimates are for the time required for the major portion of recovery to occur (no matter how incomplete or disappointing it may be). Except in cases of penetrating injury or focal damage from closed head injury, physical sequelae are typically least severe and most rapidly remitting.

Pre-morbid Characteristics and Behavioral Sequelae

While there is no doubt that head injury can produce deficits of intellect and ability, the issue of the relationship of other factors in the patient's life contributing to the development of more than transient emotional disturbance continues to be debated. Aita and Reitan[1] reviewed the outcome of 500 head-injured World War II veterans. They concluded that for those patients experiencing an enduring post-traumatic psychosis this disorder was related to pre-morbid personality characteristics and was an exaggeration of preexisting tendencies. Tennent[55] believed that a constitutional predisposition was the major factor in producing any of the major psychoses following head injury. In opposition to this view, Davison and Bagley,[12] after a review of the literature, concluded that when head injury is followed by a schizophrenic illness, the

Table 19.2
Cognitive Deficits Associated with Head Injury and Approximate Time for Recovery Following Mild to Moderate Head Injury

Motor skill and speed	0–3 months
Language skill	3–6 months
Attention/concentration	6–12 months
Memory/learning	6–24 months
Complex problem solving	6–24 months
Mental stamina	6–24 months

trauma may be a direct etiological factor and not simply a precipitant.

Bond,[8] in his usually thoughtful and scholarly fashion, has fully utilized available data to arrive at a somewhat centrist position. He concludes that

> ... there is general agreement that mental disorders after severe head injuries are the product of both physical and psychological factors. The latter include previous environmental stresses, a genetically determined predisposition towards emotional instability shown by a personal and family history, and the effect of personality upon the pattern or response to injury and disability.

Bond focused on overall social disability which includes work, leisure pursuits, and family cohesion. He concluded that social disability was related to all other head injury-related factors, including physical defect, neurological dysfunction, and mental impairment. He noted, however, that family cohesion was more negatively affected by mental decline than by physical disability.

One approach to understanding the nature of the patient's difficulty involves the joining of cognitive with personality functions under the term mental or neuropsychological. This avoids many of the difficulties which arise from this largely artificial separation of personal attributes. Complaints by relatives of "personality change" are frequently found to derive from failure of the patient to accomplish tasks which is, in fact, more the result of disability than disinclination. "When brain damage is responsible, the personality change will often be but one aspect of the dementia which ensues, and cognitive defects of some degree will be in evidence."[39] Even mild and clinically invisible decreases in cognitive capacity can significantly alter a patient's ability to perform tasks at a subjectively adequate level. Statements by physicians and other care givers that intelligence appears normal or that the patient is able to lead a full life are nothing short of additional irritants to the patient who is uncomfortably aware of his decline from his premorbid state. A "full life" without creativity, resilience to stress, or ability to compete at previous levels is hardly full enough. Such changes, when gradual and due to the process of "normal" aging, require effort for satisfactory acceptance. When they occur suddenly, to a previously healthy individual, in the early stages of life when keenest capacity is usually most demanded, the fullest appreciation by his caregivers of his actual losses and remaining strengths are crucial to optimal adjustment. The importance of understanding the integration of personality and disability was underscored by Eson and Bourke,[12] who held that psycho-social changes are a result of changes in ability to cope with all aspects of life and that "cognitive functions are primary and the personality changes are derivative or secondary."

Seizures and Behavioral Sequelae

Seizures represent a much discussed residue of head injury, which may occur early and only once, after a delay of years or may be a continuing part of the recovery process. The presence of seizures can have a strong influence on behavioral aspects of recovery. The impact of seizure frequency and the age at onset of cognitive functioning has been the subject of several recent papers from our laboratory.[45, 51, 52] These and other reports indicate that early onset has more negative implications than late onset and that reduction in frequency of seizures is associated with cognitive brightening. Dikmen and Reitan[15] reported that, in the absence of abnormalities on the neurologic exam, patients with post-traumatic epilepsy performed significantly worse on a series of sensitive neuropsychological measures of higher cognitive performance than patients with a history of head injury without seizures.

Black et al.[5] reported a much greater incidence of seizures with penetrating than closed head injury. They also found that children less than age 2 and adults had a higher incidence of late as compared to early post-head injury seizures. Children age 2–5 had an opposite pattern with a relatively high incidence of early seizures and a low incidence of late attacks. They reported that 13% of head injured children

had a seizure within one week of injury. Jennett[30] reporting on adults found a relationship between post-traumatic amnesia and seizures. With post-traumatic amnesia greater than 24 hours, seizure rate was 12% while it was 5% for those with post-traumatic amnesia less than 24 hours. He also noted, however, that when patients with focal brain damage were excluded (hematoma or depressed skull fracture) the rates fell to 1.5 and 1%, respectively. Black et al.[3] pointed out that for patients with early seizures there was a 12% risk of recurrence while the risk was only 3% for seizures among those patients who did not experience early seizures (see also Chapter 11).

Predictors of Behavioral Sequelae

One behavioral indicant of future limitations on recovery may be agitation in the acute stages during coma or the transition to alertness. Levin and Grossman[34] reported that combativeness, truncal rocking, thrashing, screaming, and signs of sympathetic activation were frequently associated with aggressiveness, hallucinations, delusions, and an eventual pattern of agitation, anxiety, thinking disturbance, depression and "generally increased psychopathology as compared with patients who were relatively inactive and unaroused during the stages of coma and stupor."

More subtle deficits in mental function, frequently requiring specialized procedures to document even when serious enough to disrupt day-to-day performance, have been identified by Kløve and Cleeland.[32] They reported that persistence of positive findings on the EEG or the physical/neurological exam augur poorly for full recovery as does the presence of an intracranial hematoma.

Post-traumatic amnesia (PTA) was cited by Fahy et al.[19] as the best single yardstick of head injury severity and its use has been popular, at least in part, due to its consistency over time.[50] PTA describes a period following head injury which the victim is unable to remember. Some authors use the earliest valid post-injury memory to measure the length of PTA. Unfortunately, "islands of memory" have been reported and these, surprisingly, tend to occur in the first one-third of the overall PTA period.[23] Post-traumatic disorientation has also been shown to be related to recovery of memory function,[47] and was suggested by Russell to be useful as an indicant of length of post-traumatic amnesia. Gronwall and Wrightson,[23] however, demonstrated that some patients are fully oriented within the PTA period while others remain disoriented after the PTA period has terminated. Lishman[39] suggested that PTA greater than 24 hours was associated with a very high likelihood of at least some permanent mental deficits. He claimed that PTA less than 24 hours was consistent with "complete intellectual recovery" in a "fair proportion" of patients. Such a rule of thumb provides little certainty for any single patient and represents considerable over-optimism based on clinical rather than specific neuropsychological type of evaluation. Oddy et al.[44] found a weak but positive relationship between PTA and time to return to work and number of suggestive symptoms of a congitive-personality nature reported by patients.

That these and other investigators[8, 43] should find a relationship between lasting problems with memory which are likely the result of diffuse brain damage or bilateral brain stem damage[56] and all forms of peritraumatic amnesias is hardly surprising. Given the very general nature of the behavior described on both sides of this relationship the rather low correlations are also understandable. Furthermore, Gronwall and Wrightson[23] have demonstrated that PTA is not as stable as was once believed. They found that 25% of PTA reports changed on re-interview. They used exceedingly careful criteria and measurement procedures not typical of most prospective studies and utterly impossible when chart data is used after the fact. Even with this degree of care, they recommended two interviews, separated in time, to assess PTA. Certainly, this crude index will continue to be found useful for severely injured patients whose PTA exceeds 24 hours. As a considerable majority of patients have far briefer PTA, however, more sensitive measures will be required.

The bulk of sequelae of a physical-medical nature following head injury are related,

in understandable fashion, to severity of brain damage and the area of the brain involved. Visual field defects, hemiparesis, and hemiplegia and persisting aphasia have obvious behavioral implications. Nevertheless, behavioral recovery can be quite satisfactory in the presence of all but aphasia. Conversely, significant behavioral deficit is frequent without any readily detectable or outward manifestation of the past trauma.

BEHAVIORAL SEQUELAE OF MILD HEAD INJURY OR CONCUSSION

In 1787 Benjamin Bell[4] described concussion:

> Every affectation of the head attended with stupefaction, when it appears as the immediate consequence of external violence, and when no mark of injury is discovered, is in general supposed to proceed from commotion or concussion of the brain; by which is meant such a derangement of this organ as obstructs its natural and usual function, without producing such obvious effects on it, as to render it capable of having its real nature assertained by dissection.

Grunthal[24] was the first to carry out a longitudinal study of patients with head injury whose disorders in behavior and function were frequently diagnosed as emotional in nature. His follow-up spanned several years with repeated clinical examinations. At autopsy he obtained evidence supporting his clinical findings of brain impairment in 16 of 17 cases. Windle et al.[59] found that 30 seconds after trauma, minimal brain changes were present but by allowing survival they found significant nerve cell degeneration by days six to eight.

Gennarelli and his colleagues[21] have developed a model for acceleration-induced head injury which has produced identifiable damage in diffuse areas of the brain (see also Chapter 6). Utilizing this method of acceleration to produce head injury without a blow to the head, Jane has discovered similar damage. The injury produced loss of consciousness of less than two minutes, blood pressure and heart rate changes and corneal reflex absence for less than thirty seconds, after which the monkey returned to normal behavior. Gross examination revealed a normal brain without edema or herniation. Fink-Heimer stains, however, revealed pronounced degenerative changes in axons and their terminal arborizations in the reticular and vestibular nuclei and dorsal regions of the medulla.[27]

A quote from an outstanding and strikingly current treatise on mild head injury and its effects by Symonds summarizes the implications of these studies.

"As a result of concussion of any degree there may be permanent loss of neural function, the amount of such loss being in proportion to the severity of the concussive effects. They suggest also that diffuse loss of neurons may be present after concussion without any symptoms being apparent either to the subject or to experienced observers.

It is reasonable to assume that the number of available neurons is ordinarily greater than that required for normal functioning. We may therefore surmise that in the patient who has been concussed and recovered, some fraction of his reserve neurons has been lost; and, if the process is repeated, it will only be a question of the number and severity of the injuries before the reserves are exhausted and permanent symptoms appear. The earliest symptoms to be expected from such a diffuse cerebral loss would be of the kind most difficult to measure—subjective difficulty over intellectual problems, and slight personality changes. In this connection it is worth noting how often after apparent recovery from severe concussion the near relatives may often state that the patient has never been quite the same person since the accident."[53]

Obviously these comments were made without knowledge of the work of Gennarelli et al.[21] and Jane.[27] Instead they reflect data that have existed for over 40 years[54] and strongly suggest that the complaints of patients who sustain mild head injury are real and not neurotic or induced by desire for financial gain.

Several points deserve further comment. One is the postulated cumulative nature of head injury and another is the similarity of mild head injury to the aging process. Important, too, is the suggestion that more specialized and sensitive measurement devices may allow direct appreciation of the intellectual-behavioral changes of which relatives and patients complain.

If, as Symonds and others have postulated, mild head injury can produce damage to various portions of brain, one must inquire how mild the injury may be. While this question is currently under investigation, considerable data exists for the occurrence of concussion without loss of consciousness. Windle et al.[59] suggested the possibility of neural damage in such mild injuries. Teuber[56] noted lasting dysphasia and significant decline on tests of mental ability in patients without retrograde or post-traumatic amnesia and even "in the absence of documented loss of consciousness." Roberts[49] reported that permanent disability could result from multiple concussions or repeated trauma without loss of consciousness. Levin et al.[35] reported disruption of neuropsychological functions in patients with very mild closed head injuries with very brief coma and even in the absence of coma. If this is indeed the case, the next question is: which head injury am I treating? If head injury of such mild nature can, in fact, cause brain changes, is it not possible that when a patient appears in the emergency room or even in the consulting room with recent head injury that the eventual sequelae may depend as much on how many unnoted head injuries the patient has had as on the one currently in question?

Data documenting that the effects of mild head injury are, in fact, cumulative make such a question important before a patient's complaints are dismissed as neurotic because the current head injury appears too trivial to cause short-term, let along lasting, difficulties. Roberts,[49] in a study of boxers with multiple closed-head injuries without loss of consciousness, documented that mental deficits extending to permanent disability can be produced. Windle et al.[59] found that two sub-concussive blows produced as much chromatolysis as a single mild concussion. Gronwall and Wrightson[22] found that following a second concussion, patients were more seriously impaired and took longer to recover than did those recovering from their first closed-head injury. It is apparent, then, that the sequelae of head injury depend on both the severity and number of head injuries experienced.

The severity and number of concussive events interact with the patient's age at the time of head injury. For patients in their middle and late years, the likelihood of disruptions in previous ability is high after an injury mild enough to allow return to a normal *neurological* condition. Cooper[11] said "the change that takes place in the intellect from injuries to the brain is very similar to the effects of age. The patient becomes, as it were, suddenly old." Symonds'[53] concept of neural reserve mentioned earlier is relevant in this context. With advancing age this reserve diminishes; not only is mortality from head injury higher but sequelae among survivors is more serious. The diminishing cerebral reserve makes even a minor additional loss all the more likely to have clinical significance.

The effects of exceedingly mild head injury can be appreciated through behavioral evaluation. These effects can be demonstrated to persist in some form even when, to relatively sophisticated examination, they may appear to have resolved. The apparently recovered patient who, without specific concerns such as memory loss, still complains about a reduction in mental stamina or energy, especially when tired or when under stress, is a distressingly common phenomenon. Ewing *et al.*[18] studied university students who had closed head injuries and measurable, albeit subtle, cognitive deficits from which recovery was both rapid and seemingly complete within 6 months. They were compared to normal colleagues, three years after head injury, under usual examination procedures and found to be as able as peers on even the most complex tasks. When both groups were placed in a hyperbaric chamber at a simulated altitude of 3,800 feet, however, the performance of the head-injured students, on tasks of memory and vigilance, was clearly impaired. If such minimal stress presented to young, mildly injured and apparently recovered students three years after injury can result in residua, the con-

fidence with which one can dismiss a patient's complaints as neurotic has at least been shaken. Symonds[53] appears to be correct when he stated: "It is, I think, questionable whether the effects of concussion, however slight, are ever completely reversible."

What was approached in the past as a simple and clearly self-limiting disorder from which full recovery was the norm has emerged as a far more complex entity. Careful neuropsychological examination reveals deficits quite consistent with the areas of function claimed by patients to be impaired. The expectation that recovery follows a one-way course beginning with a very rapid early improvement with gradual slowing over the period of six to eighteen months followed in turn by either stability or, in some cases, continued very slow further improvement, while still widely accepted, has been challenged.

Studies in France and the United States suggest that at least some patients may actually regress 18 months to 3 years after a period of good recovery[38, 57]

POST-TRAUMATIC SYNDROME

The term traumatic neurosis was originated by Oppenheim.[46] Because neurosis can occur without any injury at all, Miller recommended the term accident neurosis.[42] Oddy *et al.*[44] compared the complaints of head-injured patients with other patients admitted to the hospital for disorders unrelated to the central nervous system. They found that after any illness and absence from home and work there are certain psycho-social consequences. Even though these investigators failed to examine carefully the patient's cognitive skills, they did find areas of specific head injury-related deficits such as restlessness, irritability, impatience, and social isolation. They failed to find a relationship between delay in return to work and pending litigation in their head-injured patients. Despite the existence of some patients who are obvious malingerers, the number of such individuals has been overestimated.[48]

Dizziness, headache, fatigue, irritability, anxiety, and memory and concentration problems are the principal symptoms of the post-traumatic syndrome. Sir Aubry Lewis[37] referred to the syndrome as: "That common dubious psychopathic condition—the bugbear of the clear-minded doctor and lawyer." Lishman's[39] excellent review points out that neurotics can have head injuries and head-injured persons so disposed can manifest significant neurotic symptoms after their concussion which can, in fact, be quite disabling. While these can make clear diagnosis more difficult, the types of symptoms discussed in this context are quite different from the primarily cognitive ones focused on in this chapter which can also produce secondary emotional distress. In fact, it is this far larger group of patients with real and documentable, albeit mild, deficits who require but commonly fail to receive proper referral and examination so that their condition can be appropriately treated.

EVALUATION OF BEHAVIORAL SEQUELAE OF HEAD INJURY

The presence of behavioral-mental deficits which can be identified on the routine mental status examination is not a reliable indicator of type and severity of post-traumatic behavioral disorders. These deficits can only be discovered by more complex psychological testing.[15, 36, 56] For at least two decades, neurologists have recognized that a battery of neuropsychological tests is essential for appreciation of the patient's mental status.[13] Wechsler[58] indicated "no neurological status is complete without a mental examination" and "a complete mental examination can take several hours." The elements necessary for an adequate appreciation of mental deficits following mild head injury seem reasonably well agreed upon by clinicians approaching the problem from clinical or research, theoretical or empirical points of view.[6, 17, 36] The major elements of such examination are listed in Table 19.3.

These nine elements may be summarized as follows: 1) The use of a *standard psychometric device* such as the Wechsler Intelligence Scale will often provide data suggesting the patient's IQ is in the average

Table 19.3
Aspects of Human Behavior Recommended for Minimum Examination to Determine Sequelae of Head Injury

Psychometric intelligence	Wechsler intelligence scale
Academic achievement	Reading, spelling, arithmetic
Motor skill	Speed and coordination
Attention and concentration	Brief and sustained
Perception	Visual, tactile, auditory
Language	Word naming/fluency
Memory	Modality-material-length
Information processing	New learning, simultaneous problem solving, cognitive manipulation, resistence to interference
Personality	Coping style—resilience to stress

range. However, average psychometric IQ's are in no way synonymous with normal intelligence broadly understood and, when used alone, are entirely inadequate as a measure of mental functioning after any type of brain impairment in adults. Nevertheless, as part of a more complete battery of tests, they can provide useful information.[6] 2) Measures of academic achievement are important for issues of re-training and return to work and school. 3) Tests of *motor skills* are useful in assessing recovery and work potential and add an index of the patient's motivation in areas where deficits can be expected to be slight barring focal brain lesions.

4) Tests of *attention and concentration* are standard in almost all psychological examinations, even though the concepts of attention and concentration are themselves poorly understood. This segment of the examination attempts to assess that mecha-

nism necessary for use of all other mental skills. If there is a defect here all aspects of more complex mental activity are likely to be disrupted. 5) *Perception* of forms, faces (visual), environmental sounds (auditory), and tactile stimuli are so routine in life as to be often overlooked during behavioral examination. Deficits in any of these areas can be easily missed in observing the patient. Yet, such deficits may serve as disruptive factors when the patient attempts activities as complex as drafting and playing music, and as common as driving a car or as basic as recognizing neighborhood and friends. Deficits in such areas can make the patient act and feel quite abnormal without identification of the nature of the problem as related to ability rather than emotional and motivational difficulties. 6) *Language* disorders which are recognizable on brief mental status screening usually resolve quickly. One could easily recommend and defend a complete aphasia examination for every patient. This is true because language deficits, even mild "sub-clinical" ones, can disrupt many other higher level mental activities involved in school and occupational activities. Many aphasia batteries actually include tasks of problem solving, learning, and memory and thus provide a more comprehensive evaluation than their title suggests. Short of such time-consuming examinations, however, a test of some length (50 items) of naming skill seems the mandatory minimum. Dysnomia is seen in a variety of conditions producing brain damage and may be present in the absence of other signs of aphasia or lateralized cerebral damage. It is not the kind of deficit associated with neurosis or malingering except when the effort to fail is so obvious as to be immediately recognizable.

7) *Memory* is another term that encompasses what is known and what is yet to be learned. Any neuropsychological examination should cover verbal and non-verbal material, auditory, visual, and tactile modalities, and the immediate, short-term, long-term, and historical lengths of memory function. As with all aspects of the amnestic process, diffuse cortical and subcortical lesions appear to produce disruption here. Patients so impaired may score well on IQ and standard interview tests and yet, to themselves and others, seem strangely different, less efficient and less organized for reasons that can be clarified only if a proper examination is performed. 8) Problem solving and *information processing* involve assessment of mental process rather than relying upon examination of mental content. Such tasks are different from the usual clinical-psychological tests and are far more sensitive to the types of previously invisible deficits that produce the bulk of the cognitive and subsequent emotional disruption after apparently benign head injury. Such tasks require an ability to learn, to switch sets flexibly, to deal with unfamiliar information efficiently, and to maintain a train of thought against interference or to maintain two aspects of a situation in mind simultaneously while alternately responding to each. It is on such complex tasks, when added to more standard neuropsychological batteries[7] or used alone[17, 23] that the pattern and rate of recovery, its extent and limitations, can best be assessed. Such procedures when employed alone for research or in the context of a complete evaluation for clinical purposes allow early appreciation of the presence of deficits. 9) *Personality* evaluation is performed to provide the fullest possible understanding of the nature of the patient's reaction to the head injury. Levin and Grossman[34] documented the increases in personal disruption that correlated with more severe injuries. Their findings, using structured interview techniques, were comparable to those obtained on the Minnesota Multiphasic Personality Inventory in showing that even mild head injury leads to increased anxiety and somatic concern.[14] They found thinking disturbances, emotional withdrawal, and blunted affect suggesting additional areas in need of early intervention with family members so that such reactions do not produce greater harm than the head injury itself. In Lishman's[39] words "what is virtually certain, however, is that the mental sequelae outstrip the physical as a cause of difficulty with rehabilitation, hardship at work and social incapacity and in terms of the strain thrown on the families to whom the head injured patient is returned."

MANAGEMENT OF BEHAVIORAL SEQUELAE

Management of behavioral sequelae for most acute care physicians involves conveying realistic information to the patient and his family and appropriate and early referral for the evaluations necessary to obtain that data. A clean bill of health offered on the basis of adequately documented evidence of absence of deficit is a welcome outcome of such referral. The consequences of such reassurances based on absence of evidence of deficit due to lack of proper evaluation may become the most disruptive aspect of the head injury and its care.

When deficit is documented, two courses are open and can be pursued individually or in combination: 1) fixing, 2) coping. Fixing is the one option all would chose were it available, but frequently, it is not. Three recent reviews of interventional approaches to behavioral sequelae of neurological disorders suggest that the scientific basis for rehabilitation, enhancement of neurologic recovery, and deficit repair has yet to be established.[3, 10, 16] This is not to say that physical, occupational, and speech therapies are without benefit. Rather, the specific relationship between types of brain damage, type of intervention, and even timing of that intervention (how early to begin, when to end) has not been subject to sufficient study. Moreover, the evidence that these or other behavioral therapies can actually influence brain recovery or return of function has yet to be demonstrated.

Nevertheless, avoidance of pathological linguistic, physical, and emotional responses to the initial deficit clearly result in the patient's being able to benefit from his own natural recovery process. Furthermore, techniques based on our understanding of the behavioral consequences of brain damage with regard to learning new material greatly enhance the chance that what the patient can learn will be learned with greatest efficiency and least discouragement. In this way, avoidance of even further harm through development of negative attitudes, discouragement and even depression can be accomplished. This is no small accomplishment even if it does fall short of an actual "fix."

Coping involves far more than "putting up" with the unfixable. The first step in coping is *understanding* the situation as it actually is—not just as it appears and not just the acute surgical aspects. Results of the EEG, CT scan, and neurological examination provide no behavioral data; when normal, they provide no guarantee that a patient will not be temporarily or even permanently functionally impaired. A careful neuropsychological evaluation, while also unable to prove the negative (no deficit), approaches the issue of behavior directly and with sufficient sensitivity to assess the sequelae of even relatively mild head injuries. With such data in hand, the physician is in a position to discuss with the patient and/or family the areas in which the patient is likely to seem different, experience difficulty, and pose an extra burden on others. Areas where failure is likely can be anticipated and avoided. A return to challenging tasks can be guided by data from initial and repeat evaluations suggesting, along with the patient's experience, the proper rate of expectation and challenge for the individual.

A patient who attempts to return to work or school too soon may experience unexpected and atypical difficulty and failure which may lead to two additional problems. First, failure at previously well-managed tasks, in the absence of a known reason, results in anxiety, loss of self-esteem, even depression. Second, a reduction in the quality of performance when unexplained is most commonly assumed to be due to a defect in motivation rather than to a lack of ability. The combination of increasing anxiety, self-doubt, and the desire to avoid threatening situations or tasks when coupled with the dissatisfaction or anger of family or colleagues can be easily seen to contain all the necessary ingredients for an "emotional" disorder or "personality change." Such reactions are frequently treated without awareness of their etiology and, for that reason, treatment is prolonged and frequently unsuccessful.

On the other hand, knowing the existence of deficits, even when upsetting and not readily accepted at first telling, aids the patient, family, and employer to know the most appropriate pace of return to function to avoid negative secondary reactions described above. Early consultation with follow-ups as requested is far more cost-effective and beneficial to the patient than prolonged therapy for a disorder that was avoidable to begin with. Such early knowledge and preventive treatment applies to children and adults alike. Klonoff *et al.*,[31] in an excellent five year follow-up, have demonstrated that recovery continues in some children for 5 years and perhaps longer. Failure to recognize that all is not regained in 6 to 12 months or when the child "looks and talks okay" can lead to a degree of school mismanagement more harmful than the original deficit. Levin and Eisenberg[33] confirmed these findings and stated "neuropsychological evaluation in this study identified deficits with obvious relevance for education and overall adjustment in children and adolescents. Recognition of specific problems in language, memory, and other ability after head injury would facilitate the planning of the patient's education and provide indications for special services such as remedial instruction, speech therapy, and physical therapy."

Families who are told of the likelihood of cognitive and personality deficits and changes very frequently react with their best effort. Families surprised by such changes tend to react with rejection and anger until an explanation is given. Patients who know they are "different" would far rather have these differences recognized than denied leaving them to wonder whether they have become suddenly lazy or even crazy. Knowledge of one's limitations, even new and possibly temporary ones, can be managed. Failure to know and be helped to accept these limitations can produce no end of mischief for all involved.

Return to employment, while not necessarily more critical than return to family, presents even greater management problems. Frequently, the patient does not want his employer to know of his intellectual impairments. This leaves the physician to aid the patient in gradually increasing challenge, responsibility, and use of advanced skills in a situation out of his control. Requests for reduced duties, reduced time at work, retraining or temporary supervision may represent red flags jeopardizing the patient's situation as surely as unsatisfactory performance.

For persons in very mentally demanding positions who may seem at most risk from mild memory problems, the tendency of such jobs to be evaluated on the basis of meeting long-term goals rather than day-to-day production represents something of a cushion. Conversely, a person seemingly safe from harm due to the routine nature of his employment may find himself penalized for even a day or two of reduced efficiency in hourly production which can easily be monitored.

In summary, unless the complex issues of adequate evaluation and intervention are considered in the context of what is now known about the sequelae following even mild head injury, the best care cannot be provided.

References

1. Aita, J.A., Reitan, R.M.: Psychotic reactions in the late recovery period following brain injury. Am. J. Psych. 105:161–169, 1948.
2. Annegers, J.F., Grabow, J.D., Kurland, L.T., Laws, E.R.: The incidence, causes, and secular trends of head trauma in Olmsted County, Minnesota, 1935–1974. Neurology, 30:912–919, 1980.
3. Barth, J.T., Boll, T.J.: Rehabilitation and treatment of central nervous system dysfunction: a behavioral medicine perspective. In: Medical Psychology: A New Perspective, C. Prokop, L. Bradley, Eds., Academic Press, New York, 1981.
4. Bell, B., A System of Surgery. C. Elliot, Edinburgh, 1787.
5. Black, P., Shepard, R.H., Walker, A.E.: Outcome of head trauma: Age and post-traumatic seizures. In: Outcome of Severe Damage to the Central Nervous System, R. Porter, D.W. Fitzsimons, Eds. Elsevier, Amsterdam, Ciba Foundation Symposium 34, 1935.
6. Boll, T.J.: Diagnosing brain impairment. In: Clinical Diagnosis of Mental Disorders, B.B. Wolman, Ed. Plenum Publishing Corp., 1978.
7. Boll, T.J.: The Halstead-Reitan neuropsychology battery. In: Handbook of Clinical Neuropsychology, S.B. Filskov, T.J. Boll, Eds. John Wiley & Sons, New York, 1981.
8. Bond, M.R.: Assessment of the psychosocial outcome of severe head injury. Acta Neurochir., 34:57–70, 1976.
9. Caveness, W.: Incidence of cranio-cerebral trauma

in the United States. Trans. Am. Neurol. Assoc., 102:136–138, 1977.

10. Cleeland, C.S.: Biofeedback as a clinical tool: Its use with the neurologically impaired patient. In: Handbook of Clinical Neuropsychology, S.B. Filskov, T.J. Boll, Eds. New York, John Wiley & Sons, 1981.

11. Cooper, A.: Principles and Practice of Surgery. London, 1836.

12. Davison, K., Bagley, C.R.: Schizophrenia-like psychoses associated with organic disorders of the central nervous system: a review of the literature. In: Current Problems in Neuropsychiatry. R.N. Herrington, Ed. British J. Psych., Special Publication No. 4, 1969, pp. 113–184.

13. DeJong, R.N.: The Neurologic Examination. New York, Hoeber, 1967.

14. Dikmen, S., Reitan, R.M.: Emotional sequelae of head injury. Ann. Neurol., 2:492–494, 1977.

15. Dikmen, S., Reitan, R.M.: Neuropsychological performance in posttraumatic epilepsy. Epilepsia, 19:177–183, 1978.

16. Diller, L., Gordon, W.A.: Rehabilitation and clinical neuropsychology. In: Handbook of Clinical Neuropsychology, S.B. Filskov, T.J. Boll, Eds. John Wiley & Sons, New York, 1981.

17. Eson, M., Bourke, R.: Assessment of information processing deficits after serious head injury. Presented at the 8th Annual Meeting of the International Neuropsychological Society, 1980.

18. Ewing, R., McCarthy, D., Gronwall, D., Wrightson, P.: Persisting effects of minor head injury observable during hypoxic stress. J. Clin. Neuropsychol., 2:147–155, 1980.

19. Fahy, T.J., Irving, M.H., Millack, P.: Severe head injury: a six-year follow-up. Lancet, 2:475–479, 1967.

20. Field, G.H.: Epidemiology of Head Injuries in England and Wales. Her Majesty's Stationary Office, London, 1976.

21. Gennarelli, T.A., Adams, G.H., Graham, D.I.: Acceleration induced head injury in the monkey: the model, its mechanical and physiological correlate. Acta Neuropathol. Suppl., 7:23–25, 1981.

22. Gronwall, D., Wrightson, P.: Cumulative effect of concussion. Lancet, 2:995–997, 1975.

23. Gronwall, D., Wrightson, P.: Duration of posttraumatic amnesia after mild head injury. J. Clin. Neuropsychol., 2:51–60, 1980.

24. Grunthal, E.: Euber die erkennung der traumatischen hirnverletzung. Karger, Berlin, 1936.

25. Jacobson, S.: The Post Traumatic Syndrome Following Head Injury. Charles C Thomas, Springfield, Ill., 1963.

26. Jagger, J.: Epidemiology of central nervous trauma: Preliminary findings. Presented to the American Public Health Association 107th Annual Meeting, New York, November, 1979.

27. Jane, J.: Personal Communication.

28. Jennett, B.: Scale, scope, and philosophy of the clinical problems. In: Outcome of Severe Damage to the Central Nervous System. R. Porter, D.W. Fitzsimons, Eds. Ciba Foundation Symposium 34, Elsevier, Amsterdam, 1975.

29. Jennett, B., Teasdale, G., Knill-Jones, R.: Prognosis after severe head injury. In: Outcome of Severe Damage to the Central Nervous System, R. Porter, D.W. Fitzsimons, Eds. Ciba Foundation Symposium 34, Elsevier, Amsterdam, 1975.

30. Jennett, W.B.: Epilepsy After Non-Missile Head Injuries. Heinemann Medical Books, London, 1975.

31. Klonoff, H., Low, M.D., Clark, C.: Head injuries in children: a prospective five year follow-up. J. Neurol. Neurosurg. Psych., 40:1211–1219, 1977.

32. Kløve, H., Cleeland, C.S.: The relationship of neuropsychological impairment to other indices of severity of head injury. Scand. J. Rehab. Med., 4:55–60, 1972.

33. Levin, H.S., Eisenberg, H.M.: Neuropsychological outcome of closed head injury in children and adolescents. Child's Brain, 5:281–292, 1979.

34. Levin, H.S., Grossman, R.G.: Behavioral sequelae of closed head injury. Arch. Neurol., 35:720–727, 1978.

35. Levin, H.S., Grossman, R.G., Kelly, P.J.: Impairment of facial recognition after closed head injuries of varying severity. Cortex, 13:119–130, 1977.

36. Levin, H.S., Grossman, R.G., Rose, J.E., Teasdale, G.: Long-term neuropsychological outcome of closed head injury. J. Neurosurg., 50:412–422, 1979.

37. Lewis, A.: Discussion on differential diagnosis and treatment of post-contusional states. Proc. Roy. Soc. Med., 35:607–614, 1942.

38. Lezak, M.D.: Recovery of memory and learning functions following traumatic brain injury. Cortex, 15:63–72, 1979.

39. Lishman, W.A.: The psychiatric sequelae of head injury: a review. Psychol. Med., 3:304–318, 1973.

40. Maciver, I.N., Frew, I.J.C., Matheson, J.G.: The role of respiratory insufficiency in the mortality of severe head injuries. Lancet, 1:390–393, 1958.

41. Merritt, H.H.: Textbook of Neurology, 2nd Ed., Lea & Febiger, Philadelphia, 1959.

42. Miller, H.: Accident neurosis. Br. Med. J., 1:919–925, 1961.

43. Milner, B., Corkin, S., Teuber, H.L.: Further analysis of the Hippocampal Amnesic Syndrome: fourteen year follow-up study of H.M. Neuropsychologia, 6:215–234, 1968.

44. Oddy, M., Humphrey, M., Uttley, D.: Subjective impairment and social recovery after closed head injury. J. Neurol. Neurosurg. Psych., 41:611–616, 1978.

45. O'Leary, D.S., Seidenberg, M., Berent, S., Boll, T.J.: The effects of age of onset of tonic-clonic seizures on neuro psychological performance in children. Epilepsia, 22:197–204, 1981.

46. Oppenheim, H.: *Die Traumatischen Neurosen.* Berlin, Hirschwald, 1889.

47. Parker, S. A., Serrats, A.F.: Memory recovery after traumatic coma. Acta Neurochir., 34:71–77, 1976.

48. Rimel, R.W., Giordani, B., Barth, J.T., Boll, T.J., Jane, J.A.: Disability caused by minor head injury. Neurosurg., 9:221–228, 1981.

49. Roberts, A.H.: Brain Damage in Boxers. London, Pittman, 1969.

50. Russell, W.R., Nathan, P.W.: Traumatic amnesia. Brain, 69:280–300, 1946.

51. Seidenberg, M., O'Leary, D.S., Berent, S., Boll, T.: Changes in seizure frequency and test-retest scores on the WAIS. Epilepsia, 22:75–84, 1981.

52. Seidenberg, M., O'Leary, D.S., Giordani, B., Berent, S., Boll, T.J.: Test-retest IQ changes of epilepsy patients: assessing the influence of practice effects. J. Clin. Neuropsychol., 3:237–256, 1981.

53. Symonds, C.: Concussion and its sequelae. Lancet, 1:1–5, 1962.

54. Symonds, C.P.: In: Injuries of the Skull, Brain and Spinal Cord, S. Brock, Ed., Springer, New York, 1940.

55. Tennent, T.: Mental disorder following head injury. Proc. Roy. Soc. Med., 30:1092–1093, 1937.

56. Teuber, H.L.: Recovery of function after brain injury in man. In: Outcome of Severe Damage to the Central Nervous System, R. Porter, D.W. Fitzsimons, Eds. Ciba Foundation Symposium 34, Elsevier, Amsterdam, 1975.

57. Vigouroux, R.P., Bourand, C., Naquet, R., Chament, J.H., Choux, M., Benayoun, R., Bureau, M., Charpy, J.P., Clamens-Guey, M.J.: A series of patients with cranio-cerebral injuries studied neurologically, psychometrically, electroencephalographically and socially. In: Proceedings of an International Symposium held in Edinburgh and Madrid, April, 1970, Churchill Livingston, Edinburgh, 1971.

58. Wechsler, I.S.: Clinical Neurology. Strauss, Philadelphia, 1963.

59. Windle, W.F., Groat, R.A., Fox, C.A.: Experimental structural alterations in the brain during and after concussion. Surg. Gynecol. Obstet., 79:561, 1944.

20

Prognosis and Outcome in Severe Head Injury

STEVEN L. GIANNOTTA
JOHN M. WEINER
BARRY B. CERVERHA

It appears to me a most excellent thing for the physician to cultivate Prognosis; for by foreseeing and foretelling, in the presence of the sick, the present, the past, and the future, and explaining the omissions which patients have been guilty of, he will be the more readily believed to be acquainted with the circumstances of the sick; so that men will have confidence to intrust themselves to such a physician. As he will manage the cure best who has foreseen what is to happen from the present state of matters. For it is impossible to make all the sick well; this, indeed, would have been better than to be able to foretell what is going to happen; but since men die, some even before calling the physician, from the violence of the disease, and some die immediately after calling him, having lived, perhaps, only one day or a little longer, and before the physician could bring his art to counteract the disease; it therefore becomes necessary to know the nature of such affections, how far they are above the powers of the constitution; and, moreover, if there be anything divine in the diseases, and to learn a foreknowledge of this also. Thus a man will be the more esteemed to be a good physician, for he will be the better able to treat those aright who can be saved, from having long anticipated everything; and by seeing and announcing before-hand those who will live and those who will die, he will thus escape censure.[41]

Hippocrates can perhaps be pardoned if he emphasizes inordinately the physician's public image as a cardinal reason for developing the ability to prognosticate. He may have foreseen the recent medical malpractice crisis we have experienced in the United States. His writings, however, raise other important points that are germane to the discussion of prognosis in severe head injury. For as he states, " . . . it is impossible to make all the sick well. . . ." This concept is especially true of central nervous system trauma with its resultant severe disabilities which frequently are out of proportion to the volume of tissue that is damaged. As modern medicine continues to strive for the perhaps unattainable goal of "making all the sick well," the resulting technical advances in treatment inevitably lead to financial, social, and ethical problems for society to solve.

The brain-injured patient is a particular burden on our social structure and raises significant problems. Consider the young severely head-injured patient resuscitated in an acute care institution with all the modern means of therapy available. Biological life is rescued at an astronomical monetary cost only to have the patient succumb following several years of a vegetative existence and further financial and emotional cost to the family, not to mention the loss of a productive individual from our society.[54] Retrospectively, we ask ourselves, "Was it worth it?" "Might it have been better for all concerned had the patient not been resuscitated?" "Could the situation have been predicted and somehow avoided?" "Was there a new treatment available that could have improved the outcome; was the cost too high?" Judging by the recent literature, society's spokesmen are voicing these questions with increasing regularity.[1, 5, 39, 44, 54, 79] Studies are needed to ascertain the magnitude of the problem and potential solutions must be explored.

Of critical importance in attempts to lighten this public health burden on our social structure, is the acquisition of accurate data regarding the morbidity and mortality of head injuries. As we shall discuss, until recently there has been much confusion about the mortality rate of head injury, due mostly to the lack of an accurate system of classifying patients and information. With such organization, knowledge of the frequency and severity of disability, number of fatalities, as well as the number of patients who have a good outcome give focus to the work of increasing survival without increasing the number of those who remain vegetative.

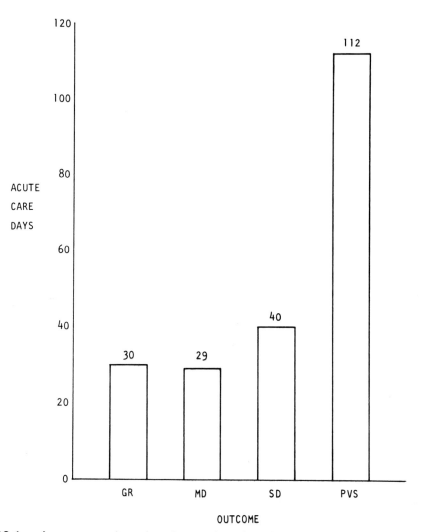

Figure 20.1. Average number of acute care inpatient days versus outcome from severe head injury. (*GR*, good recovery, *MD*, moderate disability; *SD*, severe disability; *PVS*, persistent vegetative state).

As a public health problem, head trauma may be attacked from a number of positions. Potentially, the most significant modality, but also the most difficult to implement, is prevention. Although it is not relevant to the present discussion, physicians involved in the care of trauma must recognize their responsibilities with regard to aiding society's programs in this endeavor. Better methods of treatment must continually be developed. Here, again, accurate prognostic data must be available so that the efficacy of newer treatment regimens can be evaluated. This knowledge will pay dividends by allowing physicians to discard those treatments not documented to increase survival.

Since no society has unlimited funds to extend the most advanced medical care to every ill person, reallocation of manpower and money may be another method of reducing the problem of brain trauma. As the cost of medical care rises, the price in itself becomes an all-consuming problem.[49, 61] Direct and indirect costs due to head injuries on a yearly basis exceed 2.5 billion dollars in the United States.[15] One small step in reducing those costs may be to identify those patients known to have no chance of survival and reallocate resources along more productive lines. This concept presupposes that such a group of patients can be accurately identified. Hence, the need to identify those factors related to poor survival becomes acute. Together with data on survival, a prognostication system should be developed to identify those who by today's medical means will not survive or who will survive but lead a useless, totally dependent existence.[40]

A quick example will graphically present the economic catastrophe of the severely brain injured. Figure 20.1 represents the number of days spent in the hospital for 12 randomly selected head-injured patients treated at LAC/USC Medical Center between 1977 and 1978. Glasgow Coma Scale was 8 or less upon admission. It is easy to see that the amount of time spent in the hospital and consequently total hospital bill is inversely proportional to the outcome of the patient. Those patients surviving in a vegetative state will, of course, go on to accrue further astronomical expenses for custodial care.

Other reasons for developing a method of calculating prognosis have been discussed (Table 20.1) and simply add further emphasis to the necessity of a reliable system.[44] The two most important reasons remain 1) the ability to judge the effectiveness of new treatment regimens, and 2) the deployment of economic resources and personnel in an efficient manner. The former reason assumes more importance in light of recent reports suggesting that such modern practices as respiratory support, steroids, and control of intracranial pressure may not have manifestly reduced mortality rate.[20, 28, 34, 51, 55] The latter reason is buttressed by the government's mandate to reduce the cost of medical care.

Over the past 10 years great strides have been made in developing a system to measure outcome and determine prognosis in the head injured. The most important step was taken by Jennett and his colleagues in organizing an international data bank to collect and categorize cases of head injury for the ultimate purpose of developing the power to prognosticate. This work will be discussed in detail as will the work of other authors who have investigated factors

Table 20.1

Uses for a Mathematical Model for Predicting Outcome in Head Injury

Utility of Predicting Outcome in Head Injury
Allocation of resources
Deployment of personnel
Deployment of equipment
Distribute elaborate but limited treatment regimens
Reduce cost of care
Evaluation of therapeutic advances
Efficacy of new practices
Limit established practices with little efficacy
Increase understanding of pathophysiology
Aid in management decisions
Reduce mortality
Reduce number of hopelessly disabled
Reduce uncertainty
Aid in counseling family
Aid in counseling medical team
Prepare convalescent or rehabilitation programs

which may not only affect outcome, but may be, in some way, predictive of outcome. Inevitably all facets of the care of brain-injured patients will be touched upon since aspects of the neurologic exam, methods of management, general physiologic status, associated injuries, laboratory data, and even demographic data may all be important in prognosis.

We will briefly look at what was known about the sequelae of acute head injury prior to the 1970's. This will provide some insight into the problems facing us today, especially the lack of a suitable method for organizing old head injury data so it can be analyzed in light of newer developments.[87] Several statistical methods for attempting to predict outcome will be presented along with possible areas to explore in the future if an easily applicable and accurate method is to be developed.

UPDATING PROGNOSIS OF HEAD INJURY

In 1978 Langfitt reviewed the head injury literature and concluded that since the turn of the century very little useful information on mortality and morbidity was available.[51] Several reports in the first decade of this century set the mortality rate in the range of 50–60%, although rates as high as 90% have also been reported.[21, 68, 71] Little was then written concerning the outcome of head injury until the 1950's when Maciver suggested that aggressive pulmonary management with intubation and mechanical ventilation could reduce the mortality rate from 90 to 40%.[55] However, in later reports mortality rates for severe head injury continued to hover around the 50% mark. Carlsson et al.[14] collected 196 patients who were unconscious for over 24 hours. Thirty-five percent of those patients died. His series did not include cases of intracranial hematoma, emphasizing the problem of lack of comparability among different series. Reports by other authors at about that same time continued to suggest that the mortality rate was still about 50%.[10, 23, 24, 35, 38, 65, 67, 69, 92]

Several important conclusions can be drawn from the head injury literature prior to the mid 1970's. First, it appears that despite significant advances in care of the critically ill, the mortality rate for acute injury reported in the previous 80 years had not changed dramatically. One possible explanation, foreseen by a number of early authors, was the lack of comparability of the reported series due to the lack of a definition of severity and the lack of a uniform method of classification. Phelps put it quite succinctly in 1909 when he said, "There is no class of injuries in which the issues are at all times so uncertain and so surprising."[68] In essence, these early investigators were all talking about different populations. Another possible explanation for the lack of significant change in mortality is that no treatment modality has been introduced that can significantly influence outcome. Again, this may be a reflection of a lack of uniform population in which to test various therapeutic agents.

It becomes apparent after reviewing past efforts, that before any advances are made in determining or predicting the individual patient's prognosis from a severe head injury, a universally acceptable method of classifying cases is necessary. Such a system should take into consideration the severity of the brain injury as well as those variables which influence the eventual outcome. Furthermore, any classification system must not only identify those who die and those who make a good recovery, but it must also identify gradations of disability, since much of our efforts must be directed at improving outcome in this group. In 1968, a concerted effort was made to gather a large volume of data for the purpose of categorizing injury and outcome in an acceptable way. These attempts are the subject of the following discussion.

GLASGOW COMA STUDY

In 1968 under the direction of Bryan Jennett, the Institute of Neurological Sciences in Glasgow instituted an international data bank. The purpose was to collect information from several trauma centers about those patients who suffered severe head injury. Two centers in the Netherlands were added in 1972 and finally Los

Angeles County Hospital was added in 1974 to complete the cohort.

A standard method for reporting data was employed by all reporting centers, and ultimately led to the development of a method of assessing the severity of brain damage, for monitoring progress, and finally for uniformly describing outcome. Once these objectives were met, the data bank would be used to compare the results of different methods of management in single or separate centers, as well as to be able to accurately predict prognosis in individual head injured patients.

The success of this data bank depends, in part, on a simple and accurate method of recording serial observations by hospital personnel in describing various states of impaired consciousness. In 1974, Teasdale and Jennett described a clinical scale assessing the depth and duration of coma.[85] This has come to be called the Glasgow Coma Scale or Score. This scale examines three aspects of behaviour independently; eye opening, motor response, and finally verbal response (see Chapter 2). The range of possible scores is from 3 to 15. Coma, which was defined as the state in which patients are unable to open their eyes, verbalize coherently, or are unable to follow simple commands, is by definition any score of 8 or less. Employing this system, different observers were able to elicit similar scores with a high degree of consistency, thus diminishing the likelihood of ambiguous and inconsistent reports. Aside from the obvious ease of use by medical personnel, the scale afforded a more objective means for assessment of the depth and duration of coma.

The next objective of the data bank was to formulate a standardized means for describing the ultimate outcome following head injury. Existing classifications of survivors were too general in description, subjective and optimistic in character, and often failed to estimate the extent of the mental handicap present. In 1975, the Glasgow Group reported a practical outcome scale which enabled surviving patients to be classified into five categories according to overall social outcome, thus considering both the persistent mental and physical

sequelae (Table 20.2).[43, 86] The classification is as follows: DEATH (D)—Directly related to the head injury or the consequences thereof; PERSISTENT VEGETATIVE STATE (PVS)—Patients without awareness or speech who do not respond to external stimuli, but who have cycles of wakefulness and sleep; SEVERE DISABILITY (SD)—Patients who are totally dependent because of cognitive or physical handicaps. They may or may not be institutionalized. MODERATE DISABILITY (MD)—The patients are independent in the chores of daily life, i.e., self-care, cooking and utilization of public transportation. Disabilities may include aphasia, hemiparesis, ataxia, etc.; and GOOD RECOVERY (GR)—The patient resumes a normal life despite minor neurological or psychological deficits. The pursuit of leisure or occupational goals is possible but not mandatory. Practical application of this scale has subsequently been employed for some years and a good measure of agreement between observers has been found.

The information acquired by the international data bank was ultimately used to report the progress of 1,000 patients whose clinical features of brain dysfunction during the first week following severe head injury were related to outcome six months later.[45, 48] In addition to the Glasgow Coma Scale, serial examinations of pupillary reactivity, spontaneous eye movements, and oculovestibular reflexes were performed. Because of the dynamic nature of severe head injury, the best and worst responses were noted at 24 hours, 2–3 days, and 4–7 days after the onset of coma. It was not uncommon to see early improvement in the level of consciousness, brain stem reflexes, and pupillary reactivity following fluid and oxygen resuscitation. As it turned out, the best response was a more reliable indication

Table 20.2
Glasgow Outcome Scale

Good recovery (GR)
Moderate disability (MD)
Severe disability (SD)
Persistant vegetative state (PVS)
Death (D)

of prognosis. In one-quarter of the patients studied, the 24-hour coma score was higher than that obtained at admission. Thus, to be included in this study, the patient had to remain in coma for at least six hours (coma defined previously as a state in which patients are unable to open their eyes, verbalize coherently, or follow simple commands). Those patients who died or became brain-dead within the 6 hour limit were excluded. Data accumulation contained through 1976 and a follow up was reported in 1979.[45]

Table 20.3 summarizes certain characteristics common to the patients upon their introduction into the data bank. Distribution of most parameters was fairly uniform among the centers despite the geographical disparity and differences in referral systems. The mean age for the cohort was 34 years, variance between the centers being no more than 2 years. Almost one-half of the total cases harbored intracranial hematomas and slightly more than one-quarter of the cases demonstrated a lucid interval. Over one-half of the patients had a coma score of 5 or greater.

It can be seen from Table 20.4 that al-

Table 20.3
Selected Patient Characteristics from 1000 Cases in International Head Injury Data Bank[45]

Characteristics	%
Lucid interval	29
Intracranial hematoma	48
Extracranial injury	40
Coma sum 24-hr.	
3/4	18
5/6/7	55
Unreactive pupils	23
Impaired eye movements	42

Table 20.4
Outcome at 6 Months (International Head Injury Data Bank)[45]

Outcome	%
Good recovery	23
Moderate disability	17
Severe disability	10
Vegetative	2
Dead	48

Table 20.5
Outcome at 6 Months *vs.* Best Coma Sum at 3 Days Following Injury[45]

Coma Sum	D/PVS%	MD/GR%
3/4	97	0
5	79	11
6	61	21
7	41	38
8	28	61

most 50% of the patients died of their injuries. This figure is in keeping with results from other less elaborately analyzed studies, suggesting this figure as somewhat of a threshold value.[10, 23, 35, 38, 65, 67, 69, 92] Table 20.5 compares eventual outcome with coma score at three days following injury. No patient whose best score was 3 or 4 at this time following injury made a satisfactory recovery. Well over one-half of those cases with a score of 8 attained a moderate or good recovery. The presence of an intracranial hematoma negatively affected outcome. It should be noted that only patients who remained in coma for 6 hours following evacuation were included in the study, thus eliminating some favorable cases.

An exhaustive analysis of factors influencing outcome was performed by the organizers of the data bank. The influence on outcome of such divergent factors as age, coma score, autonomic abnormalities, cause of injury, extracranial injuries, and various clinical neurologic abnormalities was calculated and published. These relationships formed the basis for the development of a sophisticated means of prognostication for individual patients. Statistical methods developed by several of the most important contributors to this work will be discussed. We hope that sample calculations will show the utility of such methods.

PREDICTING OUTCOME IN THE INDIVIDUAL PATIENT

The collaborative International Head Injury Study and its resultant data bank brought sorely needed organization to an unwieldy and often anecdotal body of information. Outcome data resulting from this effort can now be realistically used as a comparison for outcome from new forms of therapy. Aside from a standardized method of classifying head injuries according to severity of brain damage, other important contributions have been mostly methodological. The study demonstrated the feasibility of a multi-centered, cooperative investigation, it confirmed the influence of clinical factors in differentiating outcome and explored the importance of these factors with newer statistical approaches. Lastly, the study stimulated research by other groups so that a number of points have become well established thus setting the stage for nwer developments.

PREDICTION FROM CLINICAL CHARACTERISTICS

This method, as outlined by Jennett and Teasdale,[85] relies exclusively on clinical observations in selecting features with prognostic power. The rationale for using only clinical parameters was that such data was universally available regardless of the center in which the patient was treated. Also, it was determined that such indicants as eye signs and motor responses can be recorded with little interobserver error. As an example, four classical predictors and their relation to outcome are shown in Figures 20.2 through 20.5. Outcome is expressed in terms of the Glasgow Outcome Scale with five categories ranging from good recovery to death. In these analyses, good recovery and moderate disability patients are pooled and patients with persistent vegetative state are added to those who died. The resulting two categories D/PVS and MD/ GR comprise better than 90% of the total patients in the data bank.

Age

Figure 20.2 plots the outcome from head injury of three distinct age groups in the data bank, and shows that outcome is significantly different (p < 0.05). The data

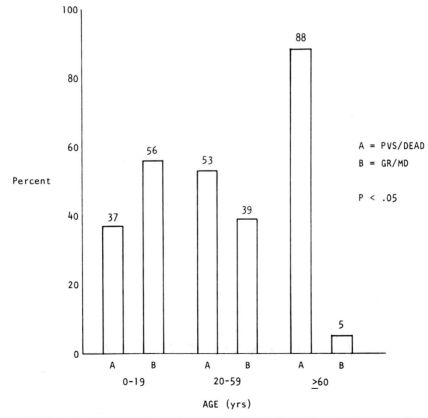

Figure 20.2.   Three age categories and their relationship to extremes of outcome.

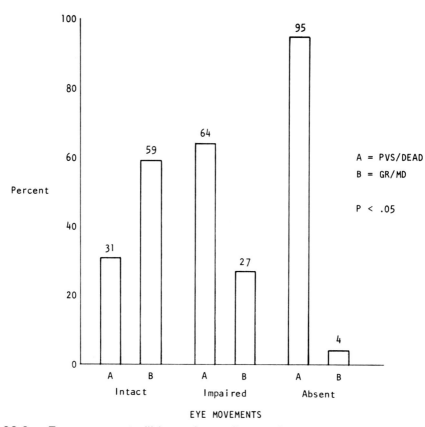

Figure 20.3. Eye movements (lid opening, reflex, and spontaneous ocular responses) and their relationship to extremes of outcome (24 hour best response).[45]

show that 88% of those patients aged 60 or older experienced a poor outcome, while only 5% were in the good outcome group. Thus, by subtraction, 7% of those 60 or older were in the severe disability group. Comparing the three age groups shows that, as age and poor outcome increase, age and good outcome decrease. Thus, 56% of those less than 20, 39% of those aged 20–59, and 5% of those over 60 experienced a good recovery or moderate disability.

Age has been considered an important factor in influencing survival in central nervous system injury for a considerable time. Russell in his study of 200 cases of head trauma in 1932 found that mortality was higher in older patients.[74] The fifth decade seemed to be a cutoff point after which mortality rapidly rose. Pazzaglia and associates[67] demonstrated a clear relationship

between age and outcome. Patients less than 20 years at injury recovered completely, while patients over the age of 60 died. The proportions showing these responses were statistically significant.

The evidence linking the aged nervous system to potential for recovery from structural damage is drawn from experimental work in animals; and while it supports the concept that age is an important prognostic factor, it has not led to new therapeutic approaches or to a clearer understanding of the clinical course.[9, 35] Carlsson and his colleagues[14] from Sweden contrasted patients who died as a direct result of their brain injuries with a group who died from extracranial complications. Their results showed that complications occurred almost exclusively and increasingly in the higher age groups. Thus, the possibility exists, supported by the work of others, that age may simply label those patients with an increased likelihood of having associated injuries and complications.[10, 12, 20] This concept does offer management potentials. Further studies describing these complications accurately and completely may lead to further therapeutic advances.

Eye Movements

Figure 20.3 demonstrates a statistically significant relationship between eye movements and outcome using data from the international data bank. Poor outcome (D/PVS) increased from 31% in patients with intact function, to 64% in patients with impaired function, to 95% in those with absent eye movements. Good outcome patients (GR/MD) showed a negative relationship to eye movement dysfunction.

Fifty-nine percent of those with intact eye movements experienced a good outcome in contrast to 4% with absent eye movements.

Neuroanatomical pathways responsible for eye movements are adjacent to brainstem areas controlling consciousness, making eye movement evaluation important in assessing the extent of coma. In comatose patients, voluntary cortical control over eye movements is lost and oculocephalic reflexes become brisk. Lesions of the brainstem producing destruction or compression of tissue produce oculocephalic reflex abnormalities. So the constellation of eye movement responses can serve to estimate location, if not severity, of central nervous system trauma. Heiden's results reinforce the concept that poor eye movement reflexes are a negative prognostic factor.[37] Only 4% of his patients made a good recov-

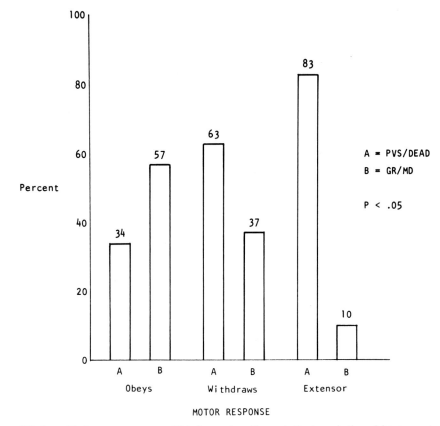

Figure 20.4. Motor responses (24 hour best) and their relationship to extremes of outcome.[45]

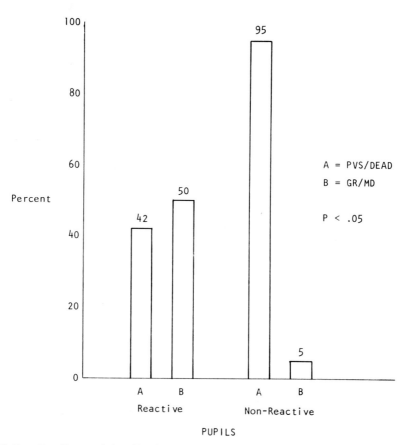

Figure 20.5.   Pupil reactivity (24 hour best) and its relationship to extremes of outcome.[45]

ery when oculovestibular reflexes were absent or dysconjugate. Fifty-four percent made a good recovery when such reflexes were intact. Braakman *et al.*[8] found oculovestibular responses to be a powerful predictor of prognosis during the first week following injury. The characteristic diminished in importance later, presumably because many of those patients whose responses were severely impaired died early. Stablein's analysis selected oculocephalic reflexes as one of the 12 most influential factors in his model of predicting outcome from head trauma.[81]

In contrast to age, this variable is a specific measure of the extent of damage and as such is an indicant in its own right of outcome. There are circumstances which can reduce the prognostic value of eye findings. The predictive power is negatively influenced by sedative or antiepileptic drugs. There may also be errors in recognizing or reporting the responses; a formal study of interobserver agreement revealed more error in recording all three types of eye movements than when recording motor response or pupillary reaction.[3, 46, 85] Part of the problem lies in the interrelationship between voluntary, oculocephalic, and oculovestibular movements. Avezaat suggested that they be combined as a single eye indicant, but identification of the most important of the three for prediction may further simplify recording.[3]

Motor Responses

Motor responses (Fig. 20.4) show the same pattern of increasingly poor outcome with decreasing functional level. Only 34% of the group obeying commands showed a poor outcome, whereas 83% with extensor posturing did poorly among the patients in the International Head Injury Study. Heiden reported a similar correlation in 184 consecutive patients with head injuries resulting in coma.[37] Fully 90% of their patients with no movement or extensor posturing ended in the D/PVS category at one year. Braakman, reporting his experience in Holland, showed a 100% mortality rate in those cases who were flaccid on admission, whereas 73% with purposeful movements had a useful outcome.[8]

One of the more notable communications linking abnormal motor responses to outcome comes from Bricolo and his colleagues.[10, 12] In a comprehensive study of severely head-injured cases, they were able to identify distinct patterns of flexor and extensor attitudes and relate them to prognosis. Among six types of motor response, classical decorticate posturing (6.6% of "decerebrate series") was associated with a lower mortality rate (57%) than bilateral decerebrate posturing (84.4%).

Several important concepts emerged from this study and others like it. It was reiterated that decerebrate posturing is not always indicative of a pure brainstem injury.[40, 63, 91] Evidence for this exists in some experimental models, but also in clinical examples of patients who remained conscious or had no ocular or vestibular signs of brainstem involvement.[35] These patients were among the relatively few who survived an injury associated with decerebration.

In the presence of abnormal extensor or flexor posturing, age had little influence on outcome in contradistinction to the findings of others.[35, 91, 92] However, decerebrate posturing in combination with several other neurologic abnormalities had an increasingly devastating effect on mortality. The combination of extensor posturing and deep coma or extensor posturing and brainstem ocular signs produced mortality rates of 77.6 and 95.4%, respectively.

Pupillary Size and Reflexes

Data from the International Head Injury Study demonstrated (Fig. 20.5) that pupillary reaction also correlates with outcome. Ninety-five percent of the group with non-

reactive pupils had a poor outcome. Those with reactive pupils showed almost equal proportions of poor and good outcomes. The Los Angeles series of cases reported by Heiden shows a similar pattern and only 3% of patients achieving a moderate or good recovery had unreactive pupils at 24 hours.[37] Others report similar findings.[8, 81]

The proximity of brainstem centers controlling consciousness and vegetative function to those mediating pupillary responses make such responses valuable in assessing coma. For this reason it is not surprising that the status of pupillary reactivity correlates closely with outcome. As with the motor responses and age, the state of the pupils is not an absolute indicator of prognosis. Bilateral fixed and dilated pupils may not always indicate that an individual will succumb. Pupillary responses do provide additive power when combined with other predictive variates.

Sum of Coma Score

By the turn of the century, the relationship between depth or duration of post-traumatic coma and prognosis was becoming better appreciated. Ransohoff described three somewhat ill-defined levels of unresponsiveness: stupor, unconsciousness, and deep coma.[71] He felt there was a demonstrable link between these levels and patient outcome. Although the principle was argued by some,[21] by 1930 quantification of the length or severity of coma was felt to be a useful predictor of the quality of outcome. The total interval of disturbed consciousness was defined as that period during which the patient was unable to store new information. This became known as post-traumatic amnesia (PTA). Longitudinal investigation of patients with head trauma generally confirmed the prognostic significance of PTA duration.[74, 75]

Numerical designation of depth of coma was not common until very recently. Overgaard devised a classification of neurological dysfunction which included depth of coma, motor response, and pupillary reactivity.[64, 65] Although his scale was more qualitative than quantitative, his categories correlated well with outcome. In 1974, Teasdale and Jennett introduced their coma scale which has since enjoyed wide acceptance.[85] For the first time, coma could be expressed numerically and although its shortcomings are not insignificant, it provided a shorthand method which almost quantified coma. Other scales have been devised but the greatest significance of the Glasgow Coma Score is its widespread use.[6, 20, 28, 53, 59]

Relationships between coma score sum and prognosis can be appreciated by reviewing Table 20.5. There appears to be a linear relationship between poor result and the lowest values of the scale. Both Heiden and Braakman demonstrated similar results in the populations they studied. Heiden was able to demonstrate that a coma sum of 8 or more at 24 hours was associated with an 83% chance of a moderate or good recovery.[8, 37] Braakman and his colleagues using their quadratic penalty score to assess the power of certain variables to aid in prediction and found coma sum to be important at each of six time epochs except day 28.

Thus, the utility of quantification of post-traumatic unresponsiveness in predicting prognosis seems established. It remains to be seen whether the Glasgow scale in its present form will be influential in precisely predicting all five of the Glasgow Outcome categories.

Timing

An important methodologic issue in calculating prognosis for the individual case is the time interval between the injury and the prediction. Timing is important in at least two respects. First, it is axiomatic that the longer one waits to make a prognosis, the more information will be available regarding the patient's course. As the information increases, so presumably does accuracy. Second, as the interval between the injury and the prediction increases, the value of making the prediction diminishes. Especially when contemplating allocation of medical resources or changes in management regimens, the earlier a decision is made, the more efficient the system becomes. Optimal timing of a prediction of outcome will occur when satisfactory accuracy can be obtained without sacrificing speed.

In the framework of the Glasgow Coma Study, probabilities were calculated at 24 hours, 2–3 days, and 4–7 days following admission to the study. A probability level of 0.97 was designated as "confident." Condensing outcome categories into D/PVS vs. recovery, 45% of existing cases could be predicted accurately at 24 hours. Jennett, however, emphasizes the lability of the neurological condition in the first 24 hours following injury.[43, 45, 48] Up to 50% of their patients manifested a coma score of 3/4 at some time during the first day after injury. Their accuracy increased to 61% of cases predicted at 2–3 days, and 68% predicted at 4–7 days. Since the majority of deaths from head trauma occur during the first week, the importance of speed is again emphasized.

Braakman attempted to predict death or survival in 305 cases of head injury at admission, day 1, 3, 7, 14 and 28.[8] The confidence limit was set at 0.90. Figure 20.6 plots the percentage of predictions which reached this level at the various time epochs. At day 3, 53% of cases could be predicted correctly, while at day 7, 60% were predictable. Further significant increases in accuracy did not occur until day 28.

Stablein and his colleagues did not analyze the concept of timing of prediction in their report.[81] Their data was collected at one time epoch, "after admission and resuscitation." Again outcome was expressed in two categories: GR/MD/SD vs. PVS/D. Using their combination of clinical and laboratory indicants and their logistic model, 69% of their predictions were made at the 0.90 confidence level. Their ability to make a slightly higher percentage of accurate predictions at an earlier stage than either Jennett or Braakman, may be a result of their statistical model or their use of additional laboratory indicants including CT scan and arterial blood gas values.

From Auer's study of 130 patients which attempted to predict a no chance survival from both laboratory and clinical data, the conclusion was reached that accurate predictions could not be made before 3 days.[2]

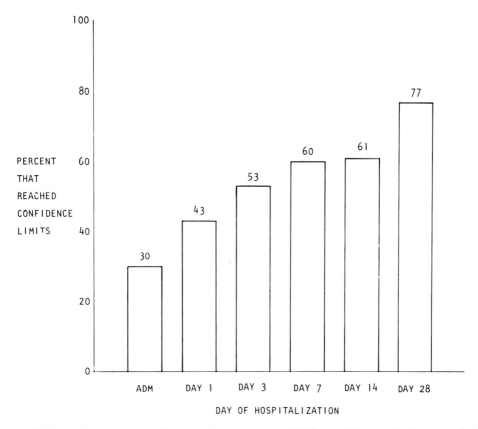

Figure 20.6.   Outcome predictions that reached 90% confidence limit at each time epoch following injury.[8]

Utilizing clinical data including coma scoring, it can be inferred that confident predictions of survival are possible at 24 hours following the injury. Further accuracy is gained at day 7 and day 28 but the trade off in delay reduces the usefulness.

MATHEMATICAL MODELS FOR PREDICTION

Bayesian Statistics

In 1976, Jennett and his colleagues, utilizing information from the data bank, attempted to develop a method of predicting outcome early in the course of a severe head injury.[46] In theory, a probability could be calculated as to which of five outcome categories (GR, MD, SD, PVS, D) a patient would most likely experience. Such a technique required the identification of the

most powerful predictors of outcome. Then in order to make a prediction, the clinical features of a given patient are compared to those of patients with known outcome (data bank) using Bayesian probability statistics. Statistical models developed by Stablein, Braakman, and others have also been effective in identifying variables important in classifying patients into outcome categories.[8, 81] The following discussion will illustrate the development of such a model based on three powerful clinical predictors using statistical tools similar to Jennett's. Alternate methods advanced by others will be included.

The basic analytic structure is shown in Table 20.6. Outcome categories are shown in vertical columns with good recovery and death representing the principal events. Variables significantly related to outcome

Table 20.6
Analytic Structure of System Relating Various Predictors to Outcome

OUTCOMES

'PREDICTOR'	DEAD/PVS	OTHER	TOTAL
I	NUMBER WITH LEVEL I and GOOD RECOVERY	NUMBER WITH LEVEL I and DEATH	NUMBER WITH LEVEL I
II	NUMBER WITH LEVEL II and GOOD RECOVERY	NUMBER WITH LEVEL II and DEATH	NUMBER WITH LEVEL II
TOTAL	NUMBER WITH GOOD RECOVERY	NUMBER DYING	TOTAL STUDIED

Table 20.7
Calculated Probabilities of Extremes of Outcome Related to Age[45]

OUTCOME

AGE	DEAD/PVS	OTHER	TOTAL
<20	106	214	320
20-59	270	259	529
≥60	131	20	151
Total	507	493	1000

$$P(\text{Age} <20 \mid \text{Dead}) = \frac{106}{507} \qquad P(\text{Age} <20 \mid \text{Other}) = \frac{214}{493}$$

$$P(\text{Age} \geq60 \mid \text{Dead}) = \frac{131}{507} \qquad P(\text{Age} \geq60 \mid \text{Other}) = \frac{20}{493}$$

$$P(\text{Dead}) = \frac{507}{1000} = .51 \qquad P(\text{Other}) = \frac{493}{1000} = .49$$

are shown as horizontal rows with categories ranging from those associated with good to poor outcome. As an example, figures from the data bank relating age to outcome (D/PVS versus other) are shown in Table 20.7. The estimated probabilities are also shown. The probability of being less than 20 years old and dying is given by the fraction 106/507 (21%) while the probability of being the same age and surviving is 214/493 (43%). The probability of dying is 507/1000 (51%) while the probability of living is 493/1000 (49%). The age relationship is seen by tracing the probabilities of age-death combinations and comparing these to the age-survival combinations. The age-death probabilities are: 21% (<20), 53% (20–59), and 26% (<60). In contrast, the age-death and age-survival probabilities are

illustrated graphically in Figure 20.7. The percentages are connected to demonstrate the shape distinctions across age.

Pupillary reaction and outcome are shown in Table 20.8. The probability of the

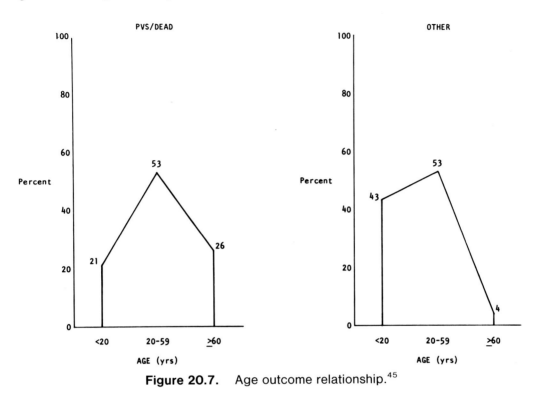

Figure 20.7.   Age outcome relationship.[45]

Table 20.8
Calculated Probabilities of Extremes of Outcome Related to Pupil Reactivity[45]

	OUTCOME		
PUPILS	DEAD/PVS	OTHER	TOTAL
Non-React	206	20	226
Reactive	292	456	748
Total	498	476	974

$$P(Pupils=React|Dead) = \frac{292}{498} \qquad P(Pupils=React|Other) = \frac{456}{476}$$

$$P(Pupils=Non-R|Dead) = \frac{206}{498} \qquad P(Pupils=Non-R|Other) = \frac{20}{476}$$

$$P(Dead) = \frac{498}{974} = .51 \qquad P(Other) = \frac{476}{974} = .49$$

combination of pupillary reactivity and death is 292/498 (59%), whereas reactive pupils and survival is 456/476 (96%). The overall probabilities for death and survival are still 51 and 49%.

The third associated variate is motor response (Table 20.9). The probabilities of the extremes of outcome (D/PVS versus other) for each category of motor responses are 122/501 (24%), 273/487 (56%), 162/501 (32%), and 29/487 (6%).

These tables then provide the necessary data to calculate the probability of a combination of characteristics—age <20, pupils = reactive, motor responses = obeys. The values are:

Probability (Combination and Death)
= Probability (Age <20 and death) × (Reactive pupils and Death) × (Motor Obeys and Death)
$$= 106/507 \times 292/498 \times 122/501$$
$$= 0.0299$$
Probability (Combination and Survival)
$$= 214/493 \times 456/476 \times 273/487 = 0.2331$$

These values when used in the Bayesian formula for estimating probabilities as described by the Glasgow group gives:

Probability of (Death and Combination) is

$$\frac{0.0299 \times .51}{0.0299 \times .51 + 0.2331 \times .49} = 0.1174$$

Similarly the Bayesian estimate for the combination —age >59 years, pupils nonreactive, and motor responses = extensor or nil—is:

Probability of (Death and Combination) is

$$\frac{(131/507 \times 206/498 \times 162/501) \times .51}{\begin{array}{c}(131/507 \times 206/498 \times 162/501) \times \\ .51 + (20/493 \times 20/476 \times 29/487) \times .49\end{array}}$$

$$= \frac{0.0176}{0.0176 + 0.000049}$$
$$= 0.9972$$

When only a few powerful predictors of outcome are used, relatively simple tables can be constructed for use in making predictions. Table 20.10 gives the probability of a poor outcome (D/PVS) given various values of age, pupillary reactivity, and motor response. For example, in patients under age 20 with unreactive pupils and extensor motor response, the probability of a poor outcome is 0.9662. Note that all of the over 59 year olds—non-reactive pupil probabilities are greater than 95% irrespective of motor response. As might be expected the lowest probability of dying is the combination—less than age 20, reactive pupils, obeys/localizes.

Table 20.10 can be used to estimate the

Table 20.9
Calculated Probabilities of Extremes of Outcome Related to Motor Response[45]

| | OUTCOME | | |
MOTOR RESPONSE	DEAD/PVS	OTHER	TOTAL
Obeys/Local	122	273	395
Withdrawal/Flexor	217	185	402
Extensor/Nil	162	29	191
Total	501	487	988

$P(Extensor/Nil \mid Dead) = \frac{162}{501}$ $\qquad$ $P(Extensor \mid Other) = \frac{2}{48}$

$P(Obeys \mid Dead) = \frac{122}{501}$ $\qquad$ $P(Obeys \mid Other) = \frac{27}{48}$

$P(Dead) = \frac{501}{988} = .51$ $\qquad$ $P(Other) = \frac{487}{988} = .49$

Table 20.10
Probabilities of Poor Outcome Related to Three Clinical Variates: Age, Pupil Response, Motor Response

MOTOR RESPONSE	AGE					
	<20		20-59		>60	
	PUPILS		PUPILS		PUPILS	
	Non-R	React	Non-R	React	Non-R	React
Obeys/ Localizes	.6812	.1175	.8179	.2191	.9638	.6373
Withdrawal/ Flexor	.8489	.2593	.9223	.4241	.9874	.8231
Extensor/ Nil	.9662	.6254	.9837	.7779	.9972	.9579

probability of a poor outcome for a new patient. To illustrate the procedure, we selected 15 patient records from our head injury data base at the LAC/USC Medical Center. Records were chosen at random within outcome categories so that all five possible outcomes would be represented. Data from our records are listed in Table 20.11. Age, pupillary reaction, and motor response determined within the first 24 hours are listed. Actual outcome and estimated probability of poor outcome are included as well.

Consider patient 21, age 59. The probabilities of poor outcome (D/PVS) for individuals 20–59 range from 0.2191–0.9837 (Table 20.11). Restricting the probabilities to the column under "pupil reactive" for this patient, the range of probabilities becomes 0.2191 to 0.7779. The finding of extensor motor response further restricts the probability to the one value in the column 20 to 59, "non-reactive" and the row "extensor/nil." This value is 0.7779. Therefore, patient 21 has a probability of a poor outcome of 0.7779 and his actual outcome was death. As another example, consider patient 10. Probabilities of poor outcome associated with his age of 27 are the same as patient 21. The findings of non-reactive pupils restricts the probability range to the column "20–59, non-reactive." The values

range from 0.8179–0.9837. Finding his motor response (obeys) in the first row produces a probability of 0.8179 for the combination of variates. This patient, however, actually achieved a good result, and illustrates the issue of timing of prediction. For example, the day 1 values of patient 10 were: age 27, pupillary reactivity (one pupil unreactive, one pupil reactive), motor response = obeys. By the next day when his pupils became reactive, his probability of a poor outcome changes from 0.8179 to 0.2191 (i.e., the next column). This is more in keeping with his actual outcome.

The estimated probabilities together with actual outcomes for our 15 patients are summarized in Table 20.11. We classified a patient as a good result if his probability value of a poor outcome was less than 0.90, and a poor result otherwise. Twelve of the 15 cases were correctly classified (80%). This level of accuracy agrees with those in other published reports, suggesting that age, pupillary reaction, and motor responses are correlated with at least the extreme categories of outcome from head trauma.[8, 46, 81] The value of 0.90 was chosen because the worst condition of each of the individual variates is associated with a poor outcome probability above this number, that is, age ≤ 60, unreactive pupils, and extensor motor response are individually and

Table 20.11

Clinical Data and Probability of Poor Outcome in 15 Randomly Selected Patients

PATIENT	AGE	PUPILS	MOTOR RESPONSE	ACTUAL	PROBABILITY DEATH/PVS
21	50	R	Extension	Death	.7779
14	55	R	Obeys/Local	Death	.2191
8	23	NR	Extensor/Nil	Death	.9837
48	38	NR	Extension	PVS	.9837
44	18	NR	Extension	PVS	.9662
43	19	NR	Extension	PVS	.9662
20	40	R	Localizes	SD	.2191
19	61	NR	Extension	SD	.9972
11	34	R	Withdraws	SD	.4241
206	40	R	Withdraws	MD	.4241
56	21	R	None	MD	.7779
36	25	R	Obeys	MD	.2191
13	19	R	Localizes	GR	.1175
12	41	R	Localizes	GR	.2191
10	27	NR	Obeys	GR	.8179

jointly associated with poor outcome. Beginning with the worst combination, probabilities greater than 0.90 emphasize these individual and joint adverse values. The probability of 0.8489 which is next largest after those greater than 0.90 represents only one adverse characteristic (non-reactive pupils). The other characteristics in that set are age <20 and withdrawal/flexor response.

Linear Logistic Statistics

Stablein and his group from the Medical College of Virginia have studied an alternate technique of calculating prognosis in patients with head injuries.[81] Their method employs the linear logistic model which is theoretically superior to the Bayesian method used by Jennett and others. The logistic can process continuous variates without creating intervals as was done in the previous examples (*i.e.*, age). One criticism leveled against the Bayesian method is that the model assumes each variate is statistically independent of other variates. The most common illustration of this concept involves the relationship of advanced age to the presence of an intracranial hematoma. It is known that hematomas occur more frequently in older patients, and that advanced age negatively affects outcome. The linear logistic method does not require independence among the variates.

The mathematical expression giving the probability of a result (in this case death or survival) involves a constant and a variable term respectively. For any value of the variable term, the logistic combines the constant and the variable value. The resulting sum is the power to which Euler's constant ($e = 2.7183\ldots$ is raised. For example, when the sum equals zero, $e^0) = 1$. When the sum is 1, $e^1 = 2.7183$. Tables for e^x are available and many modern calculators include this exponential function.

In the linear logistic, the variable term is composed of a combination of variates. Each variate is weighted to account for its importance in describing the associated probability. The weights also account for the inter-relationships between variates. Stablein using clinical and laboratory data gathered on admission, calculated the constant term for the 115 patients studied and the weights for each of 12 variates. The constant's value was 1.501. The weight for oculocephalic response is −0.0762; for pupil size is −0.8613; and for pupil reaction is −2.176. Each variate was assigned two codes, 0 representing normal and 1 abnormal or absent. The probability is calculated by entering the sum (constant plus variable terms) into the equation:

$$\text{Probability of dying} = \frac{1}{(1 + e^{\text{sum}})}$$

Where the sum is:

$$\begin{aligned}
&1.501 + (-.0762) \text{ Oculocephalic response} \\
&\quad + (-.8613) \text{ Pupil size} \\
&\quad + (-2.176) \text{ Pupil reaction} \\
&= 0.98
\end{aligned}$$

Comparison of Bayesian and logistic estimates is possible from Table 20.12 taken from Stablein's work. The first horizontal row contains the worst value for the three variates being used. The Bayesian probability is 98% and the logistic is 83%. Both are the largest values in their sets and are ranked number one (value in parentheses). Only entries ranked four and five disagree with respect to order of severity (i.e., probability of dying). The logistic, however, has a narrower range of values which is usually interpreted to mean that more information is needed. That is, the three variates are not enough to provide the full probability range. Further, ranks five and six, seven and eight, respectively, yield nearly equal probability values. This type of finding is also interpreted as insufficient information. Of course, up to 12 variates might be used to predict an outcome using Stablein's method, but the point is made that the logistic is superior to the Bayesian at least in its ability to point out unresolved issues such as a variate that does not add additional power to the prediction

For Stablein's work the logistic method obviated the relative deficiency of a small data base (115 cases). By ranking up to 12 clinical and laboratory characteristics, satisfactory accuracy could be obtained. Jennett's method using a Bayesian model relied heavily on a very large data base and strictly clinical, easily reported characteristics. Each system has its inadequacies and

Table 20.12

Comparison of Bayesian and Logistic Estimates of Outcome Given Three Clinical Variates[81]

			PROBABILITY OF DYING(%)	
OCULOCEPHALIC RESPONSE	PUPIL SIZE	PUPIL RESPONSE	BAYES ESTIMATE	LOGISTIC ESTIMATE
Impaired/Absent	Abnormal	Absent	98 (1)	83 (1)
Normal	Abnormal	Absent	93 (2)	82 (2)
Impaired/Absent	Normal	Absent	85 (3)	68 (3)
Normal	Normal	Absent	55 (5)	66 (4)
Impaired/Absent	Abnormal	Present	80 (4)	36 (5)
Normal	Abnormal	Present	46 (6)	35 (6)
Impaired/Absent	Normal	Present	28 (7)	19 (7)
Normal	Normal	Present	7 (8)	18 (8)

therefore it is not surprising that their levels of accuracy are not dissimilar. Braakman, using data from 305 head injured patients and an independent multivariate method, was also able to obtain accuracy close to that of the linear logistic model.[8]

Other Models

Other models of computing outcome in head-injured patients have been developed, but unlike those discussed above, categorization of injury and outcome are not based on a widely accepted system such as the Glasgow Coma and Outcome Scores. Stewart and co-workers presented a method using a multiple regression equation.[83] Age, pattern of consciousness on admission, and again 24 hours after the onset of coma were used to predict outcome. Outcome was defined in terms of the length of stay in the hospital (three categories) with the fourth category being death. Over 300 patients were classified with 60% accuracy. Unfortunately, in their study, coma or lack of it was taken as an absolute with no discrimination as to severity except in relation to timing of the conscious versus unconscious intervals. In terms of the Glasgow Coma Score, patients in this series may have ranged from 3 to 8 without distinction being made. They also constructed nomograms on which a given patient's data could be plotted to obtain an estimate outcome. This concept seems valid if the number of truly predictive variates remains small (Table 20.10).

Auer and co-workers[2] put together a computer program to find a pattern of laboratory values and neurological symptoms that would indicate a no survival chance of the injured. From 130 patients' coma score totals, serum osmolalities, electrolytes, blood pressure and respirations among other variates were analyzed. Although many of these factors were found to have prognostic significance, no combination could predict more than 80% of the nonsurvivors.

This work brings up at least two interesting aspects of predicting outcome. First, the concept of predicting no chance for survival may be a very realistic and useful one. If, at the present, outcome cannot be predicted in terms of distinct levels of neurologic function, it will still be of great value to be able to identify that group of patients for which no heroic effort at resuscitation should be extended. Another important aspect of Auer's study is the potential role to be played by certain laboratory values in making prognostic judgments. Such diverse parameters as serum osmolality, creatinine, blood sugar, and platelet count reach statistical significance when related to outcome. This fact underscores the principle that complicating factors other than neurological severity strongly influence prognosis and that before an accurate model is developed, a number of these variates might of necessity be included.

From the work of these authors just discussed it is apparent that the basic ingredients for a system of calculating the probability for a given outcome following head trauma are available. Currently, the methods employed by the Glasgow or Virginia groups are the most successful. In the individual case, plotting purely clinical parameters and comparing these with patients in the international data bank, a prediction can be made using either Bayesian or linear logistic statistics at 24 hours in 60–90% of cases. At three days, accuracy improves and attempts to categorize patients into several other outcome categories can be made. However, as the number of outcome categories increases, accuracy decreases until it becomes almost impossible to predict with certainty the moderately and severely disabled groups. In order to increase efficiency and accuracy of a prognostication system, new avenues must be explored. One possible direction to take may be that of defining injury in terms of new variates such as laboratory parameters. The following discussion will relate several nonclinical variates to outcome from head injury in hopes of further stimulating work in developing more accurate systems of prognostication.

NONCLINICAL MEASURES OF SEVERITY OF INJURY

Intracranial Pressure

By the early 1970's continuous measurement of intracranial pressure (ICP) had become widely accepted in the treatment of head-injured patients. Management decisions were based on both the absolute level of the ICP and on compliance testing which employed injection of small amounts of fluid intracranially with subsequent recording of the ICP response. As experience with ICP monitoring grew, investigators began to correlate the level of ICP with the amount of cerebral damage. Since the ICP was readily measured and produced objective data some felt that it might become a useful predictor of patient outcome. Relatively few reports relating ICP to the outcome in head injury are available. Unfortunately, a general consensus regarding the relationship of ICP to outcome is lacking[52, 60, 66, 73]

From reviewing the available clinical series, several conclusions are warranted.[7, 26, 28, 56–59] First, there may be some predictive power in extreme values (over 30–40 mm Hg) of ICP, but this power is overshadowed by other clinical means of assessing injury such as coma scoring. Further, as Marshall[56] has suggested, certain small subsets from the larger group of head-injured patients with elevated ICP, may derive more benefit from having their ICP lowered than others. In such a group of patients, (diffuse brain injury without a mass lesion is an example) the level of ICP may have predictive value.

Most investigators who deal with trauma patients continue to feel that ICP monitoring and control is essential to the management of head injured patients.[4] As Miller has reported, adding ICP data to patients with certain coma scores may increase the accuracy of prognostication.[58] As yet, no method of prediction has been published which includes the ICP as a variate of predictability.

Electrophysiological Measurements

Because the EEG has always been considered a sensitive index of altered cerebral function, it would seem that this modality would correlate with depth of coma and therefore be of prognostic value in the head injured patient. Unfortunately, standard EEG recordings have not proven to be of value in gauging the extent of brain dysfunction following head injury.[11, 50] However, with the advent of computerized spectral analysis and multimodality evoked responses (MER), bioelectric brain activity patterns have been found to more accurately reflect regional or global dysfunction.[82]

Evoked responses have been used to diagnose a number of central nervous system disorders including stroke, multiple sclerosis, and dysfunction of the visual pathways. Greenberg and his associates were among the first to apply this modality to the prediction of outcome from head injury.[32, 33] In 1977 they reported the findings from a group of 51 severe head injuries. Somatosensory (SER), visual (VER), auditory, and auditory brain stem responses (BAER) were catalogued at varying times following injury and correlated with clinical condition and neurological outcome. These multimodality evoked responses (MER's) were graded on a scale of I to IV (grade IV being the most abnormal) and attempts to prognosticate were made on day 3 and day 14 after injury. At day 3, SER's were found to be significantly associated with outcome, and by day 14 both SER's and BAER's had predictive capacity. Of those patients who had grade I or II MER's by day 3, 80% became responsive by day 30. Furthermore, predictions could be made as to eventual distribution and type of neurological deficit.

In another study reported by Seales *et al.*[77] BAER's were recorded in 17 comatose head-injured patients. They concluded that early in the course of the injury, abnormal BAER's may be seen even though the lesion is reversible, but BAER's taken at 3 to 6 days post-injury correspond well to eventual outcome.

As more experience is accumulated with the EEG in central nervous system disease, cerebral bioelectric rhythms may be used to precisely categorize patients according to the level and severity of brain damage. This data alone or in conjunction with clinical or other laboratory parameters may be able to be incorporated into a sophisticated prognostication system for many disease states including head injury.

Cerebral Blood Flow

Measurement of cerebral blood flow (CBF) in patients with head injuries has interested investigators for a number of years. The technique of most value to date is that of intracarotid injection or inhalation of Xenon-133 (Xe ^{133}) and subsequent evaluation of tissue washout curves. Ingvar and Ciria studied severely brain damage patients following long recovery periods and found that resting CBF values were markedly reduced.[42] They theorized that these low values represented gross cortical damage and attempted to correlate flow abnormalities with focal neurological deficits. It seemed logical to conclude that CBF may well reflect the severity of tissue damage and therefore be helpful in categorizing patients for prognostication.

Unfortunately, CBF measurements made during the acute phases of brain injury show wide variations. Patients with low coma scores may have flows in normal, hyperemic (>65 cc/100 gm/min), or low (<20 cc/100 gm/min) ranges.[62, 64] Thus, in the acute stage of injury, no reliable relationship exists between measured CBF and outcome except in one study in children.[13]

Brain trauma also has a profound effect on cerebral autoregulation and CBF response to changing $PaCO_2$ levels.[13, 19, 22, 36] It seems that in severe head injury the CO_2 response may remain intact, but as clinical deterioration occurs the response wanes. This effect is usually associated with a poor outcome or death, but again these observations do not lend themselves to a systematic method of prognostication.

CT Scan

Utilization of the CT scan in the management of severe head injury has expedited the localization of intracranial hematomas and promoted earlier surgical intervention. While angiography and ventriculography relied on shifts of normal structures to localize lesions, CT offered a means to directly visualize pathology such as contusion, edema, brainstem hemorrhage and intraventricular blood.

A number of investigators have explored the possibility that CT data may be helpful in estimating outcome from head trauma. Snoek and colleagues[80] reported on 60 patients and emphasized the negative prognostic implication of "small ventricles" and the fact that a normal appearing CT scan

was not incompatible with a poor outcome. A number of authors have underscored the importance of bilateral high density hemisphere lesions on CT, relating these findings to elevated ICP and a poor outcome.[59, 84, 93] The Medical College of Virginia group has taken the first step by using CT data in calculating prognosis in head injury.[83] They included evidence of a mass on CT as one of the scoring parameters with high prognostic ability. The Rotterdam group also attempted to gather information on the ability of the CT to aid in prognosis but could not get significant data.[8]

In the quest for a sensitive indicator of brain function for precisely determining outcome from brain trauma, CT scanning would seem to play a major role. As successive generations of equipment give better resolution, subtle lesions in strategic locations can be demonstrated and correlated with outcome. Continued neuropathological and physiological correlations with CT data in a large group of patients with known outcome may result in a scoring system which could be used to develop a method of mathematically calculating prognosis.

Biochemical Parameters

Investigators have assessed various biochemical and metabolic indices in an attempt to quantitate the degree of brain injury and to relate these values to observed clinical parameters and to outcome.

Enzymatic activity as measured in the cerebrospinal fluid (CSF) and serum has been studied in relation to prognosis.[88] It seems that with increasing severity of injury, enzymes normally found in the cytoplasm, microsomes, mitochondria, and nuclei of cells are released into the extracellular fluid, cerebrospinal fluid, and blood *via* a damaged blood-brain barrier. The higher the level of enzyme released, the more severe the brain injury.

The most sensitive enzymatic indices of brain damage seem to be lactic dehydrogenases (LDH), glutamic oxaloacetic transaminase (SGOT), and creatine phosphokinase (CPK).[30, 70, 72] In several studies to date serum or CSF levels of these enzymes have correlated with Glasgow outcome ranking

(Figs. 20.8–20.10). In general, these data are not yet specific enough to differentiate among outcome categories, so prognostic power is no greater than clinical indices of injury.

A more specific biochemical assay indicative of brain injury is the serum myelin basic protein (SMBP). Thomas and his associates found a statistically significant relationship between elevated levels of SMBP and severity of injury in 157 patients.[89, 90] The higher the level of SMBP, the poorer the outcome (Fig. 20.11).

Particularly high levels of cyclic adenosine 3',5'-monophosphate (CAMP) are present in brain and CSF. The final role of this substance is not clear, but it appears to be involved in synaptic transmission, cerebral metabolism, and hemodynamics. Fleischer reported that the clinical course of 32 head injured patients correlated well with the ventricular levels of cyclic AMP.[27, 29] Patients whose CSF cyclic AMP levels remained below 6 nM for longer than 10 days died, whereas all patients whose cyclic AMP level exceeded 15 nM recovered. Recovery was accompanied by rising cyclic AMP levels to near normal levels (22 nM). The plasma levels of cyclic AMP were found to be normal, thereby suggest-

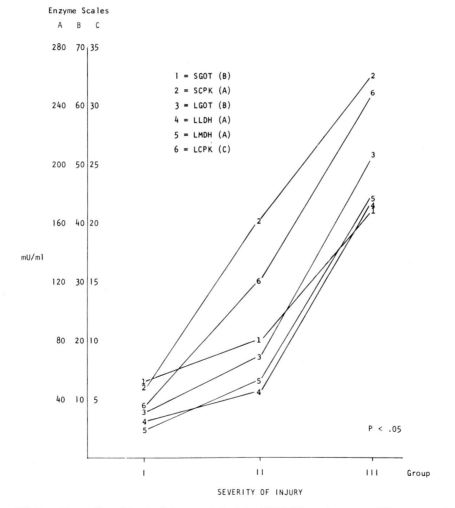

Figure 20.8. Severity of brain injury related to CSF (L) and serum (S) enzyme levels. *I*, concussion; *II*, severe injury with neurologic deficit; *III*, death.[30]

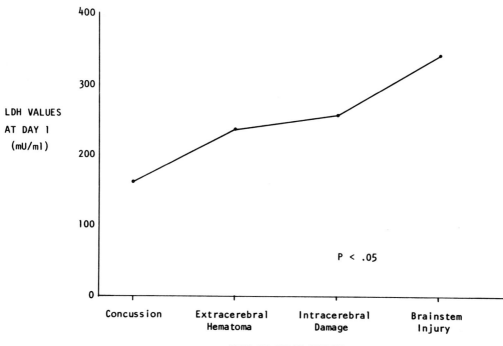

Figure 20.9. Serum LDH level related to type of brain injury.[72]

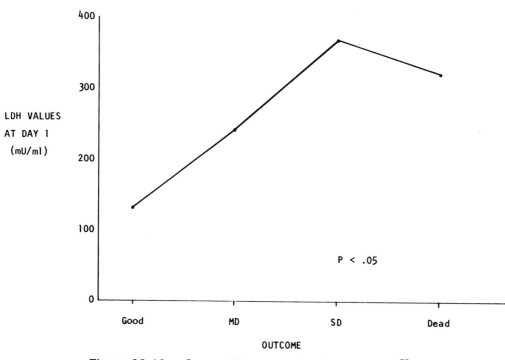

Figure 20.10. Serum LDH level related to outcome.[72]

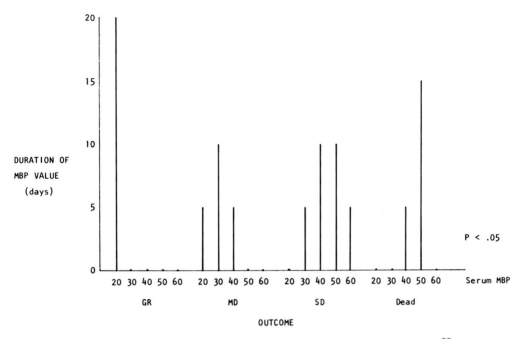

Figure 20.11. Serum myelin basic protein related to outcome.[90]

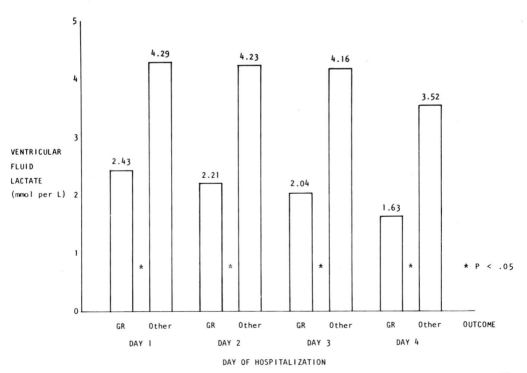

Figure 20.12. CSF lactate related to outcome at various time epochs after injury.[18]

ing that the phenomenon was not due to a transport disruption, but rather to a disorder of cyclic AMP metabolism due to head injury.

Following severe head injury, there also seems to be a significant correlation between outcome and the level of lactic acid present in the CSF.[19, 76] (Fig. 20.12). In those patients who survive head injury, there is a normalization of CSF pH and a concomittant reduction in lactate level. In those patients who succumb or remain severely impaired, elevation of lactic acid persists. CSF lactate levels seem then to be a measure of metabolic dysfunction and perhaps a means of predicting outcome. A CSF lactate level greater than 40 mg% was found not to be compatible with survival in any of the cases studied.[18]

Other Variates Related to Prognosis

Several other characteristics related to head injury have been found to have a statistical relationship to outcome. Some lend themselves easily to statistical review such as blood pressure, temperature and other vegetative functions, whereas others including social factors and background of the patient are more difficult to quantity. Despite this some of these factors are known to have a measurable effect on outcome and therefore may be important in computing prognosis. One of these variables is the type of brain injury as defined neuropathologically.

Pazzaglia recognized the heterogeneity of previously published populations of head injury and attempted, in 282 cases, to quantify the major intracranial lesions and relate them to outcome.[67] Outcome was classified in terms of re-integration into society. In general, they found that surgically treated patients had a less favorable prognosis and that it was possible to establish a scale of decreasing severity with acute subdural hematoma followed by lacerations, contusions, and extradural hematoma.

Bowers and Marshall[7] are among the very few investigators to assess the type of injury and its relation to outcome in a population categorized by the Glasgow Coma and Outcome Scores. Acute subdural he-

matoma was responsible for a 52% mortality rate in a population with an overall mortality rate of 36%. Gutterman and Shenkin[35] studied 52 patients. Because all were decerebrate, the severity of brain injury based on coma grade might be considered to be relatively uniform. They found that those patients who had hematomas evacuated had a higher survival rate than those patients who did not have intracranial masses. Heiden et al.[37] compared patients with diffuse injury with those with surgically treated hematomas. When an analysis took into account the age factor, no statistically significant differences in outcome were found. Thus, the effects of hematoma or contusion on outcome are difficult to assess, but in those few reports where a statistical method of prognostication has been presented, the presence or absence of a mass has not proven instrumental in predicting outcome.

A number of other characteristics may have prognostic power if incorporated into a system of calculating outcome. Cooper et al.,[20] in a prospective study on the effects of steroids on the outcome of head injury, included systolic blood pressure among the variables evaluated for its effect on survival. Of 11 patients with a coma score of 6 or less and systolic blood pressure of less than 90 mm Hg, only one had a good outcome. In 27 of 65 patients who were normotensive, however, a good recovery was made. Auer et al.[2] analyzed neurological and laboratory data on 130 head-injured patients to find a pattern which predicted the chance of death. Systolic blood pressure differed significantly between survivors and non-survivors. They have subsequently incorporated this as well as other factors into a computer program for predicting outcome. Stablein has also included blood pressure in his statistical method for determining early prognosis.[81] More data will be necessary before predictive values of systolic blood pressure can be analyzed.

The presence or absence of multiple injuries has a direct, but as yet unquantified, effect on outcome of head injury. Associated systemic injuries can occur in over 50% of head injured patients. The resultant systemic insults of hypotension, anemia and hypoxia in at least one series of cases were related to a statistically significant increase in poor outcome. Tofovic, after reviewing 200 autopsied cases, noted that multiple injuries were responsible for most of the mortality after 3 days from the injury.[91] Cooper's observations were not in agreement, as his results suggested that the presence of abdominal, chest or long bone injuries did not correlate with outcome.

Both Jennett and Stablein have looked at a number of vegetative parameters such as blood pressure, pulse, respirations, temperature, etc. Unfortunately, each has come to opposite conclusions about the added prognostic implications these factors might have.

Stablein included PaO_2, systolic blood pressure, and hematocrit among those factors found to be of prognostic importance. Jennett's group on the other hand feels that these factors do not increase the accuracy of prediction.

One potentially important indicator of outcome that has received little notice in the literature is the social background and environment of the head-injured patient. Gilchrist and Wilkinson[31] looked at a group of 84 people under age 40 who were being rehabilitated following severe brain injuries. Among other factors, they found that an inadequate social background negatively affected outcome as measured by the ability to find gainful employment. The study raises two important points in regard to head injury outcome. First, social and family background can be important in determining outcome and second, when more is known about the outcome of head injury, newer classifications based on long term rehabilitation and utility of function will become necessary.

CONCLUSIONS

The component parts of a system to predict outcome in head-injured patients have been assembled. The resulting machinery provides a satisfactory level of accuracy when patient data used to develop the model are recomputed to make new predictions. One further test of the system would be to prospectively add each new patient's parameters and predictions into an ongoing data bank. By this means accuracy can continue to be assessed and methods of prediction can be updated based on increased information about head trauma.

Of the various methods described, those offered by the Glasgow group using Bayesian statistics and the Medical College of Virginia group utilizing a linear logistic approach are at this point the most efficacious. Using either of these approaches, over 60% of patients can be accurately classified into two categories representing the extremes of outcome (D/PVS versus GR). Timing of the predictions, seemingly an important issue as related to accuracy, may not manifestly increase the number of patients correctly categorized. During the first day or "on admission", outcome in over one-half of Stablein's patients could be accurately predicted. In Braakman's series, 7–14 days brought about further correct predictions, but the inherent drawbacks of waiting that long are obvious.

Increased efficacy may be gained by exploring other parameters which reflect severity of injury. It seems that purely clinical parameters have taken us as far as we can go. Indicants of brain injury such as myelin basic protein or enzyme levels along with high resolution CT scanning or even PET scanning may result in an entirely new coma scale. Such a scale would be less subject to observer error, although widespread distribution of the necessary equipment and technology will take time. Everything that has been written about outcome from head injury points to the fact that the severity of brain injury governs the result. Thus, if a more precise or sophisticated measure of brain damage is discovered, more exact predictions regarding prognosis may become available.

With our present methods, accuracy is enhanced at the expense of reducing the number of outcome categories. If a more exact measure of brain injury is found, distinct classes of neurological or behavioral function may be predictable early in the course of injury. At present, the Glasgow Outcome Scale as such is not completely compatible with prognostication techniques, because collapsing of the scale is necessary for accuracy of predictions. It may be that this scale will also need some modification, with a 2 or 3 category scale reserved for early prediction, and a more diverse scale based on behavior or some other indicants of neuropsychological function for more delayed prognostication.[52, 53, 76]

After three days following head injury, brain injury begins to assume a decreasing role in causation of death, and associated injuries or complications assume increasing importance. Analysis as to which of these factors has the greatest influence over outcome, may not only result in a more exact system of predicting outcome, but also in management programs that can ultimately reduce mortality. Several recent communications suggest that "aggressive" treatment of head injuries can reduce the mortality rate from 50% to 35%. Presumably such treatment also includes aggressive management of associated injuries and complications. What effects these factors have in reducing mortality needs to be addressed.

References

1. Albrecht, G.L., Harasymiw, S.J.: Evaluating rehabilitation outcome by cost function indicators. J. Chron. Dis., 32:525–533, 1979.
2. Auer, L., Gell, G., Richling, B., Oberbauer, R.: Predicting outcome after severe head injury—a computer assisted analysis of neurological symptoms and laboratory values. Acta Neurochir. Suppl., 28:171–173, 1979.
3. Avezaat, C.J.J., Van Den Berge, H.J., Braakman, R.: Eye movements as a prognostic factor. Acta Neurochir. Suppl., 28:26–28, 1979.
4. Becker, D.P., Miller, J.D., Ward, J.D., Greenberg, R.P., Young, H.F., Sakalas, R.: The outcome from severe head injury with early diagnosis and intensive management. J. Neurosurg., 47:491–502, 1977.
5. Bond, M.R., Brooks, D.N., McKinlay, W.: Burdens imposed on the relatives of those with severe brain damage due to injury. Acta Neurochir. Suppl., 28:124–125, 1979.
6. Bouzarth, W.F., Lindermuth, J.R.: Head injury watch sheet modified for a digital scale. J. Trauma, 18:571–579, 1978.
7. Bowers, S.A., Marshall, L.F.: Outcome in 200 consecutive cases of severe head injury treated in San Diego County: a prospective analysis. Neurosurgery, 6:237–242, 1980.
8. Braakman, R., Gelpke, G.J., Habbema, J.D.F., Maas, A.I.R., Minderhoud, J.M.: Systematic selection of prognostic features in patients with severe head injury. Neurosurgery, 6:362–370, 1980.
9. Braun, J.J.: Time and recovery from brain damage. In: Recovery From Brain Damage, Finger, S., Ed. Plenum Press, New York, 1978, pp. 165–198.
10. Bricolo, A., Turazzi, S., Alexandre, A., Rizzuto, N.: Decerebrate rigidity in acute head injury. J. Neurosurg., 47:680–698, 1977.
11. Bricolo, A., Turazzi, S., Faccioli, F.: Combined clinical and EEG examinations for assessment of severity of acute head injuries. Acta Neurochir. Suppl., 28:35–39, 1979.
12. Bricolo, A., Turazzi, S., Feriotti, G.: Prolonged post-traumatic unconsciousness. Therapeutic assets and liabilities. J. Neurosurg., 52:625–634, 1980.
13. Bruce, D.A., Schut, L., Bruno, L.A., Wood, J.H., Sutton, L.N.: Outcome following severe head injuries in children. J. Neurosurg., 48:679–688, 1978.
14. Carlsson, C.A., Von Essen, C., Lofgren, J.: Factors affecting the clinical course of patients with severe head injuries. J. Neurosurg., 29:242–251, 1968.
15. Caveness, W.F.: Incidence of craniocerebral trauma in the United States in 1976 with trend from 1970 to 1975. Adv. Neurol., 22:1–3, 1979.
16. Civetta, J.M.: The inverse relationship between cost and survival. J. Surg. Res., 14:265–269, 1973.
17. Clifton, G.L., McCormick, W.F., Grossman, R.G.: Neuropathology of early and late deaths after head injury. Neurosurgery, 8:309–314, 1981.
18. Cold, G., Enevoldsen, E., Malmros, R.: Ventricular fluid lactate, pyruvate, bicarbonate and pH in unconscious brain-injured patients subjected to controlled ventilation. Acta Neurol. Scand., 52:187–195, 1975.
19. Cold, G.E., Jensen, F.T., Malmros, R.: The cerebrovascular CO_2 reactivity during the acute phase of brain injury. Acta Anaesth. Scand., 21:222–231, 1977.
20. Cooper, P.R., Moody, S., Clark, W.K., Kirkpatrick, J., Maravilla, K., Gould, A.L., Drane, W.: Dexamethasone and severe head injury. J. Neurosurg., 51:307–316, 1979.
21. Crandon, L.R.G., Wilson, L.T.: Fracture of base of skull. An analysis of 530 cases with particular reference to treatment and prognosis. Ann Surg., 44:823–841, 1906.
22. Enevoldson, E.M., Jensen, F.T.: False autoregulation of cerebral blood flow in patients with acute severe head injury. Acta Neurol. Scand Suppl. 64, 56:514–515, 1977.
23. Fahy, T.J., Irving, M.H., Millac, P.: Severe head injuries. A six-year follow up. Lancet, 2:475–479, 1967.
24. Fay, F.R.: The incidence and results of head injuries over five years (1956–1960) at the Royal Hobart Hospital. Med. J. Aust. 1:168–170, 1963.
25. Feldmann, H., Klages, G., Gärtner, F., Scharfenberg, J.: The prognostic value of intracranial pressure monitoring after severe head injuries. Acta Neurochir. Suppl., 28:74–77, 1979.
26. Fieschi, C., Battistini, N., Beduschi, A., Boselli, L., Rossanda, M.: Regional cerebral blood flow and intraventricular pressure in acute head injuries. J. Neurol. Neurosurg. Psych., 37:1378–1388, 1974.
27. Fleischer, A.S.: Prognostic Value of Cyclic Amp in Ventricular Cerebrospinal Fluid of Patients Fol-

lowing Severe Head Injury. In: Neural Trauma, A.J. Popp, R.S. Bourke, L.R. Nelson, H.K. Kimelberg, Eds. Raven Press, New York, 1979, pp. 245–252.

28. Fleischer, A.S., Payne, N.S., Tindall, G.T.: Continuous monitoring of intracranial pressure in severe closed head injury without mass lesions. Surg. Neurol., 6:31–34, 1976.

29. Fleischer, A.S., Rudman, D.R., Fresh, C.B., Tindall, G.T.: Concentration of 3′, 5′ cyclic adenosine monophosphate in ventricular CSF of patients following severe head trauma. J. Neurosurg., 47:517–524, 1977.

30. Florez, G., Cabeza, A., Gonzalez, J.M., Garcia, J., Ucar, S.: Changes in serum and cerebrospinal fluid enzyme activity after head injury. Acta Neurochir., 35:3–13, 1976.

31. Gilchrist, E., Wilkinson, M.: Some factors determining prognosis in young people with severe head injuries. Arch. Neurol., 36:355–359, 1979.

32. Greenberg, R.P., Becker, D.P., Miller, J.D., Mayer, D.J.: Evaluation of brain function in severe human head trauma with multimodality evoked potentials. II. Localization of brain dysfunction and correlation with post-traumatic neurological conditions. J. Neurosurg., 47:163–177, 1977.

33. Greenberg, R.P., Mayer, D.J., Becker, D.P., Miller, J.D.: Evaluation of brain function in severe human head trauma with multimodality evoked potentials. I. Evoked brain injury potentials, methods and analysis. J. Neurosurg., 47:150–162, 1977.

34. Gudeman, S.K., Miller, J.D., Becker, D.P.: Failure of high-dose steroid therapy to influence intracranial pressure in patients with severe head injury. J. Neurosurg., 51:301–306, 1979.

35. Gutterman, P., Shenkin, H.A.: Prognostic features in recovery from traumatic decerebration. J. Nerosurg., 32:330–335, 1970.

36. Hass, W.K.: Prognostic value of cerebral oxidative metabolism in head trauma. In *Head Injuries*, Second Chicago Symposium on Neural Trauma. R.L. McLaurin, Ed. Grune & Stratton, New York, 1975, pp. 35–37.

37. Heiden, J.S., Small, R., Caton, W., Weiss, M.H., Kurze, T.: Severe head injury and outcome: A prospective study. In: Neural Trauma, Popp, A.J., Bourke, R.S., Nelson, L.R., Kimelberg, H.K., Eds. Raven Press, New York, 1979, pp. 181–193.

38. Heiskanen, O., Sipponen, P.: Prognosis of severe brain injury. Acta Neurol. Scand., 46:343–348, 1970.

39. Hiatt, H.H.: Protecting the medical commons: who is responsible? N. Engl. J. Med., 293:235–240, 1975.

40. Higashi, K., Sakata, Y., Hatano, M., Abiko, S., Ihara, K., Katayama, S., Wakuta, Y., Okamura, T., Ueda, H., Zenke, M., Aoki, H.: Epidemiological studies on patients with a persistent vegetative state. J. Neurol., Neurosurg. Psych., 40:876–885, 1977.

41. Hippocrates: The book of prognostics. In: The Genuine Works of Hippocrates Transl: F. Adams, LL.D. The Williams & Wilkins Co., Baltimore, 1939, pp. 42–43.

42. Ingvar, D.H., Ciria, M.G.: Assessment of severe damage to the brain by multiregional measurements of cerebral blood flow. In: Outcome of Severe Damage to the Central Nervous System. CIBA Symposium 34, 1975. pp. 97–120.

43. Jennett, B.: Prognosis after severe head injury. Clin. Neurosurg., 19:200–207, 1971.

44. Jennett, B.: Resource allocation for the severely brain damaged. Arch. Neurol., 33:595–597, 1976.

45. Jennett, B., Teasdale, G., Braakman, R., Minderhoud, J., Heiden, J., Kurze, T.: Prognosis of patients with severe head injury. Neurosurgery, 4:283–289, 1979.

46. Jennett, B., Teasdale, G., Braakman, R., Minderhoud, J., Knill-Jones, R.: Predicting outcome in individual patients after severe head injury. Lancet, 1:1031–1034, 1976.

47. Jennett, B., Teasdale, G., Fry, J., Braakman, R., Minderhoud, J., Heiden, J., Kurze, T.: Treatment for severe head injury. J. Neurol Neurosurg. Psych., 43:289–295, 1980.

48. Jennett, B., Tesdale, G., Galbraith, S., Pickard, J., Grant, H., Braakman, R., Avezaat, C., Maas, A., Minderhoud, J., Vecht, C.J., Heiden, J., Small, R., Caton, W., Kurze, T.: Severe head injuries in three countries. J. Neurol. Neurosurg. Psych., 40:291–298, 1977.

49. Kalsbeek, W.D., McLaurin, R.L., Harris, B.S.H., Miller, J.D.: The national head and spinal cord injury survey: major findings. J. Neurosurg. 53:S-19–S-31, 1980.

50. Knoblich, O.E., Gaab, M.: Prognostic information for EEG and ICP monitoring after severe closed head injuries in the early post-traumatic phase. Acta Neurochir. Suppl., 28:58–62, 1979.

51. Langfitt, T.W.: Measuring the outcome from head injuries. J. Neurosurg., 48:673–678, 1978.

52. Levin, H.S., Grossman, R.G., Rose, J.E., Teasdale, G.: Long-term neuropsychological outcome of closed head injury. J. Neurosurg., 50:412–422, 1979.

53. Levin, H.S., O'Donnell, V.M., Grossman, R.G.: The Galveston Orientation and Amnesia Test. A practical scale to assess cognition after head injury. J. Nerv. Ment. Dis., 167:675–684, 1979.

54. Lezak, M.D.: Living with characterologically altered brain injured patients. J. Clin. Psych. 39:592–598, 1978.

55. Maciver, I.N., Frew, I.J.C., Matheson, J.G.: The role of respiratory insufficiency in the mortality of severe head injuries. Lancet, 1:390–393, 1958.

56. Marshall, L.F., Smith, R.W., Shapiro, H.M.: The outcome with aggressive treatment in severe head injuries. I. The significance of intracranial pressure monitoring. J. Neurosurg., 50:20–25, 1979.

57. Marshall, L.F., Smith, R.W., Shapiro, H.M.: The outcome with aggressive treatment in severe head injuries. II. Acute and chronic barbiturate administration in the management of head injury. J. Neurosurg., 50:26–30, 1979.

58. Miller, J.D., Becker, D.P., Ward, J.D., Sullivan, H.G., Adams, W.E., Rosner, M.J.: Significance of intracranial hypertension in severe head injury. J. Neurosurg., 47:503–516, 1977.

59. Miller, J.D., Gudeman, S.K., Kishore, P.R.S.,

Becker, D.P.: CT Scan, ICP and early neurological evaluation in the prognosis of severe head injury. Acta Neurochir. Suppl., 28:86–88, 1979.

60. Miltner, F.O., Halves, E., Bushe, K.A.: Prognostic aspects of electroclinical and neuroendocrine data in severe brain injury. Acta Neurochir. Suppl., 28:43–49, 1979.

61. Nygreen, N.: The Gallup survey on surgeons and surgical care. Bull. Am. Coll. Surg., 65:4–8, 1980.

62. Obrist, W.D., Gennarelli, T.A., Segawa, H., Dolinskas, C.A., Langfitt, T.W.: Relation of cerebral blood flow to neurological status and outcome in head-injured patients. J. Neurosurg., 51:292–300, 1979.

63. Ommaya, A.K., Gennarelli, T.A.: A physiopathologic basis for noninvasive diagnosis and prognosis of head injury severity. In: *Head Injuries*, Second Chicago Sympsoium on Neural Trauma. R.L. McLaurin, Ed. Grune & Stratton, New York, 1975, pp 49–75.

64. Overgaard, J.: Reflections on prognostic determinants in acute severe head injury. In: Head Injuries, Second Chicago Symposium on Neural Trauma, R.L. McLaurin, Ed. Grune & Stratton, New York, 1975, pp. 11–21.

65. Overgaard, J., Hvio-Hansen, O., Land, A.M., Pedersen, K.K., Christensen, S., Haase, J., Hein, O., Tweed, W.A.: Prognosis after head injury based on early clinical examination. Lancet, 2:631–635, 1973.

66. Papo, I., Caruselli, G.: Long-term intracranial pressure monitoring in comatose patients suffering from head injuries. A critical survey. Acta Neurochir., 39:187–200, 1977.

67. Pazzaglia, P., Frank, G., Frank, F., Gaist, G.: Clinical course and prognosis of acute post-traumatic coma. J. Neurol. Neurosurg. Psych., 38:149–154, 1975.

68. Phelps, C.: An analytical and statistical review of one thousand cases of head injury. Ann. Surg., 49:449–477, 1909.

69. Pia, H.W., Abtahi, H., Schönmayer, R.: Epidemiology, classifications and prognosis of severe craniocerebral injuries: computer-assisted study of 9038 cases. Adv. Neurosurg., 5:31–35, 1978.

70. Rabow, L., Hedman, G.: CK_{BB}—Isoenzymes as a sign of cerebral injury. Acta Neurochir. Suppl., 28:108–112, 1979.

71. Ransohoff, J.: Prognosis and operative treatment of fracture of the base of the skull. Ann. Surg., 51:796–811, 1910.

72. Rao, C.J., Shukla, P.K., Mohanty, S., Reddy, Y.J.V.: Predictive value of serum lactate dehydrogenase in head injury. J. Neurol. Neurosurg. Psych., 41:948–953, 1978.

73. Richard, K.E., Frowein, R.A.: Significance of intracranial pressure and neurological deficit as prognostic factors in acute severe brain lesions. Acta Neurochir. Suppl., 28:66–69, 1979.

74. Russell, W.R.: Cerebral involvement in head injury. A study based on the examination of two hundred cases. Brain, 55:549–603, 1932.

75. Russell, W.R., Smith, A.: Post-traumatic amnesia in closed head injury. Arch. Neurol., 5:4–17, 1961.

76. Salcman, M., Schepp, R.S., Ducker, T.B.: Calcu-

lated recovery rates in severe head trauma. Neurosurgery, 8:301–308, 1981.

77. Seales, D.M., Rossiter, V.S., Weinstein, M.E.: Brainstem auditory evoked responses in patients comatose as a result of blunt head trauma. J. Trauma, 19:347–353, 1979.

78. Seitz, H.D., Ocker, K.: The prognostic and therapeutic importance of changes in the CSF during the acute stage of brain injury. Acta Neurochir., 38:211–231, 1977.

79. Skillman, J.J.: Ethical dilemmas in the care of the critically ill. Lancet, 2:634–637, 1974.

80. Snoek, J., Jennett, B., Adams, J.H., Graham, D.I., Doyle, D.: Computerised tomography after recent severe head injury in patients without acute intracranial haematoma. J. Neurol. Neurosurg. Psych., 42:215–225, 1979.

81. Stablein, D.M., Miller, J.D., Choi, S.C., Becker, D.P.: Statistical methods for determining prognosis in severe head injury. Neurosurgery, 6:243–248, 1980.

82. Steudel, W.I., Krüger, J.: Using the spectral analysis of the EEG for prognosis of severe brain injuries in the first post-traumatic week. Acta Neurochir. Suppl., 28:40–42, 1979.

83. Stewart, W.A., Litten, S.P., Sheehe, P.R.: A prognostic model for head injury. Acta Neurochir., 45:199–208, 1979.

84. Sweet, R.C., Miller, J.D., Lipper, M., Kishore, P.R.S., Becker, D.P.: Significance of bilateral abnormalities on the CT scan in patients with severe head injury. Neurosurgery, 3:16–21, 1978.

85. Teasdale, G., Jennett, B.: Assessment of coma and impaired consciousness: a practical scale. Lancet, 2:81–83, 1974.

86. Teasdale, G., Jennett, B.: Assessment and prognosis of coma after head injury. Acta Neurochir., 34:45–55, 1976.

87. Teasdale, G., Parker, L., Murray, G., Jennett, B.: On comparing series of head injured patients. Acta Neurochir. Suppl., 28:205–208, 1979.

88. Thomas, D.G.T., Rowan, T.D.: Lactic dehydrogenase isoenzymes following head injury. Injury, 7:258–262, 1976.

89. Thomas, D.G.T., Palfreyman, J.W., Ratcliffe, J.G.: Serum-myelin-basic-protein assay in diagnosis and prognosis of patients with head injury. Lancet, 1:113–115, 1978.

90. Thomas, D.G.T., Rabow, L., Teasdale, G.: Serum myelin basic protein, clinical responsiveness, and outcome of severe head injury. Acta Neurochir. Suppl., 28:93–95, 1979.

91. Tofovic, P., Ugrinovski, J., Ruskov, P., Zoravkovska, S., Simova, M., Ancev, B.: Initial state, outcome, and autopsy findings in a series of 200 consecutive traumatic comas. A computerized analysis. Acta Neurochir. 34:99–105, 1976.

92. Vapalahti, M., Troupp, H.: Prognosis for patients with severe brain injuries. Br. Med. J., 3:404–407, 1971.

93. Zimmerman, R.A., Bilaniuk, L.T., Gennarelli, T.: Computed tomography of shearing injuries of the cerebral white matter. Radiology, 127:393–396, 1978.

Index